Born to Talk

An Introduction to Speech and Language Development

SEVENTH EDITION

Kathleen R. Fahey
University of Northern Colorado

Lloyd M. Hulit
Illinois State University

Merle R. Howard
Illinois State University

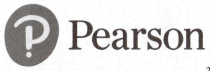

330 Hudson Street, New York, NY, 10013

Director and Publisher: Kevin Davis
Executive Portfolio Manager: Julie Peters
Managing Content Producer: Megan Moffo
Content Producer: Faraz Sharique Ali
Portfolio Management Assistant: Maria Feliberty and Casey Coriell
Development Editor: Krista Slavicek
Executive Product Marketing Manager: Christopher Barry
Executive Field Marketing Manager: Krista Clark

Manufacturing Buyer: Deidra Smith
Cover Design: Carie Keller, Cenveo
Cover Photo: FatCamera/E+/Getty Images
Media Producer: Autumn Benson
Editorial Production and Composition Services: SPi Global, Inc.
Editorial Project Manager: Jennylyn Rosiento, SPi Global
Full-Service Project Manager: Mohamed Hameed
Text Font: New Baskerville ITC Pro

Credits and acknowledgments borrowed from other sources and reproduced, with permission, in this textbook appear on the appropriate page within text or on this page.

Photo Credits: Page 1, Jupiterimages/BananaStock/Getty Images; Page 27, Syda Productions/Shutterstock; Page 62, Comstock Images/Stockbyte/Getty Images; Page 113, Michaeljung/Shutterstock; Page 180, Jules Selmes/Pearson Education, Inc.; Page 209, Comstock/Stockbyte/Getty images; Page 263, Jupiterimages/Pixland/Getty Images; Page 323, Sergey Novikov/Shutterstock; Page 363, FatCamera/Vetta/Getty Images; Page 393, Photodisc/Getty Images

Library of Congress Cataloging-in-Publication Data

Names: Fahey, Kathleen R., author. | Hulit, Lloyd M., author. | Howard, Merle R., author.
Title: Born to talk : an introduction to speech and language development / Kathleen R. Fahey, Lloyd M. Hulit, Merle R. Howard.
Description: Seventh edition. | Boston : Pearson, [2017] | Lloyd M. Hulit's name appears first in the previous edition. | Includes bibliographical references and indexes.
Identifiers: LCCN 2017040177| ISBN 9780134760797 | ISBN 0134760794
Subjects: | MESH: Language Development | Speech
Classification: LCC P118 | NLM WS 105.5.C8 | DDC 401/.93–dc23 LC record available at https://lccn.loc.gov/2017040177

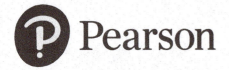

ISBN 10:   0-13-476079-4
ISBN 13: 978-0-13-476079-7

13 2023

About the Authors

Kathleen R. Fahey, Ph.D., was born in Parma Heights, Ohio. She received her bachelor's, master's, and doctoral degrees from Bowling Green State University, Kent State University, and Michigan State University, respectively. She is professor emeritus at the University of Northern Colorado. She is a speech-language pathologist with 40 years' experience in the assessment and intervention of childhood speech, language, and literacy disorders. Her areas of expertise include development and disorders of articulation and phonology, early language, and school-age language and literacy. She currently teaches undergraduate and graduate courses in an online format at the University of Northern Colorado. Kathleen is also the clinical editor of speech-language pathology and audiology for OnCourseLearning.com.

Lloyd M. Hulit, Ph.D., was born in Ashland, Ohio, and lived in several Ohio towns before his father was hired by the U.S. Agency for International Development to assist foreign departments of education establish vocational education programs in their countries. Dr. Hulit attended high school in Seoul, South Korea, and while his family lived in Benghazi, Libya, he attended the Schutz American School in Alexandria, Egypt, graduating in 1963. He attended the University of Maryland's branch in Munich, Germany. He completed his undergraduate degree, graduating magna cum laude, at Ashland (Ohio) College, with a major in speech communication and a minor in Bible studies as part of pre-seminary training. He earned his M.A. and Ph.D. at The Ohio State University with a major in speech and hearing science and a minor in instructional technology. Before attending graduate school, Dr. Hulit taught at the high school and elementary school levels and was a licensed lay minister in the Evangelical United Brethren Church. He taught at Illinois State University in Normal, Illinois, for more than 30 years. He is the author of 14 journal articles and published papers. In addition to being the senior author of *Born to Talk,* he is the sole author of three textbooks on stuttering: *Stuttering Therapy: A Guide to the Charles Van Riper Approach, Stuttering in Perspective,* and *Straight Talk on Stuttering,* now in its second edition. Dr. Hulit's professional passion was teaching. His specialties were fluency disorders, phonological disorders, and language development. Among many teaching awards, he was twice named Professor of the Year by his department, was awarded the Distinguished Teaching Award by ISU's College of Arts and Sciences, the Burlington Northern Foundation Award, and the American Speech and Hearing Association's Golden Apple Award. Dr. Hulit is married to the former Pamela Immel of Massillon, Ohio. He is the father of two extraordinary daughters, and grandfather to five beautiful and exceptionally brilliant grandchildren. In retirement, he continues another passion of his life, coaching high school and junior high school baseball, a career that now spans more than 40 years.

Dedicated to Merle R. Howard, Ph.D.

The seventh edition of *Born to Talk* is dedicated to the memory of Merle R. Howard, one of the original authors of this textbook, an outstanding teacher, a man of immeasurable personal skills, and a giant in my life as a respected colleague and beloved friend. Merle died on July 8, 2013, after a determined and courageous three-year battle against leukemia.

The first edition of this book was published in 1993, and while 20 years will seem like ancient history to most who read it, this book was actually a topic of discussion between Merle and me for more than 10 years before we actually put ink to paper and keystrokes to computer files. We had both taught a course at Illinois State University titled *Human Verbal Development,* a course designed for nonmajors who needed a background in speech and language development. Most of the students enrolled in this course were early childhood, elementary, and special education majors, but the course was a popular general education elective that attracted students from every conceivable major offered by the university. We loved teaching the course, but we were frustrated that we could not find a textbook that matched the needs of our students. Over coffee—well, coffee for Merle and diet soda for me—we talked about the possibility of writing our own textbook. The first conversations began about 1980. It was a subject we dropped and resurrected a number of times, depending on how the Chicago Cubs were faring in a given year, but about 1986, we decided to take a serious run at it. One of the publishers that eventually became part of Pearson visited our campus. We talked to a representative and shared an outline of what we had in mind. Her response was unconditionally enthusiastic, so we developed a plan of action that resulted in a book that is now an important part of Merle Howard's professional legacy.

Merle was born on August 12, 1939, in West Frankfort, Illinois. He earned B.S. and M.S. degrees at Southern Illinois University. His bachelor's degree was in speech and public address. His master's degree was in speech pathology and audiology. He earned his Ph.D. in speech pathology at the University of Cincinnati. His doctoral research and his dissertation focused on stuttering.

Merle's professional career began and ended at Illinois State University in Normal, Illinois, a career spanning 35 years. At the close of his career, Merle was the director of the ISU Speech and Hearing Clinic, but his passion was always teaching. During his tenure at ISU, he taught a wider array of courses than any other member of the faculty, but his favorite area was neuropathology. He had the extraordinary ability to make this detailed and complex subject understandable to even the most befuddled students, and they loved him for it. He was a demanding teacher, but he placed his greatest demands on himself to make sure that students in his classes understood what they needed to know about every subject he taught.

Outside of his professional life, Merle was an excellent golfer. He rode a trail bike with friends, and he spent a lot of time on his prized Harley Davidson. His favorite music was jazz, an interest intensified by his own talents playing the trumpet and by his participation as a member of The Tempos, a 14-piece jazz band at Southern Illinois University, a diversion he enjoyed during his years there as a student. Merle was married to Bonita for 50 years, and he was the father of one son, Lane.

Merle was an impressive and widely appreciated presence in this world, as a husband, a father, a friend, a colleague, and a co-author. To know Merle was to love him. It was Will Rogers who famously said, "A stranger is just a friend I haven't met yet." That too was Merle Howard. He had an incredible capacity for remembering people and their names. More importantly, he remembered their interests and facts about their lives. He was the quintessential *people person.*

Merle was rightly proud of *Born to Talk.* His contributions to this book over the years have been incalculable. I was honored to work with him on this project, but I was even more honored to be his friend. To say that I will miss him does not do justice to the void his passing has left in my life, but his influence will remain with me until I too turn my final page.

Lloyd M. Hulit, Ph.D.
Professor Emeritus, Illinois State University

Contents

Preface

Practitioners and researchers from many disciplines continue to contribute new and exciting information about human language acquisition. It is challenging to keep abreast of the complex array of topics that provides the foundation for human communication and its development from birth through the young adult period. This new edition of *Born to Talk* is suitable for students and practitioners in speech-language pathology, early childhood education, general education, special education, and related disciplines who seek a contemporary and comprehensive view of speech and language development in a reader-friendly manner.

New to This Edition

The eText for this title is an affordable, interactive version of the print text that includes videos and interactive features that provide opportunities for students to get feedback on their answers to the questions posed.

To learn more about the enhanced Pearson eText, go to: www.pearsonhighered.com/etextbooks.

New to This Edition

This edition is again available in a digital format. The seventh edition provides not only review opportunities but also application opportunities to deepen understanding.

- Several **Video Examples** in each chapter allow readers to see and hear content and examples that enhance learning of key concepts. Students read a brief description of what the video is about and watch a video that demonstrates the concept.
- The **Video Reflection** feature gives readers access to a video, a thought-provoking question that pops up from the eText, a hint for thinking about the answer, and a write-in area into which students apply content by typing a written response. Detailed feedback is provided after students submit their written response, thereby immediately providing the correct answer.
- At the end of each major section of text, students have access to a brief section quiz, called Check Your Understanding. The quiz checks comprehension of main concepts and feedback is available for each answer.
- At the end of each chapter, students have access to the Chapter Review. Feedback is available for each of these short essay format or short-answer questions.

■ A glossary is included in this edition that provides definitions for key terms in the text. These terms appear in boldface when they are first mentioned. In the eText, readers can click on the term to directly access the glossary.

■ Search terms in Surfing the Web sections at the end of each chapter encourage readers to expand their knowledge beyond the text to practical and interactive application of the concepts. The search terms provide a vehicle for extended learning opportunities for students in a multimedia context.

In addition, in this seventh edition of Born to Talk, we have

■ Added new information and reorganized information in Chapter 4 about the early language environment of parents and infants.

■ Reduced language examples and figures in Chapter 4 regarding differences in talkative versus taciturn parents, making the remaining examples the focus of the important concepts underlying their use.

■ Added a new chapter (Chapter 5) on language sampling that ties Chapter 4, about the one-word stage, to Chapter 6, regarding the development of syntax. Chapter 5 introduces and explains the process of eliciting, transcribing, analyzing, and interpreting language samples. These processes are useful for readers as they learn about the language gains children make.

■ Added examples and worksheets to Chapter 5 to encourage practice in language sampling.

■ Reorganized the information in Chapter 6 to discuss the language attainment into two, rather than four sections: Stages 2 and 3, followed by Stages 4 and 5.

■ Integrated all the information about language/cultural diversity, including social and regional dialects, bilingualism, and diversity in schools, into other chapters.

About This Text

The primary focus of this book is on *language development*. The sole purpose of Chapter 1 ("A Connection of Brains") is to pique the reader's interest in language as a unique human experience and to increase appreciation of how messages are transmitted from one human brain to another. Chapter 2 lays the groundwork for considering the impressive nature and nurture of human communication. We discuss the many perspectives involved in learning language by exploring what human communication is and how we learn it during our early years. In this edition, we also relate the three perspectives—nativist, behaviorist, and social interactionist—to how speech-language pathologists and educators use them in designing appropriate goals and intervention strategies for children with typical and atypical language development. Chapter 3 is an exploration of how the development of cognition and perception is related to language learning. In Chapter 4 we begin the journey of early interactions of parents and children that lay the foundation for language acquisition through the one-word stage. In Chapter 5 the process of language sampling is described, to help readers appreciate how language development is described and documented. Chapter 6 is a continuation of the stage model to present the journey each child takes in developing the various components of language. Chapter 7 shows how the integration of all language components, including literacy, using this real-time approach facilitates an understanding of how one aspect of language affects all other aspects. Chapter 8 explores how language is learned and transmitted from one person to another via speech production and how social and regional dialects influence speech and language. Chapter 9 provides a brief overview of developmental and acquired disorders of speech and language. Some readers will be less familiar than others with information pertaining to the anatomy and physiology of speech, language, and hearing. We include this information in the Chapter 10.

Before we get to our acknowledgments, we want to address the gender strategy we use in this book. As members of a profession that is more than 80% female, we are sensitive to the gender problem in communication. We are also frustrated by the limitations of American English pronouns. For this reason, we alternate the use of feminine and masculine pronouns, with the understanding that these pronouns are intended to be gender-neutral in all contexts. We also generally refer to the child in the singular (versus the plural *children*) in order to create an image of one child whose speech and language development we study through this book.

There are occasional personal references in this book, indicated by first-person pronouns and by phrases such as: *my sister, daughter, grandchildren,* and *father.* These references reflect the life experiences of the authors, and each is footnoted for the reader's information.

Acknowledgments

We are grateful for the invaluable contributions of several people. Pamela Hulit provided computer assistance in creating a number of tables included in the book. Dr. Jill Gilkerson from the LENA Research Foundation provided guidance in the selection of figures from LENA publications and language samples from its database. Lori Shin from the LENA Research Foundation tailored the graphic art to meet publication specifications. Taylor Weber, a graduate student in speech-language pathology from the University of Northern Colorado (UNC), assisted with the video project and created the glossary. Andy Nagel, the videographer from Mirage Video Pro, and his assistant Ian worked with us in a university and public school setting to produce the videos. We appreciate the special talents of these people, and we are grateful for their efforts on our behalf.

A special thank you is extended to the parents and their children who graciously gave their time and language interactions to the video project, Dr. Madeline Milian for her interview about learning English as a second language and bilingual education, and Carol Haworth for her coordination extraordinaire and expert speech-language pathology services in the school.

Finally, we thank the following people who reviewed the sixth edition of this book: Robin Danzak, Sacred Heart University; Stephanie Hughes, University of Toledo; Michelle Ivey, University of Houston; Donna Thomas, Southeastern Louisiana University.

To the most important people in our lives,
with immeasurable love and gratitude
Pamela, Yvonne, Carmen, Scot, John, Christopher,
Lance, Benjamin, Peyton, Brianna, Bonita, Lane, Cornelia,
Rosemary, Ernest, Daniel, Anna, Molly, Andrew, and Samantha

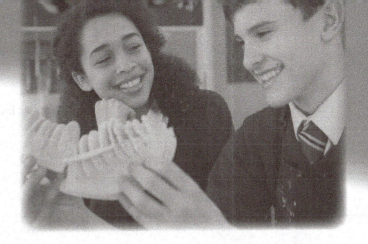

1

A Connection
of Brains

After completion of this chapter, you will be able to:
- Define and relate the terms communication, language, and speech and their components.
- Compare the design features of the human communication system.
- Examine the elements of the speech chain connecting a speaker's thoughts to a listener's understanding of those thoughts.

This first chapter is designed to pique your interest in speech and language as processes within the broader process we call communication. As a future educator, you will be in a unique position to observe and facilitate the growth of children in their journeys to be effective communicators. We define and describe these processes, and we consider how speech and language interact to produce a form of communication unique to humans. We also consider how a speaker's thoughts are conveyed to a listener's brain through a series of communication transformations known collectively as the *speech chain*.

The idea for *Born to Talk* was cultivated long before the first word of the original manuscript was written, and it was probably a good thing that there was a period of latency between the concept and the product. During that latency, I[*] observed language development firsthand in my two daughters, Yvonne and Carmen. I learned more about the power and wonder of language in observing them than I have in all the books and all the journal articles I have read over the course of my career because I witnessed their processes of discovery. I watched and listened as they made connections between the world in which they were growing up and the words and language forms that spilled out of them. They are now grown, and they have blessed my wife and me with five grandchildren, giving me five more opportunities to observe

[*]Lloyd Hulit.

speech and language development close-up and personal. Each of them has reinforced my appreciation of language as one of humankind's greatest gifts and most powerful tools.

My family has an eclectus parrot named Toby. When we were trying to teach Toby to talk in his first year, he said, "hello" and "step up." These are certainly not momentous utterances. They fall short of the magic of Abraham Lincoln's, "Four score and seven years ago . . . " and John F. Kennedy's, "Ask not what your country can do for you . . . ", but they are the beginning of speech or, at the very least, the beginning of speech-like behavior. What was fascinating about observing Toby was that the process of acquisition was so different from the process in human children, and it will always be different. His utterances, no matter how many he produces over his lifetime, will always be conditioned responses, and there is no way we will ever know if there is any connection between what is going on inside his parrot brain and what we believe in our human brains he is saying, which leads us to the power of ESP in speech and language.

Have you ever wished you could read someone's mind, or ever wished or worried that someone could read your mind? Probably each of us has wondered about mental telepathy, and perhaps some of you reading this page believe you have that gift. We would like to suggest that every person, who is able to communicate, is capable of a form of mental telepathy, because human communication allows one human brain to interact with another human brain in a wondrous and almost magical manner.

Most people give very little thought to the magic of communication through speech and language because it is acquired so naturally and used so effortlessly by humans. The purpose of this book is to explore the miracles of speech and language, to examine the marvelous anatomic structures and physiological processes we humans have adapted for talking and listening, to unravel the components of language from sounds to words to elaborate sentence structure that together help us deliver our messages, to investigate the dialectal differences in our own language, and to consider the problems that occur when speech and language do not develop properly or when something goes wrong after communication skills have been normal for a while. By the time you have turned to the final page in your journey through this book, we believe you will be convinced that words such as *magic* and *wondrous* and *miraculous* in reference to speech and language are accurately descriptive, but before we go any further, we need to address some basic terminology.

Defining Communication, Language, and Speech

In the preceding paragraphs, we used the words *speech* and *language* in a manner implying that they are not the same thing, which is correct. They are separate but related processes in the larger process called communication. To understand any of these processes, you must understand all of them and how they are interconnected.

Communication is the sending and receiving of information, ideas, feelings, or messages. To appreciate the breadth of communication, consider just some of the methods by which human beings communicate. We transmit messages of all kinds by talking, writing, using codes (Morse code, text messaging, semaphore flags, Braille), using facial expressions, gestures, art, music, dance, the distances we maintain when we interact, vocal variations, the clothes we wear, hairstyles, our natural and purchased odors, and more. We send hundreds, perhaps thousands, of messages every day. Some of our communications are intended, but many are not. We hope that most of what we send is received according to our intent, but unfortunately this is not always the case. The fact is, we humans cannot stop communicating even when we want to. You may decide to say nothing, but your saying nothing may be saying more than your saying something. Even when you are asleep you may be sending messages. You may talk in your sleep, of course, but even in the silence of unconsciousness, you may communicate restlessness by the way you thrash around in your bed, or you may communicate a basic insecurity by the way you curl into the fetal position, or you may transmit a message of utter tranquility by the relaxed and peaceful expression on your sleeping face. Do you get the point? Communication is so much a part of the human experience that we are constantly sending and receiving messages.

 ### Video Reflection 1.1: Use a Child's Nonverbal Signals to Understand the Child's Needs

Watch this video of a speech-language pathologist (SLP) using the nonverbal signals of a student to assist her in using her communication device, then answer the question.

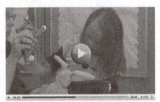

Educators develop a keen sense of the communication strategies of their students. You will notice that some students let you know that they understand or do not understand a particular idea through nodding or shaking the head, smiling or frowning, shrugging shoulders, raising an eyebrow, asking another child for help, or giving that blank stare! These communication signals are quite important as we gauge the speed, amount, and complexity of our messages.

Language is a more difficult phenomenon to describe, so we will build a definition by first looking at some of the characteristics of language and then trying to piece them together. Language is an expression of an ability that is innate in all humans. We are born with the capacity to use language in the same way a spider is born with the ability to weave webs and a bird is born with the ability to make a nest. To use language is instinctive in humans, but the capacity is realized differently in people according to the specific languages to which they are exposed. A child reared in a family of English-speaking adults, who hears only English during the language acquisition period, *will* speak English. You might be surprised that the logic of that observation escapes some people. Children do not know they are German, French, Russian, or Japanese when they are born. They speak the language they hear, but the innate capacity for that language is the same, no matter where they are born and children speak the language of their families.

It is important to understand that language and the expression of language are two very different things. Language exists in the mind, and it exists whether or not it is expressed. When we think through an idea or listen to others and understand what they are saying or asking us to do, we call this **receptive language**. When we decide what we want to say and then actually speak it, sign it, or write it, we call it **expressive language**.

It is useful to understand language as a system of abstract symbols organized according to basic rules that seem to be common to all the languages known to humankind. In other words, at the deepest, most basic level, all languages share common components and each of these components use rules that allow the members of the language community to understand each other.

 Video Reflection 1.2: Parent Strategies for a Child's Use of Polite Language

Watch the video of a parent using strategies to encourage the use of polite language from her child, then answer the question.

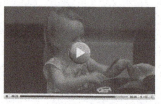

Let us look at the most functional component of language—the ability to use language as a social vehicle for establishing and maintaining relationships with others. We call this component **pragmatics**. Consider how we socialize children in our families and in early childhood settings. In Western culture, adults use a combination of obvious instructions, such as, "Wait until I finish talking before you speak," "Say please," "Ask Joey for that toy nicely," and subtle cues, such as holding up a hand to signal waiting or withholding the snack, until the child uses a polite request.

Other cultures use varying degrees of verbal and gestural cues as they socialize their children. Pragmatics involves not only using language according to socially established standards but also nonverbal behaviors, such as maintaining an appropriate distance between speakers, establishing and maintaining eye contact, and using body language appropriate to the situation. Most children learn pragmatics through daily routines and we expect that youngsters come to school with well-established social communication patterns. When a child comes to school without age-appropriate pragmatics or if pragmatics skills vary considerably from the cultural expectations of the classroom, it doesn't take long for teachers and other students to notice.

Another component of language is **semantics**. When we communicate, no matter what medium we choose, the goal is to convey meaning. Each language has rules for using words and for combining them into meaningful arrangements. Consider the following exercise. Write three nouns and then create sentences that convey different ideas. The example words in the following sentences are *flowers, vase*, and *morning*.

In the morning, I go to the garden and pick flowers for my vase.
This morning, I knocked over the vase of flowers.
The flowers in my favorite vase were dead in the morning.
The deliveryman arrived this morning with a beautiful vase of flowers.
Do you want to get your friend a vase of flowers this morning?

As you can see, semantics involves the meaning that we wish to convey, even when we are using the same topic words. It involves our use of vocabulary to construct ideas through relationships between words. Children benefit from lots of activities about words. We will explore this idea at length in subsequent chapters.

Ideas can be conveyed rather simply through three-to-five simple word combinations and even non-verbally, but humans develop rules for putting together words in complex arrangements to boost the power and efficiency of their language. We can get a lot done by speaking in an organized and clear manner. We use grammar to connect different types of words and the rule structure for these combinations is called **syntax**. In the sentences on the previous page, it is necessary to connect the nouns with other parts of speech, so that the meaning occurs. Imagine if we did not have rules for combining words. How would we make sense of messages if we only had nouns, for example? Read the sentences aloud using only the three nouns and you will get the point about the importance of syntax.

The arrangement of words is important for stating our meanings, and each word is considered a **morpheme**—a unit of meaning. But we also have small units of meaning that we add to words to enhance our messages. For example, the word *flowers*, in the example is not one, but two morphemes. *Flower* is the name of the object and we use the *s* at the end to convey that there is more than one. Thus, the *s* is a plural morpheme. We will discuss morphemes in greater detail in Chapters 4 and 5.

The fact that we do not all speak the same language suggests that some aspects of language are learned. Languages are different in many ways. They use different words and different rules for organizing words into grammatical sentences. English, for example, stresses word order in its grammar system, but other languages, such as Latin, place greater emphasis on word endings than on order to indicate grammatical relationships. That is, all languages have rules for making sentences grammatically correct, but the means by which correctness is achieved vary. We can conclude, therefore, that although the capacity for language is innate, and although all languages share very basic rules, the specific conventions of any given language are learned. The child who will speak English, for example, must learn the sounds of English as well as its vocabulary and grammar.

Now, let us put some of these pieces together into a definition. Language is a system of abstract symbols and rule-governed structures, the specific conventions of which are learned. The symbols of language may be sounds that are combined into spoken words, or letters that are combined into written words, or even the elements of sign language that are combined into larger units. It is important to note that whatever the symbols, they are arbitrarily established by the conventional usage of a given people. Furthermore, the symbols or their combinations will change over time because language is a constantly evolving phenomenon. Much more needs to be added to this definition (and will be in the chapters that follow), but this will serve as a starting point.

We can now define speech, a relatively simple task if we understand communication and language. Very simply, speech is the oral expression of language. Sometimes people use the terms *language* and *speech* as though they are interchangeable, but they clearly are not. If they were interchangeable, one could not exist without the other because they would be one and the same thing. In fact, speech can and does exist in the absence of language, and language exists in the absence of speech. Consider Toby the parrot or mynah birds that can mimic human speech, often with remarkable clarity. These birds produce speech, but they do not have language. That is, they can produce strings of sounds with the acoustic characteristics of human speech, and human listeners recognize the sequences of sounds as words, but the speech of these birds is devoid of meaning and, therefore, is not the oral expression of language. They have speech but not language. Some human beings, most notably those with severe cognitive challenges, may have the ability to imitate speech perfectly even if they do not fully understand the language underlying the speech. They have speech that reflects language abilities they do not have. Even normal children, between the ages of 18 and 24 months, often produce a form of speech known as echolalia, which is an imitation of words, phrases, or even whole sentences in the absence of an understanding of what they are saying. I[†] vividly recall a 3-year-old boy named Jerry, who arrived for his language therapy session. Jerry had very little verbal language, but he frequently used echolalia. When I said, "Hello, Jerry," he responded "Hello, Jerry." Then he pointed at the sign at the top of the door saying, "E-X-I-T. For more information call 1-800-234-6824." He echoed what I said and then recalled what he heard on a television commercial.

[†]Kathleen Fahey

Language can also exist independently of speech. Children who are born deaf, for example, may never learn to speak, but their deafness does not preclude their use of language. If these children have no other problems and receive proper stimulation and appropriate educational opportunities, they can develop language abilities just as sophisticated and complete as those of the hearing child who speaks. The child who is deaf and who does not have speech must learn a different way to express language, most likely through signs and gestures. In addition, the child who is deaf can receive and express language through the written word.

We can best understand speech as a highly complex physiological process requiring the coordination of respiration, phonation, resonation, and articulation. Some of the movements involved in producing even the simplest utterances are simultaneous and others are successive, but the synchronization of these movements is critical.

Consider what happens in the production of the single word *statistics*. The tip of the tongue is lifted from a resting position to an area on the roof of the mouth just behind the upper teeth called the **alveolar ridge** to produce the *s* sound. The tongue is pressed against the alveolar ridge hard enough to produce constriction but not so hard as to stop the airflow altogether. As the speaker slowly contracts the muscles of exhalation under precise control, air is forced between the tip of the tongue and the alveolar ridge. Leaving the tongue in the same area, the speaker now presses a little harder to stop the airflow and then quickly releases the contact for the production of the *t* sound. The tongue drops to a neutral position and the vocal folds in the larynx vibrate to produce the vowel *a*. The speaker turns off the voice and lifts the tongue to the alveolar ridge for the next *t*, then vibrates the vocal folds for the vowel *i* while the tongue stays in a forward but slightly lowered position. The speaker turns voicing off again and moves the tongue to the alveolar ridge yet again to produce the controlled constriction for the next *s*, followed by increased pressure to stop the airflow and release it for the *t*. The voice is turned on one more time and the tongue lowered to a neutral position for the *i*, and then turned off as the tongue arches to the back of the mouth, where it contacts the velum, or fleshy part of the roof of the mouth, for the *k*. Finally, the tongue tip darts to the alveolar ridge for the production of the final *s* sound.

All this occurs in the production of *one* word! Imagine what occurs in the production of a long sentence produced at an average speed. In addition to the production of each sound, we use **suprasegmental** aspects of speech. The syllables in each word are produced with varied degrees of stress. We also use intonation to emphasize certain words over others to convey meaning, and we modulate our pitch and phrasing to make speech interesting. Think of someone you know who speaks too fast, speaks in a monotone, or doesn't have a smooth rhythm. When you consider how many intricate adjustments are made so quickly in the speech mechanism and the suprasegmental aspects that we use to make our speech flow, it is difficult to imagine that anyone learns to speak at all. But we do learn to speak, and we do it easily and naturally over a very brief period of time.

Speech and Language Rejoined

Now that we have established that speech and language are separate, although related, parts of the communication process, we will reconnect them for the remainder of our analysis. For practical purposes, in people with normal communicative abilities, they are not separate. Speech is commonly understood as oral language, and that understanding will serve our purposes well. It is certainly clear to anyone who has studied the development of communication in children that speech and language develop together, but we should always remember that they do not develop at the same pace. Most of what a child will ever know about language is acquired before entering school, but some speech sounds are not mastered until age 7 or 8. Even within language itself, not all dimensions are acquired according to the same schedule. Rules pertaining to the structure of language are acquired early and most of the basic vocabulary of a language is learned early, but we continue to add vocabulary as long as we live, and most of us are developing our knowledge about how to use language well into adulthood during speaking and writing.

From this point on, however, we will consider speech and language as integrated parts of the same process in the same way that pictures and sounds are integrated parts of television. You can certainly have television without pictures: It's called radio. And you can have television without sound: That's called network difficulty. But television as we expect it includes not only pictures but also sound. Speech as we expect it in normal human beings combines phonated and articulated noises and the rule-governed structures of language.

Check Your Understanding 1.1

Assess your understanding of communication, language, and speech by completing this brief quiz.

The Unique Characteristics of Human Speech

To appreciate the power of oral language, we can compare it to the communication systems of other animals. Other animals do communicate, of course, but there is much we do not understand about their systems. Some animals seem to communicate very general messages in simple ways. The beaver, for example, slaps its tail when it senses danger. Dogs bark when they are frightened or excited. Other animals are able to communicate more elaborate messages. Bees dance to tell their fellow bees where flowers are. Other insects use their antennae to instruct or inform. There is a great deal of interest in the communication systems of dolphins and singing whales because they seem to be much more elaborate than the systems of most other animals (Herman & Forestell, 1985; Janik, 2000; Schusterman, 1986; Tyack, 2000). Recent research provides fascinating information about the communicative abilities of other species (see Table 1.1). But, no matter how much we discover about the abilities of other

Table 1.1 Animal Communication Signals

Animal	Communication Signals and Abilities	Purpose of Signal/Effect of Signal	Researchers
Monkeys (vervet)	Snake chutter	Warns other monkeys that snake is nearby/monkeys surround snake	Akmajian, Demers, and Harnish (1984)
	Aerial predator call	Warns other monkeys that eagle is overhead/monkeys seek cover on ground	
	Terrestrial predator call	Warns other monkeys that leopard is nearby/monkeys climb trees and go to ends of branches	
Marmots	Alarm signal	Intensity based on amount of risk present in situation	
Bonobos and chimpanzees	Use of symbols	Symbols represent objects or actions; limited combinations of symbols to create new meaning	Corballis (2007)
Dogs	Conative signals; play bow	Invites other dogs to play	Hauser, Chomsky, and Fitch (2002)
Bottlenose dolphins	Distress whistle	Signal for "help!"/dolphins in area arrive and raise distressed animal to the surface	
	Recognizes self in mirror	(Not evidence of theory of mind)	Akmajian, Demers, and Harnish (1984)
Birds	Aerial predator call "seet"	Warns other birds that predator is overhead/take cover in bushes and stay still	Gallup, (1982)
	Mobbing call "chink"	Warns other birds that stationary predator is nearby/surround (mob) the predator	
	Terrestrial song	Warns other male birds to keep away; invites uncommitted females to come to his location	
Chickadees	Four distinct sounds repeated in limited arrangements	(Not evidence of recursion)	Akmajian, Demers, and Harnish (1984)
Starlings	Count different sounds in sequences and match them for similarities and differences	(Not evidence of recursion)	
Nutcracker	Memory for where it stored food	Locates food in future (not evidence of recursion)	
Western scrub jay	Memory for when and how long food is stored	Locates food in future (not evidence of recursion)	Hailman and Ficken (1986)

animals to communicate, we remain convinced that no animal has a communication system as powerful as human speech.

One of the first linguists to take a detailed, analytical look at the characteristics of human speech in comparison to the communication systems of other animals was Charles F. Hockett (1960), who wrote a classic essay entitled "The Origin of Speech," in which he describes what he calls "13 design-features" of language. Although many animals share some of these features in their communication systems, Hockett believed that when taken together, his 13 features effectively separate human speech from other forms of animal communication. Since Hockett wrote his essay, new theoretical interpretations of animal communication and research data supporting these interpretations suggest that other species share many of the 13 features Hockett believed differentiated human communication from animal communication. Based on what we now know, only a few of Hockett's features are not found in the communication systems of other animals. Interestingly, we have found features beyond those identified by Hockett that can be ascribed to human communication. Nevertheless, "The Origin of Speech" remains an important and interesting part of the literature on human language, because it challenged linguists at the time to think about language and the humans who use it in revolutionary ways. We will examine Hockett's original 13 design features as a way of understanding the power of human communication, but we will also attempt to compare and contrast human communication with the communication systems of other species. We will then take a look at some design features that did not make Hockett's list. Table 1.2 shows that eight characteristics are present in humans and other species. Four characteristics are present in human language, but quite rare and limited in nonhumans, and five characteristics are particular to human language.

From Mouths to Ears

Hockett's first design feature is the **vocal-auditory channel**. That is, human beings communicate by forcing air through the vocal folds of the larynx and breaking the vibrating airstream into sounds of speech, which are organized into words and sentences. The listener's ear receives these sounds. This feature is so obvious that we may need to note that other channels can be used in communication and are used by other animals. Bees, for example, communicate by dancing, and that can be described as the visual channel. In fact, human beings who cannot hear use the visual channel when they produce and receive sign language. Still other animals communicate by touch or by odor. The primary advantage of the vocal-auditory channel for humans is that it leaves our hands free to do other things while we are communicating. We can build or repair, for example, while giving or receiving instructions. Imagine what it would be like for a construction crew building a house if everyone had to put down their tools every time one person needed to communicate with another through the gesture-visual channel. There is no question that vocal-auditory communication is convenient and allows us to be efficient in all tasks that involve communication in conjunction with other physical activities. This feature, of course,

Table 1.2 Characteristics of Communication in Humans and Other Species

Communication Characteristics	Definition
Humans and Other Species	
Vocal-Auditory Channel	Production of sound through mouth that is heard by listener's ear
Broadcast Transmission and Directional Reception	Vocalizations heard through sound waves
Rapid Fading	Vocalizations bound by time
Total Feedback	Producer and receiver recognize the message
Specialization	Vocalizations designed for communication
Arbitrariness	No relationship between the sounds and their meanings
Discreteness	Variations in sounds but limited in number and distinctiveness
Traditional Transmission	Instinctive and biologically acquired
Humans but Rare and Limited in Other Species	
Interchangeability	Unlimited exchanges of communication independent of age and gender
Semanticity and Indexicality	Specific messages that convey variety of meanings using background knowledge, situational contexts, nonvocal information, and dialect
Productivity	Communication through creative combinations of symbols
Displacement	Communicating about things remote from time and space
Humans	
Duality of Patterning	Combining sounds in infinite number of arrangements to produce words and sentences
Recursion	Creating and using words in complex and embedded arrangements and to store expressions that do not follow standard rules
Prevarication	Using language to deceive and to invent forms for artistic expression
Reflexivity	Using language to reflect on and talk about language
Learnability	Learning language from the environment, cognitive abilities, and social contexts

is not unique to human beings. Many other animals communicate by using the vocal-auditory channel. As indicated in Table 1.1, for example, monkeys and birds use this channel to communicate alarm and dolphins produce whistles to signal distress.

Sending and Receiving Signals

The second design feature involves **broadcast transmission** and **directional reception**, which are obviously related to the first feature. Two characteristics of speech are involved in this feature. When speech is produced, it radiates in all directions and can be received by any listener who is in range. In addition, a listener with two good ears can compare the loudness and timing of the signals reaching each ear and can determine the direction from which the sound is coming. If communication is visual, reception is much more limited.

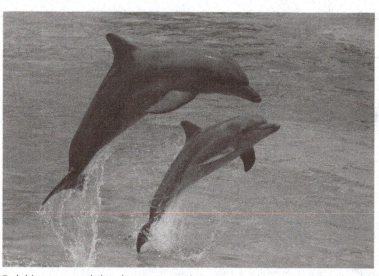

Dolphins use vocal signals to communicate.
Source: FourOaks/ iStock/Getty Images

For instance, an individual who is deaf may use sign language. The signs can be received only by someone close enough to the sender to see the subtle details of the gestures, and the receiver must directly face the sender. When Hockett wrote about this feature, he focused solely on the broadcasting and receiving of speech signals, but we must acknowledge that the general concept of sending and receiving is not unique to human speech, and it is not unique to communication that uses the vocal-auditory channel. Certainly, animals that use the vocal channel can send their messages to others of their species that have the capacity to receive them, but other animals that use gestural or even odor signals send and receive their messages as well. Starlings, for example, can communicate their location to other starlings. Vervet monkeys can send messages of warning, and ground squirrels can even communicate the degree of danger to other ground squirrels. Red-winged blackbirds signal dominance or aggression. Any form of communication produced by a particular species can be sent to and received by other members of that species.

Hear Today, Gone Immediately

Rapid fading means that speech signals are transitory. They do not linger. Humans have developed writing to put language information into a more permanent form, but writing is a relatively new ability for human beings in comparison to speech. We have also developed electronic means for preserving speech, but each time a sample of speech is produced live or on stored media, the signals are broadcast and rapidly fade. We cannot freeze-frame speech and study it in the same way we can read and study the written word or primitive paintings by prehistoric people on cave walls.

Rapid fading is common to many forms of animal communication—to those that depend on the vocal-auditory channel, of course, but also to those that are gesture-based. The difference between human speech and these forms of communication lies in the structure of the messages. Human speech is composed of speech sounds arranged in words and sentences. Other animals rely on vocal tones and cadences to form messages that sound "musical" to our ears. Crickets chirp, elks bugle, birds sing, and coyotes howl. In each case, as in human speech, the signals are transitory. They are produced, they convey their messages, and they fade away.

I Said it and I Meant It

Total feedback means that human speakers have the capacity to monitor what they say and how they say it. We hear ourselves, of course, but we also receive information from the musculature of speech about what we feel as the articulators move and contact one another. This feedback component allows a speaker to make constant adjustments so that output is as finely tuned as possible in terms of accurately conveying thoughts. Feedback also provides controls for the mechanics of speech in the sense that speech errors are caught and corrected or even anticipated and avoided. The fact that the feedback system includes information from several sensory sources also protects a speaker from communicative disaster if part of the system fails. Adults who lose hearing, for example, can maintain reasonably good speech by attending more closely to how speech feels. If we lose some of our ability to monitor the motor aspects of speech, we can concentrate more intently on what our speech sounds like.

Although it may not be directly comparable to the kind of feedback we associate with human speech, there is evidence that other species use feedback to monitor their communications as well. At the very least, members of a given species produce and recognize signals that belong to their communication system, and they recognize that other communicative productions do not belong. A bird, for example, knows the difference between bird songs and a wolf's howl.

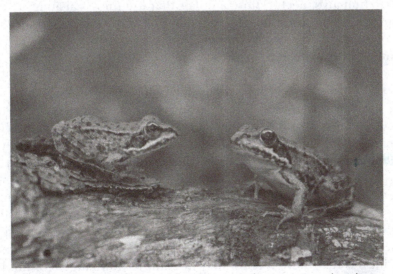

Male frogs use deep voices, and females respond to accept or reject these advances.

Source: Icefront iStock/Getty Images

Speech Is for Talking and Listening

The feature of **specialization** suggests that speech is specifically designed for communication and serves no other purpose. In Chapter 10, you will discover that the physical processes of speech are actually the secondary functions served by the structures involved. That is, human beings have adapted structures that serve more basic biological purposes for speech. Nevertheless, it is true that speech itself is a specialized human function. We speak to communicate and for no other purpose, although we may speak when no one is listening, and sometimes when we speak, we do not communicate successfully.

Consider the tongue, the structure many people most closely associate with speech. The primary biological purpose of the tongue is to aid humans in swallowing. The tongue captures food and/or liquid and moves it back toward the pharynx, where it flows into the esophagus and eventually the stomach. Obviously, this biological function is crucial to our survival as a species, but the tongue is also critical to speech. We touch the tongue to the alveolar ridge to produce sounds like *t, d, n,* and *l*. We touch the tongue to the velum to produce the sounds *k* and *g*, and we configure the tongue in a specific manner to produce the sound *r*.

In considering how the design features fit together, we should remember that speech is broadcasted, but it is also received. The perception of speech sounds and patterns of speech sounds is also highly specialized in human beings. These perceptual abilities are innate in humans, wired into our brains before we are born. Humans at birth can distinguish sounds from one another, and they show a preference for sounds that are speech-like from the beginning of their lives.

Although it is true that the communication systems of other animals are not as *specialized* as the human system, it's fair to note that specialization is not unique to human speech. Those animals that use the vocal-auditory channel use structures that have more basic biological purposes, including the same eating process we observe in humans. The bee uses its wings to produce its communicative dances, but the primary biological purpose of its wings is to fly.

Because We Say So!

One of the reasons languages differ so broadly across groups of people on Earth is that the words used to refer to the people, things, events, and concepts in human experiences do not directly reflect their referents. There is an **arbitrariness** about language. That is, there is nothing inherent in a spoken word to account for its meaning. We call the piece of furniture on which a person may sit a *chair,* not because it screams out to be called a chair, not because there is a connection between the nature of a chair and the word, but because someone at some time, for reasons of no interest to most people living today, arbitrarily decided to call it a chair. The obvious advantage of arbitrariness is that there is absolutely no limit to how language can describe anything and everything. Languages have different vocabulary because the naming of the bits and pieces that make up our environment has been done by different people in different places and at different times.

Do other animals demonstrate arbitrariness in their communication systems? We know that other species make sounds or use other communicative signals to warn, to play, and to attract other animals. These signals are arbitrary in the sense that there may be no obvious relationship between the sound or gesture and the message it conveys. We have no evidence that other animals *decide* which signals they will use to convey particular messages. It seems more likely that their innate abilities, their instincts, shape their signals in the most effective manner possible to convey the messages they need to survive.

The Limits of Speech

Discreteness is a feature that can be applied to human speech in at least two ways. Although the speech mechanism can produce an incredibly wide range of noises, each language is limited to a finite or discrete number of sounds. Furthermore, each sound used in one or more human languages has very specific characteristics so that each sound is discrete. Adult speakers adapt so completely to the specific sounds of a given language that they often have great difficulty breaking out of these patterns to produce sounds found in other languages but foreign to their own. Speakers whose native languages do not contain *l* or *r*, for example, struggle to produce these sounds when they are learning to speak English, and many of us who speak American English almost choke trying to produce certain French vowels. The flexibility we have as infants to produce virtually all sounds known to all languages is quickly lost when we begin to narrow our range to the discrete sounds of our own language.

Although other animals do not appear to have repertoires of signal choices to match the repertoires of sounds, words, and language rules that support human speech, they do demonstrate some variations in their communications. It would be fair to say, therefore, that other animals have sounds and/or gestures that are discrete in number and that have limitations in terms of how they are used or combined to create messages. The frog, for example, has only one croak, but dogs can produce different sounds—bark, whine, growl—to create different messages, and even the bark is not homogeneous. My[*] dogs, for example, produce quite different barking sounds to signal danger than to signal "let's play" and yet a different bark to signal that "we need to go outside. We REALLY need to go outside!"

Born to Talk

The suggestion involved in traditional transmission is that speech is instinctive in humans. We have a genetic or biological capacity for language so powerful that few environmental factors can stop the acquisition of speech, although they may affect the rate at which it is acquired and they may affect the quality of the language we use. Although the capacity for language is genetic, the details of a language, including vocabulary and structural rules, are learned.

---

[*]Kathleen Fahey.

Other animals do not talk, but whatever communication systems they use are genetically and biologically determined. It's also important to note that while humans can adapt to biological deficiencies in their natural communication systems by finding alternative methods for sending messages, similar abilities do not exist in other animals. A person who is deaf, for example, will have challenges in using the vocal-auditory channel for speech, but this person can use signs to effectively send and receive language messages. A monkey born blind in the wild that cannot see a predator or a deaf monkey that cannot hear an alarm call will not survive long in its natural environment.

Another reasonable comparison between humans and other animals involves innate ability in concert with exposure. The human child is born with the capacity for spoken language but will not produce speech unless exposed to it. In 3 of 27 orders of songbirds, songs are acquired as a consequence of exposure by parent birds. Just as experience facilitates language competence in human children, experience facilitates fine-tuning in the communicative abilities of other animals. As a vervet monkey develops, it tunes its alarm calls. Furthermore, the development of dialects in the vocalizations of some species is the product of innate capacity and exposure to the productions of other members of that species in a particular region.

If You Can Say It, I Can Say It

One feature of human speech that we may take for granted is **interchangeability**. This means that any human being can say anything that is said by any other human being. Children can and do imitate the speech of adults. Female humans can produce the same speech forms produced by males. Interchangeability removes communication barriers and is largely responsible for the unlimited exchange of information that characterizes human speech for both sexes and all ages.

Among other animals, this feature is rare. In courtship rituals, for example, the male of many species produces gender-limited communications, and the female produces gender-limited responses. The male frog, for example, emits a call to attract females for the purpose of mating. Female frogs are attracted to male frogs with deep "voices" because they will provide the best DNA for producing viable offspring. Female frogs produce a distinct sound to signal that they are not receptive to specific mating partners, the equivalent of letting those loser boys know that they have no chance. In most varieties of birds, males produce gender-specific songs to let other male birds know that they have staked out particular territories, and they produce songs designed to attract females.

Sending Messages Loud and Clear

One of the remarkable aspects of human communication is the ability to produce very specific messages with words having relatively stable relationships with the people, things, events, actions, and concepts they represent. These relationships allow us to share information effectively and easily, but there are times when a listener needs clarification from a speaker to correctly interpret a message. As you know from your own communicative experiences, there may be several requests for clarification before a listener is satisfied that the proper message has been received. In truth, the listener or the speaker sometimes gives up in the process, or the listener may believe that the proper message has been received even when it has not. In other words, communication, no matter how well intended, no matter how carefully crafted, is not perfect. The feature describing the ability to use human speech to convey specific messages is **semanticity,** but more than speech is needed in most cases to ensure the specificity of messages. Perconti (2002) asserts that situational context is also important in establishing meaning in our communicative attempts. He uses the term **indexicality** to describe the rich use of *presemantic, semantic, postsemantic,* and *extrasemantic* information in human communication.

Presemantics allow communicators to use their past and current experiences to help determine the meanings of words as used in a specific context. Consider, for example, a third-grade teacher who is discussing the band instruments she has given to each student. The teacher says, "It's time to play." The students know that it is time to play their instruments, not time to break for recess. The interpretation of the utterance depended not just on the words produced, but also on the human ability to use context and knowledge of phrasal stress to help establish meaning. Research indicates that other animals learn to establish meaning by observing the communication practices of other members of their species, and there are even dialectal differences in the communication systems of members of a given species, depending on where they live, but we have no evidence that other animals are able to use presemantic context to establish meaning as humans do.

When most of us think about *meaning*, we think about the most traditional use of the term *semantics*, using specific words in specific grammatical configurations to convey specific messages. Other animals appear to have limited inventories of signals they can use to shape their messages, but their messages lack the indexicality that explicitly specifies sender and receiver, and they do not appear to have the ability to establish different receivers of a given message in different situations. A dog will bow by lowering its front legs to invite another dog to play, for example. That's a fairly specific message as far as *doggie communication* is concerned, but it falls far short of the specificity inherent in human speech. Some primates have been taught to use signs to refer to specific things and actions in laboratory settings, but they do not appear to use signs to refer to particular objects or actions in the wild. Again, there is evidence of communicative specificity, but not to the extent we observe in human communication.

One of the most powerful aspects of specificity in human communication is the ability to analyze messages to determine the truth, reality, and completeness of the utterances produced in a given situation. This is what is meant by *postsemantic information*, and this ability appears to be uniquely human. Perconti (2002) uses the example, "It is raining" to show how this aspect of human speech works. In this simple sentence, the verb *is* signals the dimension of *time*, but there is nothing in the sentence to indicate *place*. The receiver, using contextual information, must determine the place to establish whether the statement is true.

Extrasemantic information includes social and psychological factors that can shade or shape meaning. If you are at a party with your best friend and something unpleasant happens to her, you can determine quickly and with a fair degree of accuracy what happened to upset her. How do you assess the situation? You listen to her words, of course, but you also take into account her voice, including stress and intonation. You react to the rhythm of her productions, to pitch fluctuations, and rate variations. Taken together, all this information helps you determine her state of mind. Your assessment of the party crisis may not be completely correct, of course, because you are hearing only one side of the story, but you will have a pretty good sense of how your friend feels. There is evidence that other animals also use context-dependent factors to shape their reactions to messages. If one member of a species communicates danger or alarm, other members will certainly become more alert, and they may flee. If the danger signal occurs in the context of a clearly visible approaching firestorm, the message is enhanced and the fleeing may be considerably more urgent. There is no doubt, however, that human communications are far more sophisticated, far more detailed and specific than those of other animals in terms of using context to interpret the social and psychological factors that help make messages complete and meaning-rich for senders and receivers.

The Creativity of the Mind and Mouth

According to Hockett (1960), **productivity** is one of the most important design features of human speech. Humans have the amazing ability to be creative in their communication efforts. We can say things that have never been said before, or we can put old messages in brand new language forms. We use words in speech in much the same way sculptors use clay. A sculptor can take a mass of clay and make everything from a bowl to a bust. We can use a finite collection of sounds and words to shape an infinite variety of messages, some simple, some profound, some old, some new. No matter what the message is, however, if we obey the rules of our language, the message will be understood by anyone who shares the language we speak. Just imagine that on this very day you may say something that no one has ever said before and perhaps no one will ever say again in exactly the same way. The productivity or creativity of language gives human speakers a communicative power that is not shared by any other species.

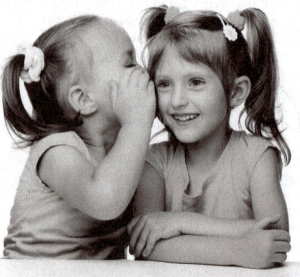

Giving and receiving information through language.

Source: Serhiy Kobyakov/ 123RF.com

It's well established that other animals have been trained to use symbols, to associate these symbols with words, and to combine them to signal meaningful messages. Most notably, some primates have developed fairly extensive repertoires of visual symbols and words used in reference to objects, people, places, and basic actions. These primates are able to understand simple commands. They can combine symbols to create messages that suggest meaningful sentences. No one is arguing that these accomplishments reflect the kinds of innate language abilities we see in humans, but by using teaching/learning paradigms that incorporate many repetitions of specific symbol–meaning combinations and by systematically rewarding their subjects' efforts and accomplishments, researchers have facilitated communicative abilities, comparable to human language, in these primates that we could not have imagined 20 years ago. Dolphins, responding to visual commands, have also performed actions that reflect the word order, or syntax, of the commands they are given. As is true of nonhuman primates, dolphins' learning depends heavily on repetition and reward, and in all cases, we have no evidence that they can use these acquired abilities to *create* their own language-like combinations, but what they have achieved is remarkable. Most importantly, this work suggests that we have grossly underestimated what other animals can do in the arena of communication—naturally or learned.

Back to the Future

One of the most intriguing features of human speech is **displacement**. That is, humans can talk about things that are distant in time or space. We can talk about what is going on in places across vast oceans or even across the infinite expanses of space. We can talk about events that occurred hundreds or thousands of years ago, and we can talk about things that have not yet happened. We know that bees dance to let other bees know about a food source that is removed in space, but this is a very limited displacement ability. It's probable that this feature does not exist at all in the communication systems of most animals.

Many Wholes From a Few Parts

Part of the creativity that is characteristic of human speech is made possible by another design feature, **duality of patterning**. Although a given language is restricted in the number of sounds it uses, these sounds can be combined in an infinite number of ways to produce an infinite variety of words, and the words of a language can be combined into an infinite variety of sentences. Every year of your life you will be witness to the creation of new words that are the product of this duality of patterning. Many of these new words reflect neverending advances in science and technology. Before there were telephones, there was no word *telephone,* but the sounds making up the word have existed for as long as human language as we know it has existed. It remained for someone to arrange this particular collection of sounds into this specific word to refer to that object. Just think for a moment about all the words that have been invented as a result of the explosion of computer-related technology. The patterning of sounds into words and words into sentences will end only when humankind ceases to communicate, and that is likely to happen only when humankind ceases to exist.

We have no reason to believe, based on research conducted so far, that duality of patterning, as described by Hockett, exists in the communication systems of other animals. Some trained animals demonstrate patterns in their communicative productions, but those patterns are limited to what their trainers specifically teach and specifically shape.

I Think, Therefore I Am

According to Hauser (2007), **recursion** involves a human's ability to use acquired knowledge to create language, to imagine what others may be thinking, to engage in mental time travel to the past and the future, to think about and gain understanding of *self*, and to relate to a divine being in the development and demonstration of spirituality. Recall that displacement, the ability to talk about things and events that are remote in time and space, is an aspect of recursion. (Hauser argues that recursion may be the singular characteristic that distinguishes humans from all other creatures. With respect to language specifically, recursion underlies the ability of humans to use words and phrases in complex and embedded arrangements, as well as to store linguistic expressions, such as idioms and other constructions, that do not follow standard syntactic rules. As we have already noted, other primates, notably chimpanzees and bonobos, have been trained to use symbols to represent objects and common actions, but they have very limited abilities to combine symbols to create new meanings. Starlings and chickadees produce and perceive a few distinctive sounds in sequence, but the emphasis is on *few*. They do not demonstrate anything that remotely resembles human recursion. As would seem reasonable, given its definition, recursion is not limited to language (Jackendoff & Pinker, 2005). It is also evident in visual processing, suggesting that it is a generalized cognitive phenomenon, not just a language phenomenon. We will certainly learn more about recursion as the debate and the subsequent research examining it continue.

Speaking Is an Art Form

Prevarication is a feature that often, though not always, addresses a darker side of human communication. Prevarication refers to the ability of humans to intentionally deceive others in their communications. This feature might be unique to humans. Other animals engage in deceptive practices for the purpose of survival, but these tactics appear to be the products of instinct, not of specific communicative intention. That is, other animals might lure prey or evade predators through deception, but we have no evidence that animals *lie*, as humans do, in order to deceive (Anderson, 2004). In fairness, prevarication is not always malicious in human beings. It can also be used to invent creatures, objects, and events for the purpose of storytelling or for other forms of artistic expression. Imagine what J. K. Rowling's Harry Potter stories would have been like without her ability to prevaricate. Used for good or ill, prevarication adds an important and unique dimension to human language.

Talking About Talking

According to Anderson (2004), **reflexiveness**—called *metalinguistic ability* by other linguists—refers to the ability of humans to use language to talk about language. Although we admit that reflexiveness is probably a product of language rather than one of its defining characteristics, it is nevertheless a characteristic of human communication not found in nonhuman communication, so we include it as another possible design feature.

Recipe for Language

Anderson (2004) also suggests **learnability** as a possible design feature of human communication. He differentiates learnability and Hockett's traditional transmission by suggesting that learning should be understood beyond the usual "interaction with the environment" concept. That is, learning occurs when we combine a person's innate capacity for learning, a learning environment, and some stimulus for learning that comes from the learner himself. Learnability suggests that cognitive structures interact with experience to produce learning. In language development, for example, environmental input, innate cognitive abilities, and the human motivation to pursue social relationships interact to produce language learning. The environmental input will shape the specific learning that occurs. If the environment includes English models, the child will learn English. If the environment includes French models, the child will learn French.

Not All Features Are Created Equal

As shown in Table 1.1, there has been considerable evolution in our thinking about human communication in comparison to animal communication since Hockett wrote his classic essay. The research since 1960, and especially since the 1980s, makes it clear that the differences are not nearly as stark as Hockett postulated. Hockett tried to identify the features of human speech that provide its communicative efficacy and power, and to determine to what extent those features can be found in the communication systems of other animals. When we look at the net result of the research conducted since Hockett's essay was published, we can conclude that most of the 13 design features he found in human speech are also found in the communication systems of animals. The traditional transmission of a system as complex as human language and duality of patterning has not been found in the communication systems of non-human species. As indicated earlier, the honeybee dance to indicate the location of a food source is an example of displacement, but it is an exceedingly limited form of displacement. Most importantly, when we look at Hockett's work, we can conclude that no nonhuman species has a communication system that incorporates all 13 of Hockett's design features. We believe that human language, as an extraordinarily complex and powerful communication system, is unique in the animal kingdom even as we concede that other animals are able to communicate much more than Hockett imagined in 1960.

   In addition to conceding that other animals communicate more, and more effectively, than we once believed, we need to point out that there are some features Hockett missed.

We have considered a range of features that, taken together, help us understand what human communication is, how it compares to the communication systems of other animals, and how it is unique among these systems. We certainly should appreciate that there are some common denominators when we compare human communication to nonhuman forms of communication, but we cannot help but be impressed by the spectacular differences that separate human communication from other systems in the animal kingdom, especially the differences reflected in features such as productivity, displacement, semanticity, indexicality, duality of patterning, recursion, prevarication, reflexiveness, and learnability that contribute to the powerful creativity that drives human language. As theorists and researchers continue to explore these subjects, we will be reminded that our understanding of human communication, nonhuman communication, and how they compare is far from complete.

Video Example 1.1

Watch the video to see human language characteristics in action. As you watch this video of first-graders talking about how animals move, notice the dynamic ways they think about the topic, react and share with each other, use gestures to enact concepts, and apply information. Review reflexivity, recursion, productivity, and duality of patterning as you consider their interactions.

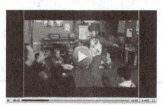

Check Your Understanding 1.2

Assess your understanding of the design features of the human communication system by completing this brief quiz.

Speech: The Tale of Two Brains

We are now ready to return to the query that opened this chapter or, more specifically, to a more complete response to that question. All human beings who are able to speak are capable of using a kind of mental telepathy because speech allows two human brains to connect.

This connection is described in another portrait of human speech contained in a book entitled *The Speech Chain* (Denes & Pinson, 1993). A summary of this description will show how the brains of a speaker and a listener connect in a communicative sense.

The speech chain (Figure 1.1) has six steps or links. In the first step, you the speaker sort through your thoughts, decide which of these thoughts to

Figure 1.1   The Speech Chain

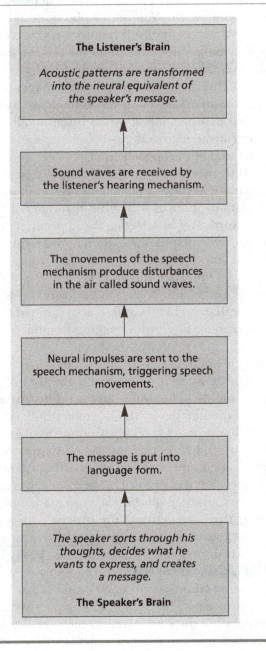

express, and make some decisions about how to express them. Although this process occurs very quickly, within seconds or fractions of a second, it is actually very complex. If, for example, a friend wearing the most atrocious dress you have ever seen asks you, "What do you think of my new dress?" you have some serious decisions to make. Your brain is filled with conflicting thoughts as you consider your response. You know that this article of clothing is an affront to anything resembling good taste. You must also consider that your friend must have liked it because she did, in fact, actually give someone real, government-green money for it. You want to be honest, but you do not want to hurt her feelings. What do you do? What do you say? Well, you sort through all your thoughts. You make a decision about the relative merits of honesty and compassion, and you finally decide what to say. Incidentally, this step is much easier for very young children, who typically spend very little time arranging and editing their thoughts. The 3-year-old is likely to say the first thing that comes to mind, which may be tactless and unintentionally hurtful. One of the aspects of communication acquired most slowly is the ability to make good decisions in the first step of the speech chain.

Regardless of how the decisions are made in the first step or whether they are appropriate decisions, the second step remains the same. You as the speaker put your message into language form by leafing through your mental dictionary to pick out the right words and by selecting the appropriate rules of grammar to create the correct word forms and place them in the right order. This step also occurs so quickly that you cannot monitor yourself doing it unless you cannot think of the right word. Only when the process is interrupted by this kind of failure do we begin to appreciate just how easily and naturally we translate thoughts into language. Notice that the first two steps are confined to the brain. We may think of speech as flapping lips and a wagging tongue, but even the simplest utterance begins in the gray matter of the brain.

In the third step, the brain sends instructions, in the form of neural impulses, to the muscles of speech. Keep in mind that these are not just the muscles of the structures in the mouth. The brain must send instructions to the muscles of respiration and to the muscles of the larynx and pharynx, as well as to the muscles of the face that support speech with nonverbal expressions, and even to the muscles of the arms, hands, fingers, and perhaps even the legs and torso, which provide additional nonverbal support to the speaker's words. The complexity of this operation is unbelievable and becomes even more amazing when you consider the speed at which all the parts are made operative.

In the fourth step, the movements of the structures of speech interrupt and constrict the flow of vibrating air from the larynx, setting up minute pressure changes in the air surrounding the speaker's mouth. These patterns of air pressure changes are called **sound waves**. Sound waves cause air particles to bump into each other, creating compression between some particles and spaces and rarefactions between others. The bumping, compression, and rarefaction of air particles continue until the sound waves reach the listener's ears.

As the air particles bump into the listener's eardrums in the fifth step, the listener's hearing mechanism is activated. As you will discover in more detail in Chapter 10 at the end of the book, the ear has the capacity to transform the mechanical energy of vibrating air particles into hydraulic energy in the fluids of the inner ear and eventually into neural energy that travels along the acoustic nerve to the brain.

Finally, in the listener's brain, the neural impulses are analyzed and interpreted so that the listener recognizes the speaker's message. Consider what has happened in the speech chain. Thoughts have been transformed into language forms, which have been transformed into neural signals, which trigger the structures of speech, which by means of their movements disturb air particles and transform them into sound waves, which bombard the listener's ears, which transform the sound waves into neural patterns, which are received and decoded by the listener's brain. Incredibly, the message is not lost or changed. The listener may not always understand what you intended to communicate, but if he is within hearing range and if you speak clearly, he will receive precisely the same pattern you sent.

Speech does indeed give us the power of mental telepathy. It allows brains to connect. Speech is so much a part of the human experience that we truly take it for granted, but it is a wondrous human gift. The next time you engage in a conversation with one or more people, consider the speech chains that connect speakers and listeners. Marvel at the speed involved in the sending and receiving of messages. Notice how quickly speakers become listeners and listeners become speakers in a ballistic communication give-and-take that almost defies understanding. Now consider that human beings know much of what they will ever know about language and have the basic skills involved in speech by the time they are just four or five years old! How does this happen? In the remainder of this book, you will take a closer look at many of the elements in the speech chain. You will consider what a child must know to be a competent language user, and explore the acquisition process along important dimensions of speech and language. You will learn much is still unknown about human language. The experts argue about almost every major topic, but much more is known about speech and language today than was known just 30 years ago. The purpose of this book is to help you understand what is known, to recognize what is not known, and, most important, to appreciate the almost mystical nature of this uniquely human talent.

Check Your Understanding 1.3

Assess your understanding of the speech chain by completing this brief quiz.

SUMMARY

Human communication is a complex phenomenon with unique features as compared to how other species communicate. Speech and language abilities allow us to socialize, get things done, and learn about our world as we send and receive information to others.

▌▌▶ Surfing the Web

If you are interested in exploring topics discussed in this chapter in more detail, search for one or more of the following relevant terms online.

animal communication
bird communication
canine communication
dolphin communication
feline communication
Hockett's design features of language
primate communication
speech chain

Chapter Review 1.1

Recall what you learned in this chapter by completing the Chapter Review.

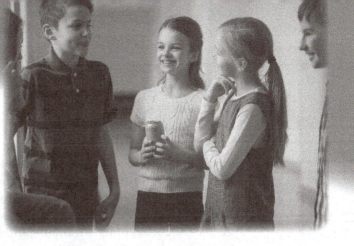

2

Language Acquisition: A Theoretical Journey

LEARNING OUTCOMES

After completion of this chapter, you will be able to:

- Summarize the nativist interpretation of the role biology plays in language development.
- Discuss the behaviorist interpretation as it relates to the role of nurturing language acquisition.
- Relay the tenets of the interactionist perspective in understanding cognitive, social, and interactional influences on language.

This chapter is designed to facilitate comprehension of the evolutionary changes that have occurred over the past 50 or more years in the theories of language acquisition. It considers the contributions made by each major theoretical view along the evolutionary continuum to furthering an understanding about how the various components of language emerge.

The Nativist Theories of Language Acquisition

People probably have argued about how human talents are acquired from the earliest days of our species. Is an artist born or made? Does the musician inherit talent, or is it shaped by hours of rehearsal? Is the great athlete destined to become a physiological virtuoso because of genes, or is athletic skill the product of teaching and practice? Even the casual observer must understand that in most nature-versus-nurture arguments, the truth does not come down on only one side. The master artist must surely be born with the ability to paint or sculpt, but it is only through study, training, and practice that an artist's skills are developed and refined. The child born with the genetic makeup to become a gifted athlete will realize that potential only when provided the opportunity to learn and perfect the skills of the game she chooses. In other words, most human talents are both born and made.

Even human traits, while widely considered to be purely genetic, can be influenced by the environment. A child might be smaller than his genetically determined size because he is malnourished. A child born with great intellectual capacity might function at a normal or below-normal level because she has not been provided adequate opportunities for learning. Sadly, if the poor diet continues long enough, the small child will remain undersized, and if the educational opportunities are withheld long enough, the intellectually gifted child will lose her gift. Sometimes, of course, environment can affect nature's outcomes in less-dramatic and less-permanent ways. A child born brown-eyed can have blue eyes by wearing tinted contact lenses. A short child can wear elevator shoes. The adult with naturally brown hair can have blonde hair by using peroxide. The list of environmental manipulations of natural conditions becomes longer with each generation of humans.

Theories designed to explain how language develops address the nature-versus-nurture debate at various points along the continuum, and you will note that each theoretical view addresses certain aspects of language more directly than others. Some theories, for example, focus primarily on the function of language. Others are more concerned with the structure of language. Others consider the connections between cognition and language, and still others attend to environmental factors as facilitators in the acquisition process.

Until about 1960, most people who studied the development of speech and language in children assumed that oral communication skills are learned. During the first half of the 20th century, much emphasis was placed on parents teaching their children to talk, even though there was concern that parents were not very good teachers. Van Riper, as late as 1964, made the observation that, "children learn to talk. Their parents do the teaching, and it is usually very poor" (p. 92). Many experts during this era believed that children learn to talk not because of their parents but in spite of them.

The nature-versus-nurture argument in speech and language became heated during the 1960s and early 1970s when theorists called *nativists* or *biological nativists* suggested that children are genetically predisposed to talk. That is, oral language is instinctive (natural) in humans and, like instincts in other animals, speech is behavior the child produces with minimal environmental involvement. It is a genetically coded behavior and is as natural for the child as walking.

What is sometimes lost in discussions about this debate is that neither side completely discounts the other. Those who believe language is learned or nurtured (behaviorists) recognize that a child must have the right anatomical equipment and maturation and must be ready to acquire language in terms of mental capacity, and the ability to use the senses to take in and interpret information. Their emphasis, however, is on environmental influences. They argue, for example, that a child reared in a stable home with parents who provide good language models has a distinct advantage over one reared in an economically, culturally, and socially impoverished home by parents who provide few and inadequate language models.

Nativists accept the fact that environment plays some role in the acquisition of speech and language. That is, the child must be exposed to language models, but nativists view these models as mere triggers for a natural, biological acquisition process. They argue that the innate drive for the development of language in humans is so powerful that even a poor environment will not prevent the child from talking.

As the debate has continued, the extreme views have moderated, and there is a general understanding that what the child brings to language development genetically is important, but so is the environment into which he is born. Differences among theorists still exist concerning the importance they place on nature or nurture, and given the history of this ongoing debate about all aspects of human development, it is unlikely the experts will ever agree.

Research has added to our understanding of how both human biology and human interaction contribute to language acquisition. Those who enter the debate about how children become expert users of language have a wealth of information to draw on to support their perspectives. We review some findings from this research as a backdrop to our discussion of the theories.

Human Biology and Language

In Chapter 1 we considered the varied communication systems of some non-human species, where we discovered several different but intricate and interesting ways in which non-humans interact. Recall that the nature and extent of animal interactions are primarily biologically based for their survival. Some species also seem to engage in social interactions that have a limited but important role in their communication. Consider, for example, the discovery of certain birds that appear to develop local dialects in their calls based on the use of the dialect in their immediate environment. The interaction between the biological system and the environment may account for variations in bird calls from one locality to another. Now we turn our attention to the nature of human biology as one way to look at how children learn language and interactions within cultures.

Psycholinguistic researchers in the 20th and 21st centuries have uncovered compelling evidence about how the human brain is specialized for language. In Chapter 10 of this book, we provide a brief account of the major cortical structures involved in language. Figure 10.13 shows a schematic drawing of the left hemisphere. **Wernicke's area** in the temporal lobe assists speakers with the formulation of language. When you have an idea to convey, you use this area to put your ideas into a form consisting of words and phrases. As a listener, you receive the speaker's information and use your knowledge of words and grammar to understand the meaning of the message; in other words, you comprehend it. Language information is transmitted to Broca's area from Wernicke's area via a bundle of nerve fibers called the **arcuate fasciculus,**. **Broca's area** is in the frontal lobe and has the role of assigning and organizing the motor sequences for the sounds of speech. When you speak words and phrases, Broca's area develops the program whereby the commands for each sound in a word are sent in the appropriate order to the **motor cortex**, which sends the neural messages to carry speech and language information to the muscles involved in producing speech. Beyond the broad areas of specialization in the temporal lobe, such as Wernicke's area, Broca's area, and the **primary motor strip** in the frontal lobe, neuropsychological and neuroimaging studies have added significantly to our understanding of the complexity and particularities of how animal and human brains respond to non-linguistic and linguistic information.

For example, a very interesting finding emerged from the study of monkeys as they engage in actions such as grasping, holding, and tearing objects. The neurons that fire during these actions are found in the ventral (anterior and lower) premotor (front) part of the monkey's inferior area (area F5). Researchers also discovered that these same neurons fire when the monkey observes these same actions performed by another. Such neurons are called **mirror neurons**. Rizzolatti and Arbib (1998b) propose that mirror neuron activity represents actions that can be used not only for imitating actions but also to recognize and determine differences in the actions of others. This feedback is used for responding appropriately in situations. They conclude that mirror neurons provide the link between the sender of a message and the receiver of it. Researchers have also discovered that mirror neurons exist in humans, as shown by experiments (Fadiga & Craighero, 2006; Rizzolatti, Fadiga, Gallese, & Fogassi, 1996) where, during observation of various actions, selective increases of motor evoked potentials (electrical responses) occur in the muscles that the subjects use to produce the actions. The presence of mirror neurons in humans may explain why we enjoy watching others slide across the ice, run the football down the field, or water or snow ski, or even why we spend several hours each week watching other people cook! In humans the area of the brain that is analogous to F5 in the monkey is Broca's area in the inferior frontal gyrus. Researchers (Rizzolatti & Arbib, 1998b) contend that the mechanism for recognizing the actions of others was the neural underpinning for the development of speech. In addition, they suggest that humans have an innate ability to match action observations with the execution of the actions. This ability coupled with rapid learning and cultural influences support the evolution of language. These exciting findings offer strong support for the nature end of the argument regarding language acquisition.

Recent research regarding the importance of mirror neurons as it relates to communication demonstrated differences in the mirror neural system (MNS) between typically developing children and children with autism spectrum disorder (ASD). Dapretto and colleagues (2005) studied ten children with high-functioning autism between 10 and 14 years and their age-matched controls using fMRI while imitating and observing emotional expressions. They were shown 80 faces expressing anger, fear, happiness, neutrality, or sadness for 2 seconds in a random sequence. One task required each child to imitate the faces, while the other task required only observation. All the children were successful with each task during a practice session. The fMRI results for typically developing children showed extensive neural activity in several premotor regions, motor regions, limbic structures, and the cerebellum. Strong activity was observed in both hemispheres, especially in the right inferior frontal gyrus, where the mirror properties are most concentrated. The children with ASD showed robust activation in the visual cortices, demonstrating that they attended to and imitated the emotional expressions; however, they did not demonstrate any activity in the mirror neuron area. Dysfunction in the MNS may explain why children with ASD show deficits in understanding the emotional state of others. Indeed, the researchers found that children with ASD who have better social functioning had more activity in the MNS than did children who were weak in the social domain.

The human brain also has a dynamic ability to change constantly as individuals learn, an ability known as **plasticity**. Plasticity provides the brain flexibility and adaptability, resulting in the **self-organizing neural network**. Consider, for example, research showing that the brain organizes the way it responds to words in relation to how the words function within the language. Thus, nouns, verbs, and other categories show different patterns of neural activity during listening tasks (Li, 2003; MacWhinney, 2001; Miikkulainen, 1993, 1997; Ritter & Kohonen, 1989). Our ability to categorize words, as you can imagine, allows us to select and use words from our memories with great speed and accuracy.

This ability to learn, store, and retrieve words is critical to normal language development. An example of the workings of the self-organizing neural network can be found during the vocabulary spurt that children experience between 18 and 20 months. A child who had the ability to name items in her environment suddenly finds herself having some confusion in naming these known objects, people, and events. This brief period has been called the **naming deficit**. It is thought to occur for one of two reasons: either because the densely packed representations stored in memory during rapid vocabulary growth also produce competition in word selection (Gershkoff-Stowe & Smith, 1997), or because the words are undergoing reorganization, causing confusion about words that have strong semantic relationships (Bowerman, 1978, 1982). The result of either or both of these processes is short-term difficulty with word recall. Consider this scenario. A child might be very excited to discuss playing with the dump truck in the sandbox with his day-care aide. In his excitement, he might repeatedly call it a tractor even though he knows all about dump trucks. Because both the dump truck and the tractor are in the sandbox and the child is using both to move dirt around, the words to distinguish one from another may be elusive.

An additional research finding regarding the brain's neural response to language input is known as the **age of acquisition effect**. Words that are learned early show faster retrieval during naming and reading tasks than words learned later (Ellis & Morrison, 1998). This phenomenon is explained in terms of plasticity in learning. As new learning occurs, the neural network needs to retain its plasticity and its stability in word representations so that word learning increases efficiently across time.

The self-organizing neural network has been used in discussions about language learning as an interconnected system where learning in one language domain, such as the sound system, cannot help but affect other language domains, such as grammar. These interconnections also may explain why such variability and widespread difficulties exist across the language system among children who have language problems (Zera & Lucian, 2001). This connectivity also helps interventionists to plan and deliver language programs targeting multiple learning goals.

There is a substantial body of literature that verifies genetic influences on language development and the occurrence of language disorders. Paul (2007) provides a review of family aggregation studies, pedigree studies, twin studies of typically developing children, and twin studies of children with language disorders. The summary statements relative to findings from many studies (see Figure 2.1) offer strong support for the genetic transmission of language capability. Specifically, individuals in families are more likely to have speech and language problems when other members of the family have them, and language disorders appear to be heritable when only one parent (autosomal dominant inheritance) has a family history of these disorders. Our growing knowledge of the human genome shows that specific regions in the human brain contain important genes that make it possible for offspring to have normal language abilities, or that result in disorders with the acquisition and use of the language system.

Biologically speaking, humans not only have the neural mechanisms that support language learning and use, but these abilities are also genetically transmitted to their offspring. But of course, genetic makeup is only one of the ingredients in successful language development. We will explore the evidence about how our environment influences language learning later in this chapter. For now, we will focus on some theories about how biology relates to language development.

Figure 2.1   Genetic Influence on Language Development and Disorders

- The mean incidence of a positive family history for speech and language problems across studies is 46% in families of children with specific language impairment and 18% in controls (Stromswold, 1998).

- An autosomal dominant inheritance pattern was found for children with specific grammatical language impairments (van der Lely & Stollwerck, 1996).

- Gene-mapping studies show that genetic region SPCH1, chromosome 7q31, is linked to severe motor dyspraxia, expressive grammar delay, written language problems, and intellectual deficits (Fisher, Vargha-Khadem, Watkins, Monaco, & Pembray, 1998).

- The human gene subregion CFTR within SPCH1 in the frontal lobe has been linked to specific language impairment causing problems with expressive language delay, severe articulatory disturbance (verbal dyspraxia), and moderate cognitive impairment (Fisher et al., 1998).

- Studies of typical children show that rapid receptive vocabulary acquisition at 14 months and expressive vocabulary acquisition at 20 months are influenced by genetics due to fast mapping of phonological forms to objects and the vocabulary spurt (Kay-Raining Bird & Chapman, 1998).

- Twin studies of children with language disorders reveal a strong role for genetic influence in the variation of language ability between normally developing and language-impaired twins (Bishop, North, & Donlan, 1995; Lewis & Thompson, 1992; Tomblin & Buckwalter, 1998).

The Extreme View of Nature's Contribution to Language Development

As the name of this view suggests, nativists stress the idea that language is innate or biologically based. They argue that human beings are born with a species-specific capacity for language, a capacity that is realized with minimal assistance from the environment. Nativists stress competence or knowledge that leads to performance. In other words, you must have the goods in order to deliver.

The theorist most closely associated with the nativist view is linguist Noam Chomsky. Chomsky (1968) expresses one of the basic assumptions of nativism in this declaration: "Anyone concerned with the study of human nature and capabilities must somehow come to grips with the fact that all humans acquire language" (p. 59). The idea that language is universal among humans and unique to humans is the foundation of the nativistic interpretation of language acquisition. These theorists point out that unless there are severe physical or mental limitations, human beings will acquire language, and that the innate drive to acquire language is so powerful that many humans talk in spite of what may seem to be insurmountable limitations. They also argue that only human beings are capable of acquiring and using language as we know and understand it.

Do other species learn language? The earliest attempts to teach chimpanzees to speak failed, but when Gardner and Gardner (1969, 1971, 1975) began their research with Washoe, a 10-month-old female chimpanzee, they tried a different language avenue. They taught Washoe how to use American Sign Language (ASL), one of the manual communication systems used by people who are deaf. Washoe eventually learned more than 100 signs and, according to the Gardners, spontaneously produced combinations of signs to express basic requests such as, "Listen dog" and, "Give me food." The fact that Washoe brought her hands to a resting position only after a series of signs was produced was interpreted to mean that she intended to combine these signs. There is no question that what Washoe accomplished was beyond what linguistics would have imagined possible, but even those most excited about attempts to teach chimpanzees to use language have recognized some important limitations. There is no evidence, for example, that Washoe learned any rules of grammar as reflected by consistent or meaningful word order. Some have suggested that this failure to acquire grammatical rules may be a function of ASL, which is not bound by the strict word order rules used in spoken and written language. On the other hand, it may simply be that chimpanzees do not have the ability to learn syntax, a conclusion that seems to be supported by the findings of Terrace (1980), another researcher who specifically analyzed his chimpanzee's signed utterances to determine whether there were any word order consistencies. He found none.

Efforts also have been made to teach language to pygmy chimpanzees, as well. (Savage-Rumbaugh, MacDonald, Sevcik, Hopkins, & Rubert, 1986). Pygmy chimpanzees are reportedly more intelligent and social than those used in earlier experiments, and the preliminary evidence suggests that they have a greater capacity for language-based communication skills. According to their trainers, these chimpanzees have acquired symbols simply by observing their human trainers, and they have used these symbols spontaneously in apparent attempts to communicate with humans. There is also evidence that they can combine these symbols to create more complex utterances, and they seem to understand some spoken words.

One of the most remarkable primates studied by Georgia State University researchers is Kanzi, a bonobo or pygmy chimpanzee, born in October 1980. *Kanzi* is the Swahili word meaning "treasure," an appropriate name for an animal that has been a treasure trove of discovery for those who care for him and study him. Kanzi is the first primate, other than human children, to acquire language not by direct teaching, but by being reared in a language-rich environment. As is true of human children, all his interactions with his caregivers, from the time he was born, have been framed in language. It is significant to note that Kanzi understands not just words, but even word order. When given the instructions, "Put jelly in the milk" and, "Put milk in the jelly," Kanzi carries out the instructions appropriately, an accomplishment dependent on understanding word order (Rumbaugh & Beran, 2003; Savage-Rumbaugh, Shanker, & Taylor, 1998). As impressive as Kanzi's abilities are, it must be acknowledged that chimpanzees, including the pygmy variety, so far have not shown the ability to acquire adult-like syntax, but we must not overlook the fact that these primates seem capable of acquiring and using the kind of language expected of very young human children (Greenfield & Savage-Rumbaugh, 1984; Savage-Rumbaugh, 1990; Savage-Rumbaugh, MacDonald, Sevcik, et al., 1986).

All the research conducted with apes must be understood in the context of the criticisms raised about the general methods used. Skeptics have noted that whatever "language" is learned is the result of extraordinary efforts to teach on the part of human trainers—the kind of constant and powerful teaching that is not necessary for humans to acquire language. Critics also suggest that the successes noted are more the result of imitation and prompting than of any natural capacity for language (Terrace, Pettito, Saunder, & Bever, 1979).

Based on all the data now available, we have no reason to believe that nonhumans are capable of acquiring and using language, at least not a language directly and completely comparable to human language. Even if we accept that chimpanzees and other animals can acquire symbols and combine them, and that they can understand some spoken words, we have no evidence that they can acquire the rules for combining words into grammatical structures, engage in conversation, or use language creatively. Language learning goes beyond vocabulary to include structure, the layering of meanings, the transformations of word forms to indicate things such as plurality, possession, and tense changes, the use of language as a pragmatic tool, and the creativity that allows even young children to formulate utterances never produced or heard before. Premack (2007) examined the evidence across eight cognitive abilities in humans: teaching, short-term memory, causal reasoning, planning, deception, transitive inference, theory of mind, and language. He concluded that while animal competencies are adaptations for a single goal, such as bringing dead prey to the young to teach them to hunt, human competencies are far-reaching cognitive attainments and allow us to pursue numerous goals.

Another basic assumption of the nativist perspective is that because language is acquired so quickly and so early in the child's life, learning alone cannot adequately account for acquisition. Nativists argue that caregivers do not provide language models that are designed to teach progressive understanding of language forms. In fact, nativists would question whether caregivers teach language at all. Children are *exposed* to language forms of enormous complexity, variety, and inconsistency, and they are typically not given specific feedback about whether their utterances are correct or incorrect (Pinker, 1984, 1987; Wexler & Culicover, 1980). If language is learned, nativists argue, we would expect the teacher to provide models that allow children to develop progressively more sophisticated hypotheses about the rules and forms they are learning, and we would certainly expect the teacher to indicate clearly when a child's productions are right or wrong.

One of the most compelling arguments for the nativist perspective is that language is essentially the same experience for all human beings no matter what language they speak, where they live, or how they interact with their language models. As listeners and speakers of languages, we may be most impressed by their differences, but when languages are studied carefully, we discover many commonalities. All languages, for example, have rules for organizing words into grammatical sentence forms. They do not all use the same rules, of course. Some languages, such as English, stress word order in conveying meaning through grammatical sentences. Italian, on the other hand, allows more freedom in word order because the inflections on verbs carry much of the information for meaning.

Nativists stress the common ground, however. That is, all languages have rules to indicate the structural relationships among words in sentences. All languages distinguish between subjects and predicates and allow the embedding of one sentence structure in another to create an elaborated sentence representing both original structures. All languages have rules to indicate changes in tense and plurality, and draw sets of speech sounds from a common pool of sounds, and the list goes on. These commonalities or *linguistic universals* are evidence, say the nativists, that language is an ability humans possess, not by virtue of specific learning or teaching, but by virtue of their humanness.

All of these assumptions led to the creation of a concept that underlies the nativist's understanding of language development: the **language acquisition device**, or **LAD** (Chomsky, 1965; Lenneberg, 1967). The LAD is an innate language reservoir filled with information about the rules of language structure. Nativists contend that it should be understood as a real part of the brain, that part specifically designed to process language. The LAD takes the syntactic information provided by the child's models and generates the grammar of that child's native language. Because no child is predetermined to speak any specific language, the LAD is driven by knowledge common to all languages. As you might imagine, the existence and certainly the nature of the LAD have been widely debated (Bohannon & Warren-Leubecker, 1989).

As you may have sensed in this discussion, nativists believe that the structure of language is somehow independent of its use. In fact, they view structure as being independent of meaning and almost every other aspect of the total language package. The rules for structuring sentences determine, for any given language, that some forms are grammatical and allowable and others are not. There is a finite, or specifically limited, number of rules for a given language. These rules allow the speaker to create an infinite number of grammatically acceptable sentences. The rules should be understood not in a prescriptive sense but in a descriptive sense. In other words, these rules do not tell the speaker what she should do but what she does do. They are rules that describe the regularities of a language. Once the speaker knows what these rules are, she can create an unlimited number of grammatical sentences, including the possibility of sentences that have never been produced by any other human. Language acquisition, therefore, is a matter of discovering and applying the rules or regularities of one's native language.

Transformational Generative Grammar

Chomsky (1957) devised **transformational generative grammar** to account for the production of an unlimited number of grammatically acceptable sentences. This grammar suggests that language is processed at two levels, and two kinds of rules describe what is occurring at each level. **Phrase structure rules** describe the underlying relationships of words and phrases, the level of structure referred to as **deep**. These rules are universal and operate in all languages. **Transformations** are rules that describe the rearrangement of deep structures as they are moved to the next level of structure, referred to as **surface structure**. These rules are not universal. Each language has its own set of transformations, although the basic principles that operate in transformations are much the same in all languages. A complete description of transformational generative grammar is beyond the scope of this book, but the reader should understand how the grammar works to appreciate Chomsky's point of view about language. Figure 2.2, shows the relationships between deep structure, transformational rules, and surface structure.

Figure 2.2   Transformational Generative Grammar

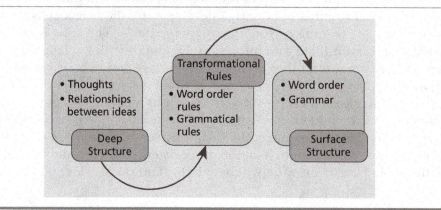

If we take a simple sentence such as, "The little boy hit the white ball," we can identify three basic phrase structure rules that operate to create this kind of sentence:

1. *Sentence = Noun Phrase + Verb Phrase*. Our sample sentence consists of the noun phrase (*The little boy*) and the verb phrase (*hit the white ball*).
2. *Verb Phrase = Verb + Noun Phrase*. The verb phrase in our sentence consists of the verb (*hit*) and the noun phrase (*the white ball*).
3. *Noun Phrase = Modifier(s) + Noun*. There are two noun phrases in our sentence. In the first noun phrase, there are two modifiers (*The* and *little*) and the noun (*boy*). The second noun phrase also has two modifiers (*the* and *white*) and the noun (*ball*).

Keep in mind that Chomsky was devising a grammar to account for the production of an infinite number of grammatical sentences with a finite number of rules. By using just these three rules, it is possible to create an unlimited number of sentences. The example here is an English sentence, but these same rules can be used to describe the deep structure of similar sentences in any language.

Think of deep structures as the origins of a sentence in the brain before it is spoken or written. Phrase structure rules describe the relationships of the most basic elements of sentences while they are thoughts, before they become spoken or written sentences. To move these deep structures to the surface, we need transformations (rules that determine how words are shaped and organized to make sentences grammatical). Each language has its own set of transformations.

In English, for example, we can understand the creation of a grammatically correct question by understanding what happens as we move from the deep structure of a particular sentence to the surface. Let's assume that you want to know whether Marco is going to the library. At the deep structure level, the origin of the question is something like this:

"Marco is going to the library."—Question?

The rule in English for transforming this deep structure into a grammatically correct interrogative form is fairly simple. You rearrange the words, reversing *Marco* and *is* to create the surface structure: "Is Marco going to the library?" The rule for rearranging the words to create a question is a transformation. If you are thinking:

"Marco is going to the library."—No!

you can use a negative transformation to express that idea on the surface. In this case, you insert the word *not* between *is* and *going* to create the grammatically acceptable sentence: "Marco is not going to the library." The transformation describes what you do on the surface to express what you have thought at the deep level.

It is also important to understand that every sentence has a deep structure and a surface structure. Notice, for example, that "The boy hit the ball" and "The ball was hit by the boy" mean the same thing. That is, they have the same deep structure. They differ only on the surface. The transformation used to change the first sentence into the second is called the **passive transformation**.

Notice the reordering of words necessary to transform the active sentence into the passive sentence. Once you understand the rule, you can transform any active sentence into its correct passive version. Try it on sentences such as, "The beautiful woman rode the aging horse" or, "The vicious cat chased the frightened dog under the porch." If several people try the same transformation, assuming basic competence in English, the resulting sentences will be the same:

> The aging horse was ridden by the beautiful woman.
> The frightened dog was chased under the porch by the vicious cat.

How did you do? You have just demonstrated something many nativists believe supports their view. That is, you know what you know about language even if you do not know what you know. Think about that for a few seconds. The point is, you might not have known what the term *passive transformation* means, and if asked how to make a sentence passive, you might not have been able to explain it; but by changing active sentences that you have never seen before into passive versions, you have demonstrated your knowledge of not only the deep structures of these sentences but the rules for surface structure as well. Nativists would argue that if language were purely learned, you would have a more conscious understanding of what you are doing when you create sentences at the deep level and as you move them to the surface. Instead, they contend, your LAD provides you with innate knowledge of deep structures and the ability to easily acquire the rules for surface structures for your native language, an acquisition that comes by exposure to models, not direct teaching.

Chomsky significantly expanded and extended his theoretical views regarding the acquisition of grammar to emphasize the limited hypotheses about language structure that the learner can formulate. These revisions include the government binding theory and several subtheories that explain constraints, principles, and rules involved in language acquisition. We must save this discussion for another time and place.

Review and Reflection on the Nativist Perspective

Nativists are clearly at the nature end of the nature/nurture continuum. They believe human beings are born with a capacity for language—that given exposure to language, human children will talk, even if environmental conditions are not favorable. Nativists contend that the universality of language among all human beings, the striking commonalities in how language is acquired, and the schedule by which it is acquired, regardless of cultural or other environmental variations, are evidence of the innateness of language. They believe children are born with a language acquisition device (LAD), a neurophysiological entity filled with language knowledge. The LAD provides children with the knowledge they need to understand any language at the deep structure level and provides them with the ability to acquire easily and quickly the surface structure rules specific to the language they will speak.

James (1990) notes that it is difficult either to confirm or to refute the nativist perspective, although several of its basic assumptions have been challenged. The assumption that language is unique to humans has been challenged, however inconclusively, by attempts to teach chimpanzees and other animals to use language. The assumption that language acquisition is essentially complete by the time the child is four or five appears to be overstated. There is evidence that significant language acquisition occurs well beyond five years, and that some complex language forms are not mastered until adolescence. For example, Nippold (1998) discussed the emergence and specific use of adverbial conjuncts (e.g., *moreover, nevertheless*) and other connectives (e.g., *because, during*), abstract or rare words, slang, idioms ("The girl threw him off the track"), analogies (*feather* is to *bird* as *wheel* is to . . . .), and metaphors ("Life is like a bowl of cherries") well into the high school years and beyond. The argument that language must be innate because parents and others provide models that are too complex and ambiguous for progressive learning also appears to be incorrect. Although it is true that adults talk to other adults in language that is often confused, incomplete, and grammatically ambiguous, evidence indicates that adults use a different kind of language with children. That is, adults tend to provide input to children that is relatively short, simple, and grammatically correct, but their input also adds a degree of complexity beyond the child's current level in order to facilitate continued language learning. Do not forget, however, based on the evidence gathered so far, that we have not ruled out the nativists' basic contention, which is that human beings are born with an innate capacity for language. What remains in the debate is to determine the relative importance of this innate capacity in comparison to the influence of environmental factors.

How might a nativist perspective influence how a speech-language pathologist or a teacher thinks about and provides intervention for children with language disorders? Is it possible to create environments and activities that directly improve an individual's biological response to information? Some practitioners do believe that the nature of the input matters and that we can indeed improve individuals' reception of information.

▶ Video Example 2.1

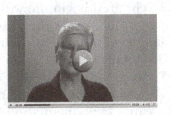

The nativist perspective is used to plan and implement intervention for children with communication disorders. As you watch the video, consider the importance of the input in designing interventions for children with hearing loss, language problems, and limitations in cognitive functioning.

✓ Check Your Understanding 2.1

Assess your understanding of the nativist perspective of language acquisition by completing this brief quiz.

The Behaviorist Theory of Language Acquisition

The proponents of the behaviorist perspective focus on observable behaviors in children to explain language development. They look for patterns of language that children demonstrate, such as the way English-speaking children combine two nouns (*daddy cookie*). Based on both observation and measurement, they then draw conclusions about the relationships between the environment and the regularities in children's language. These relationships allow predictions of the continuing course of language development across all children within the particular culture under observation (Bohannon & Warren-Leubecker, 1989). Behaviorists do not emphasize mental activities, such as attention and memory, because these activities cannot be observed directly in language learning, although they do acknowledge their existence and their important connection to language development.

Using Watson (1924) and Skinner (1957) as examples, Bohannon and Warren-Leubecker (1989) make the point that behaviorists believe language is learned because they do not believe language is unique among human behaviors. Watson (1924) categorizes language in its earliest stages as a behavior no more complicated than a habit used to influence or control the behaviors of others. Behaviorists argue that language is something humans *do,* not something they *have,* and it should be understood, therefore, in the same context of learning as other behaviors humans do, such as brushing their teeth or tying their shoes. They contend that language is learned according to the same principles used in training animals and that, like trained animal behaviors, language behaviors are learned by imitation, reinforcement, and successive approximations toward adult language behaviors. Recall from Chapter 1 the limitations found in training an animal to learn symbolic communication to appreciate the learning that is required for human language to emerge and develop.

One of the more controversial aspects of the behaviorist view is that children are passive during the process of learning language (Bryen, 1982). That is, children begin life with their "language tanks" on empty. They become language users as their tanks are filled by the experiences provided by the language models in their environments. This is not to say that children are totally inactive, of course. They are active in the sense that they imitate language forms, but they do not initiate these behaviors on their own, and the shape of their emerging language is determined not by self-discovery or creative experimentation but by the selective reinforcements received from their speech and language models.

This leads us to the key assumption underlying behaviorist views of language development. Although behaviorists have differing opinions about exactly how the process of learning occurs, they all agree that environment is the critical and most important factor in the acquisition formula. While nativists stress the *similarities* that occur in the language development of children, behaviorists stress the *differences* that are explained by the widely varying environments of children during the language acquisition period. The behaviorists focus on the external forces that shape the child's verbal behaviors into language. They see the child simply as a reactor to these forces (Bryen, 1982).

Speech and Language as Operant Behaviors

The theorist most closely associated with the behaviorist interpretation of speech and language development is B. F. Skinner. It is not surprising that Skinner (1957) viewed speech as learned behavior, because he viewed virtually all behaviors as learned according to operant conditioning principles. To understand Skinner's explanation of speech and language development, therefore, one must understand the basic principles of operant conditioning.

An **operant** is any behavior whose frequency can be affected by the responses that follow it. If a target behavior's frequency of occurrence increases as a consequence of the response that follows it, **reinforcement** has occurred. If the frequency decreases, the target behavior has been **punished**. Very often people try to understand operant punishment in terms of aversiveness or unpleasantness, but these judgments may interfere with an understanding of the principle involved. If a target behavior's frequency of occurrence decreases as a consequence of the response that follows it, punishment has occurred whether the organism being conditioned perceives the response as unpleasant or aversive. In other words, reinforcement and punishment are defined on the basis of their effects.

Consider the following example of these concepts. Sara, age 3, has her eye on a book about butterflies (stimulus). Sara says, "Daddy, give me the book, please." Daddy says, "Here you go, Sara. I like how you asked me for the book." Sara's request (the target or operant) is likely to occur again in the same polite manner because her dad's comment (response or consequence) was so positive. He not only gave her the book, but also used the opportunity to praise her (reinforcement). Now here is an example of how punishment decreases a behavior. Frank is a five-year-old who loves to go to the park (stimulus). He asks his parents repeatedly to take him (operant), to the point where they need to decrease his requests to maintain their sanity! They decide to tell Frank that he can go to the park only once each day after school and once on Saturday and Sunday morning (response). If he asks for more trips to the park, he will not be able to go at all the next day (punishment). Punishment (a decrease in the behavior) does not have to be negative. We might take the suggestions of a friend to decrease our amount of talking (operant), and when we do (response), we find that those around us like to talk to us more (punishment)!

In operant conditioning, the events that follow target behaviors are critical to learning, but the events preceding the target behaviors are also important, because they can come to control whether or not these target behaviors will be produced. During the learning period, a parent may, consciously or not, give the child a certain look as she is receiving a gift, a look that reminds the child that she should say "thank you." We call this look a **discriminative stimulus**. Now notice the sequence. The child receives the gift. The parent gives her the look. The child says "thank you," and the parent praises her for her gratitude.

Over time, the look or discriminative stimulus comes to control the frequency with which the child says "thank you."

There are other preceding events. The **delta stimulus** is a signal indicating that reinforcement will not follow a particular response. Joseph loves an audience. He practices on his skateboard when other children are present to cheer him on and when they go home, he stops practicing. The delta stimulus is the attention the other children give him. When they leave, he stops practicing because he receives no attention. An **aversive stimulus** warns that there will be an unpleasant consequence for a particular behavior. You can imagine the variety of statements that parents use to warn their children, such as, "Do not be late coming home, or you will lose your iPad time tonight!" It is very important to remember, however, that these preceding events have only as much power to control behaviors as provided by the strength and consistency of the events that follow targeted behaviors. A parent or teacher might try to use an aversive stimulus by threatening time out if the child produces a certain behavior, but if that behavior is never followed by time out, the preceding event will have no power to control. This is why parents are counseled not to make empty threats. Behavior in children and all other organisms can be managed by operant principles only if preceding events are connected to following events, at least part of the time. In other words, behavior management is effective only if efforts to manage are consistent and if the manager follows through on the promises or threats inherent in the preceding events.

Sometimes the behavior we want must be **shaped** in small steps that gradually approximate the target behavior. When the child is learning to say *water*, she might begin by saying *wawa*. The adult accepts this production as a step toward the target behavior and reinforces it, perhaps by giving the child a drink when she says *wawa*. As the child gets older and expectations for her speech rise, she might be reinforced for saying *wada* but she is no longer reinforced for saying *wawa*. The next approximation might be *wata* and finally *water*. In each step of the shaping process, what is reinforced is closer to the target. Productions that are not advanced or are perceived as regressions are ignored.

Many behaviors, including speech behaviors, occur in sequences. These sequences are learned through a procedure known as **chaining**. A child sees his mother getting ready to go out and thinks she looks pretty. He says, "You sure look pretty, Mommy." The mother, flattered, responds, "Well, thank you! That was a nice thing to say." The child says, "You're welcome." Seeing his mother looking pretty is the discriminative stimulus for the child's initial comment, which is followed by the mother's response and the child's response to her response, each reinforcing the preceding utterance.

It is not too difficult to understand how Skinner and others have applied these basic principles to speech and language development. In general, behaviorists claim that children acquire language as a result of caregiver models and selective reinforcements they provide. Children imitate the models and those most closely resembling the models are reinforced by the caregivers when they give the children what they want, when they respond with another comment, or when they give the children adoring attention. Over time, the children will cease to use productions that have not been reinforced and will continue to use those that have been reinforced. Stringing words together into sentences occurs as the result of chaining. Imitation, important throughout the learning process, undergoes a change as children move from single words to sentences. Staats (1971) suggests that a child's parents introduce this new version of imitation as their expectations for her speech increase. The child produces a single-word utterance. One of the parents, believing she can produce a longer utterance, expands this single word into a sentence and withholds reinforcement until the child imitates the expanded form.

Remember that behaviorists stress the idea that language is a doing or performing phenomenon more than a knowing phenomenon. Skinner (1957), for example, argues that verbal behavior serves one of five specific functions defined according to what they do: echoic, tact, mand, intraverbal, and autoclitic. Table 2.1 defines each of these functions and the examples illustrate how they differ and Figure 2.3 shows the relationships that the stimulus, response, and consequence have to each other.

As language structures become more complex, however, it is more difficult to explain them on the basis of learning alone. In reference to autoclitics, for example, Fey (1986) says there is the implication that only strings of words that have been specifically reinforced can be produced. We know, however, that all speakers, including young children, produce strings of words that have never been produced or heard before. In other words, operant principles cannot adequately account for the creativity that is a dominant characteristic of language. Additionally, operant principles alone fail to account for the acquisition of meaning in novel utterances.

Table 2.1 Conditioned Verbal Behaviors

Verbal Behavior Function	Definition	Example
Echoic	Imitation of a model when objects or ideas are present	Parent holds up cookie and says, "cookie." Child responds, "cookie."
Tact	Verbal behavior that associates the name with an object, action, or event	Parent holds up cookie. Child responds, "cookie."
Mand	Verbal behavior used to request or demand	Child says, "Me want drink."
Intraverbal	Social talk freely associated in situational contexts	Parent says, 'Daddy went to work." Child says, "Go outside and play now?"
Autoclitic	Linking words into sentences based on observations and experiences	Child comments, "Billy hitting the ball."

Figure 2.3   Speech and Language as Operant Behaviors

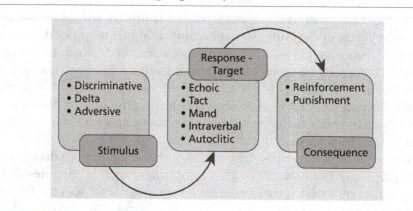

Another variation on conditioned learning is called **classical conditioning**. Staats (1971) believes we must include classical conditioning principles to explain language acquisition, especially the meaning component. In classical conditioning, an originally neutral stimulus is paired with an unconditioned stimulus that elicits an unconditioned response. In the famous Pavlovian experiment, the dog hears a bell just before seeing food, which elicits the unconditioned response, salivation. After a number of trials, the bell alone, now a conditioned stimulus, will elicit salivation, now a conditioned response. That is, the dog has learned or been conditioned to salivate upon hearing the bell. Staats argues that a word is, in the beginning, a neutral stimulus that acquires meaning only as responses are classically conditioned to it. The word *sit* develops meaning as it comes to represent the physical act associated with it through the process of conditioning. At first, when the child hears his parent say, "Sit!" there is no reaction, but if the word is paired with the physical act of being placed on a chair, the word alone, after enough trials, will elicit the act of sitting and will be understood to represent the act.

The chaining of behaviors.

Source: Rossario/Shutterstock

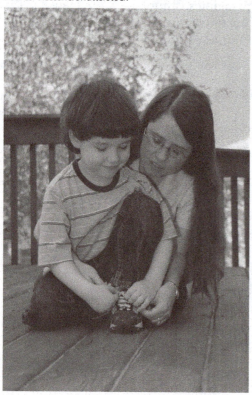

Review and Reflection on the Behaviorist Perspective

Behaviorists stress the importance of environment. The child is viewed as an empty vessel to be filled by the experiences provided by the important people in his life. The child is typically viewed as having no knowledge about the rules of language. His parents and other speakers are credited for "teaching" language by providing models that the child imitates. By selective reinforcement, the parents shape the child's utterances into adult forms.

Obviously, the behaviorist perspective of language acquisition has not gone unchallenged. James (1990) provides an excellent and succinct summary of some of the problems and criticisms. The role of imitation has been questioned, for example. As noted earlier, children produce sentences they have never heard before. This may mean that they produce sentences that are more creative and elaborate than their models, but it also means that they produce utterances that are simply not produced by adults because such utterances are infantile. The child will typically say things such as, "Daddy goed work" and, "That mine milk;" productions that are clearly not imitations of sentences produced by parents. Perhaps more importantly, the frequency of imitation decreases dramatically after the second birthday, but there is still a lot of language to be acquired beyond age 2. Some children, even from the beginning, imitate very little. If imitation is as important as the behaviorists argue, we would expect to see imitations more consistent with the models provided, and we certainly would expect to see imitation play a major role in acquisition throughout the learning period. James also notes that because parents are more likely to correct children for the content of their utterances than for the grammatical accuracy of their sentences, syntactic development cannot be explained solely on the basis of selective parental reinforcement.

Whatever the problems with the behaviorist perspective, there seems little doubt that learning explains some aspects of language acquisition. We know that language changes over the course of a person's lifetime, well beyond the age range identified by the nativists as the critical acquisition period. General learning principles best explain these changes. An innate capacity for language, for example, cannot account for how humans learn the nuances of language, such as when to use *who* and when to use *whom,* and environmental influences seem to be very important in changing a person from an adequate user of language into an exceptional user of language. We also know that behaviorist principles are used effectively in educational and therapeutic settings, especially when the learner is engaged in developing a new skill or learning new information.

Video Reflection 2.1: Behaviorist Teaching and Learning

Watch the video to learn about how practitioners apply the principles of behaviorism when teaching students, then answer the question.

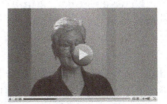

Check Your Understanding 2.2

Assess your understanding of the behaviorist perspective of language acquisition by completing this brief quiz.

Interactionist Theories of Language Acquisition

The most current view of language learning is a combined approach in which biology (neural substrates and genetics) and participation in the native linguistic environment work in tandem for language growth. Evidence supporting interactionist viewpoints shows that children learn language structure (grammar) in piecemeal fashion across many years, with a co-occurring accumulation of vocabulary. This gradual growth in language occurs through meaningful interactions between the developing child and those who communicate with her in everyday interactions. Further, we know that there are wide variations in the rate of language acquisition among children, even though they follow a predictable path. It is also clear that there are several ways in which particular aspects of language can be impaired. What accounts for this variability?

There is no clear answer to this question, except that children develop at differing rates in correspondence with many factors, including the amount of exposure and opportunities to engage in interactions with others. We know that adults do not intentionally teach language to children, but they do provide various degrees of language input. This input can be well formed, responsive to their child's communicative attempts, well adapted to their child's current focus of attention and understanding, and rich in adult modifications (contingent reformulations) that model correct forms (Paul, 2007). All of these components interact to promote language growth. On the other hand, some adults may provide little language to their children. Unfortunately, the lack of well-formed, responsive, and interactive language places children at a disadvantage for language growth and development. A fascinating study published by Hart and Risley (1995) showed a remarkable connection between the amount of talking between parents and their children in the first three years and the children's academic success at nine years of age. Notably, the more talking that occurs from infancy through three years, the more likely the child will do well in school later in life. We will describe this study and the major findings of similar studies in Chapter 4.

Cross-linguistic studies comparing one or more aspects of language provide us with very rich information on the ways in which language learning is influenced by the particular input received from those in communication with the learner. It is clear that children develop the language of their families and there are at least 6,909 spoken languages across the world (Anderson, 2010), according to the Linguistic Society of America. Languages share many commonalities, but they differ greatly in structure. A few examples will help illustrate this point. In English, nouns and verbs are inflected through the use of morphemes to convey meaning. We use the plural form *s* to indicate multiple nouns, such as *houses*, *cats*, and *books* and we use the past tense marker *ed* to reveal that an action happened in the past, such as when we say that we *poured* the lemonade or we *danced* at the party. Other highly inflected languages include Italian, Turkish, and Finnish. Some examples of languages that have few inflections are Russian and Serbo-Croatian. The point is that children who speak English must learn how to inflect nouns and verbs, whereas children who speak some other languages do not learn inflections to the same degree.

Researchers have also noted that the nature of the language input (the native language) has a strong influence on the learning of that particular language. It makes sense that the exposure and practice of the native language will be a strong determinant in the way in which a child will learn the language. Thus, English children learn to use inflections gradually, Turkish children learn inflections more quickly, yet Russian and Serbo-Croatian children have a protracted development into their sixth or seventh year. Studies led by Bates and Marchman (1988) conclude that the native language influences the route that children take in their acquisition of grammar.

Another observation from cross-linguistic studies is the way in which children learn to use verbs. English-speaking children initially avoid verbs by combining associated nouns (e.g., daddy cookie) because of the complexity of verb forms. They gradually learn to use the verbs and add inflections. However, this pattern of verb omission does not occur in all languages (MacWhinney & Bates, 1978). For example, in Hungarian, subject nouns and objects carry the inflections; therefore, verb inflections are not required. Other languages omit objects and subjects depending on the meaning conveyed by other words in the sentence. According to Bates and Marchman (1988) each language carries or maps the information to the particular structure of the language and children are predisposed to find the information salient. Infants do this very early, in the first year of life before they can speak (Kuhl, 2000). Children also seek and find important clues to word and sentence meaning through word order (Devescovi et al., 2005). Paul (2007, p. 7) states, "the specific language and conceptual understanding of events interact to give weight and cue value to particular aspects of meaning and form." Thus, word order is an important way to convey meaning. The variations in the acquisition of grammatical morphemes directly relates to the saliency (perceptual relevance) of the inflections the children are learning. In other words, children focus on the perceptually relevant aspects of their language. Children apply their perceptual and cognitive strategies in concert with their native language to the task of learning the language of their families.

Daniel Everett documented one of the most dramatic demonstrations of language variation within a cultural context. He lived for over six years with the Pirahã, a group of Brazilians who speak their language using severely constrained grammar (Everett, 2005). A striking aspect of Pirahã is the restriction of communication to the immediate experience of those engaged in conversation. This lack of perfect and future tenses, which had been thought of as a core aspect of grammar in a universal grammar framework, has caused linguists to revise the notion of universal grammar. The language does not include descriptive terms, such as number, quantity, or color, and phrases are not embedded into sentences. Speakers use only a few pronouns and they speak about immediate experiences with little reference to history. The speech sound inventory of the language is quite small, but speakers use a variety of vocalizations, such as humming and whistling, as part of their communication. The characteristics of this language also suggest that some of the features discussed in Chapter 1 (interchangeability, displacement, and productivity) may be culturally constrained. That is, culture appears to have a very important role in shaping how we think and communicate.

Many variations in linguistic input have been documented in the literature to show that environment affects language acquisition. In later chapters, we will discuss variables such as the nature and amount of prelinguistic input, parent/child interaction, and sociolinguistic factors that contribute to language learning.

Interactionist Interpretations

The interactionist viewpoints of how language acquisition occurs in children span 40 years and offer varying degrees of support for the roles that biology and the language environment play in the acquisition process. Three views are reviewed here—semantic, cognitive, and social interactionist—but note that all interactionist viewpoints realize that meaning is the reason for and the result of language.

Semantic View

During what is known as the *semantic revolution,* theorists shifted their focus from the structure of language conveyed by grammar to the meaning that children convey through grammar as they learn about their world. Language is viewed in interactionist perspectives to be intricately related to the development of thought (cognition) and our ability to use language in the construction of meaning. Those who take the semantics view argue that for a language to be truly generative, it must generate meaning as well as structure, and that meaning in language is expressed not only in words but also through the syntactic relationships among words. If we are to understand the acquisition of language, we must account for the expression of meaning.

Fillmore (1968) developed one of the earliest and most often cited generative semantic theories. Fillmore's **case grammar** is designed to explain the importance and influence of semantics on the form of language. Fillmore suggested that there is a deeper level of deep structure than that proposed by Chomsky. Beneath deep structure is a level composed of universal concepts that determine how nouns and verbs are related to one another. These are semantic concepts, not syntactic relations, and they are independent of surface structure. Even though these semantic concepts are universal, they are not necessarily innate. According to generative semantics theorists, these concepts are either genetic or environmental phenomena (Chafe, 1970).

Fillmore suggests that sentences have two components: modality and proposition. **Modality** is concerned with sentence characteristics such as verb tense or the expression of negation or interrogation. The second component, proposition, is more critical to the semantic theory. **Proposition** is concerned with the relationship between nouns and verbs in sentences. The relationship between the noun and verb in a given sentence determines the meaning underlying that sentence. Each proposition represents a type of sentence that includes a verb in combination with a *case* or a set of nouns. In the context of this view of language, certain categories of verbs require certain cases. *Case* refers to a specific semantic role or function that can be filled by a particular type of noun phrase. Fillmore identifies seven universal cases. They are displayed in Table 2.2.

Note that there are not exclusive sets of nouns for each case. A given noun may be used in any case if it meets the definition and requirements of that case. The word *boy* is agentive in the sentence: "The boy broke the window." It is dative in the sentence: "The woman gave a generous tip to the boy." It is experiencer in the sentence: "The boy dreamed about owning his car," and it is objective in the sentence: "The homecoming queen kissed the embarrassed little boy." In each case, the verb determines the case of the noun phrase, which means that structure can be explained on the basis of the semantic functions of nouns as determined by verbs. In short, structure is a product of semantic relations.

Chomsky and Fillmore share an important viewpoint relative to language production. Each believes that language production is a generative process and that any theory of language acquisition must account for how language is generated. The essential difference between Chomsky and Fillmore should be clear, however. Chomsky devised a theory to account for the generation of structure. Fillmore devised a theory to account for the generation of semantic relationships, which underlie and provide a foundation for structure.

Table 2.2   Fillmore's Seven Universal Cases

Case	Definition	Example
Agentive	The initiator of an action, usually animate	*Tom* hid the present.
Dative	A person or other animate being affected by the action or state of being ascribed by the verb	Sally gave *him* a generous tip.
Experiencer	A being who experiences an action or a mental or emotional state	*Jerry* enjoyed the concert.
Factitive	An object or being that is the product of an action or state ascribed by the verb	They built the *house*.
Instrumental	An inanimate object that is the means by which an action occurs	She made the fire with *charcoal*.
Locative	The place where the action or state ascribed by the verb occurs	He went camping in the *forest*.
Objective	A noun phrase whose role in the action or state ascribed by the verb is determined by the specific meaning of the verb	Dad kicked the *ball* to me.

Source: Fillmore (1968).

Based on Bloom's (1970) experiences in analyzing the meanings of early utterances using contextual, sematic information, she asserted that both structural analysis and semantic analysis can be used to draw conclusions about the underlying structure of an utterance because the information comes from the context of the situation. This context must take into account linguistic and nonlinguistic information, such as body language and tone of voice, because the communications of your children contain not only words, but also their intentions and feelings during interactions with others. This analysis goes beyond the speaker's words to take into account environmental and other nonverbal factors that contribute to the total message. You will see the importance of context when we discuss language sampling later in this text.

Cognitive View

At about the same time that the semantic revolution was under way, there was renewed interest in Piaget's cognitive theory and its relationship to language acquisition. Theorists considered specific connections between Piaget's stages of cognitive development and stages of speech and language development, with special emphasis on Piaget's sensorimotor period. This stage of cognitive development extends from birth through two years, the period of time that, not coincidentally, is critical for early speech and language development. In other words, it is easy to understand why linguists would be intrigued by possible, and highly plausible, connections between cognitive development and language acquisition. We will discuss this theory in depth in Chapter 3.

It should be noted that all theorists accept that a relationship exists between cognitive development and language development. What separates cognitive theorists from others is their belief that language does not hold an absolutely unique position in overall development. They believe that language itself is not innate, even though the cognitive precursors for language *are* innate. They also believe that language is not learned as behaviorists suggest it is learned. Language emerges, in the cognitive view, not because children are specifically genetically predisposed to produce language and not because learning principles shape language; language emerges as a product of cognitive organization and development. Language is one of several abilities the child develops for the purpose of forming concepts, remembering them, and manipulating them in order to think and to talk. All of these abilities emerge as a consequence of cognitive maturation. They emerge when there is an imbalance between the child's existing cognitive structures and new information he is receiving from his environment. These theorists agree that the child's cognitive abilities differ from the adult's in terms of how much information is processed and how effectively it is processed. But no matter where a person is in cognitive development, he adds new information to existing cognitive categories or, if the new information does not fit, he extends, combines, or creates new categories. The process of language acquisition, according to this view, is not separate from but related to cognitive development; it is one part of, and fully integrated into, cognitive development.

Cognitive theorists have noted a number of correlations between language use and other cognitive behaviors, correlations that may help us understand how language is acquired. There certainly seems to be a relationship, for example, between children's understanding that words represent people, places, things, and ideas and the cognitive behavior known as *symbolic play*. There seems to be a connection between understanding that language can be used to get things done and the cognitive behaviors involved in solving problems with tools. Imitation is an important behavior in overall cognitive development, and imitation is clearly an important behavior in speech and language acquisition.

Another cognitive view that has its roots in the workings of the mind is the information processing theory. This view suggests that a human processes information in much the same way a computer does. The information processing system gathers information from the environment and puts it into symbolic codes including but not limited to words and numbers. The system interprets these codes, holds them in memory, and allows for the retrieval of stored information. Language acquisition occurs when a child experiences and gathers language in the productions of her speech and language models and uses that evidence to make fundamental changes within her personal information processing system. According to this view, children are not born with an internally wired system for language. Rather, they are born with a potential for all kinds of connections between symbols and the things and ideas symbols can represent. Some connections are firmly established because they are repeated over and over again, and other possible connections eventually fade away because children do not experience the evidence to activate them. It is the constant input of language that allows children to internalize language structures and meanings.

The information processing theory suggests that the processing patterns responsible for the acquisition of language are *parallel* rather than *serial*. Parallel patterns occur at many levels at the same time. By contrast, serial patterns, which are suggested by Chomsky's linguistic view, occur in a kind of vertical sequence. That is, deep structures are generated and are then transformed in a highly predictable sequence into surface structures. Information processing theory suggests that the order in which language forms are acquired is determined by what these forms accomplish. Those language forms that show up most often in a child's language models and that tend to serve the same purpose are acquired first. If, for example, a child's earliest language evidence is filled with examples of structures that make requests, language structures that fill the requesting function will emerge early.

Those who take the information processing view try to explain what occurs in children's minds when they acquire language. They suggest, as already mentioned, that the child processes language information at a number of levels at the same time, a form of processing known as *parallel distributed processing* (PDP). The competition model of Bates and MacWhinney (1987) is an example of a PDP system. A basic premise of this model is that children are born not with an innate understanding of language but with a powerful

PDP device that has the capacity to process many different forms of information, including language information. In the earliest stages of language development, the PDP device does not differentiate among words, phonological patterns, and language forms in terms of their ability to represent communicative functions or meanings. This situation changes, however, as children's experiences with language increase and become more differentiated. Words, phonological patterns, and language forms that are experienced repeatedly activate and strengthen connections in the PDP device. Other connections weaken. As the name of the model suggests, the patterns or connections that are most consistent with the language evidence the child is gathering win the *competition*. They are retained within the child's communication system. Patterns that do not match the evidence lose the competition and are discarded.

So, is the information processing view (and therefore the competition model) a nature or a nurture view of language acquisition? You have probably already surmised, correctly so, that this view includes elements of both extremes. Bates, Bretherton, and Snyder (1988) suggest that children are innately predisposed to acquire language, just as they are innately predisposed to acquire other behaviors. In this sense, they believe that there is a biological, or innate, basis for language acquisition, though they do not believe that it necessarily accounts for language universals. In terms of nurture, they assert that each child uses biologically based abilities to learn language creatively. They point out, for example, that there are significant individual variations in language acquisition among children within the same culture as well as across cultures. Within the context of the competition model, these differences are the result of varying experiences resulting in differentiated connections within the PDP system.

Social Interactionist View

The evolution in theoretical interpretations relative to language acquisition eventually led theorists to explore a middle ground. This is what usually happens in nature-versus-nurture arguments, so the emergence of a compromise view was probably inevitable, although it has emerged later than some might have expected. This middle-ground view is known as **social interactionism**.

According to the social interactionist interpretation of speech and language development, both biological and environmental factors are important in the acquisition process, although not necessarily equally. Some interactionist theorists are closer to the nature end of the continuum in that they understand language development as a product of general cognitive development (Bates & MacWhinney, 1982). Others place more emphasis on the contributions of the environment, but all agree that the interaction of biological abilities with environmental influences accounts for language acquisition, and they note the importance of children's interaction with their parents or other caregivers. This basic assumption about the importance of both biology and environment has led to other basic interactionist assumptions about language development.

For example, these theories assume that language acquisition is a product of children's early social interactions with the important people in their life. In fact, Jerome Bruner (1983) proposed that a **language acquisition support structure (LASS)** is necessary for children to learn language as a result of interactions with others. Proponents of this viewpoint believe that children communicate and interact socially with other people before they are able to produce language forms. They believe that language develops as a natural consequence of these interactions. That is, children's attempts

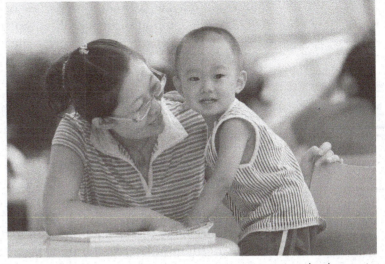

Language development is facilitated by social interaction.

Source: Bo1982/E+/Getty Images

to communicate and socialize prompt their parents and other caregivers to provide the language appropriate for these exchanges. Lev Vygotsky (1962) describes the zone of proximal development (ZPD) as the opportunities that family and others have to provide the help children need to make steady progress in their development. As children develop language, their communicative and social skills increase, allowing more mature and sophisticated interactions. These more mature interactions prompt more complex language forms from the parents, and the cycle continues until children's language systems and corresponding social skills reach adult levels.

James (1990) provides an excellent example of this progression. She suggests that a nine-month-old child requests a cookie by reaching for it and vocalizing with an utterance such as "Uh, uh, uh" while making eye contact with her mother. The mother, recognizing the communicative intent, might provide a language form as she gives the child a cookie; "Do you want a cookie? Say, 'Cookie . . . cookie.'" By the time the child is two years old, she might make the same request by saying, "Mommy, want cookie," an utterance met with a cookie and an expanded language form modeled by the mother; "Say, 'Mommy, I want a cookie.'" By the time the child is four, she will have learned, on the basis of her social and communication experiences, to ask for the cookie by hinting. She might say, "You know, Mommy, I haven't had a cookie for a long time." Notice what happens in this progression. The child is able to make a request from the beginning, before she has any language, and she certainly is able to interact with other people before she can speak. As she acquires language, however, her communicative and interactive abilities improve, and she is able to make her request known in more socially appropriate, more adult-like ways.

James's (1990) example illustrates another emphasis in the interactionist perspective. Unlike the nativists, who stress structure independent of communicative function or intent, interactionists focus on language use known as pragmatics. The intent to communicate leads a child to interact with people who can respond to his intent. The intent shapes his initial attempts to communicate, no matter how crude or unsophisticated these attempts may be. The recognition of the child's intent and associated communicative attempt prompts the caregiver not only to meet the intent but to provide an appropriate language model to support the intent. It may be that the model is given only to provide the child an opportunity to confirm or deny the intent, but the model is provided nonetheless. Over time, even though a given intent remains constant, the child acquires more sophisticated language forms by which he can make the intent more immediately and clearly known to his caregivers.

Interactionists emphasize the importance of parents or caregivers in the language acquisition process and they believe that children are active participants by virtue of their involvement with their parents. In fact, they initiate communication and social interactions as often as they receive them. Children have innate cognitive and linguistic abilities, but their interactions with the important people in their environment are the most important factor in the acquisition of language. Interactionists do not ignore grammar, but they try to discover common forms of structures in a variety of languages and cultures (DePaulo & Bonvillian, 1978) and how structures contribute to the use of language in getting things done. They believe, however, that these forms are fairly simple imitations of models to which children are exposed in social interactions (Moerk, 1975).

James (1990) notes that studies of caregivers' speech have revealed that the language forms adults use with young children are very different from the forms they use with other adults or even older children. According to James's review of the relevant research, when caregivers talk to young children, they speak in simple sentences while referring to objects or actions that children are engaged in. They add redundancy to their language by repeating what they say, but they also repeat the child's utterances to give extra feedback and to maintain turn-taking. Adults make statements of course, but they ask questions and state commands in their conversations. They vary the pitch of their voices in an exaggerated manner and use longer pauses between utterances.

This style of speech has been given several names, but perhaps the most popular and descriptive is **motherese** and more recently **parentese**. It should be noted, of course, that adults use this general style when they talk to young children, although there may be some gender differences. Ratner (1988) has found, for example, that although mothers and fathers use the same vocabulary in talking with young children, fathers are more likely than mothers to include the less commonly used words in that vocabulary. We will explore the role of parentese in language development in Chapter 4.

Interactionists believe that parentese is ideally designed to help children acquire language. It can be argued that repetition, for example, provides multiple models and, depending on the nature of the communicative exchange, several opportunities for the child to practice a particular language form. The use of short, simple sentences seems to provide the child with models she can reasonably expect to imitate. The use of pauses may help her recognize where utterances begin and end. The use of emphatic prosodic patterns might direct the child to those words or structures that are most important. Talking about

what is present and readily observable helps keep the communicative process concrete, which in turn probably helps hold the child's attention. The use of questions and commands seems to have the effect of keeping the child active in the communicative process.

On the basis of some research (Barnes, Gutfreund, Satterly, & Wells, 1983; Cross, 1978), one facet of parentese that seems to be related to language acquisition is the use of a technique known as **expansion**. Expansion occurs when the adult repeats what a child has said but adds additional words and/or structure (see Figure 2.4). For example, the child might point to a passing vehicle and say, "Truck!" The parent might respond, "That's a fire truck." Parents and other caregivers frequently use expansions when they talk to young children, and they seem to do it naturally, without instruction. Because caregivers use expansions more frequently with linguistically advanced children, and because the use of this technique seems to be associated with an increase in the mean length of children's utterances, it is reasonable to conclude that expansion probably facilitates language development. It is important, however, not to take the conclusion too far. There is, as yet, no evidence suggesting that this technique is essential for normal language development.

Figure 2.4   Parentese in Action

Imagine a toddler walking through a zoo with her mother. She is seeing animals she has never seen before, and she is very curious about these new and different creatures. Imagine the rate, pitch, and intonational patterns of the child's speech as well as the mother's speech. In the following exchange, notice some of the typical characteristics of parentese: a topic selected by the child's attention; short, simple sentences; repetition of key elements of the child's utterances; the use of questions to prompt additional responses; and expansion of the child's utterances into more complete, adultlike productions.

Child (pointing to a monkey):	Mommy, what's that?
Mother:	That's a monkey. Can you say *monkey*?
Child:	Monkey!
Mother:	Yes, *monkey*. What's the monkey doing?
Child:	Him eating.
Mother:	What's he eating?
Child:	Him eating banana.
Mother:	Do you eat bananas?
Child:	I like bananas!
Mother:	The monkey likes bananas, too . . . . What's he doing now?
Child:	Him swinging by his tail.
Mother:	Can you swing by your tail?
Child:	No. I don't gots a tail.
Mother:	No, you don't have a tail like the monkey.

Social interactionists recognize that an infant is a communicator from birth with family and other caregivers responding to cries and later to babbling and facial expressions. Caregivers assume infant sounds have meaning; thus they respond as if they are intentional attempts to communicate. Interactions become more elaborate as children grow. For example, some parents read to their children long before they can talk. Such interactions form social bonds and provide rich language input. Speech-related social games such as peekaboo are highly structured routines allowing children to participate by predicting what is going to happen (Bruner, 1978). These games are fun, but they also provide opportunities to experience all aspects of verbal and nonverbal communication while experimenting with some of the components of language they are acquiring.

A child's reaction to parent input allows the parent to assess the child's understanding and affords the parent opportunities to modify the input so that the child gains understanding. A mother may shorten her sentences, use more gestures, or repeat previous information. In any case, the interaction between the child and the adult is what drives the acquisition process.

Speech Act Theory: A Focus on Pragmatics

The last interactionist perspective reflects the evolving nature of theories about language and the acquisition process that children engage in to learn language. Pragmatics is the study of the functions served by communication. The pragmatics revolution of the 1980s and 1990s had its origins many years earlier in work completed by Austin (1962) and Searle (1969). Austin's primary assertion was that when speakers produce utterances, they are doing more than saying words organized by conventional language rules. They are also using these words to get things done. Searle, a student of Austin's, suggested that every speech act consists of three separate acts: (1) the locutionary act; (2) the illocutionary act; and (3) the perlocutionary act.

The **locutionary act** is the most obvious part of the utterance because it is the part that strikes our ears. It is the expression of the words. If you say to a friend, "You've lost some weight," the locutionary act is limited to the utterance itself. It is the sentence the speaker speaks and the hearer hears. The locutionary act, because it is a sentence, consists of a subject and a predicate. Beyond the words, however, consider the possible reasons for your making this observation, and you will get some sense that there may be more to your utterance than meets the listener's ears.

The **illocutionary act**, or *illocutionary force* (Searle, 1976), is concerned with the motive or purpose underlying an utterance. When someone says, "I know what you said, but I want to know what you meant," she is asking the speaker to identify his illocutionary act. Using the earlier example above, if you say to a friend, "You've lost some weight," you could be telling him that he looks good, but you could also be saying that he looks sickly. Your motive might be even more contrived. You might believe that your friend should be losing a lot of weight, and you hope that saying that you have noticed some weight loss will motivate him to lose more. Consider the purpose that might be served by what Searle (1975) calls an *indirect speech act*. If a woman says, "It's a little drafty in

here," it is not likely that she is simply making an observation about the wind currents and the temperature level in the room. It is more likely that her comment is an indirect way of saying, "Close the window!"

The **perlocutionary act** takes the listener into account. It is concerned with the effect the locutionary act might have on the listener, an effect that may or may not be consistent with the speaker's communicative intention. If you intend to compliment your friend by saying, "You've lost some weight," but your friend knows that he has, in fact, gained a few pounds, he might be offended by the comment, believing you are being sarcastic. Communication works best, of course, when the listener's reactions match the speaker's intentions in terms of communicative content (locutionary act) and purpose (illocutionary act). When this happens, the speaker and listener agree that they are "on the same page," communicatively speaking. When they are not on the same page, communication can be very frustrating. The speaker may be frustrated because he knows what he is trying to say, but no matter how he tries to say it, the listener does not seem to get it. The listener may be frustrated by a sense of communicative paranoia that may or not be justified. The disconnection between speaker and listener, relative to communicative purpose, is not pleasant for either party, and it causes the process of communication to break down.

Review and Reflection on the Interactionist Perspective

Although there are several ways that theorists and researchers have considered language development from an interactionist perspective, all of the views share some common ideas. Figure 2.5 shows the relationships between three main ideas. First, these views recognize strong interactions between the nature and nurture contributions to language. Second, they place language learning in the environment of the child as an active participant. Parents respond readily to their children's communication attempts and children respond to the input that parents provide. The whole context is taken into account in

Figure 2.5   Interactionist Relationships

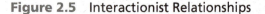

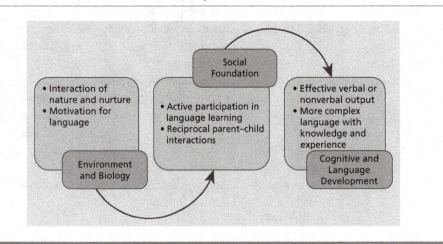

these dialogues because the outcome is effective communication regardless of whether it is verbal or nonverbal. The social underpinning of language learning drives both the desire to communicate and the scaffolding that parents use to give language input that fosters development over time and with repeated exposure in natural contexts. Of course, language is only one of many skills children learn through their interactions with parents and other caregivers. Thus language simultaneously develops with other cognitive abilities, allowing for increasingly complex meanings. The language structure becomes more complex as well, because it is the vehicle for the expression of ideas. Language from this view is to get things done and to connect in meaningful ways with others. Refer to Table 2.3 for a view of how language acquisition theories evolved.

We considered how teachers and practitioners used nativist and behaviorist theories to inform their work with children in their quest for language and literacy acquisition. It should be no surprise, therefore, that there are applications of this theory to our work with students in classrooms and in therapeutic environments. After all, students interact with each other and adults throughout each day, so the goal of effective communication is of the utmost importance.

Table 2.3   Tracing the Evolution of Theories of Language Acquisition

Theory	Primary Architect	Essential Idea	Primary Focus
Behaviorist	Skinner (1957)	Language is learned by selective reinforcement	General
Nativist	Chomsky (1957)	Language is processed by universal and innate rules governing deep and surface structure	Syntax

Interactionist
1. semantic view
   case grammar
   role of context
2. cognitive view
   information
   processing
3. social view
   speech act
	Fillmore (1968)	A level beneath deep structure includes universal semantic concepts that determine relationships between nouns and verbs	Semantics

		Context is conveyed in linguistic and nonlinguistic intentions	Semantics
	Bloom (1970)	Language and thought develop as parallel processes in cognitive organization	Structure by function
		Language processing results from repeated and patterns in environment	Function, not grammar, generates language structure
	Piaget (1963) Bates and Mac-Whinney (1987) Bruner (1983); Vygotsky (1962); Searle (1969)	Language develops through social interaction and construction	Structure by use
		Language develops through its use in interactions	Pragmatics

Video Reflection 2.2: Interactionist Teaching and Learning

Watch the video to learn how the interactive perspective is used in speech-language therapy, then answer the question.

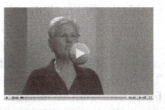

New Perspectives in Language Acquisition

Where does the evolution in theories of language acquisition stand in the 21st century? It would be inaccurate to say that the experts have reached a consensus about how children acquire language, but it would also be erroneous to conclude that we have not made progress in our considerations. Some are still convinced that language is a uniquely human and innate ability that only needs an environmental trigger to emerge, almost magically, according to a biologically predetermined schedule. Some still believe that language is almost entirely the product of environmental influences and that human children do not "develop" language as much as they "receive" language from their caregivers by virtue of their selective reinforcement and shaping of their initially random language-like behaviors. There seems to be growing support, however, for the middle ground in this nature-versus-nurture argument. As suggested in the opening of this chapter, this kind of compromise was almost inevitable. The interactionist perspective, therefore, is likely to have an increasingly greater voice in how theorists describe language acquisition and in formulating the questions researchers will attempt to answer about human language and its development.

Recall that one interactionist perspective favored the role of cognition in language acquisition. This role is being discussed more fully today. Tomasello (2003) advanced the usage-based theory of language acquisition, where language learning is considered a part of the cognitive abilities of children. He explains that human biological systems must be flexible to allow for differing inputs children are exposed to across the many languages in our world. Thus, children must learn language from those directly in their environment. Tomasello also described two sets of skills that appear important for the development of language. The first set includes the child's ability to gain and share attention to objects and people, follow attention and gestures from others, direct attention through showing and pointing, and imitate intentions of others. These skills are referred to as "intention-reading" abilities.

The second set of skills focuses on categorization through being able to detect patterns. For example, infants will form categories based on how things look or sound. They form sensory-motor schemes as they learn to move around in their environment, and they find patterns in the utterances their parents use on a daily basis. Tomasello described these skills as domain-general because they allow children to categorize all the different kinds of stimuli in their worlds, including language.

The usage-based linguistic theory posits that children recognize patterns in the sequences of symbols their parents use to communicate. These patterns become the grammar of the language as children gradually master them. There are structured, concrete patterns and there are abstract ones that allow for learning idiosyncratic expressions. A collection of patterns allows children to generalize them for use in different utterances. This view does not recognize a universal grammar, but rather emphasizes the intention-reading and pattern-finding abilities that allow children to learn all the constructions that underpin their native language.

The dynamic systems theory has been applied to the acquisition of languages and the learning of second languages, whereby variables in the environment interact over time. This dynamic interaction of variables is what makes each person learn language in a unique way and what makes for variations among individuals (De Bot, Lowie, & Verspoor, 2007). We will discuss this theory as it relates to cognitive attainments more thoroughly in Chapter 3.

In this book, we trace the development of language from the preparation stage through late childhood, primarily from the interactionist point of view, with references to other explanations where appropriate. For people who are just beginning to explore language and its development in children, it is particularly important to take the broadest possible view. Humans are complex beings who do not live in vacuums and certainly do not grow up in vacuums. To a large extent parents and other significant caregivers shape children within the context of their environment. At the same time, do not lose sight of the enormous power of genetic talent. Who does not marvel at world-class musicians and athletes? These people have worked hard to develop their considerable skills, but without the right genetic stuff a woman cannot high-jump seven feet, no matter how much she practices, and without the appropriate genetic gift, a pianist will never do justice to great music, no matter how many hours he spends at the keyboard. Language, like many other human abilities, is acquired as a genetic gift shaped by environmental forces. Which is the greater factor, heredity or environment? Let's not go there!

Check Your Understanding 2.3

Assess your understanding of the interactionist view of language acquisition by completing this brief quiz.

SUMMARY

This chapter provided an overview of the three perspectives that theorists, researchers, and practitioners use to think about how children acquire language abilities. The nativists explore the origins and acquisition of language through a biological lens, focusing on the structure and function of the specific areas and neuronal connections in the brain. Humans have a capacity for using linguistic rules to learn one or more languages. Although nativists recognize that environment plays a role in language acquisition, they believe that it is not sufficient for language learning. Behaviorists are at the opposite end of the nature-nurture debate. They focus on language as a learned behavior, just as there are other learned behaviors through exposure and conditioning from the environment.

Those who ascribe to theories that combine the views of biological and learning approaches recognize that brain structures and functions in tandem with language input, interaction, and feedback are necessary for a complete picture of how children learn language. In particular, the social interaction between children and their caregivers provides the context, motivation, and opportunities for meanings to be mapped onto the structure of the native language.

▐▌▶ Surfing the Web

If you are interested in exploring topics discussed in this chapter in more detail, search for one or more of the following relevant terms online.

theories of language development
nativist theory of language development
mirror neurons and language development
behaviorist theory of language development

interactionist theory of language development
information processing theory
culture and language
Pirahã language
David Everett
cross-linguistic studies and language development

Chapter Review 2.1

Recall what you learned in this chapter by completing the Chapter Review.

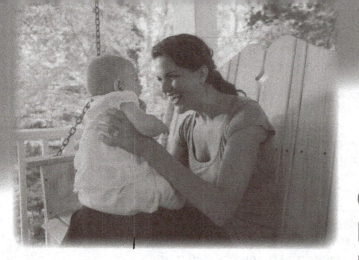

Cognitive Development: Building a Foundation for Language

LEARNING OUTCOMES

After completion of this chapter, you will be able to:

- Define concepts and behaviors central to intellectual functioning and development in Piaget's theory, including distancing, object permanence, causality, means/ends, play, and communication.
- Explain the tenets of Vygotsky's theory of cognitive development and the dynamic systems theory and contrast them with Piaget's theory.
- Distinguish the role of perception and executive functioning in the acquisition of knowledge and language.
- Summarize the role of the executive functions, attention, and memory in language and theory of mind.

What is the role of intellectual development in language development? This is one of the most interesting and challenging questions to be addressed in a study of human communication development. Because language is a means by which people express what they are thinking, the relationship between cognition and language is certainly connected, but the precise relationship has been the subject of debate throughout the ages.

This chapter focuses on varying views of the relationship between cognition and language. We will explore some theoretical positions on this topic, considering how different accounts explain early intellectual development, with special attention to the implications relative to child language development. We will also consider the perceptual basis that underlies early cognitive and language development, as well as the mental processes that contribute to thinking, knowing, and using language.

Chapter 2 examined a number of theories of language development that can be arranged along a continuum representing the possible influences of nature and nurture on the language acquisition process. The basic question that has driven the developers of these theories can be framed as follows: "Is language genetically or environmentally determined?" The answer, as you discovered, is not to be found at either extreme, but the question provides an appropriate segue into this chapter.

Are you ready for another question about language for which there is no answer or, more accurately, no easy answer? Well, ready or not, here it is.

How do language and cognition relate to each other? Unfortunately, we don't remember ourselves as infants and toddlers. In fact, this lack of consciousness about our early years tells us quite a bit about our limitations during that time regarding both language and cognition. How did we think about things then, and how is our thinking different now? What was the driving force that enabled us to learn language, and how did language development assist us in our thinking? The important point of these questions is that for many thought processes, it is not possible to separate thinking and language. As you read the words on this page, you are processing language to interpret your thoughts, and as you consider what we mean, you are manipulating your thoughts in some kind of language form. You might not use complete and grammatical sentences in your inner language, but they are in language form.

At the same time, human beings can and do think in ways that do not involve language. When Beethoven wrote his music, he thought in terms of music. When artists paint, they think in colors, forms, and visual messages. Football coaches design plays by thinking about arrangements of Xs and Os, and mathematicians think in numbers and formulas. Although we are able to use words to describe our emotions, images, sounds, and smells, words often fail to do them justice. A contemporary theorist, Howard Gardner, recognized our ability to know about and interact with our world and proposed that humans have several types of intelligence. Gardner's theory of multiple intelligences (1983) has significantly influenced educational practices by recognizing that children learn differently and through many avenues. The seven types of intelligence he initially described have expanded to eight, and two additional types are sometimes included (spiritual/existential and moral) as Gardner, other researchers, and educators continue to explore ways of thinking and knowing. Table 3.1 is a summary of the eight intelligences. You can obtain full descriptions and explore your own strengths in ways of knowing on various websites about multiple intelligence. As you review the descriptions, consider the numerous ways in which children must interact with their environment. Such variability in how children approach learning provides a compelling explanation of the great diversity among people.

As the eight types of intelligence show, language is only one of many ways that humans interact with the world, yet it is a very important aspect of thinking and knowing. In particular, language is necessary in our interactions with others, a critical aspect of learning and being a social member of our communities.

Table 3.1 Multiple Intelligences

Ways of Knowing	Description
Linguistic	To be sensitive to the meaning and order of words; learn languages; use language to accomplish goals
Logical-mathematical	To think using numbers; analyze problems; use deductive reasoning; investigate using scientific or mathematical thinking
Musical	To understand and appreciate music; compose or perform music with skill
Spatial-visual	To think in terms of pictures and to recreate the world in the mind and on paper or other media
Bodily-kinesthetic	To use the body as self-expression to achieve a goal or solve a problem
Interpersonal	To perceive and understand the moods, desires, and motivations of others; work effectively with others
Intrapersonal	To understand one's own emotions, fears, and motivations; regulate the self
Naturalist	To recognize and classify flora, fauna, and animals; draw upon certain features of the environment

To facilitate an understanding of the critical relationship between cognition and language, we will examine some theories of cognitive development. We will consider research evidence that supports each view, scholarly ponderings that these theories have generated, and what each theory suggests about the role of language and cognition in development.

Piaget's Theory of Cognitive Development

Jean Piaget is well known in the United States as a child psychologist, but his field of study was genetic epistemology, the study of how knowledge is acquired in living things. Thus, his work led him into both education and psychology. Piaget's original passion was biology, a passion born and cultivated at a young age. By the time he was 10 years old, he had already published an article describing a partly albino sparrow. This intellectually gifted boy earned his bachelor's degree at age 18 and his doctorate at 21, by which time he had already published 25 professional papers. Piaget's early studies of mollusks caused him to believe that development was not simply the product of biological maturation guided by genetics, but that it was also affected by environmental factors. During his professional career, this conclusion led him to understand that cognitive development is also the result of both nature and nurture components.

The Elements and Processes of Cognitive Organization

It is important to remember what Piaget learned from his work as a biologist. He came to understand that many actions of living creatures are **adaptations** to their environments and that these actions help creatures **organize** their environments (Wadsworth, 1971). He applied this understanding in explaining children's cognitive development by assuming that cognitive acts organize children's environments and are the result of children's adaptations to their environments. How does adaptation occur, according to this theory? We will use an example of George and his computer to introduce and explain several concepts involved in this process. Table 3.2 provides an overview of these concepts.

George is a businessman who uses his computer to create, organize, store, and retrieve his business reports, letters, appointments, budget, addresses, and so forth. In order to put his information in a certain place where he can find it, he must use a **schema** (a category) or computer file for each category. Thus, when George needs to process new information, such as adding to his budget, he must open the budget file, enter the new information, and save that file. He will not be successful in his work on the budget if he cannot find his file or if he opens another file, such as his letter file. In much the same way, we use our schemata to process, identify, store, and retrieve information in our brains. When we encounter new information, we must locate and use our existing schemata to be able to relate effectively to the new information at hand. This process of using existing schemata to include new information is called **assimilation**.

What happens when some new information does not fit an existing schema? George is a prolific letter writer, so after a few years of producing and saving letters, his letter file becomes very large. Because he writes many different kinds of letters, his file becomes unmanageable and disorganized, with family letters, letters to friends, business correspondence, and love letters to his wife, Betty. Finally, George creates new files according to new schemata. When people develop new schemata to allow for the organization of information that does not fit existing schemata, we call this process **accommodation**. Thus, we change our organizational strategy as we learn new things that do not fit easily into our current cognitive structures.

It should be noted here that some schemata, even for the most intelligent adults, are never completely accurate. An adult, for example, who has little

Table 3.2 Piagetian Concepts Underlying Cognitive Organization and Adaptation

Concept	Description
Schema	A cognitive structure that helps children process, identify, organize, and store information
Assimilation	A cognitive process whereby a new stimulus is fitted into an existing schema
Accommodation	A cognitive process whereby new schemata are created for information that does not fit existing schemata
Equilibrium	A cognitive process to maintain a balance between existing schemata (assimilation) and the creation of new schemata (accommodation)

interest in football might have a schema for a football player that is incomplete. He may not understand the specialized responsibilities of the various players on offense and defense or the difference between a nose guard and a linebacker. The point is, we are all ignorant in our own ways, and our ignorance is reflected in how our schemata are shaped and cataloged through our experiences.

We are now ready to consider the final basic concept, **equilibrium**. Think of this concept as a balance between assimilation and accommodation. If a person assimilates all new stimuli he experiences, he will have relatively few schemata—and these schemata will be so broadly defined that he will be unable to recognize the commonalities among the things he is trying to categorize. George will have so many different types of letters that he will not be very efficient in finding and using specific types when needed. But, if George accommodates all new stimuli, he will have a similar problem. There will be so many different categories on file that he will have difficulty recognizing their similarities. Thus, George needs a filing system that strikes a balance, being neither too broad nor too narrow.

How does this cognitive organization through schemata relate to how children learn language? Each time a child encounters a new stimulus, she either assimilates or accommodates, but she places the information somewhere. She might assimilate a new stimulus for a short time before she accommodates by creating a new schema more appropriate for that stimulus, but she does not leave her cognitive organization in disarray. It does not matter that her schemata are right or wrong in comparison with adult schemata. The child places stimuli according to her understanding of the world at any given moment in her intellectual development. In other words, she always finds her equilibrium.

Humans continually use assimilation and accommodation to accept new stimuli, reshape existing schemata, and create new schemata throughout their lives. It is fascinating to consider the ways in which we organize information and continue to reorganize it as needed.

The Stage Concept of Cognitive Development

Throughout our discussion of language acquisition and cognitive development, we will encounter stages and substages. It is important to remember that these stages are *not* like stair steps, in which moving from a lower step to the next higher step means leaving the lower step behind. Rather, one stage is carried over and integrated into the next stage. Each stage builds on the preceding stage so that development is a continuing process of qualitative changes in a person's schemata. Intellectual growth is a cumulative, integrative, expanding process.

Piaget (1963) described four stages of intellectual development from birth through late adolescence, briefly summarized here:

- *Sensorimotor intelligence (birth to 2 years).* Most of the child's behaviors during the sensorimotor intelligence stage are reflexive and motor. That is, he interacts with his environment in physical and mostly unlearned ways, especially early in the stage. He does not manipulate ideas in a conceptual sense, although cognitive development occurs in this stage and it occurs rapidly. The child at 2 is a very different creature intellectually from the child in infancy.

- *Preoperational thought (2 to 7 years).* The most rapid period of language development occurs during the stage of preoperational thought. The child begins to think conceptually, is able to categorize things in his environment, and can solve physical problems.
- *Concrete operations (7 to 11 years).* The child develops the ability to think logically in dealing with concrete or physical problems. He is able to place stimuli into categories based on order and levels.
- *Formal operations (11 to 15 years).* Cognitive abilities become fully developed. The child is able to think abstractly, to solve problems mentally, and to develop and test mental hypotheses. He reasons and thinks logically.

Remember, *these stages are not independent or absolute.* They are cumulative and integrated into one another, and they represent the ages when most normal children are experiencing the cognitive developments indicated. One child might show signs of preoperational thought at 14 months, but another child 10 or 11 years old might still be demonstrating characteristics of preoperational thought, and both children could be normal. There is a great deal of variability among children in terms of when and how quickly they pass through each stage, but, as Piaget insists, each child must pass through the stages in the order listed, and a child will not skip a stage.

With this overview of cognitive development in mind, we will now direct our collective attention to the first stage, sensorimotor intelligence. During this stage, according to Piaget, children develop those intellectual abilities that lay the foundation for symbolic behaviors such as dreaming, drawing, and language. Within the larger context of symbolic behaviors, therefore, this stage of cognitive development prepares children for the challenges and expressive opportunities inherent in speech and language development. We will consider some principles and concepts that emerge in the first two years of cognitive development.

The Principle of Distancing in Sensorimotor Development

The primary focus of this chapter is on the intellectual and perceptual prerequisites experts assume are necessary for the development of early language. Note, however, that as important as these factors are to language development, the acquisition of language is an extraordinarily complex process that depends on factors other than cognition and perception. This complexity being established, we will consider how perception works with cognition in helping establish a foundation for language. To understand this relationship, we must go back one step further to sensory input.

A person receives stimuli through the senses: touch, taste, smell, hearing, and vision. **Perception** refers to the processes by which the person selects, organizes, integrates, and interprets sensory stimuli. It should be obvious, therefore, that the child must be able to receive and perceptually process sensory stimuli to put this information into manipulable thought forms. Later in this chapter, we consider some of the child's earliest perceptual abilities, which appear to be related to his first attempts to communicate.

Before we can continue our explanation of the sensorimotor stage of cognitive development, however, we must identify and describe **distancing**, a basic perceptual principle affecting those cognitive changes that apparently precede and lay the foundation for language acquisition.

The infant relates to her environment in a very physical way. She grasps things with her hands and puts things into her mouth. In fact, parents often believe that everything goes into the infant's mouth. The infant is trying to understand her world primarily through touch, taste, and smell.

Now consider how you relate to the world, especially to new stimuli. The first time you saw a laptop or iPod, you did not put these new things into your mouth. You looked at the laptop. You looked at and listened to the iPod. You used senses that placed you at a greater distance from these new stimuli than if you had explored them by touch, taste, or smell. One can reasonably assume that you would eventually touch these items, but, unless you are very strange, you probably would not taste or smell an iPod during your first encounter. One thing that happens during perceptual development, therefore, is that children relate to stimuli from a greater and greater distance. Moerk (1977) believes that the child's long-range visual and/or auditory images of new stimuli are the forerunners of representational meaning. That is, she first relates to an object by putting it into her mouth—immediate and maximal contact. As she develops, she creates a kind of mental picture of the object based on what she sees. The visual image represents the real thing, and the child recognizes the real thing based on that image.

Consider what happens as distancing progresses. A toy truck represents a real truck. But, a child might use a block of wood to represent a toy truck, which represents a real truck. The child will then recognize a truck in a picture. Eventually, the word *truck* represents the real thing. In each progression, the distance between the child and contact with the actual object becomes greater. Language represents the ultimate perceptual distance. Words allow the child to mentally manipulate objects, people, and places more quickly and easily than these can be physically manipulated. The ability to use words in place of things is called **representation**. Distancing moves the child's experiences with her environment from her hands and mouth to her brain. This is a short trip when measured in feet and inches, but when understood in the context of cognitive development, it is a journey spanning an intellectual universe.

Concepts and Behaviors Central to Early Cognitive Development

As we progress through the six substages of the sensorimotor phase of cognitive development, we will encounter three *concepts* (object permanence, causality, and means/ends) and three *behaviors* (imitation, play, and communication) that account for increasingly advanced intellectual functioning as children change. Consider these concepts and behaviors the principal players in the unfolding sensorimotor drama. Although the roles of these six characters in our cognitive drama change from scene to scene or substage to substage, these concepts and behaviors are the forces that together, in an interactive manner, shape the child's intellectual growth during this rapidly evolving first stage of cognitive development. And now, before the curtain goes up, let's meet the players.

The first player in our drama is a concept clearly related to representation, **object permanence**. It would not be accurate to say that the infant is unaware of objects, because even the youngest child will grasp or suck the things in his environment with which he has direct contact. When an object is removed, however, the infant pays no attention to its removal and does not look for it. When an object is out of sight, it is literally out of mind. As cognitive development proceeds, the child understands that objects exist even when they are not being touched, tasted, smelled, seen, or heard. Only when the child understands that things are permanent can he represent them cognitively, perhaps first in mental pictures, but eventually in words. (See Table 3.3 for definitions of object permanence and other concepts and behaviors.)

The next member of our cast is **causality**. In the beginning, the child has no concept of cause and effect. As she develops intellectually, she realizes that certain events cause other events, and she understands that she can produce behaviors that have predictable effects. According to Bates, Benigni, Bretherton, Camaioni, and Volterra (1979), the development of causality is a significant factor in the child's social and communicative maturation. Communication is a process driven by intentions. We do things or say things to produce desired and predictable results. An early understanding of causality might be reflected in the child's pushing a spoonful of strained carrots out of her mouth with her tongue. As she develops language, she might simply say, "No!" She uses a word to represent her intention to cause the carrots to not be delivered to her stomach.

Table 3.3 **Concepts and Behaviors Central to Early Cognitive Development**

Concepts	Behaviors
Object Permanence—knowing that objects exist in time and space even if you can't see or act on them	*Imitation*—duplication of models you hear, see, or feel
Causality—understanding that events can cause other events	*Play*—child-directed activities that provide children with opportunities for learning
Means/Ends—a conceptual extension of causality; the understanding that there are ways (means) to attain a goal (end)	*Communication*—conceptual development contributing to the ever-increasing development of a child's language ability

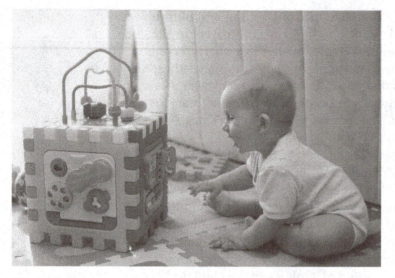

The child's first contacts with his world are physical and sensory.

Source: Ingrid Balabanova/ Hemera/Getty Images

Means/ends can be understood as a concept that extends causality. As this concept develops, the child learns to use the cause/effect concept to solve problems. The young infant's first behaviors are random and unintentional. Perhaps she sees a cookie she would like to consume. She reaches out to grab it, but it is beyond her reach. Her mother sees the child reaching, figures out what she wants, and gives her the cookie. Although the child got what she wanted, she stretched out her arms not to communicate intent but to reach the cookie. As she becomes more cognitively sophisticated, she is able to establish goals and to figure out *means* by which to accomplish these goals or *ends*. She will eventually reach for an object she knows is beyond her reach because she is intentionally signaling by this gesture that she wants the targeted object. In terms of language development, means/ends is important because language is used to get things done. It becomes a means by which many ends are accomplished. The child must learn not only that language is a means/ends phenomenon but also that adjustments in language must be made depending on who the listener is and what kind of relationship the child has with the listener. If she wants a cookie from her younger brother, she might simply demand it. If she wants a cookie from her mother, she will likely ask for it and say, "Please!" In both cases, the end is thoughtfully targeted, and the means is carefully created to maximize the possibility of success.

The fourth principal player is **imitation**. Anyone who observes young children will quickly and comfortably conclude that imitation is an important factor in cognitive development and in language development. Most of what children learn, and much of what adults learn, appears to be the result of attending to models and trying to duplicate them.

The research data concerning the acquisition of communication skills support the conclusion that imitation is an important developmental factor (Moore & Meltzoff, 1978; Rees, 1975; Snyder, 1978). Recall our discussion of mirror neurons in Chapter 2 that may be the neurological mechanism underlying the ability of humans to imitate actions, pantomime through gestures, use conventional gestures to make signs, and produce speech. It is assumed that imitation facilitates children's ability to internalize models of the behaviors of others, which they can then duplicate. Early imitations are crude, imprecise, and always immediate, but over the course of development, imitated behaviors become more accurate and sophisticated, and they occur in a delayed manner. **Delayed imitation**, or deferred imitation, is important because it allows children to produce a desired behavior even when the model is not present.

Without deferred imitation, language would not progress beyond the kind of parroted productions accomplished by talking birds. Even before children can imitate language forms, they imitate movements and gestures. Imitations of behaviors associated with objects seem to suggest some understanding of the objects themselves. For example, if the child, with or without a real comb in his hands, imitates a combing motion, we might reasonably assume that he knows something about the function of the comb. Bates and Snyder (1987) suggest that imitation is a primitive kind of labeling. That is, the child labels a comb by imitating, immediately or on a deferred basis, the action of combing. In the sensorimotor drama, imitation is a major player, as you will see.

Our next player is **play**, itself. Many adults think of playing as a frivolous activity, but professionals view play associated with child development as fairly serious business. Play is certainly a fun and entertaining activity, but it also provides children with many opportunities to learn about the things and people in their world, as well as concepts ranging from colors, numbers, and simple prepositions, such as *in* and *on,* to more complex things such as sharing and social interactions. As children grow older, language and other forms of communication become increasingly prominent and important components in play activities. Experts in cognitive and language development are especially interested in **symbolic play**, an activity in which one object represents another object. How many times, for example, have you watched children play for hours in a big box, pretending it was a house or a fort? My* youngest daughter, when she was about 2 years old, used rubber bands as bracelets and often had 10 or 12 on her wrist at one time. This kind of play has a rather obvious connection to language. In symbolic play, a child might use a stick to represent a nail-driving tool. In language, she can use the word *hammer* to refer to the same object. Both are representational activities. It is probably not a coincidence, then, that Bates, Bretherton, Snyder, Shore, and Volterra (1980) found that children who are able and willing to use objects to represent other objects progress more quickly in language development than children who are more rigid in their use of objects.

Communication is the leading character in our version of the sensorimotor drama, because speech and language are the focus of this book. Children gain an increasingly sophisticated communication system, and few would argue that imitation and play are important in helping them acquire greater conceptual understandings and the means by which to express their understandings. It is also reasonable to assume that, at some point, children use their communication abilities, especially language, to facilitate advances in their cognitive development. As we proceed through the substages of sensorimotor development, we will track changes in communication as well as changes in the other concepts and behaviors we have identified. For the sake of convenience and to allow for direct comparison of the substages, we discuss the players in the same order in each substage, however, keep in mind that the order signifies nothing about the importance of these players. The interactions among the

---

*Lloyd Hulit.

players are more important than the individual players themselves. The further into cognitive development we proceed, the more inextricably connected the players become.

The cast is set. The curtain is rising. Let the play begin.

The Sensorimotor Period (Birth to Two Years)

Scene 1—Substage 1 (Birth to One Month)

At birth and through the first three substages of the sensorimotor period, the infant is *egocentric*, which means that he sees and understands the world only as an extension of himself. Since he does not understand that he is only one thing among many other things in the environment, he does not have the concept that others can make things happen; thus, he is not able to relate to causality or means/ends. The substage 1 infant is not capable of imitation, but he does produce behaviors that seem to be imitative. McCormick (1990) describes "vocal contagion" as the phenomenon in which, when one newborn begins to cry, other newborns in the same room are likely to cry too. Piaget believed that vocal contagion is not imitation, but rather the activation of an already established response to an external stimulus. Of course, at this early stage, the newborn infant does not play and the little communication that occurs is caregiver responsiveness to his cries and sounds of pleasure and contentment. Refer to Table 3.4 for a summary of the key attributes of sensorimotor substage 1 development across the six behaviors.

As dramas go, this has not been the most exciting opening scene one might imagine. What do we have here? We have a living organism with enormous cognitive and communicative potential, but he is just sitting on the stage crying, grasping, and sucking. He pays little attention to the audience and is constantly falling asleep. This drama builds in excitement, however, so hang in there. It gets better.

Scene 2—Substage 2 (One to Four Months)

During substage 2, the infant begins to show some awareness of objects, but the awareness is sensory rather than conceptual. She reacts to objects visually and auditorially, and she is able to coordinate her visual and auditory contacts with objects. That is, when she hears a noise, she searches for the source with her eyes, and if the sound source moves within her field of vision, she follows its movement. Piaget (1954) reported that one of his daughters not only located objects visually, but also looked away from an object and then located it again. Whether a child reacts to this visual and auditory hide-and-seek activity with disappointment and expectation as Piaget suggested, it is reasonable to conclude that the child is developing an interest in objects and is using her senses to make and maintain contact with them.

Even though there is sensory interest in objects during this substage, the child still does not demonstrate an understanding that objects are separate from her. She makes few, if any, meaningful differentiations among objects and does not differentiate objects from herself, even when the objects move

Table 3.4 Highlights of Sensorimotor Development

Substage (and Months)	Object Permanence	Causality	Means–Ends	Imitation	Play	Communication
1 (0 to 1)	Out of sight, out of mind	No concept of causality	No understanding of means–ends	None	None	No communicative intent
2 (1 to 4)	Uses senses to make and maintain contact with objects	No concept of causality	No understanding of means–ends	Pre-imitation; repeats her own behavior that has been imitated by someone else	Produces behaviors preliminary to play, including grasping and looking at objects	Cries, coos, and laughs
3 (4 to 8)	Watches object move and anticipates its future position; reaches for partially hidden object	Does not understand cause/effect, behaves as though she is the cause of all actions	Produces goal-oriented behaviors but only after activity has begun	Imitates only behaviors she has spontaneously produced at an earlier time	Still very sensory but begins to interact with other people	Babbles
4 (8 to 12)	Looks for an object if he sees it being hidden	Externalizes causality, knows other people and objects can cause activities	Evidence of planning and the production of intentional behaviors	Imitates behaviors he has not spontaneously produced	Uses developing concepts in his play activities	Links gestures and vocalizations to convey fairly specific messages
5 (12 to 18)	Follows sequential displacements to find hidden object	Sees other people and objects as agents for causality in new situations	Uses experimentation to solve problems	Uninhibited imitation to facilitate her own understanding	Play reflects cognitive growth; he figures out how to make toys work	Produces first meaningful words; communication is intentional but still heavily nonverbal
6 (18 to 24)	Fully developed concept of object permanence; can now accommodate invisible displacements	Causality enhanced by ability to represent objects and cause/effect relationships in his mind	Can mentally represent a goal and his plan for achieving the goal	Deferred imitation; imitates a behavior he has represented mentally and stored in his memory	Progresses from auto-symbolic to symbolic play	Imitates and spontaneously produces multiple word utterances

in and out of her sensory fields. In other words, she is still strongly egocentric. As was true in the first substage, there is no possibility for a demonstration of causality or means/ends behaviors.

Behaviors at this stage are still essentially reflexive even though other people can modify them when they cause objects to move or make noise. Piaget (1952) contended, "Even when the child grasps an object in order to look at it, one cannot infer that there is a conscious purpose" (p. 143). In this example, it might be tempting to think of looking as the end and the grasping as the means, but because grasping is a reflexive behavior, we cannot conclude that the sequence of behaviors from grasping to looking is intentional. It just happens, and the looking is part of the reflexive sequence.

We see the beginning of imitation in this substage, although it is a specialized kind of imitation. The child produces a behavior that someone, perhaps a parent, imitates. The child then repeats the behavior. What we have, then, is the child imitating a behavior that she produced, but only after someone else imitated her. Got it? These behaviors might be gestural but are usually vocal. In a common example, the child says, "Goo-goo." The parent mimics the child, saying, "Goo-goo." The child, terribly excited by this insightful communicative exchange, repeats her original production, "Goo-goo." Piaget called this behavior "pre-imitation," suggesting it is behavior that sets the stage for true imitation. McCormick (1990) calls the same behavior "mutual imitation," which describes the nature of the exchange.

It would be a real stretch to call anything the child does in the second substage *play*, but she is engaging in sensorimotor behaviors that are preliminary to play. She is not only grasping objects but also holding them for brief periods of time and looking at them, and she is showing some interest in the sensory characteristics of objects. Even the primitive imitative responses we see in this substage are preparing the child for play activities seen in later substages. Early play activities involve very basic motor and sensory behaviors, and they often involve imitation, so the child is getting ready for play.

During the early weeks of this substage, most of the child's communications are still in the form of reflexive cries, but as the substage progresses, the child cries less frequently and develops distinctly different types of cries. According to D'Odorico 1984), at about four months the child produces three differentiated cries to signal discomfort, to call, and to request. Noncrying vocalizations signaling pleasure develop during this substage. The child begins to coo, especially when interacting with someone else. These productions are described as vowel-like to indicate that there are no consonant approximations and to suggest that the sounds produced are not true vowels. They are random, undifferentiated productions of sounds with vowel characteristics. Toward the end of this substage, at about four months, the child is also laughing (Stark, 1979), a delightful development for child and parents. The child may not be receptive to political humor or satire at this point, but she does laugh. It is, in fact, often difficult to figure out what makes a four-month-old child laugh, but if gentle pokes in the belly accompanied by funny faces and silly vocal noises make her laugh, parents will enjoy it! They have made communicative contact with their child about subjects other than hunger and soiled diapers. Refer back to Table 3.4 as a summary of key attainments in sensorimotor substage 2.

Scene 3—Substage 3 (Four to Eight Months)

The period between four and eight months is an active time in the infant's life. This is the time when sitting and crawling are attained, and the infant is highly aware of his surroundings. Infants love to explore objects during this time, but they are bound by the here and now and by objects that are in full or partial view. Thus, the child

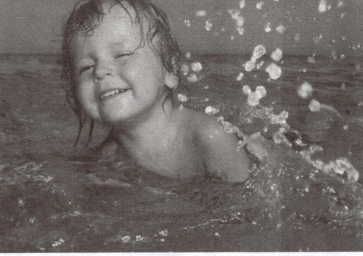

Just look what I can do with the water!
Source: Sergey Novikov/ fotolia

will follow a moving object, such as a dog running in the yard. He will watch his cookie fall to the floor, and he will reach for an object sticking out from under a blanket. However, at this stage, an object out of sight is literally out of mind. The child will not search for objects that are outside of his visual realm. Flavell (1977, p. 43,) calls this lack of *object permanence* the "essential limitation" of substage 3.

The beginnings of causality emerge during this stage. Children delight in repeating actions that capture their interest or cause pleasure. For example, a child might bang her spoon on her high chair tray simply because it feels good and she likes the noise. At this stage, the child lacks an understanding of the effects of her behavior. The idea that food is being flung far and wide is of no concern at all! It is also true that the child doesn't recognize that others can cause sounds too. Her dad might ring a bell, which could be a very enjoyable game; thus, she pushes his face to cause the bell to ring again. She does not understand that her dad's hand is the cause of the bell ringing. The child believes it is her actions that cause the bell to ring because she is, of course, the mistress of the universe.

In the third substage, there is a limited but important progression in means/ ends development. The child might pick up a new rattle, for example. In the course of examining the rattle, she shakes it and it makes a noise she finds interesting. She continues to shake the rattle. This can be construed as intentional or goal-oriented behavior, but the goals in this substage are established only after the activity has begun (Wadsworth, 1971). At this point, the child is engaging in intentional behaviors but is not yet a planner.

McCormick (1990) refers to imitation in substage 3 as, "systematic imitation." The child imitates a wider range of behaviors, including those of others. Most imitations are of sounds and physical actions, but the child will not imitate an action she herself has not performed spontaneously at an earlier time. She will imitate only complete sequences of behaviors, not isolated parts of a sequence. The child must be able to see herself perform the activity she is imitating, and if it involves sound, she must be able to hear herself or at the very least to be able to feel the movements she is making. If we put these limitations together, they mean that the child will imitate making and releasing a fist if she has previously done this on her own. If, in releasing her fist, the child spontaneously spreads her fingers, she will spread her fingers when she imitates the fist-making/fist-releasing sequence, but she will not imitate only the spreading of her fingers. She will imitate fist making/fist releasing if she can watch herself, but she will not imitate this sequence of behaviors while holding her hand behind her back.

During stage 3, we see the child engaging in activities that more closely resemble play. The child is interacting with other people and responding to models of physical and vocal activity. He is finding toys more interesting and repeats actions on toys that may or may not be appropriate. That is, he might shake a rattle, but he might also bang it on the floor or on Mom's forehead. He is still very much a sensory creature. He grasps toys, ears, nostrils, and dogs' paws, and he still tries to put all objects, including the coffee table leg, into his mouth. The child is deriving pleasure from his play activities, and they provide him opportunities for developing concepts and elaborating behaviors important for later cognitive and communicative development.

Few dramatic changes in communication occur in this substage. The child continues to produce vowel-like utterances, but we do notice the emergence of consonant-like sounds that are random and not meaningful, but have characteristics of true sounds. Toward the end of this substage, at about six to eight months, the child begins to produce productions referred to as **babbling**. These are combinations of vowel- and consonant-like sounds, resulting in utterances such as "gagaga" or "mamama." As you might imagine, parents often interpret these babbled productions as words, but until a production is used in a consistent, intentional, and meaningful manner, it cannot be considered a word. It will be a few months before the child produces true words, but she is laying the groundwork at this point by establishing control over the components of her speech mechanism (Sachs, 1989). It would certainly be a mistake to assume that the child in substage 3 is not communicating. She is using her vocalizations and gestures to communicate many things, from, "I'm not a very happy person right now because my diaper is wet—again" to, "I would like very much to have that cookie in your hand, and if you don't mind, I am going to grab it while distracting you with my devastating smile."

Scene 4—Substage 4 (8 to 12 Months)

As the child moves into the last few months of his first year, he seems more curious about his world. Part of what adults might perceive as curiosity is the further development of the object permanence concept. In the fourth substage, the child shows evidence that he remembers objects. If a playful adult hides his favorite pacifier under a pillow, he will lift the pillow to find it. In addition to understanding that objects are permanent, the child demonstrates an understanding that the shape and size of objects are constant. (We will explore shape as an important attribute in learning words later in this chapter.) If a familiar object, such as his bottle, is given to him upside down, he knows that the business end has a nipple on it, and he will turn the bottle around. In other words, he knows the shape has not changed even when his perspective of the bottle is different. He will also recognize his bottle when viewed from a distance, even though the bottle appears smaller from 30 feet away than from 6 inches. The object concept is not yet fully developed, however. For example, the child will look for an object that has disappeared, but only if he sees it disappear. The object concept is fairly complete by the end of this substage, but some gaps still exist, and we will not see a thorough understanding of object permanence until the sixth substage.

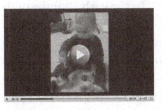

▶ Video Example 3.1

Notice in the video that this nine-month-old child is practicing his emerging ability to stack rings onto the stick. He doesn't seem particularly concerned when he misses, but he is certainly diligent in his focus on the objects and completion of the task. What sensory motor stage do you think best fits this child?

We encounter a child who is far less egocentric than in earlier substages. This shift from an egocentric view of the world is most noticeable in the child's more sophisticated understanding of causality. That is, she understands that other people and other objects can cause activities. Using the same example of bell ringing we employed in the preceding substage, we can create a very different scenario. Earlier, the child believed she was responsible for causing the bell to ring even though she did not touch the bell. Now, when the child watches Dad pick up the bell and ring it, she will push Dad's hand toward the bell to indicate that she wants him to ring it again. She understands that Dad caused the action.

In the fourth substage, the child plans behavior. She devises a means or strategy before initiating a behavior, and there is a clear connection between the strategy and the goal. Wadsworth (1971, p. 48) suggests that this behavior is one of, "the first clear acts of intelligence" we observe in the developing child. Many of the child's behaviors are now intentional, and they reflect thoughtful planning. In an earlier example related to object permanence, the child searched for her pacifier under a pillow. This same example demonstrates her more sophisticated means/ends understanding. The problem is a missing pacifier. The end is to find the pacifier. The means is to move the pillow. Eureka! There is the pacifier!

Imitation undergoes some interesting and significant changes in the fourth substage. The child now imitates behaviors he has not produced himself, although he is likely to imitate only actions or vocalizations similar to those he has produced on his own (McCormick, 1990). It is not necessary in this substage that he be able to see or hear himself while he is imitating. For example, if while holding the child on her lap, the mother sticks out her tongue, he might imitate this behavior even though he cannot see his own protruding tongue. Owens (2005) suggests that this kind of imitation requires some short-term motor memory, which has obvious relevance to the speech skills he will acquire in the near future.

It should be apparent by this point in our drama that play provides children with opportunities to use their developing concepts in activities that are pleasurable. More important, perhaps, it is through play that children discover new aspects of these concepts and demonstrate these new understandings to those who observe them. While playing with her toys, the child in the fourth substage will look for toys that are not in sight.

In the early months of the fourth substage, the child is still babbling. By the end of the substage, she may actually produce her first meaningful words. Whether or not there are true words during this time, it is evident that the child is communicating, vocally and gesturally, in an intentional manner. Even without speech, children in the latter months of this substage link gestures and vocalizations to convey fairly specific messages. Bates, Camaioni, and Volterra (1975) studied a girl in this substage who, on one occasion at least, vocalized "ha" to her mother while looking in the direction of the kitchen. When her mother carried her into the kitchen, the girl pointed at the sink, prompting her mother to give her a drink of water. The child did not use words, but she certainly communicated.

Scene 5—Substage 5 (12 to 18 Months)

Around his first birthday, the child is now capable of following sequential displacements. If Mom hides his pacifier under the pillow, he will look under the pillow. If Mom then hides it under his blanket, he will look under the blanket, and if Mom puts it in her shirt pocket, he will search for his pacifier in her pocket, undoubtedly ripping the shirt in the process. Why, then, is the concept not complete? Although the child can handle sequential displacements if he can see them, he cannot handle a displacement he cannot see. If, for example, Mom hides his pacifier under the pillow and while she has her hand under the pillow she slips the pacifier between the sofa cushions, the child will look for the pacifier under, over, and around the pillow but will not search between the sofa cushions. The object permanence concept becomes complete in the sixth and final substage, when the child is finally able to move an object from its place in the restricted physical world to the mind, where it is represented abstractly and is free of all time and space limitations.

In this substage, the child's understanding of causality becomes more sophisticated than previously in that she sees other people and objects as agents for causality in new situations. If, for example, the child is given a new toy unlike anything she has seen before, she might examine it carefully and, deciding that she does not know what to do with it, push it into an adult's hand. She is seeking the adult's assistance as an agent of causality. In essence, the child is saying, "Show me what this thing does!" In another example, we have a child who, when playing with his mother's lipstick, got the sticky red goo all over his fingers. He now approaches a fire hydrant painted the same bright red as the lipstick. He touches the hydrant and examines his fingers, expecting to see them colored red. In this example, the child is able to transfer his understanding of causality from one situation to another, and in the process learns that red does not always icky fingers make. In both examples, we see evidence that the child's understanding of external causality has increased.

Means/ends in the fifth substage can be characterized as more creative or experimental in comparison to the fourth substage. The child is becoming a problem solver, and in the process of learning to solve problems, she experiments with objects and actions. The child, for example, has a toy workbench. She uses a play hammer to drive a large wooden peg through an opening in the bench. Banging the hammer is the means by which to reach the end, defined as making the peg move. She now picks up a banana. It weighs about the same as the hammer, and it has a convenient "handle," so the child hits the peg with the banana. The banana breaks, and the peg does not move. This means did not accomplish the desired end because, as the child learned through trial and error, the banana is too soft. As her experimentation proceeds, she will learn that things other than the hammer can be used, like Dad's shoe or Mom's skillet, to drive the peg through the bench because, like the hammer, they are hard. As you might imagine, this experimentation business can be interesting and dangerous. Parents are well advised to observe their children carefully as they identify their goals and map their strategies for attaining them.

The same willingness, perhaps eagerness, to experiment—observed in means/ends experiences—is observed in imitation. The child is an excellent and uninhibited imitator in this substage. The accuracy of his imitations is limited only by his motor abilities (Owens, 2005), but he will try almost anything. Accord-

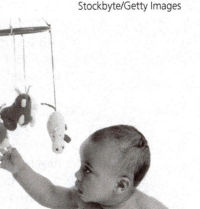

My, look at the intricate detail in this thing.

Source: Comstock Images/ Stockbyte/Getty Images

ing to McCormick (1990), this child imitates to better understand his world and the things in it. He will imitate animal noises, for example, and will attempt to imitate even complex speech productions. When my* own children were in this substage, they modeled words such as *encyclopedia, electroencephalographic,* and *diadochokinesis,* which they gladly tried to imitate. Their productions of these words were not accurate, but they produced excellent imitations of words and actions that were within their motoric capabilities.

The child's play clearly reflects his cognitive advances as he thoroughly examines his toys and quickly figures out the operative pieces. If the toy is relatively simple to operate, he figures out how to make it work through trial and error. If there is a string, he pulls it. If there is a lever, he pushes it. If there is a dial, he turns it. If he cannot figure out what to do with the toy, as mentioned in the causality

---

*Lloyd Hulit.

discussion, he hands it to someone else for consultation and demonstration. The child also combines toys in a functional manner. He might, for example, use his toy hammer to make a ball roll across the floor.

 Video Reflection 3.1: Child Attainments in SM Stage 5

Watch the video of a child who is in sensorimotor stage 5, then answer the question.

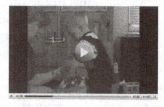

It is during this substage that we typically see children producing their first meaningful words. These words are monosyllabic (e.g., *go,no*) or duplicated disyllabic forms (e.g., *mama,wawa*). There is no question that communication during this substage is intentional. For example, the child might say, "bye-bye" to indicate that she wants to leave or wants someone else to leave. Toward the end of this substage, it is not uncommon for the child to say, "nite-nite," while shaking her head from side to side, to suggest that she has no intention of going to bed now, under any circumstances, not until *Monday Night Football* is over or until the popcorn is all gone, whichever occurs first. Communication continues to be heavily dependent on nonverbal messages conveyed by the voice, face, and gestures, but there is very little of importance, as defined by the child's own needs and desires, that she cannot communicate.

As scene 5 closes, we leave the last of the truly sensorimotor substages. The child is now ready for an important transition to substage 6, during which we will see the completion of the concepts and the elaboration of the behaviors we have been following in the first five scenes.

Scene 6—Substage 6 (18 to 24 Months)

The common denominator underlying all the significant changes in the sixth substage is representation. That is, the child's understanding of her world moves from the sensorimotor level to a level in which she is able to represent objects internally and to manipulate these internal representations of reality to solve problems. She is becoming, in a word, a cognitive thinker instead of a touchy-feely experiencer.

The child now has a fully developed concept of object permanence. Not only can she follow sequential displacements, but she can accommodate invisible displacements. If Mom moves the pacifier out of sight under the pillow and then slides the pacifier between the sofa cushions, the child will first look under the pillow but, not finding it, will continue to look in and around the area where it disappeared until she finds it. She now has a mental image of the pacifier that is entirely free of her senses and her physical contacts with it. She knows that the pacifier and all objects are permanent, do not disappear just because they are out of sight, and do not change in size or shape just because they are viewed from different angles or distances. When the object is out of sight, it is now firmly in mind. It is, in reference to the common denominator of this substage, *represented* in her mind.

The child's understanding of causality is also enhanced by this ability to represent objects and cause/effect relationships in her mind. A child in the early substages, for example, might simply react with frustration when trying to remove a pull toy with a plastic rope from her toy box, the rope of which is tangled on another toy at the bottom of the box. She cannot see what has tangled it, and she does not have the ability to conceptualize the cause/effect relationship that is preventing the removal of the pull toy. After tugging a few times, she might give up or cry, but she will not try to solve the problem by identifying and eliminating the cause. If we move this same child forward to substage 6, we see a much different performance when the same problem occurs. After tugging on the pull toy a time or two, she reaches into the toy box to discover what is tangling it. She eliminates the tangle and removes the pull toy. She was able to solve this problem because, even without seeing what was catching the pull toy, she was able to mentally represent a physical obstacle of some kind. She understood the principle of cause and effect that was operating, and she applied this intellectual understanding to the solution of a physical problem.

Means/ends, in its fully developed form, is about intentionality. The child can now represent the goal mentally, map out plans for reaching that goal in his mind's eye, and put the plan into action. In earlier substages, the child might get a cookie out of the unreachable cookie jar by pointing and grunting until someone gets the cookie for him. By the end of the sensorimotor stage, the child might push a chair to the counter, climb onto the counter, and stand on tiptoes to reach the cookie jar on the shelf his mother thought was safely beyond reach. This kind of creative planning is just part of what is waiting for parents during the stage of child development often called the *terrible twos*.

Imitation undergoes significant changes as we proceed through the sixth substage. The child produces what are called "deferred imitations" (McCormick, 1990). This means that the child can imitate a behavior modeled for her earlier, an action or vocalization that she has represented mentally and stored in her memory. Now when someone asks the child what sound the cow makes, she retrieves the model from her own mental catalog of animal noises and

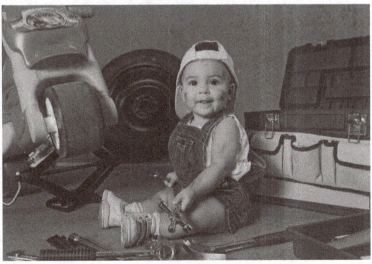

Executing an imperfect and perhaps dangerous plan of action
Source: Erllre/Fotolia.

imitates that model by saying, "Moo!" When someone leaves the house, she does not need to have someone prompt a wave by demonstration and exhortation. She remembers the action and produces it spontaneously, a deferred imitation of a model she has stored in her memory.

In addition to seeing the child apply his more complete conceptual understandings in play, we observe some fundamental changes in the nature of the child's play in the sixth substage (Westby, 1980). Early in this substage, the child might pretend to drink out of a cup or pretend to sleep, but all of his pretending behaviors are autosymbolic. That is, he limits pretending to his own actions. About midway through the final substage, he extends pretending to other objects during symbolic play, but the objects must be realistic. The child will pretend he is feeding a doll with a real or toy spoon, for example, but will not pretend that a Popsicle stick is a spoon. By the end of the sixth substage, the child will engage in play activities that represent real-life experiences. He might play house, but the toys used must still be realistic in terms of function and, to some extent, even in terms of size.

In the earliest stages of make-believe play, the child's pretending is limited to real, or at least realistic-looking, objects. At 18 months, for example, he will pretend to eat with forks and spoons—either actual forks and spoons or toy forks and spoons—but he will not pretend that a roofing plank from a set of Lincoln Logs is a fork. He is quite literal and rigid in what he uses and in the actions he performs. These initial steps in pretend play advance to pretend actions that represent what the child observes people, including himself, execute in real-life situations. Thus, as he moves beyond his second birthday, he might use Lincoln Log roof planking as a fork, or he might put a bowl on his head, pretending it is a baseball cap (Tomasello, Striano, & Rochat, 1999). By the time the child is three and well beyond sensorimotor substage 6, there need be no connection, even a visual similarity, between the object he uses in play and the object it represents (O'Reilly, 1995). He might, for example, use the bowl or the roofing plank as a car or truck.

All the changes we have identified in the sixth substage of the sensorimotor period have direct implications for what is happening to the child as a communicator as she completes this phase of her cognitive development and prepares to move forward. Imitation, especially deferred imitation, is critical to the development of communication. The essential contribution of imitation is that it helps the child develop the ability to represent behaviors internally, and eventually to produce these behaviors even when the models are not present. This is the essence of language, a system of communication based, in part, on a huge inventory of internalized models. As the sensorimotor stage comes to a close, the child is using words and combinations of words to get things done.

As a child's play progresses from a solitary, physically limited activity to a more interactive and representational activity, language plays a more important role. We have to go beyond the sensorimotor stage to observe speech as a primary play activity, but in the latter months of this first stage of cognitive development, we see communication becoming an increasingly important part of play.

As the curtain slowly falls on the sensorimotor drama, remember that this is but the beginning of the cognitive development story. Piaget's theory has three more stages, which might be viewed as sequels to the sensorimotor drama. Unlike sequels to bad movies, which typically only compound the badness of the original, however, the cognitive sequels are improved dramas, because each stage is based on and incorporates the preceding stage. We are pausing after the sensorimotor phase, not to indicate intellectual closure but to indicate that the stage has now been set for the part of the child development story that is the primary focus of this book—speech and language acquisition. We will briefly describe the other stages, but first we will review reservations about some of Piaget's views precipitated by research data gathered in recent years.

Recent Research: A Critical Review of Piaget's Sensorimotor Stage

Because the Piagetian view of cognitive development was so widely accepted and so heavily influenced the understanding of many aspects of early child development (with direct and indirect connections to cognitive development), researchers have tried to verify Piaget's observations about what happens during the sensorimotor stage and when. The results of this research suggest that children exhibit some cognitive abilities at much earlier ages than Piaget indicated. Note, however, that today's researchers understand that Piaget did not have access to modern research methodologies that would have allowed him to conduct the kinds of carefully designed and rigorously implemented studies the human behavioral research community demands today. Piaget suggested, for example, that the infant shows evidence that he is exploring his world and making preliminary efforts to control aspects of his environment when he is about four to eight months old. Using basic operant conditioning principles, researchers have demonstrated that the child is displaying this level of cognitive awareness immediately after birth. The neonate will enthusiastically suck on a nipple in order to acknowledge a wide range of sounds and sights he finds interesting. The newborn child is aware of these auditory and visual stimuli and that he is able to exercise rudimentary control to make them happen. Similar research strategies, based on operant conditioning principles, have been used to reveal what the sensorimotor-stage child knows about object permanence and mental representation and when he knows it.

Regarding object permanence, Baillargeon, Graber, DeVos, and Black (1990) concluded that the child understands object permanence even if she is not yet capable of implementing the means/ends strategies necessary for locating an object when it is moved out of sight. It is one thing, after all, to know that an object still exists even when it is no longer visible, and it is quite another to push aside, lift up, or reach behind whatever is hiding the object. The child might know object permanence, therefore, even if she is not yet demonstrating that knowledge in her searching or locating behaviors.

Piaget asserted that a child cannot represent experience until he is about 18 months old. Meltzoff (1988b) demonstrated, however, that deferred imitation occurs in children as young as 9 months old. He also found that the child at nine months retains several actions in memory at the same time. By the time he is

14 months old, he holds in memory as many as six modeled actions over the course of a week. Thus, Piaget's predictions relative to deferred imitation are much too conservative.

We also do not see evidence of mental representation, including deferred imitation and categorization in Piaget's theory, until the end of the sensorimotor period. However, it is more plausible to conclude that sensorimotor schemata and symbolic schemata develop simultaneously. This view would certainly be consistent with research findings relative to categorization, which develops incrementally from 3 months to 18 months. Children as young as 9 to 12 months look longer at pictures of things within a category than at pictures of objects foreign to that category, and they can categorize things, such as birds, food, and stuffed animals (Oakes, Madole, & Cohen, 1991; Roberts, 1988; Sherman, 1985). Eighteen-month-olds are able to categorize objects into two classes (Gopnik & Meltzoff, 1987). Thus, given a mixture of blocks and dolls, they can easily sort them.

The most significant differences between what Piaget proposed and what researchers have found center on the emergence of abilities, such as object permanence, and on how early cognitive development takes place. That is, some cognitive abilities do emerge earlier than Piaget asserted. These include the abilities we have highlighted in this discussion, object permanence and mental representation. Table 3.5 compares these cognitive attainments across researchers. A more important gap between the theory and current research focuses on *how* this development occurs. Piaget believed that in this first stage of cognitive development, the acquisition of all knowledge is facilitated by the

Table 3.5   Cognitive Abilities in the Sensorimotor Stages

Cognitive Abilities specific cognitive	Piaget	Other Researchers
Sensory awareness		
Exploration and control of environment	4 to 8 months	At birth
Object permanence		
Object that is out of sight is out of mind	4 to 8 months	3.5 months
Search last place object was hidden	8 to 12 months	8 months
Search for object hidden in several places	8 to 12 months	12 months
Mental representation		
Deferred imitation	18 months	9 months
Retain several modeled actions in memory over time	18 months	14 months
Categorization	24 months	3 to 18 months
Physical characteristics of mobiles		3 months
Pictures of objects		9 to 12 months
Objects into two classes		18 months

Sources: Baillargeon (1987); Baillargeon and DeVos (1991); Baillargeon, Graber, DeVos, and Black (1990); Gopnik and Meltzoff (1987); Meltzoff (1988a).

child's sensorimotor experiences. But researchers have expanded this idea to include knowledge from perceptual experiences including watching and listening. They also recognize that cognitive abilities are genetically determined.

Some critics believe that recent research findings suggest that cognitive development does not progress in the fairly rigid, step-by-step manner implied by Piaget's stages. According to Piaget's theory, a range of cognitive abilities develop together within each substage of the sensorimotor period, and they undergo comparable changes within each succeeding stage. The research evidence suggests that the specific cognitive abilities of a given child might be at different levels of maturity at the same time, and that when there is a change in one ability, there will not necessarily be a directly correlated change in another. Cognitive development, these critics argue, is variable because it depends on biological maturation interacting with environmental experiences.

So, where does this leave us? There is little doubt, even among the most ardent critics of Piaget's theory, that Piaget has appropriately identified the cognitive abilities the child acquires, and there is consensus that Piaget's general time frame for the maturity of cognitive abilities is, for the most part, on target. It is clear that some of Piaget's estimates about when certain cognitive abilities first appear were not correct. Children show the first signs of certain cognitive abilities much earlier than Piaget predicted. It also seems fair to conclude, based on recent research evidence, that early knowledge is not the product of sensorimotor experience only, that some cognitive abilities may be genetically predetermined, and that others may be influenced at least as much by innate perceptual abilities and experiences as by direct environmental contact. On the issue of stages, legitimate debate persists. It is reasonable to assume, however, that when the dust from this particular battle settles, we will have concluded that some semblance of a stage model is still useful in understanding cognitive development, even though any future stage model will almost certainly accommodate wide individual variations.

In closing this section on Piaget's sensorimotor stage of cognitive development, it will be useful to return to our primary focus, language. Even though, as we noted earlier, Piaget did not specifically theorize about language development, he and others who have endorsed his theory have related aspects of cognitive development, as Piaget has described it, to language. Table 3.6 contains a brief summary of key aspects of cognitive development that are related, or appear to be related, to language development. In processing this information, keep in mind that *relationship* does not necessarily mean *cause/effect*. In fact, most of the research data do not suggest that the connections between cognitive and language factors are more than correlational relationships. Nevertheless, it is intriguing to think about what these relationships might mean relative to both cognitive and language functions.

Piaget's Higher Cognitive Stages

Let us now move ahead to a brief discussion about later cognitive attainments and their relationship to language. The first two years of cognitive development and language development are formative and highly important in

Table 3.6   Sensorimotor and Language Events: A Summary

Sensorimotor Concept/Behavior	Language Behavior
Object Permanence	1. Object permanence appears to be related to early semantic functions, including nonexistence, disappearance, and recurrence. 2. Brown (1973) suggests that the understanding of object permanence reflected in substage 4 may be adequate for the acquisition of the child's first productive words.
Causality	1. An understanding of causality is a cognitive prerequisite for communication. 2. There appears to be a significant relationship between causality and the child's ability to understand verbs and semantic relations.
Means/Ends	1. An understanding of means/ends is critical to language development. 2. There is a significant correlation between an understanding of means/ends and language development during the early portion of substage 4. This cognitive ability is particularly important to the development of communicative intentionality. 3. The understanding of means/ends reflected in substage 6 appears to be significantly related to the emergence of two-word utterances .
Imitation	1. Imitation is significantly correlated with gestural development at 9 to 10 months. 2. Deferred imitation is significantly correlated with naming and with recognitory gestures (i.e., gestures that represent the functions or uses of objects). 3. When the child produces deferred imitation, we can assume that she has a true understanding of symbolic function because in deferred imitation, the referent for the imitation need not be present.
Play	1. There is a significant correlation between object play and language at 10 to 13 months. 2. Children who show a propensity for using a variety of schemes for objects in their early play experiences tend to progress more dramatically in language development than children who are more limited in their use of object schemes. 3. A child will produce meaningful words as symbols for people, things, and events before he has demonstrated complete competence in symbolic play.

Sources: Bates, Benigni, Bretherton, Camaioni, & Volterra, 1977, 1979; Bates, Camaioni & Voltera, 1975, 1979; Bates & Snyder, 1987; Greenwald & Leonard, 1979; James, 1980; Miller, Chapman, Branston, & Reichle, 1980; Snyder, 1978; Sugarman, 1978; Zachary, 1978.

future learning. This is why professionals who are involved in education view early childhood learning as being foundational for success as children become students in preschool and the early elementary grades. We will see how this foundation provides the support for the advancement of thinking and communicating.

Preoperational Thought (Two to Seven Years)

What knowledge and skills in thinking and language do preschool teachers expect children to have as they transition to kindergarten? What do children attain as they participate in first grade? One clue is to investigate the curricula offered to children during preschool, kindergarten, and first grade.

Just as families have routines, so too do teachers as they structure the day for young children. Morning routines begin with getting settled as children hang up coats and gather on the floor or in chairs around the teacher for circle time. Teachers use this opportunity to orient children to the day, weather, and the daily schedule of activities. They engage children by using their background experiences to teach new vocabulary and concepts and they remind them of the rules of the classroom as children participate in verbal exchanges about experiences, conversations about stories, and singing. Notice how preschool classrooms have lots of visual and motor tasks that children do with real objects. Because children are able to think conceptually, they categorize things and can solve physical problems. They learn words at a very rapid rate and develop sentence structures to convey ideas. We will expand on word learning and the development of grammar in Chapter 4. In short, the concrete and repetitive environment of preschool provides children with lots of hands-on practice— just what their developing brains need!

In kindergarten and first grade, students still require hands-on learning activities, but teachers introduce printed language, increase the amount of talking about ideas and events while decreasing demonstration, and gradually challenge students to solve problems that require thinking rather than doing. Students are challenged by problems that require them to take another person's perspective. Until about age 7, children are still egocentric. An egocentric child assumes that others see his own view of objects and events. He is not able to take the perspective of another person. For example, young children consider only the view of an object that is in front of them. They do not consider the view another person might have of that same object from across the table. Researchers use the "three mountains task" to demonstrate how the child's perspective prior to age 7 differs from older children's perspective. You can view demonstrations of preschool-age children performing this task on the Web.

Preoperational children are able to focus on one dimension of a problem (centering), but not on several aspects. Imagine asking a child which word is longer, *elephant* or *train*. The child in this stage of cognitive development will answer *"train."* She relates to the meaning of the word, not the number of sounds or syllables in the word.

Conservation tasks are also challenging in that they require knowledge about mass, number,and volume. A tall, narrow glass of milk is perceived as having more milk than a short, stocky glass of milk. These limitations in how children respond to their experiences do not last long as they move into the next stage.

Concrete Operations (7 to 11 Years)

Consider what happens in classrooms as students advance into second grade and beyond. One of the major efforts of teachers is to teach students to read and write while continuing to develop their verbal knowledge and skills. This goal is achievable because students are developing the ability to think logically in dealing with concrete or physical problems. No wonder there is much to learn in the curriculum about rules in reading and spelling and discussions about how things work. The limitations on thinking during the preoperational period are no longer limiting. Children are able, for example, to see the transformation of water to ice, and know that it is still water. In other words, they "conserve."

What limitations in thinking do students have during the early elementary grades? The name of this stage, "concrete operations," gives us a clue. Students do not have the ability to think abstractly. They are still bound by the manipulation of objects to solve problems. Thus, teachers continue to use contexts whereby students listen and read, but also use demonstration and provide hands-on practice time during the learning of new concepts and the application of information to different problems.

 Video Example 3.2

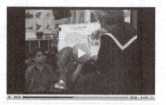

Early elementary classrooms buzz with activity as teachers engage students in learning to use their developing minds. Watch the video and pay attention to how the teacher uses demonstration of a clear bowl of water and an empty glass to discuss how air remains in the glass even when the glass is submerged in water. Children apply thinking, reasoning, and problem solving to this physical problem.

Formal Operations (11 to 15 Years)

Sometime after age 11, students are able to free themselves from objects and events. They begin to manipulate ideas in the mind. For example, rather than having to count blocks in line 1 and continue counting the blocks in line 2 to discover the total, students can do mathematical calculations without having blocks present at all. They are able to create their own ideas to make stories or to draw scenes. The perfect gift for a student in this adolescent period is one that allows him to use ideas to build something. Can you see in your own mind the tree fort that you and your neighbors built in a nearby field? Consider the thinking, planning, and execution of this task. In order to have a successful outcome, the group members also had to develop and test their mental hypotheses, all the while communicating their ideas with one another. The systematic and logical approach to building the tree house requires the characteristics of the formal operational stage.

In the classroom, teachers ask students to think about a topic and use what they already know to predict what the reading passage will be about. They ask children to discuss what they have read and to draw conclusions that may not be directly stated in the passage. Students evaluate the information they have and need in order to participate in an activity and they learn where and how to seek additional information.

Piaget gave us a lot to think about and use as we build opportunities for students of all ages. Teachers who have a good grasp of developmental milestones, from birth through adolescence, have a treasure trove available for making learning fun, productive, and developmentally appropriate.

Check Your Understanding 3.1

Assess your understanding of concepts and behaviors central to cognitive development and the sensorimotor stages of cognitive development by completing this brief quiz.

Sociocultural Perspectives of Cognitive Development

Vygotsky's Theory

The issue stated at the beginning of this chapter has significant relevance in relation to Vygotsky's theory of cognitive development: *the relationship between cognition and language.* Hold that issue in mind as this section unfolds, and try to determine how Lev Vygotsky would answer it.

Like Piaget, Vygotsky believed that the child is an active agent in her quest for knowledge. Beyond this general agreement, however, emerges a striking difference in the views of the two men. Whereas Piaget believed that the child operates independently to construct knowledge through her actions on the environment, especially during the early stages of cognitive development, Vygotsky was convinced that the child's cognitive development is heavily influenced by her environment and by her culture from the very beginning of knowledge acquisition. In fact, Vygotsky believed that the developing child interacts with her environment in order to develop cognitive abilities that will allow her to adapt to her culture. In other words, during the course of intellectual development, there is a synergistic relationship between what the child brings to the cognitive table in terms of innate abilities and self-directed exploration and what her environment and culture bring to the table.

Vygotsky's own boyhood experiences related to learning shaped his views of cognitive development. As a youngster, he did not attend a formal school. The tutor who taught him at home believed that education involved more than simply filling an empty intellectual vessel. The tutor challenged the young Russian boy to be fully engaged in the process of learning, to answer and pose questions, to process answers, to think about how one piece of knowledge is integrated with established knowledge, to consider how one question leads to another. His was a truly interactive learning experience, and he came away from this personal experience believing that knowledge acquisition and intellectual development must necessarily proceed in this interactive manner.

Piaget and Vygotsky communicated with each other between 1924 and 1929, but communication was challenging due to Stalin's dictatorial rule. Despite the political climate of their era, these theorists shared ideas through their published works and each had an influence on the other's thinking about human development (Pass, 2007). For instance, Vygotsky modified his stages of development from three to four after studying Piaget, and Piaget recognized that social and historical contexts might impact a child's learning.

One might well ask why there is so much interest in Vygotsky's views about cognitive development today. After all, this man's views about cognition were published more than 70 years ago. According to Wertsch and Tulviste (1992), the present interest in Vygotsky's theory can be traced to his belief that the child is not an independently operating agent, that the child's cognitive development is the product of an interaction between the child's innate abilities and his social experiences. It is noteworthy that Vygotsky's view of intellectual development is generally consonant with the dominant view of language development today, the social interactionist view. The marriage between a sociocultural view of cognition and a social interactionist view of language is a natural and eminently logical phenomenon.

Even though some people might be tempted to park Vygotsky at the nurture end of the nature/nurture continuum, that would be an oversimplification of his views about development. Vygotsky begins, in fact, with a nature base. He believes that human children are born with fundamental cognitive and perceptual abilities, including capacities for memory and attending, abilities that human beings share with other animals. During the first two years of the human child's life, these abilities develop and mature according to a mostly biological calendar and as a result of the child's primitive contacts with his environment. The nature of cognitive development changes radically, however, as soon as the child can mentally represent the environmental phenomena he is experiencing. This mental representation includes, as a primary component, language.

At this point, armed with naturally developing cognitive and perceptual abilities and with emerging language skills, the child is able to engage in the social dialogues that are so inextricably connected to cultural activities. The groundwork is now laid for the component of Vygotsky's theory of cognitive development most closely associated with his name, *private speech*. When the young child begins to talk to herself (**private speech**), she crosses an important threshold in her cognitive development. From this point forward, and as a direct result of the power of language, the child's mental abilities will be shaped into the higher-order cognitive processes of an intelligence that clearly separates human beings from animals with lesser cognitive capacities. That is, the child uses language to direct her actions and to learn how to get things done (Wertsch & Tulviste, 1992).

Before we take a closer look at private speech and other critical elements of Vygotsky's theory, there is another basic difference between Piaget and Vygotsky that must be stressed. Piaget, as we have noted at a number of junctures in this chapter, believed that cognitive development proceeds in a predictable stage-by-stage manner. Vygotsky's view was that cognitive development does not proceed through exactly the same progressive sequence for all children. He argued that while each child experiences progressive changes in the way she thinks and behaves as a cognitive creature, the progression is continuous rather than stage-by-stage. More important, each child's cognitive development is shaped by the influences of the important adults and peers in the social environment and by the experiences unique to her culture.

Although Vygotsky and Piaget would agree that there are systematic changes in cognitive development, Vygotsky would argue that these systematic changes

vary widely across cultures because the nature of social interactions between children and the important people in their lives varies widely by culture. The tasks around which learning occurs differ from culture to culture. In some cultures, for example, girls are taught to perform domestic tasks at a young age. In other cultures, boys are taught how to hunt and fish. In our culture, children are free of these kinds of responsibilities and are encouraged to play and "have fun." It is not difficult to imagine significant differences in the kinds of interactions that will occur between adults and children in each of these cultural situations. Children who live in cultures that place a premium on written language will face different cognitive challenges and will experience different social and communicative interactions with their significant others than children who live in cultures that depend mostly or solely on spoken language.

Vygotsky's point is that cognitive development does not occur in isolation but is a function of a person's social and cultural environment. That there are cross-cultural differences in the nature of social/communicative exchanges between young children and adults has been demonstrated by research that lends support to Vygotsky's argument (Bakeman, Adamson, Konner, & Barr, 1990; Childs & Greenfield, 1982; Draper & Cashdan, 1988; Saxe, 1988). We will now turn our attention to some of the critical elements in Vygotsky's theory, beginning with private speech.

Private Speech

Anyone who has watched young children play has heard private speech. A preschool child who is trying to construct a building out of blocks might say to himself, "This piece is too big. It sticks out. I need a smaller one." A child with a fistful of crayons and a coloring book might mutter to herself, "What color should the house be? I think I'll make it purple. No, that's not right. Houses aren't purple. It should be white. Where's the white crayon?" Yet another child, trying to put plastic pieces of varying geometric shapes into a box with holes corresponding to these shapes, might be heard to say to himself, "This one is round, so it won't fit here, but it will fit here. Whoops, it didn't fit because it's too big. I need to find the small round one. There it is!"

What is all this self-talking about? The answer to that question depends on the expert to whom it is addressed. Piaget referred to this self-directed talk as *egocentric speech,* which he believed is nonsocial, relatively purposeless, and produced by the individual child for the individual child who cannot mentally represent the viewpoints of other people. Vygotsky (1986) believed that when children speak to themselves, they are guiding themselves through their actions. Especially early in their lives, children use self-directed private speechliterally to help themselves think through problems and tasks, to help themselves choose actions that are most appropriate to doing whatever it is they are trying to do. Private speech is a first step toward more elaborate cognitive skills. It helps the child learn how to pay attention, how to memorize and recall bits of information from memory, how to formulate and execute plans in solving problems, and, in a very real sense, how to think, ponder, or muse. As the child gets older, the nature of self-directed talking changes. In the beginning, the child talks out loud. As she gets older, she might whisper or mutter

under her breath. Eventually, her private speech will be truly private. It will be silent and internalized. In short, it will become exactly the kind of private speech you use every day to think through your problems, to choose plans of actions for solving your problems, and to reflect on the meaning of life.

The most telling evidence supporting Vygotsky's view about private speech shows that children are more likely to talk to themselves when they are engaged in difficult tasks, when they are struggling with tasks and making mistakes, or when they are unsure about what they should do next (Berk, 1992,). The research also confirms that Vygotsky was correct about the changes that occur to private speech as children mature. That is, it becomes less overt and more private until it becomes essentially speech in thought form (Berk & Landau, 1993; Frauenglass & Diaz, 1985). From a cognitive development point of view, Vygotsky's most crucial assertion is that private speech provides a foundation for higher-order cognitive functions. When the child engages in make-believe play, for example, private speech is a critical element of that activity. The coexistence of these two activities suggests that private speech helps the child place the control of action within the constraints of thought (Krafft & Berk, 1998). Research indicates that children who are uninhibited self-talkers when they are confronted with challenging tasks are more attentive, more fully engaged, and more likely to complete tasks successfully than children who are more reticent self-talkers (Behrend, Rosengren, & Perlmutter, 1992; Bivens & Berk, 1990). There is also evidence that preschool children who participate in elaborate sociodramatic play, an activity that depends heavily on private speech, make more rapid progress in learning to follow classroom rules than children who are less inclined to participate in this kind of activity (Elias & Berk, 2002).

Social Keys to Cognitive Development

Keep in mind that Vygotsky believed that the establishment of higher-order cognitive functions begins in children's social interactions with the important people in their environment, interactions that reflect the culture of which they are members. This means that, from Vygotsky's point of view, we cannot talk about cognitive development without taking these social interactions into account. Children learn how to do things, and they learn how to process their thoughts in ways that appropriately reflect the culture in which they live, by interacting with adults who already know how things should be done and how to think in ways that are culturally acceptable. The child might be able to handle some tasks with which he is confronted without any direct intervention or assistance. That is, he will figure some things out, just as Piaget suggested, by independent discovery. There are many other tasks, however, that the child cannot manage on his own. He needs help from people who have greater knowledge, experience, and skill than he possesses. These tasks fall into what is called the **zone of proximal development** (ZPD). Within this zone are those tasks with which the child needs help, and the help typically comes in the form of language. As a child and an adult work together to learn a skill or

solve a problem, they talk to each other. The child retains language from these exchanges that he incorporates into his private speech. At some later time, he will use this private speech, now enhanced by the language he has garnered from these dialogues, to solve problems on his own.

 Video Reflection 3.2: The Zone of Proximal Development

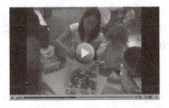

Watch the video to observe a teacher using the zone of proximal development to guide students, then answer the question.

If he had lived longer and continued to revise and elaborate his theory, Vygotsky would have probably tried to identify the features of adult/child dialogues that would most effectively facilitate the development of the child's cognitive abilities. In the absence of direction from Vygotsky himself on this subject, researchers have identified at least two attributes of these dialogues they believe are crucial in transferring the adult's cognitive competence to the child's cognitive development. The first of these attributes is **intersubjectivity**. An interaction is characterized by intersubjectivity when people work together on a common task with different levels of understanding about how the task can or should be accomplished,and manage to merge what they know into a shared understanding as the task is completed. Each partner accommodates the viewpoint and competence of the other partner. In an interaction shared by an adult and a child, the adult will convey what she knows to the child in a manner that fits what the child already knows and that does not exceed the child's ability to understand. You will recognize that this is exactly what occurs in any good teaching/learning situation even when the teacher and learner are both adults. That is, the teacher conveys her knowledge to the student by drawing on what the student already knows, by taking into account the student's abilities to understand, and by challenging the student to expand his own knowledge. In an interaction characterized by intersubjectivity, therefore, the child is challenged by the adult's dialogue and demonstrations to extend his understanding so that he develops a more mature, adult-like strategy for completing the targeted task (Rogoff, 1990).

The second attribute that characterizes facilitating dialogues is **scaffolding**(Bruner, 1983; Wood, 1989). To understand this feature of dialogues, we should first consider the literal meaning of the word *scaffold* and consider how scaffolds are used in real life. These structures are made of steel pipes that have platforms for moving along walkways at various heights. They support the workers as they perform the tasks and then are taken down when no longer needed.

How does scaffolding relate to cognitive development and to the dialogues and interactions that facilitate cognitive development? Just as a real-life scaffold is adjusted to the height necessary for the completion of a task such as washing windows, adults can provide scaffolds for the child when she is trying to reach new heights of cognitive competence. If the child has little idea about how to accomplish a targeted task, adults will set the scaffold low in the sense that they provide direct instruction. At this level, adults might try to segment the task into smaller tasks, building on what the child does know and can do, and then helping her master the next level, and then the next, until she can complete the whole task. When we teach children to write, for example, we do not expect them to move from no writing skill to adult mastery in one step. We begin by asking the children to draw vertical lines, horizontal lines, and circles, skills they already have or that they can easily master. We scaffold the skills upward from the easiest and most basic drawing skills to increasingly elaborate writing skills until the children are actually producing written letters. As a child's cognitive competence increases, her need for direct support decreases. The adult who is skilled at using scaffolds will gradually withdraw cognitive supports as the child gradually demonstrates less need for them, but will be prepared to introduce the supports again if the child's independent efforts are producing more frustration and failure than success. The general rule in effective scaffolding, therefore, is to adjust support so that it meets the changing cognitive needs of the child.

Does effective scaffolding make a difference? There is research evidence indicating that it does. In studies focusing on the possible benefits of this strategy, some mothers used scaffolding more effectively than others in the process of teaching their children how to solve a particularly difficult puzzle. The children of the more effective scaffolders used more private speech and were more successful in independently solving a similar puzzle than the children of mothers who were less skillful in the use of scaffolding (Behrend, Rosengren, & Perlmutter, 1992; Berk & Spuhl, 1995.)

During his tragically brief life, Vygotsky gave us much to think about relative to cognition, cognitive development, and the synergistic relationship between cognition and language (see Figure 3.1). Researchers continue to test the principles and concepts of his theory, and, so far at least, his views that cognitive development occurs within the larger context of social and cultural experiences, and that language directs cognition as much as cognition directs language, are holding up well to empirical scrutiny.

Second Learning Outcome: dynamic systems theory

As we continue to explore ways that children develop knowledge and thinking abilities, researchers and practitioners recognize the interactions that occur between learners and their environment. Vygotsky's social-cultural perspective is one view. Consider a young child just beginning to talk in single words. What is the driving force behind this amazing accomplishment? The dynamic systems theory provides us with a look into the complexity of each learning situation.

Figure 3.1   Key Features of Vygotsky's Theory

- Children are active participants in their quest for knowledge.
- Cognitive development is heavily influenced by the environment and culture.
- Language is a key player in cognitive development.
- Children use private speech to guide themselves through their actions.
- Children are born with basic cognitive and perceptual abilities.
- Children's cognitive abilities during the first two years of life develop and mature according to a biological calendar.
- At about two years, cognition and language influence each other.
- Children's ability to represent their environment mentally, including their use of language, facilitates cognitive development.
- Cognitive development does not proceed through exactly the same sequence for all children.

Let's look at Ricardo, a 12-month-old child who is beginning to say his first words. Ricardo is an active and curious child, who has three older siblings: 10-year-old Angela, 7-year-old Juan, and 3-year-old Maria. They are delighted with their young brother, and the household is filled with verbal chatter and play. The parents are bilingual in Spanish and English, and the children speak both Spanish and English in the home and at school. Thus, Ricardo is hearing and learning both language forms. As we can imagine, Ricardo's learning is influenced by the totality of his experiences and his own very typical physical and cognitive growth. His parents, three siblings, two languages, and interactions throughout each day create unique opportunities for his specific growth in knowledge and his organization and use of his knowledge for future learning.

Researchers consider the uniqueness of each child and his environment as being particularly important in development of cognition. Samuelson and Horst (2008) emphasize that the real-time interactions of all the components of the child and his environment have an additive effect where context-specific interactions in the past and present set up the conditions for subsequent interactions. In other words, what Ricardo has learned during the past 12 months within his family environment adds up to who he is, what he knows, and how he relates to his family members and they to him. He is truly unique and this foundation will be critical for future development. According to the dynamic systems theory, stable patterns emerge over time, but variability also occurs as changes occur in the abilities and experiences of the child. So, the child continues to use foundational abilities, but learning also continues as the child's future unfolds.

What evidence do we have that a dynamic systems theory explains cognitive growth? One example involving concept development that illustrates this perspective is known as the **shape bias**.

The rate at which youngsters acquire names of things has intrigued theorists and researchers in developmental psychology for several decades. We know that children do not and probably cannot learn each new word without being able to relate it to their previous knowledge and the contexts in which learning occurs; thus, perception and cognition are important ingredients in learning. Numerous studies have verified that young children generalize novel names to new instances that match in shape. This ability to generalize based on shape helps children learn new words (Samuelson & Bloom, 2008). Generalization is very important to learning in that it allows us to apply what we know to new information, thus increasing our ability to learn rapidly.

Dynamic systems theory may help to explain this rapid early growth as an ability to perceive regularities in language forms and the properties of objects and to categorize and organize these properties. Thus, children are able to use the information patterns, such as shape, in new word learning situations as they encounter the words within the contexts of their individual histories with language, culture, and experiences (Samuelson and Horst, 2008).

The shape bias has been observed in children as young as 15 months old following 9 weeks of training (Smith, Jones, Landau, Gershkoff-Stowe, & Samuelson, 2002), and 2- and 3-year-old children appear to use shape consistently as a feature to attend to word learning (Booth, Waxman, & Huang, 2005; Diesendruck & Bloom, 2003). Researchers will likely debate the actual mechanisms and processes that underlie the shape bias. What is important for us is the realization and understanding that multiple aspects of cognition are operating to influence learning in children. We must take advantage of our students' perceptual abilities and their ability to generalize as we design appropriate learning experiences that help them build upon their current foundations.

We have considered three theories regarding cognition and the relationship of cognition to language. It should be evident that we still have much to learn about human thought and language in developing children, but we should also have an appreciation for the many perspectives that provide us with plausible examples and explanations as to what is likely taking place within the first two years of development and beyond.

Check Your Understanding 3.2

Assess your understanding of Vygotsky's theory of cognitive development by completing this brief quiz.

The Perceptual Groundwork for Communication

Before we proceed to a detailed description of language development in the next three chapters, we must address more fully the perceptual preparation for communication, a topic briefly introduced when we discussed the principle of distancing earlier in this chapter. Perception, you may remember, refers to the processes by which a person selects, organizes, integrates, and interprets the sensory stimuli he receives. Because children must somehow make sense of the sensory information they receive related to communication in general and speech specifically before they can create their own communicative output, we should know something about what they receive and what catches their attention during the preparation period. What follows, then, is a brief summary of what we believe are children's earliest perceptual abilities as they pertain to communication.

The Relationship Between Perception and Cognition

It should be fairly obvious that perception cannot be completely separated from cognition. To understand, think, solve problems, and engage in all other activities associated with cognition, we must be able to sort through the stimuli our senses are receiving, recognize important stimuli, ignore unimportant ones, and then categorize, integrate, and interpret the stimuli we have selected. The further into perception we proceed, the closer to cognition we get, until the line between them becomes effectively blurred to the point of virtual elimination.

We know that children perceive sensory information and store and use those characteristics, such as shape, when responding to new experiences. When auditory information is heard, the loudness and pitch of the sounds may be perceptually salient. If visual information is present, children may perceive size, shape, and color. Children recognize stimuli by their sensory characteristics, but they come to understand what they are hearing and seeing and compare it to other information around them (Stern, 1977). A doorbell is differentiated from a ringing phone based on sound, but also expectations about what is to follow. Thus perception and cognition become intertwined as they develop together.

Visual and Tactile Perception

You might wonder what visual and tactile perception has to do with language and especially with speech. Actually, what children see and feel can be very important in the language acquisition process. Sachs (1989) contends that visual and tactile stimuli, "play a great role in establishing the bond between adult and child" (p. 38). This in no way minimizes the importance of auditory stimulation, but it does suggest that what the child sees and feels helps to direct and fix her attention. Presumably, once the speaker has gained the child's attention by whatever visual or tactile stimuli are required, the child will gain more from the auditory stimuli produced by the speaker. Even though we have no proof that this connection of sensory modalities is necessary for speech development, it is probably more than coincidental that infants are interested in the kinds of visual stimuli that are characteristic of early child/adult interactions.

Vision is the first sensory system children control (Tiegerman, 1989). Within hours after birth, the infant can follow movement visually (Greenman, 1963) and is able to focus on a target 7.5 inches removed, the distance at which vision achieves its optimal focus (Owens, 2005). This is potentially significant because when the child is being fed, his mother's eyes are almost exactly eight inches away, and his mother watches him almost constantly during feeding (Stern, 1977), while he returns the visual favor. It is tempting to conclude, as some observers have, that the child is genetically preprogrammed for this visual coupling, which, it is further assumed, leads to bonding between the child and mother.

By the time the child is three months old, she can control eye movements sufficiently to determine the visual information she chooses to receive. She looks at things and people she finds interesting, and she turns away when she is no longer interested. The infant prefers objects of contrasting colors, and she likes things that move (Haith, 1976). She is attracted to objects with designs of varying angles and curves, and visually complex objects that reflect light variably (Fantz, 1964; Haaf & Bell, 1967). What makes this fascinating is that the infant shows strong interest in the human face, an object that meets all these criteria for preference and interest. The face can consist of many colors when you include all the parts: hair, eyes, eyebrows, lashes, lips, and cheeks. The face is capable of almost infinite movement and has many angles and curves that reflect and shade light. Again, it is tempting to conclude that the child is born with visual interests that perfectly match the facial characteristics of her primary object of attention and affection, the caregiver.

Researchers and theorists have paid much attention to children's interest in the human face in general, to a caregiver's face in particular, and to the eye contact or gaze between child and caregiver. There has been much speculation about what **joint attention** might suggest about bonding in the child/caregiver relationship. Certainly no one questions the newborn's preoccupation with looking at his caregiver's face. So fixed is he on looking at the caregiver's face in the first few weeks of his life that it is difficult to direct his visual attention anywhere else. By the time he is just two weeks old, he may be able to distinguish, on the basis of face and voice, his caregiver from other people (Bower, 1977,). When he is three weeks old, he will respond to his caregiver's face and other human faces by smiling (Trevarthen, 1979) and at three months, the infant and his caregiver exchange gazes in a manner that suggests adult-like conversational turn taking (Jaffe, Stern, & Perry, 1973). At the very least, this is intriguing stuff. At most, contingent on more research that would allow for more confident conclusions, it might suggest that the child is genetically attuned to certain visual stimuli that are important in capturing his attention and in helping to establish a communicative relationship with his caregiver, a relationship many social interactionist theorists believe is important, if not vital, to normal communication development. The infant who does not gaze at his mother's or father's face, or who gazes but does not react to changes in expressions that accompany emotions, clearly is at a disadvantage in using this important perceptual avenue to establish and maintain the social bond with his parents. Consider also the impact that little to no visual stimuli have on the infant who is blind.

Children with autism have communication and interaction impairments. Research has shown that as infants, they frequently show disturbances of visual attention and gaze patterning. Current research at the University of Denver is focused on creating computer models of eye gaze patterns to use as an assessment tool for identifying children with autism at six months of age. Early identification of autism is highly desirable so that intervention can begin during this important developmental period (Alie, Mohoor, Mattson, Anderson, & Messigner, 2011).

Other researchers are putting their efforts into discovering the nature of eye gaze differences between children with autism, typically developing children, and those with other developmental delays. The findings from a study of 20-month-old infants showed that children with autism spent less time looking at people and more time looking at objects. They also shifted attention from one object to another more frequently than their peers. These differences in spontaneous eye shifts with social stimuli (people) and nonsocial stimuli (objects) may help to explain the abnormal pattern in social orientation that is commonly seen in children with autism (Swettenham et al., 1998).

Recall our discussion of mirror neurons in Chapter 2. As we continue to find out more information regarding eye gaze pattern differences and the neural network's response to affective information (emotions on faces), we will be able to assist families and their babies in early detection and intervention. It is an exciting time in determining the links between perception and learning.

As children mature, they continue to use their visual and tactile perceptions to gain information about objects. But it is not known precisely how children make discoveries about the properties of objects, especially when they have not fully developed reflective understanding about how access to information can assist in knowledge gains. Robinson, Haigh, and Pendle (2008) reviewed literature across 20 years that shows that young children below age 7 or 8 do not realize that input can be ambiguous; that several interpretations of information are possible; and that different people can make different interpretations. For instance, young children not only make inaccurate assumptions about partially hidden objects, but also have incomplete knowledge of how different modalities (seeing and feeling) are used to gain information, and they are poor at reporting the source of knowledge gained. It isn't until children reach seven or eight years of age that they have the reflective understanding to be able to describe how they know which are important.

We know that infants and toddlers explore objects as they see, touch, and mouth them. Parents and early childhood caregivers provide lots of opportunities for exploration, as this input is food for the brain. Preschool teachers take full advantage of children's natural curiosity and their need for concrete manipulation of objects too, and this experiential focus does not wane until children are able to think and solve problems in the mind.

Auditory Perception

Just as children seem to have a special interest in the visual characteristics of the human face, they seem to be especially attracted to sound, especially the human voice and speech. One reasonable suggestion of the localization of sound in young infants is turning the head, a behavior studied by Muir and Field (1979). Using head turning as a criterion for localizing sound, they found that infants ranging in age from two to seven days turned in the direction of a rattling noise about three-fourths of the time. This consistency allows us to conclude that newborns can determine at least the general direction of sound sources.

From the time the child is born, perhaps even prior to birth, he can make many kinds of auditory discriminations. That is, his brain responds when one sound is not the same as the previous one. Some newborn children, for example, can discriminate between a pure tone at 400 Hz and another at 1,000 Hz (Bridger, 1961), and there is evidence that they seem to make their best discriminations among frequencies characteristic of human speech (Eisenberg, 1976).

Newborns can make gross discriminations about the loudness levels of sounds. When they listen to white noise (a mixture of a wide range of frequencies) that is varied in loudness, there are noticeable changes in heart rate and in the startle reflex (Bench, 1969). Similar changes in behavior occur when children hear pure tones varied by loudness (Bartoshuk, 1964).

Although it is important to remember that we are dealing with only the broadest judgments of differences, some evidence suggests that infants respond differentially to sounds of varying durations (Clifton, Graham, & Hatton, 1968; Ling, 1972). In reference to the Ling study, Reich (1986) cautions that it, "does not demonstrate that the infant can detect these differences, only that it reacts more to signals of longer duration" (p. 15). At the least, this research indicates that infants are aware of when sounds begin and end and how long they are sustained, and it is probable that infants are able to make some discriminations concerning durations.

An Early Interest in the Human Voice and Speech

One of the most exciting general findings of the research related to the early perceptual abilities of children is that infants show a greater interest in human speech than in other noises (Eisenberg, 1976; Jensen, Williams, & Bzoch, 1975). There is evidence that a child may prefer the acoustic characteristics of a speech passage his mother recited while she was pregnant over the acoustic characteristics of something she did not read (DeCasper & Spence, 1986), and there is evidence that a child as young as three days recognizes his mother's voice and discriminates it from the voices of other mothers (DeCasper & Fifer, 1980). All of this can be interpreted to mean that, just as children are born with basic biological abilities to produce speech and language, they are born with biological perceptual abilities to receive and interpret speech and language. Whether or not a conclusion as sweeping as this is warranted, we can conclude that a newborn infant is able to distinguish between speech and non-speech sounds, that he seems to prefer speech, that he recognizes his mother's voice very early, and that he seems to be aware of differences between sounds to which he was exposed while in the uterus and sounds to which he was not exposed. These are significant perceptual abilities.

As impressive as the infant's general speech discrimination is, it is perhaps even more impressive that as early as one month, a child can discriminate among speech sounds. One of the methods used to assess this ability in infants is known as *nonnutritive sucking* or *high-amplitude sucking* and was developed at Brown University (Eimas, Siqueland, Jusczyk, & Vigorito, 1971). In this procedure, the infant sucks on a specially designed pacifier connected to a sound generator. When she sucks on the pacifier with enough vigor, she hears a predetermined sound. Because the only thing that changes in this exercise is the sound produced by the sucking, it is reasonable to assume that if the infant does not recognize the difference between the first sound and the second, there will be no change in the rate of sucking, but this is not what happens. When Eimas et al. (1971) presented "ba," the one-month-old infant sucked vigorously and quickly, but after a few minutes lost interest and decreased the rate of sucking. When a new sound, "pa," was introduced, the infant increased the rate of sucking. A number of studies reviewed by Aslin, Pisoni, and Jusczyk (1983) have shown the same reaction with a variety of speech sounds.

Because this ability is demonstrated at such a young age, it appears to be an innate ability rather than environmental. In an attempt to answer this particular nature/nurture question, Trehub (1976) tested the ability of Canadian infants and English-speaking adults to discriminate between two Czech sounds. Although the infants discriminated between the Czech sounds as well as between English sounds such as *p* and *b,* the adults had great difficulty with the Czech sounds. Trehub concluded that children are born with the ability to discriminate among sounds found in all languages. As speakers become more immersed in their own languages, they lose some of this discriminative ability.

Taking the question to the next logical level, Werker and Tees (1984) tried to determine how quickly infants lose this open-ended ability to discriminate speech sounds. They presented non-English sounds to English-speaking children ranging in age from 6 to 12 months. Infants between six and eight months had little difficulty making the necessary discriminations. Those between 8 and 10 months had more difficulty, and those between 10 and 12 months had the most difficulty. It appears, then, that the ability to discriminate a wide range of sounds representing many languages declines early in the child's life. Werker and Tees suggest that it is probably not coincidental that children's discrimination abilities become narrow as they are acquiring their own sound system and language. Environment does play a role in shaping discrimination abilities, therefore, but rather than expanding these abilities, children's environmental experiences make their discriminations more selective, more consistent with the speech sounds native to their language.

During the toddler years, remarkable advances occur in vocabulary knowledge. An eight-month-old child will gain 200 times her number of comprehended words at 16 months and another 10 times her number of words at 24 months. The period between 16 and 19 months is especially critical for word learning. A child needs only to be exposed to a new word once for learning to occur. It appears that speech perception in toddlers requires the participation of several neural systems in addition to the language systems within the temporal and parietal lobes (Redclay, Haist, & Courchesne, 2008). When the initial language spurt is over, these other systems may no longer be necessary to the same degree during passive listening, as children have a base of semantic knowledge with which to process familiar words and to incorporate newly learned words.

We must also consider the relationship between speech perception and visual perception in developing children because speech perception is not just an auditory phenomenon. In fact, children and adults use both auditory and visual information to determine speech sounds. You probably experience better understanding of someone else when you are able to see his face during speaking. The developmental influence of visual cues (lip and facial movements) helps listeners to compensate for degraded acoustic information (poor quality of information due to background noise, for example) or the tendency for listeners to fail to perceive a mismatch between what is seen and what is heard, known as the *McGurk effect* (McGurk & McDonald, 1976). For example, if a syllable is spoken /ba-ba/ over the lip movements of /ga-ga/, the perception of it will be /da-da/. This means that there is an integration of the auditory and visual information. There is also a developmental increase in how visual information affects the ability to perceive speech in the auditory and visual modes. Children ages three to five years and seven to eight years have less visual influence on their perception than do adults. One explanation for the increase in the use of visual information over time is that as children make advances in their speech articulation, they develop a better internal representation of visible speech. In other words, they know what speech sounds like and also what it looks like. Thus, as children make fewer speech production errors, they are also better at using visual cues to determine speech sounds spoken by others.

It may be tempting to assume that all humans use auditory and visual information regarding speech in the same way. We have evidence, however, that language experience impacts auditory-visual speech perception. Sekiyama and Burnham (2008) compared adults from Japanese and Australian English language backgrounds. In the first experiment the syllables *ba, da*, and *ga* were presented under three highly controlled conditions: auditory-only, visual-only, and audiovisual. English speakers relied on the visual influence more than did Japanese speakers. Both groups showed greater visual influence for nonnative stimuli, and both groups performed similarly in the auditory-only condition, but English speakers performed better in speech-reading (visual cues) on nonnative as opposed to native stimuli than did Japanese speakers. Thus, there was a weaker visual influence on auditory-visual speech perception in Japanese-speaking adults than in English-speaking adults. The researchers also timed the responses of their participants. The comparison of reaction times across groups revealed that Japanese speakers were faster in the auditory-only condition. The English speakers were faster in the visual-only trials. The authors speculate that the differences between Japanese and English response frequency data may be the result of a different time course in their auditory, visual, and auditory-visual speech processing. Japanese speakers may use auditory information first because it is faster for them, whereas English speakers may use visual information first because it is faster for them.

The second experiment involved three age groups of children (6, 8, and 11 years old) who were Japanese speakers and English speakers. The same

experiment described above revealed that six-year-olds showed relatively weak visual influence; however, this influence increased for English but not Japanese speakers at eight years of age and older. The growth was related to increased speed in auditory and visual processing for English speakers. Japanese speakers showed stronger auditory processing at six years compared to English speakers, and this auditory superiority increased across time.

What accounts for such differences? The results of these two studies show that language experience impacts auditory-visual speech perception. English speakers appear to need the integration of visual and auditory input because English has a more complex arrangement of consonants and vowels than Japanese. Specifically, English has more varied and complex syllable structures, more vowels, more consonant contrasts, syllable-initial consonant clusters, and distinct visual consonant contrasts. Note these complex arrangements of consonants (C) and vowels (V) in the following examples of one-syllable words:

CCVC – star CCVCC – start CCCV – stray CCCVC – stream CCCVCC– strand

This complexity may result in English speakers seeking extra sources of information to assist in speech perception. Japanese speakers, on the other hand, may not need to integrate visual information to the same extent because their phonological environment does not demand it.

Regardless of the native language of students, educators know that a multi-sensory environment is not only interesting to young learners, but also helpful in establishing the integration of information across modalities: seeing, hearing, touching, and moving. Teachers help students who have learning challenges derive benefit from the extra cues that come with a multisensory approach.

Executive Functions

Have you ever wondered about what is going on when you drive your car? Once we know how, driving a car is a pretty effortless task. We get into it, put the key in the ignition, and steer our way out of the parking place and down the road to our destination. Looking, steering, braking, and putting varying degrees of pressure on the gas pedal are about all that we need to do. We can even think about other things, listen to the radio or iPad, talk to someone else (preferably not on a cell phone and never texting) while driving to our destination. We even can get directions from our GPS so that planning our journey has become a thing of the past, or at least requires minimal effort. But what makes all this possible? What is under the hood and in the dashboard that frees us from so much of what is happening mechanically and electrically in our car? We'll leave it to automotive experts to explain the workings of the car. It should be obvious, though, that cars are equipped with many systems which function in spite of anything we do. We trust that everything is working on the inside so that when we act, the car does what it is designed to do. Now let's consider the control centers of our brains as being akin to the car.

Executive functions refers to a set of control processes in the human brain that allow us to maintain attention, inhibit irrelevant associations, and use

working memory. These processes develop slowly during maturation (Cutting & Denckla, 2003), and they correspond to functions involved in motor control, cognitive control, and social-emotional control. For instance, you might choose to dive off the diving board but change your mind at the last moment and jump instead. Your impulse may be to respond to something negative that someone says, but you restrain yourself from a temping retort in favor of saying nothing. Executive functions keep us on task, allow us to monitor and regulate our behavior, and definitely keep us out of trouble.

Interrelationships between executive functions, language, and academic skills are complex and not well understood, but associations have been made between executive functions and social competence, moral conduct, school readiness, and theory of mind. We will explore attention and memory in the following sections as they relate to learning language, as well as show that bilingual experience and theory of mind are related to executive functioning.

Attention and Memory

Attention and memory are highly interactive processes for learning; thus, one cannot be discussed fully without the other. We might presume that in order to learn something, a child needs to be able to focus his attention on it and then store the relevant details while inhibiting other stimuli not directly related to the learning at hand. Thus, attention and memory co-occur in any learning situation. Given this relationship, we provide some information about these processes in order to illustrate how they contribute to learning.

Controlled attention, defined by Swanson and Saez (2003), includes the capacity to maintain and hold relevant information, especially when there are internal or external distractions or interferences in the environment. Imagine yourself in a crowded airport waiting for your flight. You may become deeply involved in your science fiction novel, despite crying babies, announcements of other flights, people talking to each other and on cell phones, and the cacophony of sounds of people on the move. Wolf and Bell (2007) add that **working memory** allows for the voluntary, focused, and exclusive processing and maintenance of task-relevant information. Thus, you should be able to read and comprehend the information on one page in your novel and use it to understand subsequent paragraphs. Working memory allows us to encode, process, and retrieve information to which we have been exposed, and it is related to performance across academic and cognitive areas.

A well-supported theory of working memory views it as consisting of an executive control system that interacts with, coordinates, controls, and regulates two storage systems. The phonological loop temporarily stores verbal information that individuals use during the process of subvocal articulation. This storage area allows you to rehearse a message in your mind before you store it or speak it. The other storage system is a visual-spatial sketch pad that assists individuals in generating and manipulating mental images (Baddeley, 1986, 1996; Baddeley & Logie, 1999; Swanson & Saez, 2003). You might use this storage space to picture yourself expertly skiing, dancing, or delivering the speech you have prepared for your class assignment.

Working memory develops as children mature, along with all aspects of cognitive control during the early childhood years. Research (Wolf & Bell, 2007) indicates that young children between the ages of three-and-a-half and seven years develop these self-regulatory skills, with working memory positively associated with verbal fluency for complex spoken language in three- and four-year-old children, and phonological short-term memory associated with receptive vocabulary knowledge in four-year-olds. In other words, preschoolers and students in the early grades gain in their working memory capacity and they gain in the length and complexity of their sentences as well as their knowledge of words. Further, as children use their knowledge to practice and learn, phonological abilities and vocabulary have a reciprocal influence, whereby increases in both occur. Listening, speaking, and remembering are thus highly important skills for teachers to cultivate.

As you can imagine, difficulties in controlled attention and working memory result in poor performance when attention must be divided. Children who have attention and memory problems demonstrate weak monitoring of information and difficulty in suppressing irrelevant information. They also show weak storage and processing when verbal and visual-spatial tasks occur together. Let's consider a student in first grade with these challenges.

> Peter tries to pay attention to Mrs. Larson, but he is distracted. Sounds from the hallway, movements of other students in the classroom, and his desire to get outside for recess make it a struggle for him to listen to his teacher's lesson about short and long vowels. Peter cannot recall the vowel that the teacher talked about yesterday, so he does not have a reference point as to how the "vowel of the day" compares.

It is difficult to imagine learning anything without the ability to control attention and use working memory to process, store, and retrieve information. To extend our airport example, consider how frustrating and futile it would be to read the novel when you could nottune out other people or when you couldn'trecall what you'djust read even if you couldtune them out.

Teachers realize that attention and memory develop gradually from early childhood through middle school, so they plan their classrooms and daily lessons to correspond to these developmental trends. Students in the early grades benefit from short lessons and short periods of focused work. They need external support to establish and maintain attention. The kindergarten teacher who uses the cue "fold and focus" is instructing her students to sit quietly with hands folded and eyes on her. Teachers also help students to remember through the use of visual boards and direct teaching of memory devices, such as mnemonics. Recall how you learned the spelling rules for the words *believe* and *receive:i* before *e* except after *c*, or when sounding like *a* as in *neighbor* and *weigh*.

Executive Functioning and Bilingual Acquisition

As reported by Wolf and Bell (2007), language is highly associated with attention and working memory. But what influence does knowing two languages have on executive functioning? Do children who are bilingual have advantages

in executive functioning compared to monolingual children? Carlson and Meltzoff (2008) set out to discover the relationship between bilingual experience and executive functioning in young children. They relied heavily on Bialystok's comprehensive literature review (2001) to establish that inhibitory control over attentional resources develops more rapidly in children who are bilingual; thus, these children are more advanced in their ability to focus attention in the presence of competing information. This finding offers strong support for the cognitive benefit of being bilingual.

You may believe that bilingual individuals use their native language when interacting with one group of people, such as family members, and then switch to their second language when in the presence of another group, such as schoolmates. Guttentag, Haith, Goodman, and Hauch (1984) dispelled the notion that bilingual individuals switch from one language to the other specific to the communication situations they encounter. They found that both languages remain active during language processing, thus requiring the language user to hold the relevant language in mind while inhibiting the nonrelevant language. Daily practice with inhibitory control might thus be more developed in bilingual children. This assumption was put to the test in the Carlson and Meltzoff study of three groups of kindergarten children: monolinguals (English), bilinguals (Spanish-English), and children in an immersive language program. Only the native bilingual children showed an advantage on tasks requiring inhibitory control as compared to the other groups. The groups did not differ on tasks that require suppression of motor responses or delayed gratification that requires little use of working memory. This finding supports Bialystok's theory (2001) regarding the dual direction of influences between language and executive functioning. Specifically, exposure to more than one language enhances cognitive flexibility, allowing children to develop cognitive operations, such as inhibition and working memory, in order to be adept at language switching. The ability to make these switches is evidence of the interaction between the acquisition of cognitive functions and linguistic development. Although children who are bilingual (Spanish-English) in the United States often show less verbal ability than monolingual children, their stronger cognitive operations may provide them with the necessary capabilities for language and academic learning. Again, this is a strong endorsement for bilingual education. Later in this book we will explore the processes, benefits, and challenges of acquiring two or more languages and we will hear from an expert regarding bilingual education.

Executive Functioning and Theory of Mind

Remember in Chapter 1 our discussion about how two brains communicate? Not only do we use our eyes and ears to receive information, and speech structures to transmit messages, but we also develop the ability to know what others know and need to know and we can reflect on our own thoughts in order to understand ourselves and the other people we talk to in daily interactions. The understanding of our mentalworld—that place where beliefs, desires, emotions, thoughts, perceptions, and intentionsreside—is what we call the

theory of mind. It is probably no surprise that the development of executive functions and language have been associated with advances in theory of mind. It is also no surprise that many theories have been discussed as to how mental processes develop. Research during the past 30 years has uncovered much about how children gain knowledge. Table 3.7 is a summary of the major findings regarding their cognitive attainments.

There is some evidence that bilingual speakers have advanced theory of mind in comparison to monolingual preschoolers (Goetz, 2003). Miller (2006) tracks some precursors of theory of mind as it relates to communication

Table 3.7   Development of Theory of Mind

Age Ranges	Mental Attainments
Infancy	Respond differently to human faces, voices, and movements than to objects Seek attention from others See people as agents of action Learn that people have intentions Use pointing and vocalizing to change or direct the attention of others Follow another person's gaze Recognize that a word refers to an object being looked at by another person Recognize that a person can display emotion about an object
18 Months to 2 Years	Know that people's actions are intentional and goal-directed Reason that other people have different desires from one's own Comfort others in distress Use mental state terms, such as *want* and *see*
3 to 5 Years	Know that others see objects only when looking in that direction and when vision is not blocked Infer that a person sees something one does not and vice versa Recognize that a thing has different appearances based on each person's view of it Appreciate that attention is selective Grasp simple causal relations among desires, emotions, and actions Attribute inner feelings to people who display emotions Recognize that thinking can be about real or imaginary things Realize that others will have different ideas about objects and gradually succeed on false belief tasks
Post 5 Years	Understand that people interpret information based on previous experiences and biases Realize that information is necessary in order to make adequate decisions and judgments Recognize that thinking is an ongoing mental activity

Source: Based on Flavell (2004).

development. She includes joint attention, appreciation of intentionality, recognition that people have different perspectives, use of mental state words, and pretend play in her discussion of the first five years of development. Even as early as nine months of age, infants begin to establish that adults focus their attention on specific aspects of objects or events. Between the ages of one and five years, several areas of understanding emerge that allow children to engage effectively in conversations and play. Language development is interwoven with the development of theory of mind. We are able to talk about internal states such as thinking, knowing, and feeling. Language is the way these ideas are represented and shared with others. Pronounced deficits in theory of mind and communication are evident in children who have autism and other developmental disabilities. Educators must use much more demonstration, explanation, and experiential learning activities with these children than they use with typically developing children to assist them with the development of these abilities.

Check Your Understanding 3.3

Assess your understanding of the relationship between cognition and perception by completing this brief quiz.

Cognition, Language, and Literacy Development

As we established earlier, cognition, language, and literacy are closely related, and there are connections between them and language development. What impact does bilingual learning have on cognition and literacy?

Research suggests that bilingualism does not adversely affect cognitive development but, in fact, strengthens it. We've established that bilingual children perform better than monolingual children on a number of cognitive tasks, including selective attention, forming concepts, and reasoning analytically. In addition, children who speak two or more languages are more cognitively agile or flexible than children who speak just one language (Bialystok, 1999; Hakuta, Ferdman, & Diaz, 1989).

It is also noteworthy, especially to people who are specifically interested in the language aspects of cognition, that bilingual children are superior to monolingual children in their metalinguistic skills, that is, in their ability to use language to think about, analyze, and describe language (Bialystok, 2001; Ricciardelli, 1992). Bilingual children are more aware of the arbitrariness of words as symbols than monolingual children. They are more adept at identifying grammatical and semantic errors, and they have greater phonological awareness and metalinguistic development (Herdina & Jessner, 2002; Jessner, 2008).

Questions remain about exactly why and under what conditions bilingualism enhances cognitive function, and we do not know precisely how, or even if, the brain is organized differently when a person is fluent in two languages, but research over the past several decades has effectively dispelled the notion that the effects of bilingualism on cognition and on cognitive development are deleterious.

Cognition and a Second Language: Two Views

Even among those who accept the obvious fact that a child can acquire two languages simultaneously without a significant or long-term negative impact on cognitive function, there is disagreement about what might happen in the earliest phases of development if the child is exposed to two or more languages. According to the **limited capacity hypothesis** (Genesee, Paradis, & Crago, 2004), the child has the innate ability to acquire one language completely, but she does not have the ability to acquire two or more languages simultaneously without suffering some reduction in competence in one or both languages.

An opposing, and decidedly more positive, view is that the child does, in fact, have the cognitive capacity to acquire two languages at the same time with no ill effects. Genesee and his colleagues (2004) use a computer analogy to explain this view. The child's brain is like the hardware in a computer that gives the computer a tremendous capacity for processing information. Computer software is added to the computer to allow for complex and sophisticated multitasking. Inserting a second language into the child's brain is like adding more software. If the hardware is sophisticated enough and powerful enough, we can add many elements of software, and the computer continues to function smoothly and flawlessly. Assuming the child's brain has the vast capacity for processing information that we believe it does, adding a second language will not slow down or diminish the effectiveness of cognitive or linguistic processing.

All experts in bilingualism would agree, as we have already established in this chapter, that not all children who speak two languages are the same. They acquire their languages under different circumstances, in different social and language environments, with different expectations from their caregivers, some with formal educational assistance and some without, and at different ages. Genesee and his colleagues (2004) note another difference that might affect the impact of acquiring two languages on cognition. Even if this difference does not affect cognition, it is a difference worth noting.

Many of the children included in the studies of the early 20th century lived in what have been identified as **subtractive bilingual environments**. In this environment, a child who speaks a minority language gives up his minority language when he acquires the majority language. In the process of giving up his first language, this child gives up his heritage, his culture. The child who lives in an **additive bilingual environment** has a much different life experience. This child is encouraged to retain his first language and to embrace his native culture while he learns the majority language and embraces a second culture. What is interesting about this contrast, from a cognitive point of view, is that the research that showed negative effects of bilingualism on cognitive function was conducted primarily on children from subtractive bilingual environments. The more recent research, showing cognitive advantages derived from bilingualism, involved children from predominantly additive bilingual environments. Common sense, together with the research data, would suggest that a child's cognitive abilities, including concept formation, selective attention, reasoning, and metalinguistic abilities, would be enhanced by increasing competence in two languages, both of which are valued and both of which are used frequently, as is true in an additive bilingual environment. In this circumstance, the child simply has more language information available to him, and he can directly compare one language to the other in terms of vocabulary, grammar, phonology, and so on. Not only would this presumably enhance his overall understanding of language, all the language data would be grist for cognitive exercise. If one language is being systematically erased while another is being acquired, as in the subtractive bilingual environment, it is difficult to imagine that any cognitive advantage would accrue because language data would be lost, not gained.

Language competence is an important prerequisite to learning to read. Thus, it is particularly difficult for bilingual children whose first or second language is weak to learn to read effectively in the weak language. When the home language is strong, then reading in that language progresses more easily than when the school language is the basis for reading acquisition (Bialystok, 2007). Words must be learned separately for each language; therefore, vocabulary in the weak language will impact reading acquisition. Think about this idea of word knowledge. You have a very large vocabulary in English as a consequence of learning it over a long period and using it on a daily basis. Does this competence automatically mean that you will know the meaning of words in German, French, or Portuguese? Of course, the bilingual learner who develops comparable strength in both languages will find that ease in reading acquisition in each language will also be similar.

In addition to oral language competency, successful readers need to develop a level of knowledge about print. Learning the alphabet, making sound/symbol associations, and learning word representations through exposure and instruction lead to the ability to decode and ultimately understand written language. Just as with vocabulary, however, print knowledge is specific to the individual language. Languages that use the alphabet principle have a good deal of similarity, but languages such as Chinese use a pictorial representation that differs greatly from English. The bilingual child must learn the various ways that print knowledge is represented, which depends on the language being read (Bialystok, Luk, & Kwan, 2005). Given these differences, it makes sense that bilingual children will take longer to learn to read in one or both languages, depending on the strength of each and the exposure to and instruction in the printed forms of each language.

Knowledge of storybooks in both languages is also necessary for bilingual children through exposure to both literary registers. Herman (1996) points out that each language has specific discourse demands, structures, and nuances. Thus, children will need to have experiences with storybooks in each language so that they have the opportunity to learn these conventions individually and build up their literary register for each language separately.

Another element in learning to read is the development of phonological awareness skills. Unlike oral language competence and print knowledge, phonological awareness skills, as well as meta-linguistic skills in general, reflect general cognitive mechanisms. Bilingual and trilingual children have been shown to use metalinguistic awareness to develop divergent and creative thinking, interactional and/or pragmatic competence, communicative sensitivity and flexibility, and translation skills (Jessner, 2006). Metalinguistic skills transfer easily across languages (Bialystok, 2007; Ciscero & Royer, 1995; Durgunoglu, 1998; Durgunoglu, Nagy, & Hancin-Bhatt, 1993; Rickard Liow & Poon, 1998). Thus, acquisition of metalinguistic skills in the first language will influence further knowledge in the second language (Kemp, 2001). But it should also be noted that although such awareness is a positive factor, bilingual children must also develop the knowledge of the other characteristics and strategies particular to the second language.

The discussion about bilingualism and literacy reminds us that the acquisition of literacy is a complex process, with many factors coming into play. Research has confirmed that children are able to transfer reading ability and some of the underlying skills associated with reading across languages and systems. This cross-linguistic awareness (James, 1996) means that children can potentially benefit from the mastery of such skills in one system by applying them to the other. The ability to transfer some skills makes learning to read in two or more languages much more efficient than would be the case if every skill needed to be learned specifically for each language.

Check Your Understanding 3.4

Assess your understanding of the role of executive functioning in cognition and the relationships between cognition, language, and literacy by completing this brief quiz.

SUMMARY

In this chapter, we explored the relationships between cognitive growth and language development by considering several points of view. Children have amazing and complex strategies for gaining all types of information and progressively relating it to their world as they develop. Piaget mapped how they use their sensory and motor systems to move from thinking in the here and the now based on what objects, people, and events are present, to being able to employ distancing and mental representations to think about the world not only in the present, but also in the immediate past and into the future. We discussed the important role of others, as Vygotsky explained, in providing the social context for our interactions with the world, and how all of our experiences are similar, but unique, in the dynamic relationships that unfold in daily living. The knowledge that children are prepared to receive all the input about their world through all of their senses as they see, hear, touch, and move with their caregivers, makes learning a remarkable process. Children not only amass all the information and retrieve it on command, but they learn to attend to what is new and add it to their existing knowledge, ignore what is not important, tune in to one or several languages, and think with an increasing and agile ability to learn, become literate, and reflect on desires, emotions, thoughts, beliefs, and what others know and think.

▮▷ Surfing the Web

If you are interested in exploring topics discussed in this chapter in more detail, search for one or more of the following relevant terms online.

cognition and learning a second language

theories and concepts of cognition

Howard Gardner's multiple intelligences

Piaget's theory of cognitive development

Vygotsky's social development theory

zone of proximal development

scaffolding during instruction

dynamic systems theory

theory of mind

Chapter Review 3.1

Recall what you learned in this chapter by completing the Chapter Review.

4

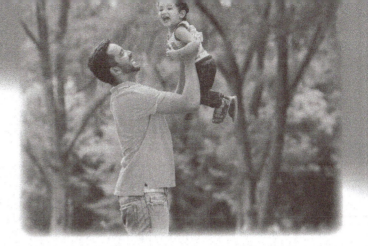

In the Beginning: Communication Development from Birth to 2 Years

LEARNING OUTCOMES

After completion of this chapter, you will be able to:

- Discuss the social and cultural factors within the language learning environment.
- Discuss the nature of interactions parents use with infants prior to and after birth to create a nurturing communication environment.
- Describe the child-directed communication strategies parents use with their children.
- Evaluate the importance of providing linguistic input to young children.
- Trace the receptive and expressive attainments of the infant's communication system.
- Describe the emergence of first words and their functions.
- Discuss the features of word combinations in early and late stage 1.

Three chapters trace language development from birth through the school-age years. In this chapter, we consider language development from birth through two years. We emphasize that the child is a communicator from the beginning of her life, and the changes in her communication system over the first two years are dramatic. She begins by crying, and by the time she is two years old, she has already been talking for a year.

As a framework for our discussion of language acquisition in this chapter and the next, we use a stage view of development. Although we focus primarily on speech and language *production*, we also consider the vital role of *comprehension* in communication development.

To the casual observer, the child's first year of life is fairly uneventful. It seems to be a succession of days marked by sleeping, eating, spitting up, crying, and soiling diapers. The more educated observer understands that much more than this is going on. The child comes into the world genetically programmed to become a whole person, a thinking, acting, reacting, speaking human being, and he does not wait until his first birthday to begin his growth into personhood. He is born with an enormous intellectual capacity that begins to develop immediately. He has fairly sophisticated perceptual abilities that he uses within the first hours and days of his life. Much of his first year is devoted to making contact with his world, first through his senses. He absorbs the sights, sounds, and textures of this new environment into which he has been hurled. He makes immediate connections to those people who will be most important in his early development. In the beginning, he does not understand his relationship to the people and things in his environment, but in a very real sense he *relates* to these people and things by looking at them, listening to them, grasping them, and putting them into his mouth. The new-born child is not a mass of tissue simply waiting to be molded. During the first year of his life, he is a vital, active, exploring, thinking creature, and from the very beginning he is a communicator.

Before we launch into our saga regarding all the wonderful attainments in language children gain during their first two years, it is important to highlight again the impact of the home environment and home language on the developing child. Of course, the impact of these for the child begins before birth, and you should recognize that the first two years are critical for language acquisition.

Throughout this book, we stress that language is a universal human phenomenon. People are born with the same genetic predispositions for language use, and although people have different experiences with their speech and language models, most are exposed to adequate samples of speech and language and have normal interactive relationships with their models. We do not have to travel very far outside our homes or neighborhoods, however, to discover that there are some significant differences in language. In some cases, of course, people speak different languages, but even within a single language, there are differences. We must consider socioeconomic factors including poverty, socioeconomic status (SES), race, and ethnicity as related to language and learning.

Social and Cultural Factors in the Language Learning Environment

Although children are born to talk, they are not born to speak a particular language or to speak a particular variation of a language. If a child is born in Paris to French-speaking parents, he will speak French. If a child is born to Korean parents, but adopted shortly after her birth by English-speaking parents,

she will speak English, and she will speak the same kind of English modeled for her by her adoptive parents. The language one speaks and the variation of the language one speaks are not products of biology. They are products of environment.

According to Taylor (1990), seven major variables influence the acquisition of language and language behaviors: (1) race and ethnicity; (2) social class, education, and occupation; (3) region; (4) gender; (5) situation or context; (6) peer group association or identification; and (7) first-language community or culture. These factors operate in an interactive manner to determine the language one speaks, the language one uses in one situation with one group of people, and the language one uses in another situation with a different group of people. This might mean, for example, that the Vietnamese child who emigrated to the United States with his family speaks Vietnamese to his parents, but speaks English to his U.S. friends.

Social Class, Education, and Occupation

Because environment is so important in shaping human language, we will consider three factors that have a direct bearing on the language development of children. We will explore the impact of socioeconomic status (SES), especially as it relates to poverty and children in low-SES families, the languages used within families that reflect race and ethnicity, and the regional, gender, and age-related factors that have an impact on language.

The language environment in American households differs in relationship to the SES of the parents. In particular, low-income households not only are disadvantaged in terms of wealth, but also are impoverished in terms of the opportunities that children need for optimal growth and development. Poverty is a complex condition; thus, we will explore it and its relationship to language development.

What does it mean to live in poverty? There are many definitions of poverty and there are guidelines for determining who is eligible for government benefits. One way to define poverty is through the use of the **poverty threshold**. The U.S. Census Bureau uses income before taxes to establish thresholds that are based on family size and composition. For example, the U.S. Census Poverty Thresholds for 2015 define the poverty threshold for one person under age 65 as $12,082; for one person over age 65 as $11,367; for a four-person family as $24,257; and for a family of eight people as $41,029. Extreme poverty occurs in households who spend less than $2 per day before government benefits (1.2% in 2011).

According to the U.S. Census Bureau (2012a) statistics, 46.2 million people, about 15% of our population, live in poverty and at least 20% of children under 18 are affected. However, poverty does not equally affect American citizens. The following breakdown provides information on national poverty rates according to race/ethnicity and age from 2007 to 2011; the data for children under 18 years is based on 2010 statistics (Macartney, 2011):

African Americans	27.4%	38.2.1% under 18 years
Hispanic/Latino Americans	25.2%*	32.3% under 18 years
American Indian/Alaskan Native	23.3%*	
Native Hawaiian/Pacific Islanders	19.4%*	
Asian	14.7%*	13% under 18 years
White	14.4%	17% under 18 years

(*Based on highest 30 cities for each group.)

The south and east regions of the United States are where children are most highly affected by poverty, although at least 16% of children in every state live in poverty. Ten states (Alabama, Arkansas, Kentucky, Louisiana, Mississippi, New Mexico, South Carolina, Tennessee, Texas, West Virginia), the District of Columbia, and Puerto Rico have 25% childhood poverty rates.

An important consideration regarding poverty is marital status and gender. In 2007, married families in poverty were estimated at 5.8%, whereas the poverty rate for single-parent families was 26.6%. Impoverished households with a female single parent comprise 75% of the total (U.S. Bureau of the Census, 2007). These statistics make it clear that single women raising children are the most vulnerable group that struggle to stay out of poverty.

Some families live in a cycle of chronic poverty that spans generations. This means that older generations who live in poverty transmit poverty to the younger generations, but the transference can occur in the opposite direction (Moore, 2001). Intergenerational poverty does not just refer to income thresholds. A person's SES includes family income, parental education, and occupation of the parents (Bradley & Corwyn, 2002). It also includes other types of capital, such as, "human, social-cultural, social-political, financial/material, and environmental/natural" (Moore, 2001, p. 2).

Human capital involves parents' investment in their children, which is influenced by their culture and is affected by parental and societal beliefs about age, gender, and birth order. Such beliefs lead to parental decisions about whether their children work or go to school, for example. Gender discrimination is one example of a negative impact brought about by intergenerational transfer (Engle, Castle, & Menon, 1996). In many countries, girls are treated differently than their brothers in regard to education, status within the family, and other opportunities throughout life.

The most important idea here is that families have relationships within their families, with other families in the community, in the marketplace, and within the country or state where they reside. These relationships allow for getting and giving resources. The low amount of capital that families who live in poverty have reduces their ability to access resources. However, it is also important to consider that some families are able to sacrifice on behalf of their children in order to break the cycle of poverty and some societal programs, such as public education, can provide the education a child needs

for success after graduation (Moore, 2001). Head Start, which has been in operation since 1965, is one example of a government-funded childhood and parent program.

Human capital includes much more than beliefs and values. The structure of households, educational attainment of parents and their children, genetic inheritance of cognitive abilities, early childhood nutrition, mother-to-child transmission of HIV in utero or through breastfeeding, and inherited or communicable diseases are some of the factors that influence poverty, especially for children (Moore, 2001). Of course, all families are different and exhibit a mix of these factors that are shared, sometimes unequally, among family members.

Families often transfer money between members in the form of gifts, loans, and inheritances according to the nature of their familial and cultural relationships. For example, in many cultures across the world, family, customs, and culture come into play when two individuals marry. Some cultures require that the bride's family pay a dowry to the groom's family, while other cultures favor having the bride's family pay for the wedding. Inheritance patterns also vary greatly around the world and in the United States, where the "last will and testament" has a major bearing on inheritance. These examples are merely illustrative; many other variations in **financial/material capital** impact families and individuals.

Another form of capital discussed by Moore (2001) is **social-cultural**. This topic has been debated in the literature since the 1950s in the form of the "culture of poverty." Essentially, views have varied widely regarding the nature of poverty. On one end of the debate are those who believe that individual characteristics, such as laziness or lack of intelligence, cause poverty. On the other end are those who think that societal structures including the lack of safety nets cause poverty. Somewhere in the middle are those who believe that a history of poverty in families is a cycle that limits the family members' ability to change the behaviors, beliefs, and attitudes that emerge from living in poverty.

Related to the other forms of capital is the **social-political** reality of being a member of a society. Individuals are born into families who have a social and political standing. A family's socioeconomic status places them in relationship to other families, community organizations, and agencies, creating a limited and relatively defined sphere of influence and access. For instance, a middle-class parent will find that she is able to work effectively in the local parent-teacher association to advocate for her child's sports program. Her social-political clout, if you will, is on par with the teacher's status in the community. Families who live in poverty do not share this status and may feel powerless regarding decisions made by others about them and their children, especially regarding education.

As stated earlier, families live within communities and some communities have limited access to resources. Factors such as climate, geographic constraints (e.g., mountains, waterways, forests), pollution, chronic poverty, and limited employment opportunities are examples of how the *environment* functions as a form of capital.

It is important to note that not all poverty is transmitted generationally. Situational poverty is another form, one that has been growing recently since the economy took a severe downturn in 2008. People lost jobs and homes as a result and unemployment and the need for public assistance grew. Individuals who experience situational poverty often have access to family and societal resources that may help to make their situation temporary (Payne, 2003).

The Impact of Socioeconomic Status on Language and Learning

Socioeconomic status (SES) is an important consideration as we work with parents and their children. SES is based on family income, parental education, and the occupation of the parents. As related to child development, SES is likely to be a strong factor in all aspects of the child's life. When children are raised in impoverished circumstances, some or many of the following factors may not only affect their health, safety, and welfare, but also put them at risk for language and learning difficulties.

Health Factors

- Poor prenatal care
- Prenatal exposure to substance abuse
- Prematurity and low-birth-weight babies
- Undernourished or poor diet of mother and child
- Untreated illnesses
- Exposure to lead and other environmental agents causing illness and birth defects
- Unclean housing
- Limited access to health care (O'Hanlon & Roseberry-McKibbin, 2004; Park, Turnbull, & Turnbull, 2002; Robinson & Acevedo, 2001; Roseberry-McKibbin, 2007)

Safety Factors

- Overcrowded living conditions
- Unsafe neighborhoods and schools
- Access to illegal drugs
- Access to weapons

Educational Factors

- Low education of caregivers
- School absences (illness, migrant relocation, transportation)
- Limited exposure to language
- Depressed oral language skills
- Limited access to literacy materials
- Behavioral difficulties (Fazio, Naremore, & Connell, 1996; Friedlander & Martinson, 1996; Hart & Risley, 1995; Qi & Kaiser, 2004; Smith, Landry, & Swank, 2000)

In this chapter we will spend considerable time discussing the importance of language stimulation for young children. Research supports findings that parents with middle-class SES raise children who have the benefits of language scaffolding during reading, exposure to literacy materials, and literacy experiences including phonics and phonological awareness on a regular basis (Dodd & Carr, 2003; Payne, Whitehurst, & Angell, 1994; van Kleeck, Gillam, Hamilton, & McGrath, 1997). Children who have the benefit of language-rich environments tend to have strong language and literacy outcomes.

Practitioners who work in early childhood environments benefit from being aware of and responsive to the needs of children from low-SES households. This means that childcare providers, preschool teachers, early elementary school teachers, teachers of English as a second language, special education teachers, and speech-language pathologists and other providers have many opportunities for action. These include but are not limited to:

- Exploring the backgrounds of children in the educational setting to confirm that low SES is a factor
- Providing parents current information about community resources for health, safety, and education
- Encouraging parents to take advantage of educational opportunities for themselves and their children
- Providing education to parents about ways to enhance language growth in their children
- Using evidence-based practices in distinguishing language differences from language disorders
- Infusing culture into educational practices
- Offering resources about cultural factors and strategies to other practitioners
- Increasing oral and written language awareness
- Targeting language and literacy skills into all aspects of the educational experience
- Assisting children as they become familiar with school routines and expectations
- Promoting early language intervention for children who are behind their age-matched peers

Video Example 4.1

Children who live in low-socioeconomic (SES) families benefit from participation in Head Start and its related programs. Watch the video to learn about these programs and their goals.

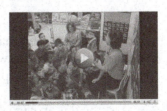

Check Your Understanding 4.1

Assess your understanding of social and cultural factors in language acquisition by completing this brief quiz.

Parent-Infant Communication Prior to and After Birth

With culture as a backdrop, let us now explore how parents and other caregivers use social experiences to interact with children from infancy through two years of age.

When is the beginning of communication between a mother and her baby? Research shows that much is going on prior to birth in this regard. Expectant mothers communicate with their developing child even when they don't intend to. Especially in the last trimester, the fetus is taking in information through listening, tasting, and moving. Let's explore what goes on inside the womb that prepares the infant's brain at birth for his environment.

- The mother's voice is amplified through her abdomen and vocal cord vibration; the fetus hears it as muffled and low in pitch (Fifer, 1994; Voegtline, Costigan, Pater, & DiPietro, 2013)
- The fetus hears the rhythms, vowels, and melodies of the native language of the mother and differing attributes of each language if the mother is bilingual; this early exposure may predispose the infant to learning the languages after birth (Moon, Lagercrantz, & Kuhl, 2013)
- When a mother produces rhymes or reads stories, the fetus hears their patterns (DeCasper, Lecanuet, Busnel, Granier-Deferre, & Maugeais, 1994; Voegtline, Costigan, Pater, & DiPietro, 2013)
- The fetus tastes spices the mother eats in foods via the amniotic fluid in the second trimester, and these experiences increase the likelihood the infant will be receptive to variety in foods (Beauchamp & Mennella, 2009)
- Smell is transmitted through the amniotic fluid and facilitates bonding between the infant and mother at birth through breastfeeding (Beauchamp & Mennella, 2009)
- Evidence suggests that fetuses experience active REM sleep by 36 weeks as well as deep NREM sleep and quiet alertness (Mirmiran, Maas, & Ariagno, 2003)
- In the last trimester fetuses move around, suck on hands, thumbs, feet, and push and pull whatever is in their path (Roodenburg, Wladimiroff, van Es, & Prechti, 1991)

We have compelling evidence that the developing fetus is busy acquiring information from the womb that establishes sensory, neural, and behavioral connections to the mother. It is with this foundation that the infant is literally "born to talk" as well as to fully participate with all his senses in his new environment from day one.

At last the day arrives when the infant is born. Immediately her senses experience new information and she quickly becomes attuned to sights, sounds, smells, and movements. As discussed early, her perceptual world is her oyster!

Before the child sends *intentional* messages, she communicates. As noted earlier, human beings communicate even when they do not intend to communicate. We cannot help ourselves! When the newborn infant cries, she is sending a message, even though she does not send it with any sense of purpose. Those within hearing distance will likely interpret this reflexive cry to mean

"I am hungry," "I am sleepy," or "I am in pain." Parents respond similarly when their infants create reflexive motor movements and facial expressions. There are no boundaries when parents use these signals, most of which are reflexive responses to specific stimuli, to connect to the child. Some adults even attach messages to noises such as sucking, gurgling, and burping—"Oh, he's telling us he's hungry" or, "She really enjoyed those strained peas!"

Chapter 3 traced cognitive development over the first two years of life and beyond and explored the perceptual abilities the child has from the earliest days of his life as he receives and processes sensory data. He uses this information to develop an understanding of objects, cause/effect, and means/ends, eventually gaining intentional communication before the end of the first year. Over the next few years, the child becomes an amazingly sophisticated and effective communicator. This chapter and the next will trace the impressive progression in communicative ability and the emergence of language that characterize the child's development through the preschool years. We begin by taking a closer look at communication development during infancy.

Creating a Communication Environment: Social Routines Involving Songs, Rhymes, and Stories

Parents, siblings, grandparents and a host of others not only fill the infant's day with conversations, but also select times to provide him with very specific types of language through songs, rhymes and stories. We discovered earlier in this chapter that some mothers begin these melodic and literacy activities during their pregnancies. What aspects of language differ from those encountered during conversations? How do these activities facilitate social, language, and literacy development?

Infant-Directed Singing

Infant-directed (ID) singing occurs in all human cultures and is considered a universal caregiving behavior (Trehub, 2001; Trehub, Schellenberg, & Hill, 1997). Lullabies and play songs are used cross-culturally and share many characteristics of motherese (Trehub, Hill, & Kamenetsky, 1997). Lullabies are soothing and often promote sleep, as they elicit an inward focus of attention, whereas play songs heighten positive emotion and increase stimulation as attention is focused on the mother.

Songs between mothers and their infants allow several aspects of human development to occur. First, mothers convey emotional information to infants during ID singing. The emotion conveyed through the melodies helps infants to either focus or shift attention. Second, singing allows mothers and infants to synchronize their emotional states, leading to modulation and social regulation (Trainor, Austin, & Desjardins, 2000; Trainor & Desjardins, 2002; Trehub, Trainor, & Unyk, 1993). These two reactions are considered essential for affect regulation. Third, ID singing may help mothers and infants establish a secure relationship that plays an important role in the development of attachment (Milligan, Atkinson, Trehub, Benoit, & Poulton, 2003). Finally, songs may contribute to language acquisition in three important ways: (1) emotional aspects may increase arousal; attention, (2) pitch contours may enhance phonological discrimination, because syllable change is often accompanied by a change in pitch; and (3) the consistent mapping of musical and linguistic structure may optimize the operation of learning mechanisms (Schön et al., 2008). The statistical learning ability that allows us to extract words from continuous speech also allows for tone sequence segmentation. Neural networks that subserve language and music perception are partly overlapping (Koelsch & Siebel, 2005; Maess, Koelsch, Gunter, & Friederici, 2001). Thus, a consistent mapping of linguistic and musical information through song may enhance learning. In short, ID singing creates opportunities for meaningful interaction between parents and children. Recent research (de l'Etoile, 2006) has demonstrated that ID singing is as effective in gaining and sustaining infant attention as interactions involving toys and books or ID speech, and it is superior to infants' responses to recorded music.

There are certain acoustical properties that characterize ID singing as different from songs not directed to infants. Mothers with infants use higher pitch, greater emotional expressions, sustained vowels, slow tempo, and gliding between pitch levels. They modify these characteristics to match or alter their infant's state. A cyclical interaction occurs as a result of the infants' behavioral responses to singing. In fact, infants show a preference for their mother's voice and higher levels of sustained attention to ID singing than to ID speech (Milligan et al., 2003; Nakata & Trehub, 2004).

The benefits of ID singing have implications for mother/infant pairs who are at risk due to infant prematurity, maternal attachment or other emotional difficulties, and special needs of the infants. For instance, ID singing has a stress-reducing effect on premature infants in the neonatal intensive care unit (NICU) (Blumenfeld & Eisenfeld, 2006), encourages a reciprocal relationship, provides a way for mothers to become intimately involved in caregiving, and increases their confidence as caregivers (de l'Etoile, 2006). Thus, ID singing may be recommended as one way in which mothers can interact with their babies in the NICU. Mothers who are less available emotionally to their children have less frequent modulation and less frequent use of motherese and ID singing, especially when their infants are distressed (Milligan et al., 2003). Teaching mothers to respond through singing to regulate their infant's state establishes the type of interaction that promotes healthy attachment. The coaching process for inclusion of ID singing should include modeling, practice, discussion, and interpretation of infant responses (de l'Etoile, 2006).

Children's songs vary significantly from the typical conversations caregivers have with infants. Songs have the special quality of continuous melody in very regular and repetitious patterns. The melody provides the frame for the words and phrases in the songs. Think of a familiar song that you might sing to an infant. You'll notice that the repetition of the melody and words provides high redundancy to the infant. Redundant information is easier to process, especially when it is presented within the same modality. Music engages the auditory channel in hearing both the music and the words simultaneously and in a repeated fashion. Thus, both the emotional/arousal and linguistic functions are fulfilled, making songs particularly beneficial to learning (Schön et al., 2008).

Rhymes

Beyond melodies that contain words, alliteration and rhymes are embedded in songs and social routines, such as nursery rhymes and simple interactive games. The patterned alliterations, rhythms, and repetitions of words in combination with sequenced actions of the parent and child provide a social structure for engaging in the routine. The interactions are typically highly entertaining, where attention is focused on facial expressions, clapping, or other sound effects, and a lot of redundancy is provided through repetition of the chorus. These characteristics serve to capture and hold the attention of children, provide prolonged joint interaction, develop coordination of the rhymes with accompanying gestures (Rogow, 1982), and contribute to the social relationship of the participants.

Alliterations and rhymes also focus infants on the variation in word structure to create new meanings. It is interesting to note that infants as young as 3 months old detect alliteration in syllables (Hayes & Slater, 2008). That is, infants focus on the beginning consonant of words (the *onset*) very early in their experiences with their native language. By six months they are beginning to comprehend some words, and they begin to segment words from the speech stream at around seven-and-a-half months. Later, they are able to attend to the vowel and final consonant (the *rime*). The ability to detect subtle changes in words is a necessary component to the development of phonological representations and awareness. Word variations for rhyming are made by maintaining the rime of the syllable and changing the onset of the syllable. For example, the rime *un* can be used to create many different rhyming words by adding a new consonant in the onset position: *fun, run, sun, won*. Rhymes for very young children typically occur at the ends of phrases in short poems or songs.

Stories

Mothers and other caregivers who tell or read stories aloud during the infant years provide similar focused language experiences to their children. Stories differ from conversations in important ways. They are typically very simple, but their complexity can vary dramatically. During story time, there is no expectation for turn taking and interaction between the mother and child is kept to a minimum. The narrative aspects of stories provide a specific type of structure. In Western culture, stories begin with the setting ("Once there was a giant dog named Gus"), lead to an event ("Gus went to a birthday party for his friend Barry the Bear"), an episode ("But when he got there, all the friends were gone"), and end in a conclusion ("He was sad, so he started to go back home, when—SURPRISE!—all his friends jumped out of the box. The party was for him! Now he was happy") and an ending ("The End"). As children listen to stories over and over, they learn the structure of stories so that they predict what is coming next and expect a similar structure in future stories. These experiences provide a framework for their future ability to tell stories and to listen effectively to more complex stories as they grow.

In summary, songs, rhymes, and stories that parents engage in with their children provide a strong foundation for the development of speech perception, for phonological structure, and, later, for literacy. The take-home message here is that parents and other caregivers should use all of these forms of language to heighten social interaction with infants and provide the necessary access to language that will assist infants in learning. Other forms of language exposure, including television, should be used only as a supplemental strategy for language exposure when children are approaching their second birthday.

Check Your Understanding 4.2

Assess your understanding of parent-infant communication by completing this brief quiz.

Child-Directed Interactions

Parents are eager to communicate with their children, often even before birth as they talk, read, or play music to their children in utero. These parents are anxious to connect to their babies to establish meaningful interpersonal relationships and they often attach messages to the movements of the child in the uterus, and after he is born, they are likely to associate meaning with every noise the child makes, from cries to burps. It is not surprising, therefore, that parents and other adults do talk to babies and eventually they talk back.

We will explore the nature of parent talk a bit later, but first it is important to reiterate that adults create a directive and responsive environment for infants. There are two essential components of preverbal behavior during the infant's first year. The first is the caregiver's interest in and intuitive adaptations of his communications to the infant's abilities. Caregivers respond to infants' feelings and actions. In other words, parents respond in a turn-taking fashion to their infant as a communicating and feeling person by mirroring what she does. The second component is the infant's corresponding interaction through motor activity and demonstration of feelings, such as smiling, laughing, or cooing. Thus, this interplay of **contingent responding** becomes linked successively and allows for mutual reciprocity and understanding (Papousek, 2007). There is evidence that when mothers encourage their infants to attend, the language development of those infants is enhanced (Karrass, Braungart-Rieker, Mullins, & Lefever, 2002). Consider a typical interaction that illustrates contingency:

Parent: Hm, those plums are really good, yes?
 Infant: Ah, um (smiles)
Parent: Looks like you like it. More?
 Infant: Ah, ah, ah, eeeooo! (shrieks and laughs)
Parent: Okay, here it comes. Hm, good plums!
 Infant: Hm. (Opens mouth for more)

Contingency is also important for the infant's development of self-awareness and efficacy. Research has demonstrated that infants actively seek contingency and by four weeks of age they are interested in gaining feedback from their own actions and detect differences in their own actions as compared to the actions of others. By eight weeks, removal of contingency from others (shown through research using the still face paradigm) was distressing for infants and even for preterm infants (Hsu & Jeng, 2007). The infants reacted to the interruption in social contingency with significant changes in the length of their social gaze (looking away from distressing stimuli) and showing signs of stress, indicating some ability to self-regulate. Preterm infants became stressed faster than full-term infants.

In another study, researchers (Reddy et al., 2007) established that infants at 13 weeks (but not as early as 9 weeks) were able to discriminate between a live video of themselves, where their own actions are mirrored in the video, and a replay condition, where their real-time actions differed from what they do in the video. This study and similar studies show that interactions with the self and others appear to be a developmental process that begins at around two months of age with advances occurring through the first several months. Social contingency and self-awareness both set the stage for caregivers to introduce the infant to others and objects in the environment.

Joint reference suggests that a caregiver and child are focusing on the same object or event at the same time. Current research on joint attention and joint reference shows that they are a basis for shared experiences and are a necessary aspect of infant development, including language acquisition. Much work has been devoted to joint attention and joint reference interactions between infants, adult partners, and external objects at nine months of age. However, this triadic relationship is, of course, a developmental process that emerges from the requisite skills of gaze-following at 2 months, shifting gaze to follow the adult's shift in eye direction at 3 months, coordinated attention and point-following, and means/ends at 5-10 months (Striano & Bertin, 2005).

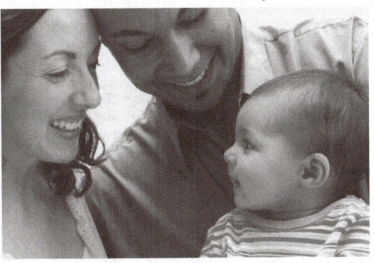

Infant–adult interaction, a precursor of communication.
Source: VStock/360/Getty Images.

Owens (2005) notes that there are four phases in the development of establishing joint reference. Table 4.1 shows the key features in the progression of this skill from four weeks to the first year.

The speech directed at infants, as you know from your own experiences, is not the same as speech directed at adults. In Chapter 2 we introduced infant-directed speech as parentese, recognizing that fathers, siblings, and other caregivers use the style as well. Many researchers believe that the unique characteristics of parentese facilitate the acquisition of language.

Table 4.1 Four Phases in the Development of Joint Reference

Phase	Approximate Age Range	Key Features
1	4–6 weeks	Caregiver places object where child can see it and calls attention to the object with a verbal stimulus such as "Look!"
	By 6 months	Child may recognize caregiver's pitch pattern as a signal to establish joint attention.
2	7 months	Child begins to demonstrate efforts to communicate intentionally; may create joint reference by pointing to an object of interest.
	By 8 months	Child may reach for an object and look to caregiver for a response.
3	8–12 months	Child uses combinations of gestures and vocalizations to indicate interest in objects.
4	12 months	Child exercises control over topic; produces names of objects and events.

Infants tune in to the speech sounds, pitch variations, stress on syllables and words, and overall melody of their parents' utterances as they engage in face-to-face interactions with their babies. Infants also tune in to facial expressions, movements, and gestures. In fact, mothers who sign to their children incorporate rhythms with their hands that are remarkably similar to the rhythms underlying the speech directed to hearing children (Fernald, 1994). There is evidence that the input provided through sign language enables children who are deaf to achieve normal developmental milestones (Petitto, 1985a, 1985b, 1986, 1987, 1988; Petitto & Marentette, 1991).

Kaye (1980) notes that mothers use considerable repetition in their speech and that each successive utterance is semantically similar to the preceding utterance. Two examples of successive utterances are highlighted in Figure 4.1. Most early topics tend to focus on objects children can see and hear (Bruner, 1975; Phillips, 1973). When children reach the sixth month of life, their mothers tend to employ an informational style of talking, a style that is less centered on objects and more centered on their infants' surroundings and behaviors (Penman, Cross, Milgrom-Friedman, & Meares, 1983).

Although there may be exceptions, parentese in most languages is produced at higher than normal pitch levels, and with intonational patterns that include greater extremes of high and low pitches than are typically used in adult-to-adult speech. These characteristics are so universal that one might believe they are the salient features in baby talk to which infants respond most positively, but that may not be the case. In one study, six-month-old babies were exposed to speech that had the stereotypical high pitch levels and exaggerated prosodic elements commonly associated with parentese, but there was no apparent *joy* or *happiness* in these samples. The babies were also exposed to speech delivered

---

Figure 4.1 Semantic Similarity in Infant-Directed Speech

Example 1—Focus is on the infant

Oh, pretty baby!
Yes, you are so pretty!
Pretty, pretty baby
Mama loves you.
Yes, I do!
Mama loves you.
Who's my baby?
Who's my pretty baby?

Example 2—Focus is on the object

Look at baby bear!
Soft, baby bear.
Oh, so soft!
Oh, so soft bear!
Just like my sweet baby.
So soft, baby bear!

---

in a typical adult-to-adult style but expressed in an obviously *joyful* manner. These babies preferred speech that was joyful or happy, even if it lacked the characteristics of pitch and highly variable intonational patterns associated with parentese (Singh, Morgan, & Best, 2002).

One specific characteristic of parentese that seems to transcend speech is rhythm. The rhythm of speech directed to babies is more regular than that of adult speech, resulting in what some researchers describe as a *singsong cadence*. In fact, a study by Bergeson and Trehub (2007) demonstrated that mothers use individually distinctive pitch patterns that may play an important role in establishing identification and preference for the mother's voice over other female voices. These **signature tunes** may be used along with other aspects of maternal speech to facilitate infants' processing of speech and to scaffold early learning. We will discuss the particular role of infant-directed singing later in this chapter. There are, of course many characteristics of speech directed to children that distinguish it from adult-to-adult speech, including those summarized in Figure 4.2.

Parents across the globe engage infants in social verbal interactions, such as parentese; however, socialization practices are culturally embedded. It is not surprising, therefore, that some differences in early dialogues between parent and child occur. For instance, Keller, Otto, Lamb, Yovsi, and Kärtner (2007) compared urban German mother/infant dyads with rural Cameroonian Nso mother/infant dyads to determine cross-cultural differences in the timing of verbal/vocal interactions during the first three months of the infants' lives. They based their comparison on the different styles reflected in

---

Figure 4.2 Parentese (Child-Directed Speech) Characteristics

- Higher than normal overall pitch level
- More frequent use of pitch extremes—high and low
- More regular rhythm
- References to objects a child can see and/or hear
- Longer-than-normal pauses between segments
- Slower-than-normal rate
- Utterances that are shorter than normal in length
- Facial expressions are exaggerated
- Sentences are simple syntactic constructions
- More utterance repetitions
- Greater loudness variation

---

independent-dialogic (urban) and interdependence-apprenticeship (rural) models of interaction observed in these different cultures. The authors measured contingent responsiveness (verbal turn taking between infant and parent). They found that German urban mothers produced more verbal turn taking in response to infant cues, but the differences were not statistically different from those of Nso mothers. However, Nso mothers responded less often than German mothers with vocal/verbal exchanges as infants increased in age. The authors state that Nso mothers rely more on body contact and body stimulation characteristic of this proximal interactional style, with verbal interactions becoming more pronounced with progressive development of their children.

When infants begin to babble, caregivers respond with contingent social feedback that provides information to them for vocal learning. Goldstein and Schwade (2008) found that nine-month-old infants modified their babbling in accordance with the type of speech sound structure present in their caregivers' contingent utterances. Specifically, one infant group increased their proportion of vowels in accordance with the nature of the feedback from their caregivers—more vowels of course—and the other group increased their proportion of consonant-vowel (CV)-structured syllables in response to this type of feedback. A control group of infants increased their number of vocalizations in response to social feedback, but they did not change the sound characteristics of their babbling. The authors emphasize the importance of socially guided learning in early vocal development as a foundational step in establishing communication development. In other words, the input that caregivers provide is the fuel that children use to experiment with language. The nature of the input is quite important and we will discuss this again later.

The infant is able to use her perceptual abilities and the social verbal context of interactions with family members to make distinctions among pitch levels, especially in the fundamental frequency range of sounds in speech. She can make at least gross discriminations among loudness levels, sounds

of varying durations, and different consonants in consonant-vowel-consonant (CVC) syllables (Moon, Bever, & Fifer, 1992). Note that infants not only prefer speech over other kinds of sounds, but also prefer parentese to adult speech (Fernald, 1985; Sullivan & Horowitz, 1983). Whether infants are innately attuned to the characteristics of parentese or prefer it because caregivers use it for social interaction is a subject for debate. Adults do tend to gain the attention of their infants more effectively through it, and it would be difficult to argue against the idea that each generation and culture learns how to use parentese by observing members of the preceding generation communicate with babies. Also note, however, that recent research with parents who have children with language delays show important differences in the outcomes of those children's language when a particular aspect of parentese (utterances that are shorter in length) is used. Children whose parents use a high degree of telegraphic speech (predominant use of content words, such as, "Baby want cookie?") develop less than children exposed to grammatical simplified input where parents use short sentences but grammatical forms are complete, such as, "Does Baby want the cookie?" (van Kleeck et al., 2010)

Even if we cannot determine whether parentese is the product of genetics or environment, we can appreciate its role in child/adult interactions. In Chapter 3, we indicated that the infant has an early and powerful interest in the caregiver's face. He has a similar interest in the caregiver's voice and speech. The caregiver quickly learns that she can use her face, voice, and speech to capture the infant's attention, and she learns the features of her child's communicative efforts that are most meaningful in their exchanges (Meadows, Elias, & Bain, 2000). On the basis of present knowledge, it might be a stretch to argue that this kind of contact is essential for speech and language development, but there seems little doubt that during special moments when the caregiver is attending carefully to all aspects of the child's reflexive and learned behaviors, and when she gazes into the baby's attentive eyes and fills his discriminating ears with the lilting, soothing sounds of speech, an important bond is being formed, a bond that certainly has the potential to facilitate communication acquisition.

 Video Example 4.2

Joint attention, contingent responding, and parentese are three ways that caregivers establish and maintain interactions with infants. As you watch the video, observe these three types of interaction strategies.

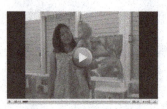

Expansions and Extensions

Keep in mind that language does not develop in a vacuum. Children bring to the acquisition process a strong biological drive to develop language, and the emergence of language is closely associated with cognitive development,

but they will not acquire language unless they are exposed to language models. There is evidence, too, that simply hearing language is not enough. The child's communicative interactions with his caregivers facilitate vocabulary acquisition (Ahktar, Dunham, & Dunham, 1991) and overall language development. When a caregiver responds to her child's early utterances, she often expands them, thus the term **expansion**. If the child says, "Mommy work," the caregiver might respond, "Yes, Mommy went to work." The caregiver does not change the order of the words in the child's utterance, and she maintains what she believes is the child's communicative intent, but she expands the utterance into a complete form. Researchers note that caregivers expand about 20% of their 2-year-old children's utterances into more syntactically correct and complete sentences, and children often respond to these expansions by imitating them (Hirsh-Pasek, Treiman, & Schneiderman 1984; Folger & Chapman, 1978).

Although it is not known precisely *what* expansions contribute to language development, Scherer and Olswang (1984) believe they assist the acquisition of language by helping the child better understand the grammatical functions of words and the rules by which words are combined, by keeping the communicative effort focused on subjects the child has selected, and by reinforcing the turn-taking aspect of conversation. Farrar (1990) suggests that the child may derive different benefits from different types of expansion in learning grammatical morphemes. For example, restating the child's utterances with added or revised grammatical morphemes may assist the child in acquiring plurals and possessives, whereas expanding the topic or general intent of the child's utterance may be more helpful in the acquisition of other grammatical morphemes, including tense markers.

Caregiver/child interactions make an important contribution to language development.

Source: Ptaxa/iStock/Getty Images

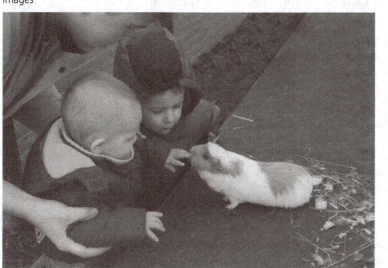

Apparently, caregivers are sensitive to the length and complexity of their own models even before they expand the child's utterances. According to Murray, Johnson, and Peters (1990), caregivers actually produce shorter utterances when they talk to toddlers than when they talk to infants. Furthermore, there seems to be a relationship between these shorter adult utterances during the second half of the child's second year and her receptive language abilities at 18 months. It appears that when adults sense that the child is old enough to benefit from speech and language models, they pay greater attention to the length and complexity of the models they provide in order to give the child clear and attainable language targets. Then when the child begins to produce her own utterances, adults provide additional assistance through various forms of expansion.

Video Example 4.3

Verbal exchanges with young children provide many opportunities for the use of expansions, extensions, and imitations. As you watch the video, try to identify each of these strategies.

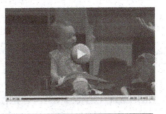

Sometimes a caregiver will do more than expand the child's utterance. For instance, the child might say, "Daddy go," and the caregiver responds by saying, "Yes, Daddy went to work." In this case, the caregiver is providing not only a more syntactically accurate model, but also additional semantic information. This kind of response is called **extension**. On other occasions, the caregiver will simply imitate what the child has said. Very often when the adult imitates the child's utterance, the child will imitate the imitation to create a simple form of turn taking. Whether the caregiver expands, extends, or imitates, the child is taking the communicative initiative, but he is being provided models that include enriched syntactic and semantic information. Of no less importance, the child is being encouraged in his language attempts and rewarded for his successful communication connections.

Conversations between parents and their children also show developmental trends. Snow (1977) described the evolution of conversation between two mothers and their babies as the babies moved from three months of age to their second birthday. Initially, the communication exchanges were simple and child-directed. When the children smiled or burped, for example, the mothers treated the sounds as though they were intentional messages, and they reacted with short, simple comments or questions. There was no expectation that the babies understood the content of the replies. As their children matured in their first year, mothers increased their expectations and demands by being more selective in their responses to child-vocalized sounds rather than noises. To maintain conversational turn taking, the mothers often imitated their babies' utterances. When the children responded by repeating their own vocalizations, these utterances were treated like appropriate turns in the conversations. Of course, these exchanges occur during everyday activities, such as mealtime and bathing, where parents establish routines for these scaffolded interactions that guide their child's learning in each situation. At the end of the first year, the communicative stakes had been raised considerably, with a stronger emphasis on speech-like behaviors in terms of what was judged to be conversationally acceptable. The mothers often interpreted their babies' utterances as real words, even when they probably were not. Because children begin to produce true words at about 12 months and begin to combine words into multiple-word utterances by about 18 months, conversation becomes much more adult-like as the second year unfolds.

Now imagine the interplay of expectations and reactions between a parent and child when more than one language is being used in the home. Quay

(2008) describes a fascinating account of a child learning to use three languages at two years of age through a study of her family's dinner conversations. The family lived in Japan but spent about a month in China and a month in the United States in the child's early years. The mother spoke fluent Chinese, Japanese, and English. The father spoke fluent English and Japanese, and he knew a little Chinese, Spanish, and German. The mother spoke Chinese to her daughter, while the father spoke English to her. The daughter attended a day-care center where Japanese was spoken. With some minor variations across time, English accounted for about 20% of the input to the child, whereas Chinese and Japanese each equaled about 40% of her input. Each parent spoke his or her native language to the child, but Japanese was spoken in the community. The parents also used **code mixing** unconsciously in unanticipated situations. That is, they used various combinations of words or phrases from more than one language. Video recordings of 20 dinner conversations revealed the following patterns:

- Japanese was used to open and close the meal. The utterances were used to socialize the child in the appropriate cultural script used in their community.
- The child was strongest in Japanese, with her parents ranking Chinese second and English third.
- The child used predominantly the language of each parent when communicating with them individually. She used Japanese, especially when communicating with both parents simultaneously, presumably because this was the shared language among the parents and child. English was used next most often, and language mixing occurred at low levels. This happened when the language being used was less familiar.

It is evident from this study that despite her dominance in Japanese, the child used the language that mirrored the language spoken by the parent in that particular interaction. The child's use of Japanese when speaking to both parents may reflect her knowledge that both parents understand and use this language; thus, communication was facilitated. Quay (2008) concludes that the interactions within the family between parent/child and parent–parent serve to demonstrate the acceptance of all three languages. The child learned the strengths of each parent, allowing her to adjust her own use of the languages in suitable contexts. This is an amazing accomplishment for a two-year-old child, reminding us of the influence of social interaction on language acquisition.

The Right Stuff for Nurturing Language

We know that quantity and quality of language input is important, especially during infancy and the toddler years. But what ingredients are necessary for young minds to develop strong foundations in language and learning? As you have seen, research tells us a lot about what parents and educators can do to establish listening and speaking environments and interactions that are rich and nurturing. Warren (2015) provides us with the basic and essential ingredients:

- Begin language interactions at birth during caregiving and play routines
- Be highly and consistently responsive to the child's interests

- Use opportunities to follow the child's lead to establish joint attention to objects, events, and people
- Use contingent responses to child-initiated interactions to maintain child attention and create turn-taking episodes
- Respond to a child's utterance with recasts where some of the child's words are repeated and new information is added to the turn that highlights new words, types of words, and more complex grammar
- Use picture books as a context for conversation about topics and to establish book routines
- Read simple stories to enhance vocabulary growth, joint book-reading routines, and exposure to story structure

There are several research-based programs available to parents, day-care staff, teachers, and speech-language pathologists that focus on enhancement of the interactions parents have with their infants and toddlers (Girolametto, Weitzman, & Greenberg, 2003). Training for adults who interact with children has been shown to have positive effects on the language outcomes of children. The LENA Foundation incorporates the above list in the LENA Start model. Other programs called It Takes Two to Talk® (Pepper & Weitzman, 2004) and More than Words®, (Sussman, 1999) published by the Hanen Center®, are particularly beneficial for high-risk families and families who have children with known or suspected developmental delays, such as autism.

Check Your Understanding 4.3

Assess your understanding of child-directed interactions by completing this brief quiz.

Child-Directed Speech Matters

Now that we have established that joint attention and conversational interactions are the hallmarks of infant/adult interactions in the context of everyday events, what evidence exists to support how often and how much interaction needs to occur for optimal development? In 1995, Hart and Risley published findings from their longitudinal study of parent/child talk in families. They studied verbal interactions in 42 families over a 3-year period, with children from 7 to 36 months of age. The family interactions were recorded once per month for one hour during the late afternoon or early evening in order to capture conversations. The researchers included groups of families in the upper, middle, and lower socioeconomic strata. Forty percent (17 families) were African American, and 55% of the participants were female.

Three key findings from the Hart and Risley study were emphasized (Gilkerson & Richards, 2008, p. 4):

1. The amount of parental talk directed to their children relates to the variation in children's IQ and language abilities.

2. The amount of talk directed to children from birth to age 3 predicts their academic success at ages 9 and 10.
3. Children who are advanced in language have parents who talk significantly more to them than do children who are not advanced in language.

Hart and Risley (1995) found that some families spoke an average of 3,000 words to their children during the hour, whereas other families spoke as few as 500 words. If one were to consider the long-term impact of this variability, it could mean the difference between 33 million words (30,000 per day) compared to only 9 million words by age 3. Today, this disparity in word use by parents to their children is referred to as the "word gap" (Warren, 2015). These researchers showed that a child's rate of vocabulary growth, word use, and IQ score related more strongly to the number of parent words spoken per hour than other factors, including parent education and socioeconomic status. Another important finding of this study was the long-term effect of early talking on children's language development. The more parents talked to their children, the higher the children's vocabulary and IQ test scores at age 3 and the stronger the children's language skills at ages 9 and 10. It is remarkable that the sheer volume of talk is such a powerful determinant of language learning.

Gilkerson and Richards (2008) reported extensively on a natural language study conducted by the LENA Research Foundation. Their Language Environment Analysis (LENA) uses a digital language processor (DLP), which captures a full day of conversation between each child and his or her caregiver. The software analyzes the conversation and computes the number of words the child hears from adults, the number of vocalizations the child produces, and the number of conversational turns the child experiences. The processor is lightweight, small, and durable. Special clothing keeps the DLP at the appropriate distance from the child's mouth and captures the naturally occurring interactions between the parent and child.

The LENA Research Foundation's researchers analyzed 12-hour-per-day recordings taken each month across a 6-month period from 329 children between 2 and 48 months of age and their parents. Eighty participants continued their involvement in the longitudinal phase of the study for an additional 6 months. Participants matched the U.S. census in terms of education level of the participants' mothers.

The vast amount of data available from this natural language study provides us with a treasure trove of information. Key findings of the data analysis (Gilkerson & Richards, 2008, p. 3), summarized in Figure 4.3, not only confirm the findings from Hart and Risley (1995) but also add important insights into aspects of parent/child interactions. Several of these state-of-the-art findings are discussed in more detail, as they provide new information that will continue to be explored and expanded on as the LENA Foundation adds to its database.

In order to determine how much talking adults use with children and what this means for language development during the first four years, review of the

---

Figure 4.3   Key Findings from the LENA Foundation Study

- Parents of advanced children—children who scored consistently between the 90th and 99th percentiles on independent standard language assessments—spoke substantially more to those children than did parents of children who were not as advanced, confirming the Hart and Risley results.

- Parents estimated that they talked more with their children than they actually did.

- Most language training for children came from mothers, with mothers accounting for 75% of total talk in the child's environment.

- Mothers talked roughly 9% more to their daughters than to their sons.

- Parents talked more to their first-born than to their other children, particularly first-born males.

- Most adult talk in the child's environment occurred in the late afternoon and early evening compared to other times of day.

- Children of talkative parents were also talkative.

- Although the average daily talk for parents who had graduated from college was higher than for all other parents, the average daily talk for the upper 50% of parents who did not complete high school was significantly higher than for the lower 50% of parents who had graduated from college.

- The more television in a child's day, the lower his or her language ability scores tended to be.

- Monolingual Spanish-speaking families were similar to English-speaking families with respect to patterns of adult talk.

- Parents of children with autism tended to talk less the more severe their child's symptoms were. Conversely, the stronger their child's language abilities, the more they talked.

- Parents are quite variable in the day-to-day amount they talk to their children, but given the opportunity to receive feedback, they are able to increase the amount of talk consistently.

Source: From *The Power of Talk* (2nd ed., p. 15) by J. Gilkerson and J. A. Richards. Copyright 2008 by the LENA Foundation. Reprinted with permission. For further information, contact the LENA Foundation at http://www.lenafoundation.org/ or info@lenafoundation.org.

data provides us with a fascinating look at what variables operate to influence increased language use.

Variability in Amount of Interaction

The amount of interaction parents have with their children is reported in Figure 4.4, which represents the range of adult word count (AWC) across a 12-hour day that occurs for children from 2 to 48 months of age. Notice that adults maintain a pretty steady amount of talking during the morning, with a sharp decline during and after lunch. There is a steady rise in the amount of talking through the afternoon, with peak talking time occurring just before dinner. When we consider the routines of households with young children, it is not surprising that the amount of talking varies considerably across the

Figure 4.4   Adult Talk Varies Throughout the Day

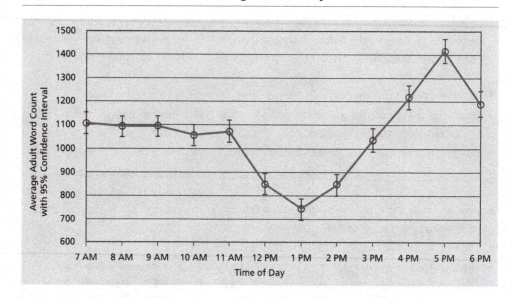

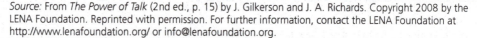

Source: From *The Power of Talk* (2nd ed., p. 15) by J. Gilkerson and J. A. Richards. Copyright 2008 by the LENA Foundation. Reprinted with permission. For further information, contact the LENA Foundation at http://www.lenafoundation.org/ or info@lenafoundation.org.

day. Toddlers often need naps, snacks, meals, changing, bathing, and play. Although cultural variations are likely to occur to some degree, the pattern of adult talk over the course of the day is similar for Spanish-speaking and English-speaking families.

Percentile norms show us that parent/child interactions vary greatly across the day from very little talking (10th to 30th percentiles) to an average amount of talking (40th to 70th percentiles) to a high amount of talking (80th to 99th percentiles). What is particularly interesting about this variability is that it correlates directly with what the children do. Notably, as the AWC increases, so do conversational turns (CTs) and child vocalizations (CVs). Thus, the amount of parent talk relates directly to the amount of child talk. In fact, parents who are average talkers lead children to more than double their talking compared to parents who are low talkers (taciturn)! Very talkative adults have a fourfold return in talking from their children. This information has implications for how language educators work with families to increase the amount of talking they do, especially to mirror the trends seen here.

To explore this relationship between adult talk and child talk, and to gain an appreciation of what it really means to have low or high AWCs, CTs, and CVs, we have included two language samples from the LENA Foundation's database. Brett is 24 months old, and his mother provides a low AWC (3rd percentile) in her interactions. Figure 4.5 shows a portion of Brett's language sample to give you a sense of what this low AWC really means in the context of natural

Figure 4.5 Brett at 24 Months with a Taciturn Mother

CHI: xxx mommy wanna get this
MOT: mm mm
CHI: xxx mom, how?
CHI: how?
CHI: mommy?
CHI: no?
MOT: no, mm mm
CHI: why mom?
CHI: what dis, what dis?
MOT: what?
CHI: huh?
MOT: huh?
CHI: more
MOT: more?
CHI: xxx
CHI: pop
MOT: more?
CHI: pop?
MOT: more?
CHI: no, pop
MOT: what?
CHI: a pop
MOT: a ball?

CHI: no
MOT: a pop?
CHI: mm
MOT: no
CHI: why?
MOT: 'cause you don't get any
MOT: want milk or water?
CHI: this
MOT: no
CHI: why?
MOT: (laughing) because
MOT: I love you to death
MOT: look at those baby toes, oh they're so cute
CHI: no
MOT: yes they are
MOT: you want milk?
MOT: more?
CHI: xxx
CHI: (vocal play)
MOT: (vocal play imitating child)
CHI: (vocal play)
MOT: here you go

Source: Retrieved February 11, 2009, from the LENA Foundation's Natural Language Corpus. Reprinted with permission. For further information, contact the LENA Foundation at http://www.lenafoundation.org/ or info@lenafoundation.org.

exchanges. Now look at Figures 4.6 and 4.7 to view the low number of adult words and the low number of CTs throughout the day.

Contrast the language sample from Brett with the sample from Trevor, who is 23 months of age and conversing with his father (Figure 4.8). It should be evident from comparing the samples of Brett and Trevor that the language input is very different. Trevor's father has a very high AWC (93 percentile), as seen in Figure 4.9, and as expected and shown in Figure 4.10, Trevor's CTs are also high.

We see these same trends for children who are older, suggesting that the input that parents provide to their children remains relatively constant. Thus, when parents interact with children with low levels of input, the children persist in responding with low language levels.

Predictability of Language Growth

What are the effects of low or high amounts of talking on the language development of children, especially during the first six months and beyond? Data on a sample of 27 children from Gilkerson and Richards's (2008) longitudinal study

Figure 4.6   Brett at 24 Months with a Taciturn Mother: AWC

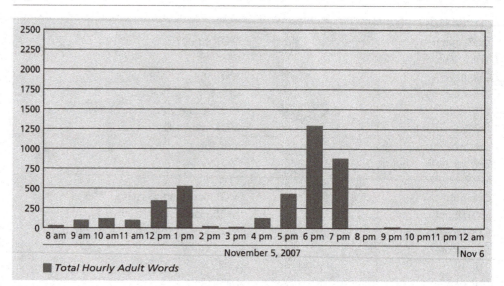

Source: Retrieved February 11, 2009, from the LENA Foundation's Natural Language Corpus. Reprinted with permission. For further information, contact the LENA Foundation at http://www.lenafoundation.org/ or info@lenafoundation.org.

Figure 4.7   Brett at 24 Months with a Taciturn Mother: CTs

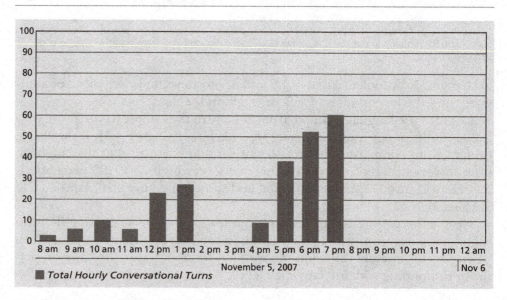

Source: Retrieved February 11, 2009, from the LENA Foundation's Natural Language Corpus. Reprinted with permission. For further information, contact the LENA Foundation at www.lenafoundation.org/ or info@lenafoundation.org.

Figure 4.8   Trevor at 23 Months with a Talkative Father

FAT: are you gunna stop are you gonna eat?

CHI: yep

FAT: alright

CHI: noodle

FAT: noodle

CHI: it noodle

FAT: there's no noodles in there

FAT: that's an onion

CHI: eat it

FAT: you can eat it

FAT: pick it up

FAT: I don't know if you'll like it

FAT: (giggle)

FAT: good?

CHI: yeah

FAT: yeah

CHI: I eat it

FAT: I don't want it

FAT: eat your potatoes

FAT: no, use your fork like a big boy

FAT: naw, eat your potatoes you don't like
that onion remember

FAT: no you don't want that

CHI: onion

FAT: you don't like the onion

CHI: onion, onion

FAT: alright eat the onion

FAT: (laughing) quit being a goober, eat it

FAT: you don't like it?

FAT: if you don't like it don't eat it

FAT: I know you like the potatoes and carrots
though

FAT: there you go

FAT: good job

FAT: that was a good one buddy

CHI: mmm

CHI: this one yum

MOT: do you like onions?

CHI: poke it

FAT: no other way remember?

CHI: my poke it

FAT: turn it

MOT: other way

FAT: turn it

MOT: there you go

CHI: mama (vocal play)

CHI: my like it (crash)

FAT: see what happens when you live on the
edge?

FAT: you fall down

CHI: my apple sauce

FAT: mmm

CHI: dad like?

FAT: I'm good thank you

CHI: xxx

FAT: I'm fine

CHI: dad like?

FAT: that's okay, thank you

FAT: (singing) Oh my love went riding she
went to the sea . . .

FAT: (singing) She went to the . . .

FAT: no other way, good job

FAT: (singing) Oh my love went . . .

CHI: (humming)

FAT: good job

FAT: (singing) She went to the . . .

FAT: you're livin' on the edge dude, be careful

CHI: dat a guy?

FAT: is that a guy on there?

FAT: not that guy, that's an "h"

FAT: what are you doing?

FAT: too big?

CHI: (vocal play)

CHI: noodles

MOT: you got noodles?

FAT: no those are onions

CHI: onions in there

MOT: onions in there

CHI: eat it

FAT: you don't like them remember?

CHI: I like them

MOT: I know you don't like them

MOT: I don't wanna eat it

FAT: no thank you

FAT: he ain't gonna eat it, trust me

CHI: onion yum yum

(continued)

Figure 4.8   Continued

CHI: ya ya yum

CHI: apple sauce?

MOT: you want applesauce instead?

FAT: you want potatoes

CHI: apple sauce apple sauce apple sauce?

FAT: apple sauce?

CHI: who did it

FAT: I think I'll get it

CHI: who did it, who did it

CHI: who did it, who did it

FAT: okay

CHI: who did it

FAT: okay well give it to dad so I can open it

CHI: good job dad

MOT: good job dad

MOT: good job Trevor

Source: Retrieved February 11, 2009, from the LENA Foundation's Natural Language Corpus. Reprinted with permission. For further information, contact the LENA Foundation at http://www.lenafoundation.org/ or info@lenafoundation.org.

revealed that the more adult words children were exposed to, the higher their language ability scores were a year or more later. This trend was also observed for CTs. These striking results suggest that the amount of talking makes a critical difference in the language development of children. During the first few months, children did not differ much in the number of vocalizations in relation to the amount of parent talk, but the difference became apparent even before children were five months old, and the gap steadily widened, especially during the first three years. Gilkerson and Richards (2008) point out that this finding supports the premise that parents have a very important role as language teachers for their children.

Figure 4.9   Trevor at 23 Months with a Talkative Father: AWC

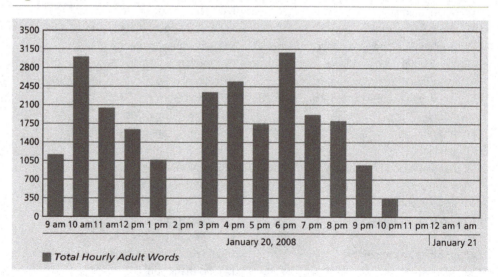

Total Hourly Adult Words

Source: Retrieved February 11, 2009, from the LENA Foundation's Natural Language Corpus. Reprinted with permission. For further information, contact the LENA Foundation at http://www.lenafoundation.org/ or info@lenafoundation.org.

Figure 4.10   Trevor at 23 Months with a Talkative Father: CTs

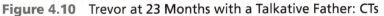

Source: Retrieved February 11, 2009, from the LENA Foundation's Natural Language Corpus. Reprinted with permission. For further information, contact the LENA Foundation at http://www.lenafoundation.org/ or info@lenafoundation.org.

Impact of the Language Environment on Language Growth

So far we have discussed the impact of the amount of talking between parent and child and typical patterns of communication throughout typical days in households. But we also must consider the types of input children receive because quality matters too. Certainly positive and engaging language interactions should be the goal, and diverse and abundant vocabulary is the way children learn new words and how to use their growing lexicon to convey their thoughts. A recent study (Sosa, 2016) demonstrated that traditional toys and books were associated with higher word counts and turns than electronic toys.

A large study with 329 participants confirmed that when the television is on, children and adults talk significantly less, as noted earlier (Christakis, Gilkerson, Richards, Zimmerman, Garrison, Xu, Gray, & Yapanel, 2009). In fact, with each hour of television exposure, children heard 500-to-1,000 less words from the parent compared to what each child normally heard. The authors commented that the reduced interactions were likely due to children watching television alone and parents being distracted by television content.

Do you know that since the introduction of programming for children under 3 years of age, 1-year-olds spend an average of 80 minutes per day in front of the television and 2-year-olds spend about 2 hours (Rideout & Hamel, 2006)? Compelling information now exists regarding the impact of television on language use in adult caregivers and their young children. Christakis and colleagues (2009) showed that caregivers decreased their adult words by 7% (about 770 words per hour) and children (aged 2 months to 4 years) significantly decreased vocalizations and conversational turns in the presence of audible television. They concluded that reduced speech for caregivers and infants is potentially harmful for language acquisition and brain development.

Until recently, little information was available regarding toddler learning from television. Researchers set out to discover whether younger toddlers (15 to 21 months) and older toddlers (22 to 24 months) differed in their ability to learn new words (fast mapping) when taught by an adult or via a television program (Krcmar, Grela, & Lin, 2007). Recall that fast mapping occurs when children know the meaning of a word after only one exposure to it in context and understand the word at a later point in time. Typically in normal interactions, children between 13 and 16 months are able to fast-map words, particularly when an adult provides child-directed speech when the object is shared (joint attention and reference) during word learning. The pairing of verbal and visual information is considered to be an important ingredient in making words salient for children.

The study confirmed that both groups of children identified target words most successfully in the joint reference condition. Higher attention to the adult was more beneficial to learning than higher attention to a children's program. Both younger and older toddlers performed the fast-mapping task when they received information from the adult, but only the older children demonstrated fast mapping when they watched the children's program. The authors explain that although young children (15 to 21 months old) attend to television and understand the relationship between the two-dimensional objects and live objects, they may not know what to focus on during a fast-mapping task. They may also have difficulty processing and storing the amount of sensory information that is typical in children's programs. Finally, these youngsters may not relate well to nonhuman characters in that their facial movements do not match their word formation, thus masking important phonological information about the new words. Thus, results of this study suggest that mere exposure to language is not sufficient for teaching new words to new language learners. They need active engagement with an adult to guide their focus, maintain their attention, and minimize the amount of stimulation they receive during learning. Once the child has a foundational vocabulary and can focus attention on television (after 22 months), some learning of new information may occur through educational media (Krcmar et al., 2007).

The reduction in interaction during television viewing highlights the importance of the American Academy of Pediatrics recommendation to reduce screen time for children younger than two years of age (2001).

Applicability of Child/Adult Interaction Data to Children with Disabilities

Researchers are using the LENA technology to study interactional patterns of children, including children who have disabilities in a wide variety of settings. These research efforts are directed toward discovering ways to identify children early who are at risk of having communication disorders and to determine the effects of working with parents and child-care providers to increase opportunities for successful outcomes. The following summary of research provides us with important information.

- Analysis of audio recordings of children at risk for autism spectrum disorder with particular attention to vocal quality (duration, pitch, and rhythm) and restrictive and repetitive vocal behaviors was effective in identifying these children with close to 90% accuracy. The LENA analysis may be an effective procedure for early identification of children with autism spectrum disorder (Warren, Gilkerson, Richards, Oller, Xu, Yapanel, & Gray, 2010).

- Specific education of parents regarding how to increase their language input to children can have both immediate and long-term effects on language learning and academic achievement. Language therapy has been shown to increase the AWC from the parent of a child with autism as compared to the AWC from the parent during home interactions. Parents can greatly benefit from first observing the amount and types of interactional exchanges during therapy and then participating directly in the therapy to increase their own AWCs and CTs with their child.

- Children with autism engage in fewer CTs than children who are typically developing; Figure 4.11 shows this contrast. In a recent study comparing children with autism to typically developing peers, children with autism showed 26% fewer conversational turns and 29% fewer vocalizations. Their average difference of 146 fewer conversational turns leads to 4,529 fewer turns per week and 236,155 per year. Children with autism also showed shorter conversational exchanges and their vocalizations were less likely to lead to responses from adults (Warren et al., 2010). The impact of these differences on active social engagement and language development is not hard to imagine.

- There is early support for the use of LENA data in preschool settings regarding the language environment of children with autism spectrum disorder. Teachers play an important role in providing the quantity and quality of language input, thus they benefit from information about their interactions and a means to monitor it, especially with children who have autism spectrum disorder. Research is needed to identify the characteristics of a high-quality language environment in preschool classrooms, which will lead to greater and more consistent efforts to optimize interventions for children with autism spectrum disorders. In addition, LENA data may also be useful for monitoring the progress of individual children in the preschool setting (Dykstra et al., 2012).

- Children with hearing loss benefit from preschool programming using an auditory-oral approach during the summer months because they receive more complex language input than they do at home and parents benefit from parental education regarding language stimulation at home (Wiggins et al., 2012).

- The amount of television children watch is linked to decreased quantity and quality of parent/child interactions. Children with hearing loss have additional challenges with television and with face-to-face interactions, as the speech signal may be degraded and inconsistent, even for children who have hearing aids. Background noise including television is one factor that reduces opportunity for word learning. Children with hearing loss benefit from reduced exposure to television viewing and television background noise. Conversational interactions with high word counts result in the strongest language outcomes for these children (Ambrose, VanDam, & Moeller, 2012).

- Neonatal Intensive Care Units (NICU) include noises from standard equipment and talking from hospital personnel. But, parent talk with pre-term infants in the Neonatal Intensive Care Unit is associated with increases in infant vocalizations at 32 and 36 weeks, suggesting the value of encouraging parent talk for high-risk infants in this setting (Caskey, et. Al., 2011).
- Parent education is an important endeavor to promote a strong linguistic environment for infants and toddlers. Researchers showed that a one-time intervention for parents that included feedback about their LENA data and ways to improve the parent-child interactions had a positive effect on the adult's language output during follow-up measures. Thus, data can be used directly with parents to teach them to increase their interactions (Suskind et al., 2013).

The mounting research findings are important not only for parents but also for professionals who will plan intervention programs for these children. They need to consider goals that involve both the parents and their children so that talking becomes a focus of the intervention program.

We have seen that children benefit from the amount of talking parents engage in with their infants and toddlers, and that the quality of the talking is important to provide the best language outcomes in children. As the LENA database continues to expand and further analysis is conducted, exciting implications arise from such language development studies. We now know much more about the interactions parents have with their children than we did after

Figure 4.11   Children with Autism Engage in Fewer CTs with Adults

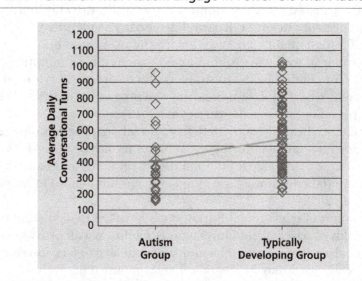

Source: From *The Power of Talk* (2nd ed., p. 25) by J. Gilkerson and J. A. Richards. Copyright 2008 by the Lena Foundation. Reprinted with permission.

Figure 4.12   Uses of the LENA Foundation Data

- Educational and counseling programming for young parents and parents of children who have suspected or known language disabilities
- Educational programming for providers of early childhood child care
- Educational programming for professionals in early childhood education, special education, and related services
- Early intervention for parents of children who have suspected or known language disabilities
- Use of the LENA System with parents and children in early language intervention to increase AWC, CTs, and CVs
- Publications that urge local, state, and federal public policy makers to promote early childhood language development
- Further research to explore the language trends and relationships for children with known language disabilities and the impact of early intervention

---

Hart and Risley's 1995 study. We know how much parents talk and how much children respond. We know that there is great variability in parent talk, but we also know that parents tend to be either high or low talkers and that this pattern influences how talkative their children become. We now understand that there are peak talking times and low talking times during the day, and this trend is evident across both Spanish-speaking and English-speaking families. Most importantly, it is evident that talking plays a critical role in the development of language, especially during the first three years. We also know that children with autism and children with hearing loss require specialized input from parents in the home and teachers in early childhood settings. With the knowledge of these outcomes, some implications for education, early intervention, public policy, and further research are highlighted in Figure 4.12.

The Hart and Risley (1995) study estimated that their professional parents used a mean of 30,137 words per day in talking to their children. The LENA Foundation study resulted in an estimate of 20,824 words. It is noteworthy that the difference between these estimates is due to very different data collection procedures. Hart and Risley collected 1-hour samples in one afternoon each month, whereas the LENA Foundation collected 12-hour continuous samples each month. No matter what data set is used to estimate language input from parents, the number of words provided by talkative parents per day is truly impressive, providing us with valuable information about how much talking is needed for children to acquire strong language and learning skills.

Check Your Understanding 4.4

Assess your understanding of child-directed speech by completing this brief quiz.

Ready for Language: Infants' Early Comprehension and Expression

The remarkable process of language development occurs when the communicative environment is rich and positive. The interactions that develop as parents and children go about their daily routines are sufficient for language to flourish in most children. Most adults recognize the first birthday as a milestone for first words, but so much is happening regarding language development prior to the child's first use of words that we must take a look at the way in which children come to understand words spoken by those around them.

Perception and Comprehension of Words

Most babies are equipped with good hearing acuity. In fact, it is estimated that only 1 to 6 per 1,000 babies are born with hearing loss (Task Force on Newborn and Infant Hearing, 1999). The ability to hear provides the infant with the opportunity to receive and perceive speech from others, a critical ingredient in learning words. As children hear auditory information, speech and language development depends on the formation of auditory patterns (Owens, 2005) through the ability to:

- Attend specifically to speech
- Discriminate the difference between speech sounds
- Detect and generalize regular patterns in the speech of others
- Store and remember the sequence of speech sounds in words
- Discriminate between words
- Compare words to a model stored in memory
- Make discriminations among intonation patterns

These abilities provide a framework for discussion of speech perception, an essential component in the process of language development. You may recognize the first two of these skills from the previous chapter. The infant not only can make gross discriminations among sounds relative to the direction of the sounds' source, pitch, loudness, and duration, but also seems to have a special and discriminating interest in speech and the human voice.

Sounds are arranged in various combinations in all the languages of the world. In fact, each language has its own collection of individual sounds, but more importantly, each language is governed by rules that allow for permissible arrangements of sounds. Such **phonotactic** rules specify which sounds can occur in a sequence. For example, you can easily think of English words that begin with the consonants *st* or *r*. But can you think of words that begin with *nd* or *lr*? Only certain consonants or combinations of consonants are acceptable in English at the beginning of words. We also have rules that govern English syllables. We can combine consonants (C) and vowels (V) in many ways. It is easy to recall examples of both simple and complex syllable structures in words, such as CVC (*bug*), CCCVC (*scream*), and CVCC (*farm,*). But, there are limits to these combinations. Each syllable is allowed only one vowel sound, and consonant sound combinations never exceed three in a row. Youngsters, who are

exposed to verbal language in the context of everyday interactions, hear these sound and syllable patterns over and over again. They also hear and respond to the intonation patterns of the native language. Their auditory systems help them receive, perceive, and store this linguistic information for interpretation and then retrieve the codes as they learn to express speech and language.

We refer often to the importance of the language input that parents provide to their developing infants. They speak about the people, objects, and events of their homes using words and sentences. Thus, during the first year, infants are awash in language from others. They have the impressive task of learning what family members mean as they speak about their surroundings. How do children learn the meaning of words from all this talk? Recall that, earlier, we reported that talkative families use a hefty 20,000 words per day. How do infants in their first year sort out the sounds, syllables, intonation patterns, and words to understand the meaning of even a few words and then continue to learn meanings at a rapid pace during their second year? The process whereby children hear and understand words is called **fast mapping**. Let's look specifically at this concept in relation to word learning.

The typical toddler accrues a vocabulary (lexicon) of more than 500 words before the age of 3 years (Fenson et al., 1994), and he does so without direct teaching of the words. Fast mapping has been observed as early as 9 months of age (Jusczyk & Hohne, 1997; Kay-Raining Bird & Chapman, 1998; Schafer & Plunkett, 1998; Woodward, Markham & Fitzsimmons, 1994); however, retention of words in long-term memory after a 5-minute delay is still rather poor in 24-month-old toddlers (Horst & Samuelson, 2008). The process of word comprehension has been explained as a series of steps that involves accessing information the child has previously stored in memory (Figure 4.13). What are these steps in word learning? To comprehend the meaning of a word, the child begins with hearing the word (auditory cue) that activates his memory about the sounds and syllables of the word (phonological representation) stored previously. Activation then spreads from the phonological level to the word meaning (semantic) level, where, given sufficient activation of the associated concept, the word is comprehended (Gershkoff-Stowe & Hahn, 2007; Stemberger, 1989; Swingley, 2010).

It is likely that beginning word learners do not have strong phonological representations, because these memories develop with experience in hearing

Figure 4.13 Steps in Word Learning

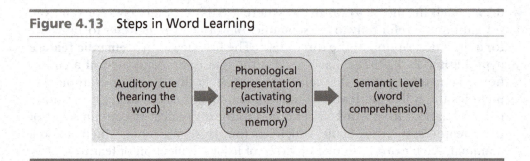

many words. You might relate to this whenever you hear a new word as you continue your studies. "Will you spell that, please?" is the cue that I get when students are not quite sure what they just heard. Thus, when the child hears the word, there is low-level activation of the phonological information and high-level activation at the semantic level. You have probably observed a parent spending considerable time and effort pointing, naming, demonstrating, and talking about an object with her child, but little time saying each consonant and vowel carefully for the child. Imagine that a parent is introducing a new food to her child. The child hears the parent say *applesauce* but then sees it and tastes it in a highly interactive and positive context. The child just learning about this new item does not have a match of this word already stored, so the semantic information (sweet, creamy, and good) is likely to prevail.

For a beginning word learner, hearing a particular word provides a temporary boost to the initially low level of activation associated with the proper phonological unit (the sounds in the word). This activation spreads to the semantic level (word meaning), where the more highly activated concept needs only a small contribution from the phonological level to become available for access. As children expand their lexicon with age and experience, improved access to phonological information occurs; thus, activation of the phonological codes becomes similar in strength to activation of semantic information. So, returning to our example about applesauce, when the child hears it, he is able to make a match from his memory of hearing that word numerous times. His phonological representation is activated along with the word meaning.

Fast mapping has been associated with the large vocabulary spurt that children achieve at about two years of age. It is also interesting to note that not all types of words are easily fast-mapped. Words that occur often in the language used at home and in other familiar places are processed faster and are less susceptible to error than low-use words (Dell, 1990; Stemberger & MacWhinney, 1986). In addition, words that are similar in phonetic and syllable structure are considered to be from high-density phonological neighborhoods, such as the words *floor, door, store,* and *more.* Essentially, children learn words that sound similar to each other. Words that are highly dissimilar (low density) are not learned as easily, such as *aluminum* and *celebrity.* Another factor in the ease of word learning is the meaning relationship words have to other words (Levelt, 1989). Thus, children learn items in a category easily, such as names of fruit, because they share an aspect of meaning.

There is not complete agreement among language experts about how children attach meanings to words, but there are three other views for our consideration that refer only to the semantics of word learning. Refer to Table 4.2 for a brief description of the three views. The first view is the **semantic feature hypothesis** (Clark, 1975). Each word is thought to be composed of a collection of semantic features that carry meaning about the word. For example, *dog* includes the following features: animal, mammal, furry, four legs, wet nose, tail, and barks. Other words that are not in the dog category contain some of these features, such as a table, which has four legs, or a zebra, which is also a mammal. Each word is unique by virtue of its own collection of features. Only

Table 4.2   Learning Word Meanings: Three Perspectives

Semantic Feature Hypothesis (Clark, 1973)	Each word has its own set of semantic features that distinguishes it from other words. Features are perceptual characteristics such as shape and size (e.g., *dog* = furry, four legs, tail, barks).
Functional Core Hypothesis (Nelson, 1974)	Early word meanings are learned primarily on the basis of the function of objects (e.g., broom-sweep, dog-bark).
Prototype Hypothesis (Bowerman, 1978)	Early word meanings are based on experiences with the object the word represents. This experience forms a model (prototype) against which the child can compare other words and the objects or actions they represent (e.g., furniture- sofa, chair, bed).

dog includes all the semantic features of a dog, and it is that particular set of features that separates "dogness" from other meanings, such as "catness, pigness," or other words that share some but not all of the semantic features.

Nelson (1974) proposed the **functional core hypothesis** to explain the acquisition of word meaning. Rather than a child categorizing things according to perceptual attributes, such as size and shape, Nelson argued that meanings of early words are based on their actions if they are animate objects or on the actions performed on them if they are inanimate objects. Recall that Piaget explained early cognitive development in the sensorimotor phase as being based on the child's sensory contacts with objects and on his manipulation of these objects. The idea here is that the concept of *ball* will be learned through observation and interaction of the ball with human actions (throwing, catching, rolling, bouncing, and even spinning) and with other objects, such as hands, a bat, the basketball hoop, and glass objects that break.

The third view of the acquisition of word meanings, offered by Bowerman (1978), combines the best of the other two hypotheses. In the **prototype hypothesis**, Bowerman contends that the child relies on both perceptual features and functions of words. A prototype can be best understood as a model or standard. Thus, the model for *dog* will likely be a cocker spaniel rather than a Chihuahua because a cocker spaniel is more doglike in size than a Chihuahua. The prototype for *chair* will likely be the usual four-legged variety, not the bean bag chair in the family room. The closer an object comes to matching the child's prototype for a given concept, the more likely she is to learn the name for that concept. Any new object or activity will be included in the concept, depending on how close it comes to fitting the prototype.

Whatever the mechanism used to learn the meaning of words initially through fast mapping, the child's initial understanding of a concept will be fairly narrow. Through experiences with the word in multiple contexts, meanings become expanded and refined. The process of expanding and fine-tuning word meanings is called **slow mapping** or **extended mapping** (Swingley, 2010).

It is a lengthy process that spans many years as words are acquired and the relationship between words develops along with cognition and linguistic attainments. We will explore vocabulary growth further in the next two chapters.

Prelinguistic Vocalizations: Sounds of Distress, Comfort, and Pleasure

Now we will turn our attention to how infants express themselves vocally and verbally from birth through the development of words. Like other aspects of development, prelinguistic vocalizations by babies occur in a predictable sequence across the first year. Table 4.3 lists and describes the attainments that characterize this period.

The first sounds the infant makes, including her first cries, are reflexive. In addition to crying, she also burps, sneezes, and coughs. These noises are sometimes called *vegetative* sounds to indicate that they are natural sounds made by a passive but living organism. At first, infant cries are undifferentiated, but, by the end of the first month, caregivers can usually differentiate among several basic cries (Wolff, 1969) to indicate hunger, pain, and anger. The unpleasant sounds that include loud, piercing wails, shrieking, or whimpers bring caregivers to the rescue. By the time the infant is two months old, caregivers notice that crying behaviors are decreasing in frequency, but cries become even more differentiated to include discomfort, calling, and requesting (D'Odorico, 1984).

The most positive change occurring at this time is the emergence of sounds communicating pleasure and comfort. By two months, the infant is cooing. **Cooing** involves the production of vowel-like sounds, but there may also be brief consonant-like sounds resembling *k* or *g*, and they often occur when the caregiver smiles during gaze coupling and says something such as, "Aren't you a sweetheart." The infant responds with, "C-o-o-o-u-u-u-u," and the caregiver

Table 4.3 Typical Development of Prelinguistic Vocalizations

Approximate Age Range	Vocalizations
0–1 month	• Reflexive cries, vegetative sounds
1–4 months	• Cooing (vowel-like sounds), differentiated crying (hunger, pain, etc.)
4–6 months	• Transitional or marginal babbling: single-syllable productions of vowel- and consonant-like sounds
6–8 months	• Reduplicated babbling (productions of the same syllable— e.g., "babababa")
8–12 months	• Echolalia (imitation of sounds and syllables—continues beyond 12 months) • Variegated babbling (changes in consonant/vowel combinations—e.g., "dadu") • Jargon babbling (intonational changes added to syllable productions to give impression of sentence-like behavior) • Vocables or protowords (productions unique to each child)

imitates the coo. This cooing-imitation-cooing exchange can sometimes continue for 15 minutes or longer, and most adults find it as delightful a communication experience as the infant. The child at four months is not only cooing but also laughing (Stark, 1979). How can you resist responding to a laughing baby?

To this point, we have emphasized the importance of *reception* in the infant's earliest communication experiences, and we have addressed the importance of infant-caregiver interaction.

Transitional and True Babbling

According to Stark (1979) and Sachs (1989), true babbling does not begin until the child is six months of age or older. Beginning at about five months, however, the infant is producing vocalizations that seem to bridge cooing and true babbling. These are single-syllable productions consisting of vowel- and consonant-like sounds, and we can think of them as transitional behaviors that extend beyond cooing and prepare the way for babbling. Stark refers to these sequences as "marginal babbling."

We traditionally use the term *babbling* to describe repeated consonant–vowel (CV) syllables, such as "mamama" or "nanana," productions that tend to appear at about six or seven months. The more specific term for this kind of production is **reduplicated babbling**. According to Stark, Bernstein, and Demorest (1993), reduplicated babbling occurs most often when the infant is investigating the environment or holding an object. The consonants most frequently incorporated into these utterances are produced at the front of the mouth—for example, *m, p, b, t, d,* and *n.* Some of the intonation contours the infant produced during cooing have disappeared (Stark, 1979), but the production of consonants suggests an increasing maturity in the child's control of the speech mechanism.

Whereas cooing is often elicited by social interaction between the infant and caregiver, the infant will often babble most when she is by herself (Nakazima, 1975; Stark, 1981). Many researchers and writers have observed that during babbling, the infant produces a wide variety of sounds, many of which are not included in the sound system of her native language. Ferguson (1978) suggests that the sounds the child produces are largely the product of the limitations of her speech mechanism. As the structures of speech mature physiologically and as the infant becomes more absorbed in the sounds of her own language, her babbling more closely resembles her native language (Rees, 1972).

In addition to babbling, the infant between 8 and 12 months produces an interesting behavior called *echolalia.* Echolalia is the immediate, parrot-like imitation of sounds, syllables, or words produced by someone else. The term *parrot-like* suggests that the infant does not understand what he is saying even though his imitations may be fairly accurate. If for no other reason, this behavior is important because it represents a change in the nature of imitation in speech and language development. In the cooing stage, communication is maintained when the caregiver imitates the infant. In echolalia, the infant imitates the caregiver. In the months and years to come, the child's imitations of the speech models he hears become increasingly important in terms of acquiring the sound system, vocabulary, and structure of his language.

During true babbling, the infant's productions become more heavily dependent on self-hearing. For this reason, infants who are deaf sound very much like children who hear until they reach this point. Infants who are deaf cry, laugh, coo, and produce some marginal babbling, but they begin to restrict their output and use fewer consonant sounds than infants who hear at about eight months of age (Oller, Eilers, Bull, & Carney, 1985; Stoel-Gammon & Otomo, 1986). This paucity of sound play can have a potential long-term effect on expressive language development in children who are deaf or hard of hearing. However, as indicated earlier, infants who are deaf and hearing infants whose parents are deaf have been observed to use their hands to mimic gestures used in sign language. Thus, they babble through the use of hand movements (Petitto, Holowka, Sergio, & Ostry, 2001). This activity is important and useful as they learn these foundations for sign language communication.

Variegated Babbling and Jargon

Beginning at about 9 months and continuing through 18 months, the nature of babbling changes in the sense that it becomes more varied within a single utterance. Instead of simply repeating the same syllable she repeated in the earlier stage, the child now produces successive syllables that differ from one another, as in "madagaba." This more advanced babbling is known as **variegated babbling**. Stark (1986) found that some variegated babbling productions are consonant-vowel-consonant (CVC) combinations, in which the consonant is replicated, and vowel-consonant-vowel (VCV) combinations, in which the vowel is replicated. That is, the child might say "Gug" (CVC) or "Ugu" (VCV). As the name suggests, variegated babbling is characterized by a wider range of sounds, especially consonants, than reduplicated babbling. It should be noted that not all researchers are convinced that the variegated babbling period necessarily follows the reduplicated babbling period (Mitchell & Kent, 1990), but there is a certain logical appeal to the progression.

The seven- or eight-month-old infant attends to the intonation contours of adult speech. It makes sense then that, as he continues to experiment with sounds and sound combinations, he begins to incorporate intonation contours into his vocalizations, producing what is called **jargon babbling**. Jargon babbling productions are distinguished by melodic patterns. In fact, this form of babbling has many of the characteristics of real speech. If you attend just to the melody of jargon babbling utterances, they sound adult-like. The child produces the rhythm, stresses, rate variations, and intonation contours of his language, even though he produces few, if any, meaningful words.

Jargon babbling is to speech as humming or "la-la-laing" is to singing when we do not know or cannot remember the lyrics. When the child produces these vocalizations, adult listeners hear what they believe are questions, commands, expressions of joy, statements of concern, and virtually every kind of communication imaginable. The son of a friend in graduate school was particularly proficient in jargon babbling. His father was a great storyteller. The son would "tell stories" in jargon babbling—some "funny," as evidenced by his laughter, and some "serious," as reflected by the tone of his voice and the look on his face—using the same speech melodies used by his father. These vocalizations were delightfully entertaining, and, if the truth be told, many of the son's stories were better than the father's!

 Video Example 4.4

Children use variegated babbling and jargon during purposeful activities. In the video, you will notice that the 1-year-old child is having a pretend conversation on the telephone, complete with the intonation of his native language.

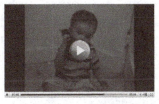

Although jargon babbling is interesting and clearly indicates that the child is paying attention to and imitating the melodic characteristics of adult speech, it is not language. Early in this same 9- to 18-month period, however, evidence suggests that the child is moving from prelinguistic communication to language. The child will not produce her first conventional words until she is about 12 months old, but by the time she is 9 or 10 months old, she may be producing what are called **vocables**. Other terms include *phonetically consistent forms, performatives,* or *protowords*. All of these terms refer to productions, unique to a given child, that are consistent patterns of sounds used in reference to particular things or situations. A child may produce the sound "e-e-e" to signal that he wants an object, and "u-u-u" to signal disapproval. These are not words, of course, but they represent an important transition from vocal play and babbling, vocalizations that are random and devoid of specific meaning, to productions that are purposive, consistent, and meaningful. Carter's (1975) analysis of vocables in one child suggests that there may be a fairly direct connection between some vocables and corresponding true words. She found, for example, that vocables beginning with *m*, accompanied by a gesture to indicate "I want," gradually evolved into the words *more, my,* and *mine*. Some evidence suggests that vocables are present in children's productions, no matter which language they are acquiring (Blake & deBoysson-Bardies, 1992). See Table 4.3 for a summary of prevocalizations.

Using Communication to Get Things Done

It is clear that parents establish meaningful connections with their baby right from the start as they anticipate and interpret what she needs without any conscious participation from the baby. The time between birth and about eight months of age is known as the **perlocutionary stage**, indicating that the infant is responding in a reflexive manner to her environment. At the end of this stage, she is just beginning to use gestures to demonstrate goal-directed behaviors described in substage 3 of Piaget's sensorimotor period. It doesn't take long, however, for infants to begin responding and initiating interactions with their parents. Because it takes time for them to develop knowledge and production of words, gestures serve as the way for babies to respond to the language used by parents and to initiate interactions with them. The use of gestures occurs from about 8 to 12 months, a period known as the **illocutionary stage**. During this stage, babies combine gestures with vocalizations to express a range of specific and recognizable communicative functions. We will focus on the development of intentionality through the use of imitation and pointing to show the advances in how infants participate in conversations with caregivers. These attainments set the stage for the beginnings of expressive language development known as the **locutionary stage**, when the child is beyond her first birthday and producing her first words. Figure 4.14 depicts the stages of the speech act (Austin, 1962; Searle, 1969).

Intentionality

A longitudinal study of 12 children from 6 to 24 months of age (Crais, Douglas, & Campbell, 2004) mapped the development of gestures used to signal intent. The purpose of the study was to document early indicators of intentionality, thus providing information about early communication skills in prelinguistic and linguistic infants and toddlers. **Deictic gestures** call attention to or indicate an object or event (similar to the phrase, "It is right here!"). As we discussed early in this chapter, infants use eye gaze to direct the attention of caregivers at around 8 months of age and use it to alter the behavior of caregivers by 12 months. Other gestures, such as reaching, pushing away, giving an object, pointing, waving, and showing can be made with or without eye contact and occur between 8 and 11 months.

Representational gestures signify some features of an object or its function, such as pretending to eat with a spoon, or they can be social in nature, such as waving good-bye. Representational gestures are often seen in infants by about one year. The developmental hierarchy of gestural development used to regulate others' behavior spans, on average, 5.5 months (looking and vocalizing) to 14.5 months (uses a word), with a lot of reaching and pointing in between. Behaviors for social interaction emerge between 6.5 months (shows interest)

Figure 4.14   Development of the Three Stages of a Speech Act

Development	
Birth	{ Perlocution
8 Months	{ Perlocution Illocution
12 Months+	{ Perlocution Illocution Locution

Source: Based on *Introduction to Language Development,* by S. McLaughlin, 1998, San Diego, CA: Singular Publishing Group.

and 1.5 years (excitement gestures), including waving, clapping, imitation of social games, dancing, and pretending to sleep. Infants between seven months and one-and-a-half years use behaviors to gain joint attention that includes looking, showing, giving, pointing, using words with rising intonation, and using gestures to clarify words. The authors stress that gestural behaviors emerge in an overlapping function, and they provide a way to assess the emergence of intentionality in infants. This information can be useful to parents and clinicians, especially when a child is suspected of having delays in learning. Gestural development can assist professionals in distinguishing between children who have symbol formation deficits and those who have deficits in language and thus provide developmental targets for intervention (Crais et al., 2004).

Imitation

The ability of infants to imitate has been used to assess infants' awareness of the mental state of others (Meltzoff, 1995), because reproducing a behavior requires an understanding of the intention of the person performing the action. Imitation has also been studied to examine age-related changes in long-term retention. Researchers have uncovered a developmental sequence to imitation that reflects infants' acquisition of the understanding of another person's goal (Legerstee & Markova, 2008) and their ability to use trace memory and to generalize what they learn (Herbert, Gross, & Hayne, 2006):

- First six months—imitates bodily movements, including facial gestures (e.g., smile), shortly after birth
- Six to nine months—imitates simple actions of the model on objects (e.g., bang spoon on tray)
- 9 months—imitates target action when tested after a 24-hour delay (deferred imitation; e.g., bang spoon on tray after delay)
- 10 months—completes the actions of the model in an unsuccessful action demonstration (e.g., roll ball but not successfully)
- 9 to 12 months—produces novel and combined action sequences (e.g., peekaboo)

Pointing

By the time infants have reached their first year, pointing becomes a way to interact further with people, things, and events in the infants' surroundings. There is some debate as to whether pointing at this age shows communicative intent or whether it is for the self only. Bates, Camaioni, and Volterra (1975) argued that when infants point without looking at their partner, communicative intent is absent. But, this interpretation has been challenged by others who show that infants point differentially as a function of different adult responses (Liszkowski, Carpenter, Henning, Striano, & Tomasello, 2004; Liszkowski, Carpenter, & Tomasello, 2007). Liszkowski, Albrecht, Carpenter, and Tomasello (2008) took this idea one step further to show that adult behavior does appear to influence pointing: one-year-old infants tailored their gestures to adults' visual availability. Infants pointed more when the adult was looking at them than when the adult was not visually available. They also repeated their pointing

Table 4.4   Early Communicative Functions

Function (Definition)	Example
*Instrumental** (to have needs and wants satisfied)	"Uh-uh-uh" while pointing at a refrigerator to get food or drink
Regulatory (to control the behaviors of other people)	"Kuh-kuh" while moving the caregiver's hands together to suggest the continuation of patty-cake
Interactional (to establish or maintain interpersonal contact)	"Muh-muh" while holding the caregiver's face to maintain attention on an object of shared interest
Personal (to express an emotion, interest, or attitude)	"Ga-ga" in angry tones while playing with a toy the child cannot manipulate properly

*The italicized terms are used by Halliday (1975).

when their communicative intent was not satisfied. In addition, when the adults did not respond, infants accompanied their pointing with vocalizations.

The ability to convey intentions through gestures opens up many possibilities for prelinguistic children to communicate in social situations. They learn quickly that what they do has immediate effects on other people. Thus, infants develop functional use of their gestures. Halliday (1975) concluded that his son Nigel, between the ages of 9 and 16 months, produced a number of non-linguistic utterances to convey four identifiable communicative intents: satisfy his wants and needs, control the behavior of others, interact with others, and express an emotion or interest (Table 4.4).

Bates (1979) used the term **protodeclaratives** to describe when a child points to the objects or events of focus (joint attention) by the child and adult. For example, a child might point to a cow only to establish that it is a fascinating creature, as if to say, "Hey, Mom, look at that big thing standing over there with a multifingered bubble on its belly!" Bates used the term **protoimperative** in reference to gestures used by the child to control or manipulate the behaviors of others. The child who points to indicate his desire for the milk bottle on the counter, or the child who vigorously shakes his head to indicate that he doesn't want to eat more strained peas, is using a protoimperative. They function like commands, such as, "Give me the milk" and, "Take those peas away."

In summary, children acquire the ability to use nonverbal behaviors and vocalizations with specific communication intentions as a result of their overall biological maturation, cognitive development, and social interaction with caregivers. They have a large repertoire of ways to get their wants, needs, and thoughts addressed.

Check Your Understanding 4.5

Assess your understanding of early comprehension and expressive language attainments by completing this brief quiz.

Beyond Infancy: The Emergence of First Words

The first birthday marks many accomplishments in development. It is often the time that children begin to walk, having spent many months mastering sitting unsupported, creeping and crawling, balancing on both feet, and taking first steps with much falling down and getting up to try again. This very active time is filled with laughter, wonder, lots of energy devoted to achieving that next skill, and a healthy share of frustration. Children are very expressive as they go about the development process, using a combination of gestures, vocalizations, and early forms of words in delightful combinations. Not coincidentally, the first words also emerge somewhere between 11 and 14 months, usually close to the first birthday and the development of walking. Note that children already know the meaning of many words used by familiar people in everyday environments. It is the use of these familiar words that we focus on now.

First Words

What kinds of words do children use at the one-word utterance stage? The child's first words are used in reference to things that matter most in her own world. She names people, objects, and actions that are of immediate interest. Think of your own household and imagine a one-year-old child in your midst. What names would she say? What objects will she be allowed to play with and encounter as she learns to walk around her bedroom, the living area, the bathroom, and the kitchen? Some possibilities include her teddy bear, blocks, a favorite blanket, a picture book, the couch, a throw blanket, her bottle, and a cookie. Children also use social greetings, such as, "hi" and, "bye-bye" or request simple actions, such as, "night-night" or, "up." Some words may not contain all of the sounds that are in the adult version. For example, "ba-ba" may be the form used for "bottle." In fact, most of the child's first words consist of one syllable ("up"), two syllables ("doggie"), or one repeated syllable ("wawa"). The words have very limited phonetic forms comprised of simple consonant/vowel combinations. Typical combinations include CV (*no*), VC (*eat*), and CVCV syllables (*mama*); however, CVC (*hot*) combinations are rare at this age because the final consonant is often omitted as a simplified strategy for word production (Owens, 2005). There are only a few consonants and vowels that children say during the first-word stage. The number of sounds and their arrangements expand across time and with experience.

Because the process of adding new words takes time, it makes sense that children in the first-word stage must use the same words to express many different meanings. One child we knew, for example, used the word "go-go" in reference to a wide range of motions, but she also used it to refer to cars, trucks, and other objects that moved. She might use the word "hot" as a noun in reference to a flame on the stove before she uses it as an adjective referring to the temperature of the object.

In our discussion of a child's cognitive development in Chapter 3, we described the processes of assimilation and accommodation. We can see the child's application of these processes in his first words. At first, the child might use "doggie" to refer to the family pet. As he sees other four-legged animals, such as horses, cows, and goats, on a family outing, he may apply his knowledge by naming them "doggie." This **overextension** of the word is a common characteristic in the language of young children.

Of course, children also are observed to be too narrow—**underextended**—in their use of a word. A child who uses the word *book* for the large, glossy book about Peter Rabbit may not prefer to use that word to refer to other literature in the family library. The child might ask for "Barney" as an example. As children sort out what should be assimilated and then accommodate when new schemata are needed, they define and apply words more accurately to adult usage.

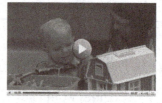

Video Reflection 4.1: Parent-Son Interaction at 19 Months

Watch the video of a parent interacting with her 19-month-old son, Sam, and then answer the questions. Sam is just beginning to acquire spoken words.

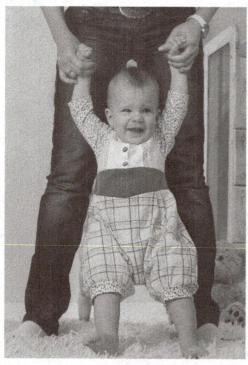

Walking and talking present many challenges.

Source: Leonid & Anna Dedukh/Fotolia.

Classifying the Child's First Words

In order to talk about how first words function for children, let's take a look at a language sample of Patrick at one year of age in Figure 4.15. In this exchange there is a combination of single words (*doggie, peas, yeah, whatsat, baby,* and *wow*), babbling, jargon, and sound effects of joy, as well as a little bit of whining. This overlap is quite common at the single-word stage. There is certainly no silence, and Patrick makes the most of lunch, as he is highly aware of the animals and people around him for social interaction.

It is tempting to ignore the non-linguistic utterances (babbling, shrieking, whining) in this sample and focus only on real words, classifying each word according to traditional grammatical categories. If we limited ourselves in this way, we could say that Patrick is using a few nouns and only one question form. Looking more carefully, however, we will discover that non-linguistic utterances and first words do not always fit into adult categories. It is important to consider the context in which these utterances occur and the function of all utterances, even those that are not true words. For example, when Patrick points and says "doggie,"

Figure 4.15   Patrick's Communicative Functions at 1 Year

ECF: Early Communicative Functions (Halliday, 1975)
CF: Communicative Functions (Halliday, 1975)
PSA: Primitive Speech Acts (Dore, 1975)

Utterance	Function
K*: Patrick, what do you have?	
K: Where's doggie?	
K: You like those grapes. Where's doggie?	
P: Doggie ("dodi")	ECF/CF: Interacting
K: Where's doggie?	
P: Points and whines	ECF: Personal
K: You want more grapes? How about more peas? Try it. Oh yum.	
P: Peas	CF: Instrumental
K: You want more peas? Here they come? Oh, good job.	
P: Points and says "dodi"	PSA: Labeling
K: (Points) Where are the doggies? They're outside. Here are more peas.	
P: Ahheee, e, o	ECF: Personal
P: Doggies ("dodi")	PSA: Labeling
K: Is that your Cheerios? Peas, ready? Good job.	
K: They're barking? Who's barking?	
P: Doggies, doggies, doggies, doggies ("dodis, dodis, dodis, dodis!")	ECF/CF: Interacting
K: Bubbles. You made bubbles. (Laughing)	
P: "Brrrr"	ECF/CF: Personal
K: A Cheerio there.	
P: babbling ("a, a-e, ya, ya, ya")	ECF/CF: Personal
K: Are you done with these peas already? Do you want another bite? Oh yea, good job.	
P: babbling ("oo, ah")	ECF/CF: Personal
K: Here's your Cheerio.	
K: What's that in there? Do you have water in your bottle?	
P: "yeah"	PSA: Answering
K: Where did it go? Did you hide your cup?	
P: screech	ECF/CF: Personal
K: Here's your cup. Did you hide your cup? Where did it go?	
P: screech	ECF/CF: Personal
K: Want me to get it? Here it comes. Yeah, here it is!	
P: babble ("dadada")	ECF/CF: Interacting
P: Whasat?	PSA: Requesting answer
P: Doggie ("dodi!")	PSA: Greeting
K: Yes, that's a doggie.	
P: babble ("dawea")	ECF/CF: Interacting
K: That's a blue one.	

(continued)

Figure 4.15 Continued

K: Are you tired?	
P: Ah! Ah! Ah! Ah! Ah!	ECF/CF: Personal
K: Patrick? Patrick	
P: babble ("be, ba, ah, ah, oo, ee, ee-oo")	ECF/CF: Personal
P: babble ("e-a, e-a, boo, boo, boo, boo, boo")	ECF/CF: Personal
P: babble ("boo, da, da, ah")	ECF/CF: Personal
K: Alright. Hah—give me that spoon back. Give me that spoon. (Laughing) That's it. Good job. You're getting a lot for lunch.	
P: Ahhhh (whining)	PSA: Protesting
	ECF: Personal
K: I know. Give me that spoon. Is that a new thing to bite your spoon. I got it! I got it!	
P: Ah (whining)	PSA: Protesting
	ECF: Personal
K: I got it (laughing)	
P: Ah! Ah! (screech)	ECF: Personal
K: Are you all done?	
P: Ah!	PSA: Protesting
	ECF: Personal
K: No, here.	
K: What happened? What happened to the blue cup? Here it is.	
P: Ah! Ah! Ah! (whining)	PSA: Protesting
	ECF: Personal
K: Wow, that's a lot of water.	
P: Baby! Baby!	CF: Interacting
P: Wow! Wowee!	ECF: Personal

*Kathleen Fahey

---

he may mean several things, depending on what is happening. Here are some potential meanings:

- That is a doggie.
- Come here, doggie. (or go away)
- I like/don't like the doggie.
- The doggie ate the food I dropped.
- That doggie is different from the other doggie.
- Here is another doggie.

Patrick is using only one word, but he is conveying several different messages. One way to classify non-linguistic utterances and single-word utterances is, therefore, by function. Recall that Halliday (1975) developed a taxonomy for classifying communicative functions based on his interactions with his son Nigel from 9 to 16 months. His initial four categories allowed the assignment

Table 4.5 Halliday's Communicative Functions

Function	Explanation	Example
Interacting	Using language to maintain contact with others	Child says, "Mama," while mother is in the room; comparable to Dore's categories of *greeting* and *calling*.
Regulatory	Using language to control the behavior of others	Child says, "Ball," in an attempt to have his mother give him the object; comparable to Dore's category of *requesting an action*.
Personal	Using language to express emotions or interest	Child says, "Whee!" as she plays with toy; comparable to Dore's category of *protesting*.
Heuristic	Using language to explore and categorize	Child sees a new toy and asks "Doggie?"; comparable to Dore's category of *requesting an answer*.
Instrumental	Using language to satisfy needs and wants	Child says, "Milk," in an effort to obtain a drink; comparable to Dore's category of *requesting an action*.
Imagine (pretend)	Using language to accompany play activity	Child says, "Up," as he puts a doll in a chair.
Informative	Using language to share knowledge with others	Child points to daddy's eye and says, "Eye"; comparable to Dore's category of *labeling*.

Source: Based on Halliday (1975).

of meaning to non-linguistic utterances (Table 4.4). He expanded this list to capture the functions of his son's single words (Table 4.5). As we can see, children express their intentions through both the illocutionary and locutionary stages in a variety of important ways. Halliday's interpretation of early communicative intents takes into account the reactions of listeners. His categories of functions are based on how well the child's communication attempts work to accomplish specified purposes.

At the same time that Halliday was documenting and classifying Nigel's communicative functions, Dore (1974, 1975) was describing communicative functions from the point of view of the child. That is, what are the child's intentions and reasons for communicating, regardless of whether they work or do not work from the listener's perspective? Dore called the single-word stage (12 to 18 months) **primitive speech acts** (PSAs). As seen in Table 4.6, a PSA might be a word, a change in prosodic pattern, or a gesture. Dore found that children could use these communication skills to label objects or events, to answer questions, to request an action or answer, to address a person or thing, to greet someone, to protest or object, to imitate or repeat, and simply to practice language.

Now let's go back to our sample from Patrick. His few words are conveying much more information than we may have originally thought. Figure 4.15 also includes an analysis of Patrick's utterances based on Halliday's early communicative functions, communicative function of words, and Dore's PSAs.

Table 4.6 Dore's Primitive Speech Acts (PSAs)

The Act	Communicative Purpose	Child's Behavior
Labeling	Identifies an object	Child points to mother's eye and says, "Eye."
Answering	Responds to caregiver's inquiry	Caregiver asks, "What's that?" while pointing to a toy dog. Child says, "Doggie."
Requesting an action	Looks at caregiver; produces a word or a prosodic change; waits for a response	Child says, "Ball," in a manner indicating that the caregiver is being instructed to give him the ball.
Requesting an answer	Asks for information from a caregiver	Child says, "Doggie?" and waits for caregiver to respond and confirm identification.
Calling	Attempts to gain the attention of a caregiver	Child says, "Daddy" in an attempt to gain his attention.
Greeting	Acknowledges a caregiver upon entering a room	Child says, "Daddy," as he enters a room.
Protesting	Rejects an object or action	Child says, "No!" when an attempt is made to give him spinach.
Repeating/ Imitating	Produces at least part of what is said by a caregiver	Dad hits his hand with a hammer and says, "Ouch!" Child responds with, "Ouch!"
Practicing	Produces a word or prosodic pattern without anyone being in the room	Child says, "Ball," while playing with a ball.

Source: Based on Dore (1975), p. 31.

At least eight different functions can be seen in this sample. It is safe to say that Patrick is well on his way to capturing the attention of others and controlling his environment to suit himself!

Words can certainly be categorized in other ways besides function. Bloom (1973) suggested that early words are of two basic types. **Substantive** words refer to objects or events that have perceptual or functional features in common. Words such as *mama, dada,* and *doggie* are substantive. These words refer to things that cause action; thus, they are called **agents**. Words that refer to things receiving action are called **objects**. **Relational** words reflect the child's understanding of object permanence and causality, as they refer to actions or states of being that can affect a variety of categories. For example, Patrick said, "whatsat?" in reference to one of the dogs. He could use that same word to ask about any object. In this case, he immediately provided the answer, but if he didn't, you can be sure that an adult would provide the name for him. Relational words most typically refer to the appearance or disappearance of objects (*allgone*) or to the location of objects. Productions such as *more, no, stop,* and *bye-bye* are common relational words in the early vocabularies of children.

Table 4.7 Categories of the First Fifty Words: The Results of Two Studies

Grammatical Category	Description	Benedict (1979); result as a percentage	Nelson (1973); result as a percentage	Examples
Nominals—specific	Refer to only one thing	11	14	"Casey" referring to the family's pet dog
Nominals—general	Refer to all members of an object category	50	51	*Doggie, girl, boy, cup*
Action words	Describe or demand an action	19	13	*Go, look, run*
Modifiers	Identify qualities or characteristics of things or events	10	9	*Hot, little, mine*
Personal–social	Express emotions or identify relationships	10	8	*No, please*
Functional	Serve a grammatical function	*Note:* Benedict did not include a Functional category.	4	*For, that, this*

Source: Owens (2005), p. 233.

Bloom discovered that when her daughter's speech was confined to single-word productions, she used a limited number of relational words and a much larger number of substantive words, but many of these were not used often and tended to drop out of her vocabulary for weeks or even months. By about 18 months of age, she was no longer dropping substantive words, and her functional vocabulary showed overall growth.

Whereas Bloom's view of early vocabulary is largely semantic in orientation because of her emphasis on the meaning of words, Nelson (1973) interpreted early vocabulary from a grammatical point of view. She placed early words into five categories based on grammatical function: (1) nominals (specific and general); (2) action words; (3) modifiers; (4) personal-social words; and (5) functional words. A brief description of each category is presented in Table 4.7, along with the results of two studies that investigated the percentage of use of each type of word (Benedict, 1979; Nelson, 1973). Notice that nominals were reported most frequently, followed by action words, with modifiers, personal-social, and functional words used less often.

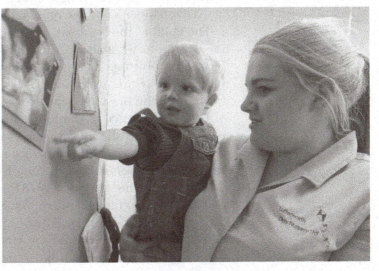

Discovering new things, words, and meanings.

Source: Jules Selmes/Pearson Education, Inc.

Although the early words of children are predominantly nouns (Gentner, 1982; Schwartz & Leonard, 1984), it is also appropriate to note that not all early vocabularies are the same. Horgan (1981) identified some children as "noun lovers" and others as "noun leavers." That is, some children use many nouns and other children use fewer nouns, but English-speaking children use more nouns than other categories of words. Early personality differences may account for the preference of some children to describe and categorize, whereas other children use language for social and personal interactions. Again, it is worth emphasizing that normally developing children do not all follow the same course. Some children acquire their first words earlier than other children, and some children add words to their vocabularies more quickly than other children. Research findings show that girls acquire their first meaningful words earlier and more quickly than boys (Bauer, Goldfield, & Reznick, 2002).

Presuppositions and Conversational Turn Taking

As the child's communicative intentions become more elaborate, the role of the child in speaker/listener relationships becomes more interesting and complex. During the single-word stage, we see evidence of what are called presuppositions. A **presupposition** is an assumption the speaker makes concerning what the listener knows about the subject of the conversation. In a typical communicative exchange, the child will provide information the listener needs and will not comment on what he believes the listener already knows (Greenfield & Smith, 1976). If the child is preparing to push a toy car, for example, he may make the presupposition that the listener knows that the object in his hand is a car. He might comment on what the speaker does not know, which is that he is about to make the car move, so he says, "Go!" while pushing the car across the floor toward Rex, the previously sleeping, now frantic and scurrying family dog. We should keep in mind, of course, that the adult's ability to interpret what the child says is made a little easier because children at this early stage of language development typically talk about the here and now (Greenfield, 1978). Most adults, given even modest communicative assistance from children, are bright enough to figure out communications that focus on what is happening in the present tense in the present place.

The child in the single-word stage is just beginning to develop presuppositional skills. As we shall see, the child at three and four years is still having difficulty with presuppositions that consider the listener's perspective. Although this aspect of communication begins to emerge early, it continues to develop throughout the preschool and school-age years.

There is evidence of communicative turn taking before the child begins to use words, but as she moves from pre-linguistic to linguistic communication, develops specific communicative intentions, and begins to use presuppositions, she begins to develop a turn-taking style more closely resembling adult conversation. By the time the child is 18-months-old, she is demonstrating some of the basic rules of turn taking in her conversations with other people (Bloom, Rocissano, & Hood, 1976). If, for example, the child's conversational partner names an object in the child's possession, the child might make a comment about the object, but she will not repeat the label already identified by her partner. She presupposes this knowledge and uses her turn to describe the object or to explain to her partner what is going to happen next. Her partner might then comment on the action the child has taken, and the child, presupposing knowledge of all that has been said before, uses her turn to contribute additional information or respond directly to her partner's comments. Turn taking, assuming knowledge, and taking into account a partner's perspective are some of the elements of adult-like conversation.

Midstage Review: What Is Happening So Far?

To this point, the child's productions have been mostly single words. Before moving to the combination phase of stage 1, it will be useful to review some of what you have learned so far about the child's earliest language efforts.

The child's first meaningful word appears at about 12 months. By the time he is 18 months old, he will have about 50 words in his expressive vocabulary, and he will understand many more than that. His first words are mostly nouns, but he does use some action words, and he uses a few modifiers such as *big, bad,* or *hot.* These first words refer to things, events, people, and actions that are of personal interest to the child. They may not be adult forms of comparable words, and they are often used with wider or narrower meanings than adult versions of the same words. The child might call a dog a *gaga,* for example. He might produce an adult-like version such as *doggie,* but he might use *doggie* to refer to all four-legged animals, not just dogs, or he might use the word to refer to just one dog, the family pet.

His first words are used for fairly specific purposes: to name objects or people, to request something, to control the behavior of someone else, or to express emotion. Even though he is typically using only one word at a time, he shows some understanding of conversation. In a limited way, he takes into account what his listener knows about a subject and tends not to repeat redundant information. He engages in a turn-taking style of communication that allows for comment and the contributions of new information on the part of both conversational partners. By using basic body language and by varying intonation, the child can indicate that he is asking questions, and he can produce a negative communication by shaking his head or using the word *no,* which is likely to show up in his vocabulary very early.

Although it is true that adults must be fairly active interpreters to determine the semantic and pragmatic messages in the child's speech, this is pretty impressive stuff for a communicator whose utterances are mostly single words. Try to imagine what will happen to the child's communicative abilities when he begins to put words together.

Check Your Understanding 4.6

Assess your knowledge of the development of first words by completing this brief quiz.

Early Syntactic Development: A Stage Model

Thus far, we have been concerned with how one-year-old children learn and then produce their first words, particularly in the framework of functional uses of those words. We will continue this discussion by exploring how children learn to put words together in meaningful ways to suit their communication needs. But first, we will describe a categorical system with which we can track grammatical development. A specific stage model was developed by Roger Brown (1973). Brown's stages are widely used by language experts to describe the development of grammar (syntax). The five major stages (see Table 4.8) provide us with important transition points to consider in language development from one year to five years of age. In this chapter, we are exploring only stage 1. Chapter 5 will afford us the opportunity to continue our journey across the remaining stages.

Brown tracked syntactic development of English by measuring the average number of units of meaning expressed in utterances across a sample of language. What constitutes a unit of meaning? We use the word *morpheme* to describe each unit of meaning. It is best to explain morphemes by using some examples. Single words are counted as one morpheme when they exist by themselves as a unit of meaning. Thus, words such as *cup, purse, lamp, window, lake,* and *Bailey* (my very cute Pembroke Welsh Corgi[*]) are all considered to have one morpheme. They are considered free morphemes because they stand alone as being meaningful.

Single words also have units that can be attached to them in order to add information to their meanings. For example, *house* can be expressed in its plural form (*houses*) to indicate that there are two of them. If Bailey is carrying his favorite small yellow ball, we can say that it is "Bailey's" ball. The possessive form of *s* alters the meaning of his name to include ownership of an object.

Table 4.8   Overview of Brown's (1973) Stages of Syntactic Development

Stage/Description	Age Range (Months)	Mean Length of Utterance (MLU)
1. Semantic roles and grammatical relations	12–26	1.0–2.00
2. Grammatical morphemes and the modulation of meanings	27–30	2.0–2.50
3. Modalities of the simple sentence	31–34	2.5–3.00
4. Embedding of one sentence within another	35–40	3.0–3.75
5. Coordination of simple sentences and propositional relations	41–46	3.75–4.50

---

[*]Kathleen Fahey.

Morphemes that are added to words are called **bound morphemes** because they must be attached to words. Bound morphemes are either **derivational** or **inflectional**. Derivational morphemes are added to the front of free morphemes, as demonstrated in the words *unbutton* and *refill*. We can also refer to these words as having prefixes. They are also added to the ends of words as suffixes and change the class or category of the word, as seen in words such as *slowly* or *sadness*.

Inflectional morphemes, which occur only as suffixes, change the meaning of words by marking grammatical adjustments for things such as plurality, possession, and verb tense. Some examples of words that have inflectional morphemes are *light sabers, girl's,* and *shouted.* Figure 4.16 will assist your learning about grammatical morphemes.

Mean length of utterance (MLU) is a calculation of the average number of morphemes a child produces in a representative sample of utterances. To determine the MLU, count the morphemes in each utterance, add the total

Figure 4.16 Morphemes: Types and Examples

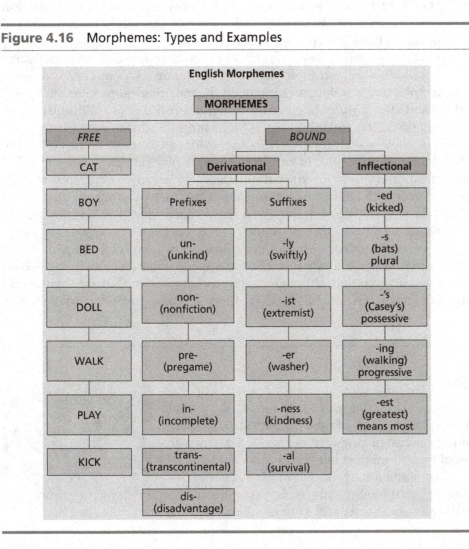

number of morphemes, and divide by the number of utterances in the sample. For example, if a child produces a total of 310 morphemes across 100 utterances, the MLU is 3.1. You will see how the MLU helps us determine the grammatical development of the child as we explore stage 1 in this chapter and stages 2-5 in the next chapter.

Early Stage 1 (MLU: 1.0 to 1.5; Age: 12 to 22 Months)

In the first stage of grammatical development, children use one-word utterances; thus, they use only one morpheme at a time. These whole words are not combined with bound morphemes at this stage. Looking back at Patrick's sample, it is evident that he is at this early stage. When he does produce a succession of syllables, it is evidence of babbling and jargon. Even when he repeats a word a few times, this is still a succession of single-word utterances. Thus, Patrick is described as a child who has a mean length of utterance at or below (because many instances of babbling occur) one morpheme. He is in the earliest of the MLU stages. Yet, it won't be long before he makes the transition to two-word utterances. In fact, we anticipate that this will happen in about 6 months, when Patrick is 18 months of age.

According to some observers, children go through a transitional stage between single-word and multiple-word productions. Bloom (1973) reports, for example, that her daughter included the meaningless production "wida" before and after a wide range of meaningful words. Some children repeat a word but vary stress and intonation. Others produce what appear to be merely strings of single-word utterances. Bloom provides an example of the child who, while looking at a picture of another child in a play car, said, "Go, car, ride." She interpreted this as three separate utterances because equal stress was put on each word with falling intonation. Patrick produced a string of words as well (*Baby! Baby! Wow! Wowee!*), but given his exclamations, it is likely that these each represent single-word utterances.

Not everyone agrees with Bloom's conclusions, however. Branigan (1979) reports that closer examination of what appear to be successive single-word utterances suggests that, although the pauses between words make them sound like distinct and separate productions, there are other prosodic variations that

---

 Video Example 4.5

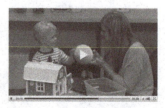

We must keep in mind that each child transitions from single words to two-word combinations within a range of time. In the video, Jackson's mother uses sign language to provide her son with visual cues to support her verbal model of two-word combinations. Jackson's mother is a speech-language pathologist and has concerns that her son is delayed in gaining expressive vocabulary and word combinations.

are more sentence-like. In some cases, not all the words end with a falling pitch, and the last word in the string is often produced with a longer duration than the preceding words. These variations suggest that the child is putting words together in some fashion, even if we cannot recognize the rules or the meaningfulness of the combinations.

Late Stage 1: Syntactic Development—Words to Word Combinations (MLU: 1.5 to 2.0; Age: 22 to 26 Months)

Whether or not there is a transitional stage between single- and multiple-word productions, we know that the child typically begins to put two words together between the ages of 18 and 24 months. These combinations represent the beginning of language structure, or *syntax*. The child discovers and applies rules for putting words together in a manner that creates meaning greater than the added meanings of the words alone. That's what makes a sentence. The meaning of any sentence is the result not just of the cumulative meanings of the individual words, but of the interactive meanings of words based on their semantic and grammatical relationships with one another, and on how they are ordered in the sentence. The child's two-word utterances do not allow for much complexity in terms of sentence meaning, of course, but they do represent the beginning of syntax and the dramatic extension of meaning made possible by putting words together. Armed with a limited vocabulary and combining only two words at a time, the child is able to make declarative statements ("Daddy go") and to express negation ("No night-night"). Whereas early in stage 1 the child expressed questions by using a rising intonation on single-word productions ("Doggie?" or "Bye-bye?") or single-word productions such as "What?" or "Where?" the child in late stage 1 creates primitive interrogative forms by combining those words with other words in productions such as "What doing?" or "Where go?" These are very simple structures to be sure, but they are the embryos of real syntax.

The significance of two-word utterances can be examined and described on three levels: syntactic, semantic, and pragmatic. We consider each level separately, but keep in mind that this separation is for convenience only. When human beings communicate, whether they are adults or children, they do not fragment their messages into structure, meaning, and purpose. The meanings of words are enriched and clarified by the structuring of words into sentences, and our communicative intentions are facilitated, if we use language well, by choosing the right words with the right meanings and putting them in correct and appropriate relationships with one another in effectively crafted sentences.

It is important to remember that some children use a combination of single, very simple word combinations and even more complex ones at this stage. Patrick's sample at 2 years, 2 weeks (26 months), which is at the end of this stage, contained a wide variety of one-, two-, and three-word combinations. He also used a few four-, five-, and six-word combinations! Since his MLU exceeds 2.0, we will discuss the characteristics of his sample in more detail in Chapter 6.

The Syntactic Level: Arranging Words Appropriately

There are at least two ways to describe syntax in two-word utterances. Crystal, Fletcher, and Garman (1976) suggest that the child chooses two words from four basic sentence constructions: subject, verb, object, and adverbial. These options allow the child to produce clause-like utterances with subjects and predicates as well as phrase-like constructions that include modifications of a subject or predicate. For example, the child might say, "Car go," a clause-like production in which *car* is the subject and *go* is the predicate. He might then say, "Go fast," a phrase-like construction in which *fast* is an adverbial modification of the verb *go*. He might also produce a phrase such as "Daddy car," in which *Daddy* is used to modify the noun *car*, indicating that Daddy has a car.

Another approach to describing syntax at the two-word level was proposed by Braine (1963). Braine suggested that the child uses a primitive form of grammar called **pivot-open grammar**. According to this view, the child has just two categories of words: open and pivot. **Open words** can be used alone and in combination with other open words, in combination with pivot words, and in either the first or second position of two-word utterances. **Pivot words** cannot be used alone and cannot be combined with other pivot words but can be used in either the first or second position of utterances. This means, then, that the child can produce the following kinds of two-word sentences: open + open ("Mommy cup"), pivot + open ("Go Mommy"), or open + pivot ("Mommy up"), but does not produce pivot + pivot sentences ("Up go"). One cannot assume that a given word will always be an open word or always a pivot word. Two children might use a given word in different ways so that the word is open for one but pivot for the other.

When Braine's grammar was first published, it seemed a promising way to describe and understand the child's early two-word utterances, but by 1970 some of the limitations of this approach were becoming apparent. One of the first language experts to express concern about pivot-open grammar was Bloom (1970), who criticized the approach because it did not take into account the meanings of the child's two-word productions. She contended that because pivot-open grammar considers only structure, it does not give children adequate credit for their language knowledge. Using one child's productions as examples, Bloom contends that in one context, "Mommy sock" was produced when the child picked up one of her mother's socks. On another occasion, when the child's mother was putting a sock on the child's foot, the child produced the same two-word utterance, "Mommy sock." Categorizing these productions as combinations of open and pivot words misses much of what is being communicated, according to Bloom. In the first case, "Mommy sock" is used to mean, "This sock belongs to Mommy." In the second case, "Mommy sock" seems to mean, "Mommy is putting a sock on my foot." The first utterance focuses on possession. The second utterance is primarily concerned with action performed by an agent (mother) on an object (sock). One of Bloom's primary contentions, therefore, is that one cannot determine how a child is using language, what a child knows about language, or what a child means

by the language she is using unless one takes **communicative context** into account. Using context to help determine the meanings of a child's utterances is referred to as **rich interpretation** (Brown, 1973). This process has helped guide much of the research on the language of children since the early 1970s.

The Semantic Level: Determining the Meanings of Early Sentences

Bloom's objections to a strictly syntactic description of the child's early word combinations, and her emphasis on taking communicative context into account, led to a semantic interpretation of early sentences. Bloom and Lahey (1978) assert that early two-word utterances reflect the child's understanding of meaning relations and rules for word order. To take this twofold understanding into account, they suggest that the rules the child uses at this juncture in development be referred to as **semantic-syntactic rules**. One might argue that when the child is producing two-word utterances, there is not much opportunity for creating language structure, just as it would be difficult to structure a wall with only two bricks. On the other hand, we have already discovered that the child is able effectively to communicate complete, and sometimes fairly sophisticated, thoughts with single-word utterances. What kinds of messages might the child be able to convey if he puts words together with meaning relationships that, when they interact, communicate far more than the additive values of their meanings?

Language experts have proposed several semantic classification systems they believe will more adequately describe children's two-word combinations. Bloom (1970) was the first expert to identify semantic relations in the early language productions of three American children. A few years later, Brown (1973) examined semantic relations in the early productions of children acquiring a range of languages from English to Samoan. Brown suggests that these early productions reflect what children know about the things and actions in their lives and that the meanings they express are consistent with the level of their intellectual development. The eight amalgamated meanings in Table 4.9 were typical of those produced by the late stage 1 children who were the subjects in Brown's study.

Other researchers have identified additional two-term relations (Bloom, 1973; Schlesinger, 1971). For example, the child might use a recurrence + production if she wants something to occur or appear again, as in, "More juice!" She might use a nonexistence/disappearance production such as, "Allgone juice" to proudly announce that she has finished her drink, that it has disappeared, that it no longer exists. She might use a rejection production such as, "No 'tatoes!" when she exercises what she thinks is her right to refuse an order to finish her helping of mashed potatoes. She might use a denial production such as, "Not kitty" in response to her mother's incorrect reference to the family dog as a, "kitty."

Among the forms children use to express negative semantic relations, nonexistence/disappearance is used more frequently than rejection or denial. The use of denial involves some fairly complicated cognitive and perceptual

Table 4.9   Two-Word Semantic Relations

Semantic–Syntactic Relation	Example
demonstrative (*this/that*) + entity	*That ball*
entity + attribute	*Kitty nice*
possessor + possession	*My dolly*
entity + location	*Dolly chair*
action + location	*Put table* (object is being placed on a table)
agent + object	*Baby shoe*
agent + action	*Doggie sit*
action + object	*Drink juice*

manipulations. That is, the child must compare the object or being described by the caregiver to his own perception and understanding of that object or being in order to make a judgment about the validity of the caregiver's observation or question. If the caregiver points to the family dog, for example, and asks, "Is that a kitty?" the child must compare his understanding of what he sees with his understanding of what a kitty is. If there is a mismatch between what he is being asked and what he knows, he produces the denial, "Not kitty!" (Hummer, Wimmer, & Antes, 1993). Researchers have noted that because this kind of production depends on fairly sophisticated perceptual and cognitive processing, it emerges at about 20 to 25 months, somewhat later than other productions that are otherwise comparable in terms of meaning and function (Bloom, 1970, 1973; Choi, 1988; Vaidyanathan, 1991).

Research has provided some information about the developmental order of a few semantic relations. According to Wells (1985), for example, when children express *entity + location,* they generally refer to the location of a static or stationary entity or object before they refer to the movement or action of placing an object *in* or *on* something. That is, the child will typically say something such as, "Doggie chair" to indicate that a dog is sitting on a chair before she manages a comment about an activity in progress involving the movement of an object from one place to another. Caregivers must patiently wait for the child to make a statement such as, "In box" to indicate that she is in the process of dumping a spoonful of mashed potatoes into her mother's sewing basket. This kind of utterance, in addition to creating a sense of excitement for the mother, expresses an entity + location semantic relation in which there is the movement of something (mashed potatoes) from one place (the child's plate) to another (the mother's sewing basket). Wells's (1985) findings suggest that the child will produce location relations by 21 months, and the typical child will be using two-word combinations to express attribute (attribute + entity) by the time she is 2 years old.

Using this kind of analysis, one might reasonably conclude that the child is able to talk about things, where they are, what actions they perform, what actions are performed on them, and who creates these actions. He is also able to identify characteristics or attributes of things, and he can express

---

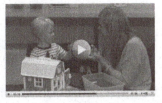

Video Reflection 4.2: Semantic Relations at 21 Months

Watch the video of a parent teaching her child to produce two-word semantic relations, then answer the questions.

---

ownership or possession. We should not lose sight of the fact that the child in early stage 1 can use single-word utterances to express relations such as **existence**, **nonexistence**, **disappearance**, and **recurrence**, but the successful communication of these relations during early stage 1 depends heavily on the interpretative powers of adult listeners. When the child begins to use two-word combinations, interpretation remains difficult, but it is somewhat less murky because the child is now employing syntactic rules for ordering words in combination with the stress patterns of his language to help convey his intended meanings. Interpretation is also facilitated by context. That is, if the adult takes into account what was said before the utterance was interpreted, and if she considers the nonlinguistic circumstances surrounding the production, she is more likely to interpret the meaning of the child's message correctly.

As the child develops into late stage 1 (22-to-26 months), she continues to make steady, if not always dramatic, progress in terms of semantic-syntactic relations. There is evidence that the child will begin to produce three- and even four-word combinations at approximately 24 months. Only about half of her productions at this point are two-word utterances (Owens, 2005, p. 255). Productions such as, "Baby push truck" (agent + action + object) and, "Daddy put box" (agent + action + location, to indicate that Daddy is putting something in the box) are not uncommon utterances for the late stage 1 child.

The Pragmatic Level: An Emphasis on the Functions of Early Sentences

Throughout this chapter, we have cited the work of Dore (1974, 1975) and Halliday (1975) to trace the development of communicative intents during stage 1 of language development. Before the child begins using words, he is able to express four communicative intentions, according to Halliday. When the child uses words, he expands his repertoire of intentions to about seven. When the child begins to put words together, between the ages of 18 and 24 months, we see additional changes in communicative intentions. The child now engages in what can properly be considered dialogue. He understands that in two-way communication, the participants fill and exchange certain roles. One speaks and the other listens; then the listener speaks and the speaker listens. When one speaks, the other sometimes responds to the message expressed by the speaker, sometimes by simply acknowledging the message, sometimes by adding information, sometimes by agreeing or disagreeing. Sometimes the speaker is a questioner and the listener is a responder. There are many roles to be filled in communication, and even with a limited expressive vocabulary and only single-word and two-word utterances, the child is able to fill these roles.

The functions or intentions we identified earlier from Halliday's work are now combined and modified into at least three new functions: pragmatic, mathetic, and informative. The pragmatic function of language is undoubtedly the most basic. The child uses language to get things done. She uses language to make requests and demands, and to satisfy needs to interact with and control the behavior of other people.

The **mathetic** function of language is manifested in communications concerned with learning. The child uses language to learn about herself and about her world. She comments, questions, predicts, and remembers. She uses language to express her developing understanding of how people, things, and events are connected. Her language, however limited, is a reflection of her intellectual development.

The **informative** function emerges when the child uses language to give new information to others. Adults often think of the informative function as the most basic function of language and probably the first to emerge, but it is actually one of the last. Why? We cannot use language to inform until we know something others do not or until we think we know something we assume others do not know. In the beginning, everyone knows more than the child! Before stage 1 ends, however, the child is more than happy to use language to tell others what she knows, even if what she "knows" is incorrect, incomplete, or irrelevant. She uses language to inform the dog, brothers and sisters, Mom and Dad, Teddy Bear, and anyone else who cares to profit from her wisdom. This is one of the most delightful functions of early multiple-word utterances. When this child speaks, listen, learn, enjoy, and be prepared to be amazed.

A child at this stage abides by some of the basic rules of conversation. He will address his conversational partner by name to gain his or her attention before speaking. He will listen before he responds, and he understands the turn-taking aspect of conversation. His primary limitation as a conversationalist is a short attention span. He will usually stay on the same topic for only a few turns before he is ready to move on to something else (Bloom, Rocissano, & Hood, 1976). We will see a dramatic change in this aspect of conversation after the child passes his third birthday. It's quite possible that you have already encountered a three-year-old who wanted to talk about a topic long after your knowledge and/or interest was exhausted.

Comprehension and Production: A Critical and Evolving Relationship

Before concluding this description of language development in stage 1, we need to include a brief review of what children comprehend at this time. Expressive blanguage cannot be separated from receptive language, of course. As children mature, what they understand dramatically impacts what they are able to express and how they express it.

For as long as people have systematically studied language and language development, there have been questions about the relationship between comprehension and production. There is appealing logic in the assumption that comprehension must precede production, and many linguists have held that view. In fact, one notable linguist, Ingram (1974), made the clear assertion that, "comprehension ahead of production is a linguistic universal of acquisition" (p. 313). Others are not sure that the relationship is this simple. Bloom (1974b), for example, argues that although we do not know the precise character of the relationship between comprehension and production, we know it is a relationship of shared dependence.

Whatever the true nature of this relationship, it seems clear that it changes as language develops, and it is not the same for all components of language. As we noted in this chapter, the infant comprehends differences among speech sounds, sequences of speech sounds, and intonation patterns long before he produces sounds and superimposes intonation patterns on sequences of sounds. These discriminations are made within the first half of the first year (Goodsitt, Morse, VerHoeve, & Cowan, 1984; Kessen, Levine, & Wendrich, 1979), while comparable productions do not occur until after the first birthday.

When the child begins to produce his first meaningful words, we see a changing relationship between comprehension and production. The child produces words *before* he has a complete understanding of them. We have already noted, for example, that the child might use the word *doggie* to refer to only the family pet, or he might use *doggie* to refer to any four-legged animal. There is some comprehension associated with this production, of course, but it is not complete comprehension according to adult standards. Only after the child experiences sufficient intellectual development to understand *doggie* as a category that includes all dogs but only dogs and only after he acquires additional words to reflect this understanding will his comprehension of *doggie* be complete. In the meantime, the child's ability to understand is greatly influenced by all the non-linguistic cues that surround the words spoken to him. Because adults often fail to take this non-linguistic information into account, they may overestimate what the child really comprehends in the words spoken to him, and they may overestimate, based on the child's language production, the child's real language competence.

According to Benedict, (1979), comprehension does precede production to a significant extent for the first 50 words. The 8 children in her study comprehended about 50 words before they were able to produce 10 words. They comprehended 50 words at 13 months, but did not produce 50 words until they were 19 months old. Their receptive vocabularies increased by about 22 words per month, but their expressive vocabularies grew by only 9 or 10 words each month. Based on these findings, it is reasonable to conclude that in early language development, the gap between comprehension and production is substantial.

The child's first understandings of words are based on nonverbal insights about things, actions, and the relationships among things and actions (Huttenlocher, 1974). Paul (1990) refers to this type of understanding as "knowledge based on routines," or "scripts of events," in which repetitions of the event itself in combination with adults' repetitive linguistic and non-linguistic behaviors associated with the event facilitate word comprehension. The child understands important and basic categories of things such as food, people, and pets. She understands basic actions such as eating or sitting and obvious relationships such as putting food into the mouth. The child conceptualizes these things, actions, and relationships apart from language, but as she hears certain sequences of sounds produced in connection with these mental representations, she associates the sequences of sounds, or words, with the things, actions, and relationships. When the connections become established, the words serve to help the child recall the things, actions, and relationships to which the words refer. It is important to notice the sequence in comprehension Huttenlocher is suggesting. The child first understands aspects or characteristics of things and actions in her environment. She then creates mental pictures or concepts of these things and actions, and she gradually associates these mental pictures with spoken words. The words help her to retrieve the mental pictures.

As one might guess, children comprehend names for things and people before they comprehend words that describe actions and relationships. As one might also guess, children understand words for things and people in the here and now before they understand words for things and people that are absent in time or space. The findings of a study of children between the ages of 10 and 21 months by Miller, Chapman, Branston, and Reichle (1980) suggest a fairly consistent sequence of comprehensions. All of the 12-month-old subjects understood names for people in sight, and about half understood words for things in their presence. Words describing actions were understood by most of the subjects older than 15 months. A little more than half of the children between 19 and 21 months understood words referring to people and things not present. Only children over 18 months understood semantic relationships in two- and three-word utterances. Among the semantic relationships studied, the most often understood was possessor + possession, as in, "My doggie" or, "Mommy shoe."

Just as adults may overestimate the child's understanding of single words, they may overestimate what the child is able to comprehend in the sentences he hears. Chapman (1978) suggests that when the child responds to utterances, he may use comprehension strategies that give the impression of greater understanding than the child actually possesses. For example, when an adult says, "Throw the ball," the child might pick up the ball and throw it. The adult assumes that the child understands the words *ball* and *throw* and the relationship between them. If the adult then says, "Hide the ball" or, "Kiss the ball" or, "Hit the ball," the child is likely to throw the ball again. If the child has selected the ball from among several objects, it might be safe to assume that he understands the word *ball*, but he may not understand the rest of the words in any of these sentences. What he does know is that balls are for throwing, so whenever he hears *ball* in an utterance, he throws it. His comprehension strategy, therefore, is to perform the action on an object most commonly associated with that object. Assuming he understands the words *milk, cookie,* and *ball*, he *drinks* milk, *eats* the cookie, and *throws* the ball, no matter what other words happen to surround the words he knows in sentences spoken to him.

Huttenlocher (1974) asserts that when the child *comprehends* language, she uses a word to retrieve the mental image of an object, person, or action. When she *produces* language, she recognizes an object, person, or action and must retrieve the matching word. Comprehension involves an easier or more direct association between object and word than production, according to Huttenlocher, because the child's understanding of objects, people, and events is more complete than her understanding of the words used to represent them. Adults often have a similar experience with a foreign language. It is easier to comprehend a new language than to speak it because when we listen to the vocabulary of the new language that is not well known, we move to the vocabulary of our native language, which is well understood. When we try to speak the language, we must move from the known to the incompletely known, a much more difficult task. During language development, this difference seems to be reflected in the occurrence of overextensions. The child tends to overextend the meanings of words in production but not in comprehension. In the example we have used several times, the child overextends the word *doggie* to include not only dogs but also cats, horses, cows, and many other four-legged animals. The same child who produces *doggie* to refer to a cow would likely point to the correct animal if, while looking at a cat, dog, and cow, an adult produced each animal's name. In other words, it is easier for the child to retrieve her mental image of an object than to retrieve the word that represents the object.

Check Your Understanding 4.7

Assess your understanding of word combinations in early and late stage 1 by completing this brief quiz.

SUMMARY

Stage 1 began with the production of first words and ended with the production of combinations of words. The child produces her first word at about 12 months and begins to combine words at about 18 months. Her expressive vocabulary grows from 1 word at the beginning of the stage to 200-to-300 words by the end of the stage. Her first words are mostly nouns used to name people or objects. By the end of the stage, she is producing two-word and even some three- and four-word utterances to make statements, ask questions, express negatives, and make demands. She is using language to get things done, manipulate the behaviors of other people, and exchange information in a rudimentary form of conversation, complete with turn taking and presuppositional skills, although these skills are just beginning to emerge and are quite primitive by adult standards (see Table 4.10).

During the remaining stages, the child will learn to produce a greater variety of sentences and to make them more elaborate. She will learn how to put simple sentences

Table 4.10   **Stage 1 Highlights,**

Typical Age Range: 12–26 Months

MLU: 1.0–2.0 Morphemes

Role of Caregiver

- Provides models for language development and opportunities for communicative interactions.
- Assists by expanding and extending the child's utterances.

Uses songs, alliteration, rhymes, and stories to focus the child on emotional information, phonological structure of syllables and words, phrase contours, and story structure.

First Words

- Do not always sound like adult words.
- Used in reference to things of greatest importance to the child: people, objects, actions of immediate interest.
- Most are single-syllable words or single syllables repeated.
- May infrequently exhibit overextended or underextended meanings.

Pragmatics

- Uses nonverbal and verbal communication to satisfy needs and wants, control the behavior of others, interact with others, express emotion or interest, explore and categorize, imagine, and inform.
- Demonstrates primitive presuppositional and turn-taking skills.

Multiword Productions

- The combining of two words typically begins at 18-to-24 months.
- Three-word and some four-word combinations appear when about half of the child's utterances are two-word productions.
- These productions can be interpreted at three levels: syntactic, semantic, and pragmatic.

Sentence Types

- In early stage 1, the child uses a rising intonation on single words to pose *yes/no* questions and may use approximated forms of *what* or *where* to ask questions.
- In late stage 1, the child combines two and three words, but still using a rising intonation to pose *yes/no* questions, as in "*That* + _____?" *Wh*-interrogative words are still limited to *what* and *where*.
- In early stage 1, words such as *no, gone*, and *allgone* appear. One of these words may be used in combination with another word negative + _____).
- In late stage 1, the words *no* and *not* are used interchangeably at the beginning of word combinations (e.g., "No bye-bye!").
- In early stage 1, declarative statements are limited to two constructions: agent + action and action + object.
- In late stage 1, the child forms declarative statements by combining subject + verb + object.
- In late stage 1, the prepositions *in* and *on* are embedded in a sentence.
- In late stage 1, the child uses *and* to form conjoined sentences.

Comprehension

- Comprehension probably precedes production for the first 50 words.
- Understanding names for things and people precedes understanding of words describing actions and relationships.
- Understanding of early words appears to be facilitated by knowledge of event routines or scripts.

together to produce compound sentences and how to put sentences into one another to make complex sentences. She will also become a more sophisticated conversationalist, and, of course, her vocabulary will grow, and her understanding of the meanings of words and word combinations will increase. As exciting and full as stage 1 has been, the child's language development has truly just begun!

▐▐▶ Surfing the Web

If you are interested in exploring topics discussed in this chapter in more detail, search for one or more of the following relevant terms online.

Brown's stages of syntactic development
Child-directed speech
Early gestures to convey intentions
Early pragmatic functions
English morphemes
Learning first words
Learning new words from birth to age 2

Parent-infant communication prior to birth
Prelinguistic vocalizations
Relationship between comprehension and production
Semantic relations
Socioeconomic status and language
Social routines involving songs, rhymes, and stories

Chapter Review 4.1

Recall what you learned in this chapter by completing the Chapter Review.

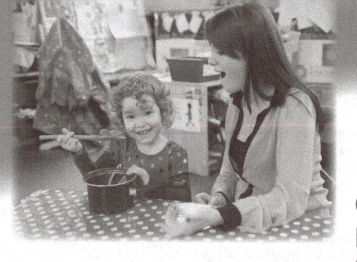

Children Learning Language: Participating in Language Samples

LEARNING OUTCOMES

After completion of this chapter, you will be able to:

- Explain the purposes of language sampling.
- Describe the methods researchers and clinicians use to obtain language samples from children.
- Discuss the analysis and interpretation of morphology, syntax, semantics, and pragmatics within language samples.
- Use a sample to practice analyzing and interpreting language sample information.

How do parents, teachers and others in a child's environment know that child is acquiring language on par with other children? The most obvious answer to this question is that they rely on their daily interactions with the child and observations of the child's communication with other children. As each typical day unfolds into the events, situations, places, and people that abound, they participate in brief exchanges, extended interactions, laughter, explanations, commands, songs, and all the other ways we exchange social communication. Thus, within homes, schools, churches, community shops, and recreation sites, children are observed learning language.

It makes sense that the best way we can know how a particular child is doing on his language journey at any moment in time is to take a careful look at his expressive language. What he says and how he says it will speak volumes about what he knows and the development of his sounds, vocabulary, grammar, expression of meaning, and social use of language during communication.

We will not know everything about a child's language through one brief encounter, or even several interactions, but researchers and clinicians use some basic strategies to obtain, analyze, and make inferences from language samples. These strategies give them a lot of information, that they are able to determine if the child is developing within the time frame and patterns of typical children, or whether the child appears to be lagging behind and/or demonstrating patterns that are not typical. This knowledge is especially useful when the child needs some help on her developmental journey.

Purposes of Language Sampling

There are several purposes and benefits of sampling a child's language. The first purpose is to document the child's abilities at a particular point in time. The benefit of capturing the child's interactions via an audio or video recording and then creating a written transcription is so that researchers and clinicians are able to study it. The sample may be analyzed to determine the child's abilities as compared to typical peers. If the child is not developing in a typical and timely fashion, intervention may be needed.

Another purpose for sampling a child's language periodically is to describe the nature and extent of the child's progress as an outcome of intervention. Caregivers and clinicians may note the child's use of new words and longer sentences, but a detailed analysis allows for documentation of progress and planning for continued intervention. Routine samples also help clinicians confirm the acquisition of new language skills needed for the child to continue on her path without direct support.

Researchers use language samples to select children who qualify for studies about language acquisition. Well-designed studies often match children by age and their language abilities to compare treatment strategies. Research about how children with language impairments learn language has given practitioners valuable information about the nature of language impairments and how to remediate them.

Another benefit of language sampling that you will soon discover is thinking about the language forms and meanings of every utterance. This activity will help you learn so much about your English language—more than you thought possible! Our primary purpose of this chapter is to provide you with the tools you need to explore language sampling. This knowledge will help you understand the attainments children make that are described with great detail in Chapters 6 and 7.

✓ Check Your Understanding 5.1

Assess your understanding of the purposes of language sampling by completing this brief quiz.

Obtaining Reliable and Valid Language Samples

If we are going to go to the trouble of obtaining and analyzing language samples, we must concern ourselves with two concepts. The first concept is reliability. Suppose you spent an hour with a child in her home right after she woke from her nap. The child seemed very quiet and needed lots of coaxing from her mother to name some pictures as you talked with her about a book. When you asked the mother near the end of your hour whether the sample was typical, the mother said, "Oh my heavens, no. My little girl jabbers all the time. I was surprised she was so quiet!" You decide that your sample was not reliable. Given another time of day and the chance to know you, the child will likely talk much more. Sure enough, you schedule another appointment at a different time and behold, you get a much different language sample that is more representative of what this child is able to do.

A related concept involves getting a sample that truly provides a glimpse of the full range of a child's language skills. In a word, the sample must be valid. Suppose you intended to use the child's toy farm set to stage interactions, only to find that the child loves to sing "Old MacDonald." While singing is great fun and the child is engaged with you, songs do not provide you with a good picture of his productive language because songs are learned through repetition and do not contain the grammar and meaning used in conversational utterances. So, singing is not a valid representation of his language. Let's imagine that after the songs, the child has a wonderful time interacting with you about the horses, cows, chickens, sheep, and pigs as they wander into and out of the barn, around the fences, and through the gates, and are eating, drinking, and playing in the barn yard. Now you have captured a child at play using language to express his ideas.

Another important consideration during the collection of a language sample is to be sure to get enough language from your interactions with the child. How much language is enough to be a representative snapshot (reliable and valid) of a child's expressive language? At least 50-100 utterances is the minimum for any sample, but there are more important considerations to insure reliability and validity. It is often necessary to eliminate sections of the sample, so you should seek to have 75-100 usable utterances for analysis. For example, at the beginning of the interaction, the child may be shy and his parent may prompt the child to talk. He may say his name, count to 10, name a few pictures, and answer yes/no questions. These utterances will not be analyzed, so don't include them in your count. Strive for 100-150 utterances at the outset, so that you end up with a strong data set. The utterances should be successive except for any groupings that reflect rote language (e.g., counting, singing, reciting chants or poems), unintelligible words or phrases, or repetitions of a word, phrase, or sentence. We will review in detail some rules about these later.

It is a challenge for many clinicians to let the child lead the conversation and do most of the talking. Learning to wait for the child to initiate her ideas takes practice and patience, but the rewards are great. Children have a lot to say, but they need the time and space to talk. Avoid asking the child a lot of questions, such as, "What is this? What color is it? What do you do with it?" Rather, as the child makes comments, you can engage in strategies that facilitate interaction.

[Margin notes:]

Time matters with children and their schedules.

Don't rely on songs/music for evaluations.

The conversation must be child lead for a valid eval.

Facilitating Interaction

Spending some time with the child prior to collecting the sample will be time well spent. Just 10 minutes can make all the difference in insuring a reliable and valid sample. Whether you interact with the child in his home, at a child center, or in your office, it is good practice to have a conversation with the parents ahead of time to note the child's interests and favorite activities, toys, and books. It is fine to ask parents to bring some favorite items to the session or to gather them in the home. Most children love to show and tell their favorite things. You should also plan to have several materials available so that a variety of topics will be shared during the sample. For example, a farm set, snack time, and a high-interest book offer good variety of vocabulary, actions, and events. If you are able, moving around to different settings affords opportunities to experience the child interacting in natural environments. Playgrounds, parks, stores, a kitchen, anyplace where the child is able to talk freely will yield lots of language. My recent trip to the grocery store provided a glimpse into a wonder-fully positive and productive exchange between a preschooler and his dad. The father involved the child in finding the food on the shopping list. "OK, let's see if we can find the bananas. You show me where they are. Mom said we need a bunch. What does she mean?" The young boy was quite enthusiastic about this treasure hunt and talked a lot as he moved down the aisles! Consider the child's age when selecting materials for your interaction. Children who are one to two years old respond to toys and household objects, whereas two- and three-year-old children are able to engage in pretend play and talk about experiences they have had with family and friends. For older preschoolers, description of objects, pictures, and personal experiences will be advantageous. School-age children who are developing language in a typical fashion will have very rich and complex language. But children who have language disorders often have reduced sophistication with language. Nevertheless, it is important to engage the child in materials and language activities that are age-appropriate. School-age children like to retell stories or make up stories from pictures (Shipley & McAfee, 2009). Narratives not only provide clinicians with observations about connected discourse, but also allow for analysis of knowledge about stories that develop during the preschool and school-age years (Heilmann, Miller, Nockerts, & Dunaway, 2010). Another way to engage children in conversation is with questions or statements that encourage a topic. For example, "Pretend I've never had _____. How do you make it?" or, "Have you ever been to _____? Tell me about it." (Shipley & McAfee, 2009).

It is a very good idea to practice eliciting language samples with children before you collect one for analysis. It may seem pretty simple to interact with a child in such a way as to get a representative sample, but it is not simple at all. If you have access to a child between two and six years, you have a good opportunity to hone your language sample elicitation skills. If you do not have access to a child, role-playing with another adult will be useful too. The goal of practice is to try out your techniques of waiting, listening, prompting, avoiding a lot of questions, and avoiding the "name game." Asking the child to name people, objects, pictures, places, and events will yield one-word responses. This outcome is not reflective of the child's abilities. The best results are obtained by prompts, such as, "Tell me about that truck," "It's your turn to make something and tell me about it," "What should we do next?" Picture sequences or pictures that have lots going on may also serve to prompt the child to talk about them. "What is going on here?" Let's talk about what this family is doing." "I wonder what will happen to this dog?" will be effective conversation starters.

Video Example 5.1

Watch the video of a father's conversation with his three-year-old son, Micah. Notice how the parent uses open-ended questions and a conversational style to prompt Micah to talk about hard jobs.
https://www.youtube.com/watch?v=KDC9HinpcaI

Recording the Language Sample

It is necessary to audio record or video record the language sample session. Recording the sample allows you to capture exactly what happened during the collection of the sample, provides a record for transcription, and facilitates verification during the analysis. In addition, the recording provides the context for each utterance and a video recording allows you to see subtle shifts in the situation or materials. A child may, for example, glance out the window and make a comment that is not related to the materials on the table. When talking about Spiderman, he may shift topic to say, "Oh, that is the dog next door. His name is Sam." Without the benefit of context, this comment would be strange, indeed. Recordings do present technology into the sample environment, so the recording device should be unobtrusive. If the child becomes interested in it, some time playing with it usually is enough to satisfy curiosity and it is soon forgotten. Be sure that your batteries are fresh and your recording device is working. Always check that you have activated it prior to the start of the your language sample. It is very unfortunate for everyone if you discover during or after the sample that you forgot to turn it on or it didn't work!

Transcribing the Sample

The goal of transcription is to accurately transfer the contents of the recording to a written document. Once the content of the sample is written, it can be analyzed. The person who collected the sample should transcribe it if possible. This is because the context of each utterance is important, as well as the nuances of communication that may not be apparent to someone who was not present and when you transform the recording into written text.

Transcription is an important step in creating a written record of the child's language for analysis. It involves several components that taken together

---

Figure 5.1 Creating a Language Sample Transcription

Decide on the format of the transcription. A form that has space for the adult utterances, child utterances and context notes is very useful. Appendix A is a sample form.

Listen to the recording in full and determine any sections of the recording that will not be included in the sample due to signing, chanting, naming items, counting, etc. Determine if you will use the beginning utterances, as these are sometimes not representative of the child's communication abilities.

Use one line for each utterance made by the adult and another line for the child, moving down the page in the appropriate columns. Number only the child utterances.

An utterance is determined by a thought. It is tempting to transcribe all the verbage in a turn as one thought, but it is typically many. For example, "My daddy and mommy and Jimmy went home/and we ate pizza/and daddy had three pieces/and I have one" is actually four utterances. You may have several successive adult or child utterances, so be careful that you parse these out. The goal is to have at least 75 to 100 usable utterances for analysis.

Do not number utterances that contain one or more unintelligible words.

Transcribe everything the child says, even if she repeats words or phrases.

Nonfluent speech, such as repeating the first sound in a word, should be transcribed, but rules for counting morphemes will be used.

Refer to Appendix B for a sample transcription.

---

produce a document that maintains reliability and validity and allows the clinician a structure that will facilitate the application of procedures.

Transcribing is a time-consuming and detailed process, so be sure you have a quiet working space and headphones. Figure 5.1 contains steps that will guide you to achieving the written transcript. A form that has space for the adult utterances, child utterances, and context notes is very useful. Appendix A is a sample transcription form. It may be necessary to listen to an utterance several times to ensure accuracy. Children who have sound errors may be more difficult to understand via the recording. Some clinicians repeat the child's utterances during the sample to make sure they know what the utterance is. This **glossing** technique can be distracting to the child because it is not a part of natural interaction with children. The clinician should use discretion to employ this technique during the collection of the sample only when necessary.

Check Your Understanding 5.2

Assess your understanding of the methods used to obtain language samples from children by completing this brief quiz.

Analyzing the Language Sample

The purpose of the analysis of a language sample is to describe the child's productive language during conversational exchanges. We want to know several

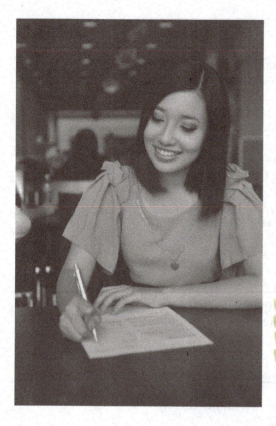

things about all aspects of language relative to a child's age. As you know, language abilities increase with experience and age; thus, age is an important guide to what individual children should be demonstrating in their language. Of course age isn't the only factor and we must be mindful of each child's life journey and characteristics that make him who he is. We will discuss some language development stages in the chapters to come, so you will see how age assists us in mapping out what most children do as they gain language skills.

In addition to finding out how sophisticated the child's language is relative to her age, we want to know what advances she has made in her ability to put words together in phrases and sentences. In short, we want to describe her grammar.

==Grammatical structure gives us one perspective on the complexity of the child's language skills, but he must be able to communicate his ideas in meaningful ways both for social communication and for formulating and expressing his thoughts.== Recall the important connection between thought and language discussed in Chapters 2 and 3. Knowledge of words and the ability to retrieve them and combine them with other words is necessary for us to convey our ideas. Thus, semantic analysis is a way to determine what the child knows from what he says.

Social communication is an important aspect of language growth. Families must be able to understand one another to get things done, but also to share their feelings, opinions, thoughts, and daily exchanges that help bond people to one another. Pragmatic analysis assists us in determining whether the verbal exchanges between the child and others is appropriate and functional.

With transcript in hand, let us begin to analyze a language sample. Refer to Appendix B for a transcript. We will use this transcript as a step-by-step guide to analyzing the syntax, semantics, and pragmatics of three-year-old Carrie. We will not analyze her speech sounds, because our primary focus is about language.

Grammatical Analysis

Children learning language start with understanding and speaking a few words. Then they begin to combine words into phrases. Expansion of phrases into sentences takes time and practice; thus, this process is a protracted one from about two years of age through five years of age and beyond. One way that we can determine a child's progress is to count the number of words she says in each utterance. For example, in the sentence, "*My doggie is barking,*" the child has produced four words. But the number of words does not tell us the whole story. Language sophistication involves the addition of meaning to words. We call these meaningful units **morphemes**. Recall our discussion of morphemes in Chapter 4 and revisit the types and examples in Figure 4.16. In this sentence, the child added information to the verb *bark,* using the present progressive form *is + ing.* While this sentence does indeed have four words, it also has five morphemes. We now know that this child is able to expand the verb to a phrase that shows active voice and present tense.

Counting morphemes requires a systematic procedure so that our results are consistent and valid from one sample to another for any given child and from one child to the next. Rules exist that assist us in determining the number of morphemes per utterance. Table 5.1 shows 14 grammatical morphemes and an example of their use. Figure 5.2 is the list of rules we follow to count them.

The number of morphemes can be easily added to the end of each utterance. For example, here is Carrie's morpheme count for her first 10 utterances.

1. I want to build too	5
2. Let me do it	4
3. That a red block	4/5
4. Here, let me show you how	6
5. My birthday blocks?	4
6. Uh hum	1
7. My mommy and daddy gave them for my birthday	9
8. Oh look at my tower	5
9. It big. (laughs)	2/3
10. Me too, mommy!	3

Table 5.1   14 Grammatical Morphemes and Examples of Use

Grammatical Morpheme	Example
Present progressive	She runn*ing.*
In (preposition)	Milk *in* cup.
On (preposition)	Doggie *on* bed.
Regular plural	Girl*s* playing.
Irregular past tense	Mommy *went* work.
Possessive	Billy*'s* ball.
Uncontractible copula	Billy *was* bad.
Articles (*the, a*)	Daddy eating *the* cookie.
Regular past tense	Mommy look*ed.*
Regular third person singular	She *eats.*
Irregular third person singular	Daddy *has* cookie.
Uncontractible auxiliary	I *was* eating.
Contractible copula	Billy*'s* bad.
Contractible auxiliary	He*'s* running.

Figure 5.2   Rules for Counting Morphemes

Count as one morpheme

Whole words including nouns, pronouns, verbs, articles, prepositions, etc.

Auxiliary and model verbs, such as *is, are, have, had, may,* and *should*

Uninflected verbs, such as *go, buy,* and *sit*

Semi-infinitive forms, such as *gonna, wanna, hafta*

Diminutive forms, such as *horsey, kitty,* and *daddy*

Inflections on nouns

> Plural –s (e.g., dogs, houses, apples, elephants)
>
> Plurals that have no singular form (e.g., they, water, herd)
>
> Possessive –s (e.g., mom's book, horse's tail, baby's bottle)

Inflections on verbs

> Present progressive –ing (e.g., laughing, singing, playing)
>
> Irregular past tense (e.g., fell, bought, ate)
>
> Regular third person singular verb (e.g., sits, eats, writes)
>
> Regular past tense verb –ed (e.g., walked, climbed, jumped)
>
> Contractions when the segments do not occur alone in the sample
>
> (e.g., we'll, shouldn't, can't)

Gerunds and participles not a part of the verb phrase, such as *Dancing is good exercise* or *The girl was flabbergasted.*

Unintended repetitions of part or whole words, such as *I-I-I like pie* or *W-w-what is your name?*

Compound words, like *cupcake, rainbow,* and *airplane* and proper names of people, places, and things, such as George Washington, New York, and the Eiffel Tower

Learned reduplications of a word or phrase, such as *night-night* or *bye-bye*

Count as more than one morpheme

Inflected nouns, pronouns, verbs, adjectives, participles of the verb phrase, and adverbs.

Contractions when one or both parts occur by itself elsewhere.

Word repetitions if the word is clearly produced for emphasis.

Do not count as a morpheme

Incomplete utterances and utterances containing unintelligible words

Direct imitations of a model

Songs, rhymes, counting, listing or any rote productions

False starts, such as *Once when we, One time we, On vacation we drove to Ohio.*

Fillers (e.g., um, oh, you know, like um) and noises or sound effects

---

Based on Chapman, R. (1981), Lund & Duchan, (1993) and Owens, R. (2004).

Notice that Carrie omitted a morpheme in utterances three and nine. The number of morphemes present in the utterance is first and the number required is second.

This designation makes it easy to spot the utterances where grammatical errors have occurred, which is important for further analysis. As indicated earlier, the goal is to analyze 75 to 100 utterances. It is necessary to determine the morpheme count of each utterance according to the rules. When all the morphemes have been counted, add them all up. In our example, we have a total of 43 morphemes and 10 sentences. Divide the number of morphemes by the number of sentences to obtain the average (mean) number of morphemes in the sample (4.3). Let's pretend that Carrie's total morpheme count for 100 utterances is 430. Her Mean Length of Utterance (MLU) would still be 4.3. Now go to Appendix C to see what Carrie's MLU is for 75 utterances.

What does the MLU tell us and what inferences can we make about the development of the child? This question is an important one, as MLU is used as an indicator of language development during an initial assessment and as a measure of progress during language intervention. It also is a goalpost for establishing the outcomes of therapy. MLU is most valuable for children between two and five years or up to an average of five morphemes when grammatical forms are developing for the creation of sentences. However, it can also be useful for children who are older and still acquiring sentence constructions.

When children begin to expand the noun phrase and verb phrase in sentences, MLU increases. Researchers have discovered that this fairly predictable journey can be divided into some stages. We included this information in Chapter 4, Table 4.8. The table shows each stage and the corresponding age ranges of advances in syntactic development.

The grammatical forms and the arrangement of these forms within utterances tells us quite a lot about the child's language growth. We will see the emergence of the 14 grammatical morphemes in words and word combinations from simple two-word utterances to fully formed sentences with embedded phrases and sentences. Mapping out which forms and combinations the child uses reveals his current sophistication and provides us with information on incomplete development.

The example of Carrie's language shows two instances where the verb "to be" as the main verb is absent. This verb form should be mastered between 27 and 39 months. Carrie is 36 months, so we would expect some emerging use of this verb in her language sample. Refer to the complete analysis in Appendix D to see what other grammatical forms are omitted or used incorrectly.

Beyond grammatical morphemes, the syntactic analysis will also provide us with information on the development of simple, compound, and complex sentences. We expect these attainments when a child is using clausal structures and conjunctions to connect sentences during stages 4 and 5. Carrie is at the simple sentence stage, so no compound or complex sentences are observed.

Semantic Analysis

We emphasized earlier that meaning is the crux of language no matter what the child's ability level is. For children who are in the single-word and two-word stages, there is very little in the way of grammar to analyze. But meaning is certainly being conveyed in these short utterances, and semantic analysis affords us the opportunity to document the types of meaning being conveyed. Researchers have outlined what meanings can be ascribed to simple one-word utterances. As we saw in Chapter 4, Table 4.5 shows Halliday's Communicative Functions and

Table 5.2 Some Common Three-Word Semantic Relations

Semantic Relation	Example
Agent-Action-Object	Teacher make cookie
Agent-Action-Locative	Mommy go upstairs
Action-Object-Locative	Drink juice here
Possessor-Agent-Object	Daddy's bike
Attribute-Entity-Action	Green ball roll
Demonstrative-Attribute-Entity	That big house
Negative-Action-Object	No go home

Table 4.6 reveals Dore's Primitive Speech Acts. These allow us to interpret the meaning of the child's language from the context of the exchange. The context is highly important in the interpretation of what a child means.

When children are producing word combinations, the semantic analysis must account for the meaning of each word in the utterance. Just as we might describe the sentence *Mommy go car* as noun + verb + noun during grammatical analysis, we would describe it as Agent + action + object during semantic analysis. Refer to Table 4.9 in Chapter 4 for some common two-word semantic relations. Table 5.2 lists some common semantic relations for three-word utterances.

Pragmatic Analysis

The use of language in situational contexts allows children to relate effectively to those they interact with for a variety of purposes. Just as maturity in grammar and meaning develops over time, so too does the child's understanding and use of social rules. Pragmatic abilities during the formative years of language growth allow children to participate fully in interactions with family and others. Some of these functions are displayed in Figure 5.3. It is evident in Carrie's language sample that she is a highly engaged communicator.

Figure 5.3 Pragmatic Functions

Pragmatic functions increase with age and language abilities

Gain listener attention

Request objects and actions from others

Obtain information by asking questions

Respond to questions and comments of others

Produce verbal responses and decrease gestures

Maintain topic

Engage in conversational turn-taking

Attempt conversational repairs

Use polite forms in situational contexts

Check Your Understanding 5.3

Assess your understanding of the analysis and interpretation of morphology, syntax, semantics, and pragmatics within language samples by completing this brief quiz.

Sample Analysis and Interpretation

The analysis of Carrie's language sample (Appendix D) shows Carrie's grammar focusing on her use of morphemes and errors in verbs, pronouns, and possessive forms. Notice that the number of morphemes Carrie produced in each utterance is the first number reported, followed by the number of morphemes she should have used. Most of the time these numbers differ, especially due to omitted morphemes, but in some utterances (e.g., 19, 23, 25), the number of morphemes is reported twice. This is to show that an error occurred on the morpheme, but the count is not altered. In utterance 19, Carrie used the present tense singular verb *have* when the correct form was *has*. Notice here that each of these verbs count as only one morpheme because the verb is not inflected.

Carrie's MLU is 4.92. She has utterances that range from 1 (lower bound) to 9 (upper bound) morphemes. Her MLU determines her to be in Stage 5 based on Brown's stages of syntactic development (1973). See Table 4.8 in Chapter 4 for an outline of Brown's stages. Notice that Carrie's stage is appropriate for children who are in the 41- to 46-month range. Carrie is 36 months, so she is doing just fine in her language development regarding utterance length. How is Carrie doing in her development of grammatical morphemes? Examine the age range for mastery of particular morphemes in Chapter 6, Table 6.1. As you can see, Carrie is making very common errors for her age, and it is likely she will add the use of omitted forms within the next six to nine months. She will sort out the use of objective and subjective pronouns, produce full verb forms containing the verb "to be," and use infinitive forms and modals. She will learn to ask questions using *do* and *does*.

We have provided Carrie's sample and analysis of grammar as an example of how to go about the process of collecting, transcribing, and analyzing the syntax of this three-year-old child. Now let us turn our attention to the semantic and pragmatic features of Carrie's language sample.

We mentioned some early semantic roles earlier in this chapter for children who are in the single-word stage. Carrie's use of multi-word utterances requires us to use tools that suit that purpose. The goal of the semantic analysis is to determine if the child is able to convey a variety of meanings. Children do this through the use of many different words and word combinations.

Using Table 5.2, we see that Carrie is using common semantic relations as she combines words. Her utterances alone tell us that she is communicating a lot of ideas that relate to objects and people, their actions and reactions. Some examples from her sample show the diversity of meanings she conveys through sophisticated word combinations.

That a red block – Demonstrative + Attribute + Entity
Daddyridehimbiketowork – Agent + Action + Possession + Object + Locative
Go to the barn horsey – Action + Locative + Object
Him no drink water – Agent + Negative + Action + Object

One procedure to determine word diversity is called the Type-Token Ratio. It is determined from the number of different words in the sample divided by the total number of words. A ratio is a proportion, so it tells us if a particular child has variety in his word choices. A typical ratio is about .50 during early childhood. So, about half the words a child uses are different words and about half are the same words (Nelson, 2010). We can consider vocabulary diversity by identifying the number of different words in a 75- to 100-utterance sample. Figure 5.4 is the worksheet for Carrie's use of words. Let's see what Carries sample tells us about her vocabulary diversity. First, Carrie produced 144 different words in 75 utterances. Data from research studies show that children who are 5 years old produce between 156 and 206 different words in 100-utterance samples (Leadholm & Miller, 1992), so it is reasonable to say that Carrie's diversity is adequate given her age. She also has a Type-Token Ratio of .43, which is within an acceptable range. The 75-utterance sample may be the limiting factor here. An additional way to consider vocabulary is to look at the different types of words the child is producing. You can see that Carrie has many nouns, pronouns, modifiers, locatives, action words, and function words, and some *Wh-* question words. This is important because they can be combined into many different sentences in order to convey meaning.

The goal of a pragmatic analysis is to decide if utterances are appropriate in function: Do they serve a variety of purposes? We don't have to do an analysis to see that Carrie is conveying her thoughts in an appropriate and diverse manner. However, for some children we will need a tool to guide our observations. The items in Figure 5.5 can be used as a checklist during observation of a child in his normal environment. A clinician may set up situations to observe any of these skills if they do not occur during the language sample.

Carrie demonstrates appropriate communication skills for her age. Within her language sample she used 1a, 1b, 2a, 2b, 3a, 3b, 3c, 4a, 4b, 5a, 5b. A few items are not listed, such as 1c and 1d, because we cannot tell they occurred from the written transcript.

It should be evident that three-year-old Carrie is well on her way to being a skilled speaker of English. She has several more years to expand her utterance length, as we will see in the chapters to come.

Figure 5.4   Type-Token Ratio

Objects/People/Places	Pronouns/Demonstratives	Modifiers	Locatives	Action/State
Block // (3)	I //////// (9)	Red	For ///// (6)	Want / (2)
Mommy ///////////// (13)	Me /// (4)	Birthday / (2)	At /// (4)	To / (2)
Daddy /// (4)	It //////// (9)	Big	In /// (4)	Build
Tower	You / (2)	Kitty	To //// (5)	Do
Puzzle	My ///////// (7)	Pretty	On	Show
Room	Them	Green	Up /// (4)	Gave
dolly	This // (3)	Blue	With / (2)	Look // (3)
dress	That // (3)	Yellow	Of	Go /////// (8)
Red ! (2)	Her	Lots	Over // (3)	Find
Green / (2)	His	Mad	Outside	Have
Bike / (2)	Him ///// (6)	grape	out	Like / (2)
Work	He /// (4)	sippy		Ride
Dog / (2)	Your	some // (3)		Walking
TV	You	all / (2)		See
Stairs	We	first		Gonna
Friend / (2)	Let's / (2)	sleepy		Play
Buttons	They	other		Is
Water //////// (8)		more		Drink(s) /// (4)
Floor		silly		Splash
Drink				Get ////// (7)
Juice / (2)				Slip
Cup				Falled
Sink / (2)				Wipe
Breakfast /// (4)				Can / (2)
Cheerios / (2)				Have // (3)
Toast				Put / (2)
Animals // (3)				night-night / (2)
Barn / (2)				sleep // (3)
Horsey //// (5)				come
Nap				made/make (2)
Bed				eat // (3)
Sheep /// (4)				help
Chicken / (2)				
Cows / (2)				
One / (2)				
Time / (2)				
Table				
Kitchen				
Pancakes ///// (6)				
bucket				

Question Words	Function Words, Negatives, Polite Forms
What	To / (2)
Where // (3)	Too / (2)
Why	Let / (2)
	A /// (4)
	Here ////// (7)

(continued)

Figure 5.4 Continued

Question Words	Function Words, Negatives, Polite Forms
	How
	Uh hum
	Oh / (2)
	Not
	Maybe
	Yeah //// (5)
	The //////////// (14)
	Probably
	And //////// (9)
	All // (3)
	Sometime
	Please
	OK
	No //// (5)
	There
	not
	Total Number of Words = 335
	Total Number of Different Words = 144
	Number of Different Words/Number of Words = .43

Figure 5.5. Pragmatic Skills

1. Attends to communication
   a. Establishes joint reference to people and objects
   b. Maintains attention during communication
   c. Shifts attention between communication partners
   d. Makes eye contact at appropriate intervals during communication

2. Makes requests
   a. Gestures, speaks or writes to gain objects
   b. Gestures, speaks or writes to request an action
   c. Asks others to communicate

3. Responds to requests, questions or commands
   a. Brings objects, follows directions, or obeys commands
   b. Answers questions, gives verbal or gestural responses
   c. Greets others
   d. Responds to a greeting

4. Takes turns
   a. Waits to take verbal turns
   b. Doesn't interrupt others

5. Maintains topic
   a. Stays on topic for at least two turns
   b. Shifts topic at appropriate time

✓ Check Your Understanding 5.4

Assess your understanding of the analysis of language sample transcripts by completing this brief quiz.

SUMMARY

Language sampling and analysis is one technique that reveals much about a child's language. Researchers and clinicians use language sampling to determine the progress a child has made in grammatical forms, semantic relations, and pragmatics. Because children advance in language in predictable ways, it is possible to document an individual child's progress as he moves from one stage to another.

We discussed the procedures for facilitating language in young children, collecting the sample and transcribing it, and analysis procedures that focus on grammar, semantic, and pragmatic sophistication. These basic procedures will allow you to practice language sample analysis and interpretation. Try these procedures on the sample provided in Appendix E. Use information in Chapter 4, Chapter 5, and Chapter 6 to make decisions about this child's language forms, meanings, and how he uses language in conversation.

▌▶ Surfing the Web

If you are interested in exploring topics discussed in this chapter in more detail, search for one or more of the following relevant terms online.
language sampling
reliable language samples
valid language samples
transcribing language samples
glossing utterances
mean length of utterance
grammatical analysis
semantic analysis
pragmatic analysis

✓ Chapter Review 5.1

Recall what you learned in this chapter by completing the Chapter Review.

Appendices

Appendix A

Sample Language Transcription Form

Child's Name:		
Participant's Name:		
Participant-Observer:		
Date:		
Location:		
Context	**Adult**	**Child**

Appendix B

Sample Language Transcript: Three-Year-Old Child

Child's Name: Carrie Bartman

Participant's Name: JoAnn Bartman (J)

Participant-Observer: Rosemary Strand, Speech-Language Pathologist (R)

Date: November 28, 2017

Location: Home

Context	Adult	Child
Bag of blocks dumped on the floor.	J: Let's play with these blocks, Carrie. I'm going to build a tower.	I want to build too. Let me do it. That a red block. Here, let me show you how.
	J: OK. You like to play with these? R: I didn't know you got them for your birthday.	My birthday blocks? Uh hum. My mommy and daddy gave them for my birthday. Oh look at my tower. It big. (laughs)
Carrie shifts attention to a puzzle piece on the floor.	J: Ok, I'm gonna knock mine down. J: Now I have to build it again. R: I think it is a piece to a puzzle.	Me too, mommy! What this? That not a block. Where it go?
	J: That is a piece to your Kitty puzzle.	Where my Kitty puzzle? I go find it, mommy. Maybe it in my room.
Mother redirects child to a doll	J: Well, stay here and play with me and your doll. J: I like her dress. It has lots of colors. R: What is your very favorite color, Carrie.	My dolly! Look mommy. Her have a pretty dress. Yeah, green, blue, yellow. Red

	J: OK, I like red too. R: Yes, I like red but blue is my favorite.	Mommy you like red?
	J: That's true. He got that green bike for his birthday.	Daddy like green. His bike green.
	J: No, not today because he was late leaving this morning. R: Where do you think he is going? R: Do you have a dog?	Daddy ride him bike to work? Look at the dog on TV. He walking up the stairs. Oh, probably to see him friend. He gonna play with him friend. Yes! Buttons is my doggie and he in the backyard.
	R: What does Buttons like to do?	Uhm, Buttons likes to play with him ball and drink lots of water. He splash water all over on the floor. Mommy get mad at all the water. It all over and sometime I slip and fall.
	R: Well, yes because she has to clean it up.	
	R: That's dangerous so you have to wipe it up.	Wipe it up, yeah. Can I have a drink, Mommy?
	J: Sure. Do you want water or grape juice?	Grape juice, please. My sippy cup in the sink. I dranked some at breakfast. And I have Cheerios.
	J: When did you use it?	Daddy have Cherrios too and toast.
R shifts focus to the bag of farm animals	R: OK, let's see if we can set up this farm. Here is the barn. Now what should we do? R: Well, that's a lot. How about if we decide which ones should go there and which should stay outside.	Put all the animals in the barn. OK, I go first. Go to the barn horsey. He up here for a nap. Night-night horsey. Him sleepy, mommy.

		This horsey bed. No sheep, mommy. Sheep go outside over here.
	J: The sheep has its own bed here?	
		Yeah it go sleep here. Night-night sheep. This chicken can sleep with the other chickens. Where the cows go to sleep? I put one here and one here.
	R: Is it morning? What are all the animals going to do?	
		It time for breakfast! Get up animals. Time for your breakfast. Come out to the table.
	J: Who is going to make breakfast for all these animals.	
		You make breakfast, mommy.
	J: Wow, let's have pancakes.	
		Get my kitchen, mommy. We make pancakes for all them animals.
	R: Can I help you set the table?	
		Yeah, I want to eat pancakes. Here pancake for cow and sheep. Horsey eat pancake (gobble noises). Pancake him eat. No more pancake horsey. Him no drink water. Why there no water in the bucket?
	R: We had better put some water in that bucket for the animals.	
		Let's go to the sink and get some. Let's go get some water. Help me get water, mommy.
	J: Do you think they want grape juice?	
		No, that silly, mommy. They drink water, not juice.

Appendix C

Language Sample Transcription— Counting Morphemes

Child utterances numbered and grammatical errors identified.

Utterance	Morphemes
1. I want to build too	5
2. Let me do it	4
3. That a red block (That *is* a red block)	4/5
4. Here let me show you how	6
5. My birthday blocks?	4
6. Uh hum	1
7. My mommy and daddy gave them for my birthday	9
8. Oh look at my tower	5
9. It big (laughs) (It *is* big)	2/3
10. Me too mommy!	3
11. What this? (What *is* this)	2/3
12. That not a block (That *is* not a block)	4/5
13. Where it go? (Where *does* it go?)	3/4
14. Where my Kitty puzzle? (Where *is* my Kitty puzzle?)	4/5
15. I go find it mommy (I *will* go find it, mommy)	5/6
16. Maybe it in my room (Maybe it *is* in my room)	5/6
17. My dolly!	2
18. Look mommy	2
19. Her have a pretty dress (*She has* a pretty dress)	5/5
20. Yeah, green, blue, yellow	4
21. Red	1
22. Mommy you like red? (Mommy, *do* you like red?)	4/5
23. Daddy like green (Daddy *likes* green)	3/3
24. His bike green (His bike *is* green)	3/4
25. Daddy ride him bike to work? (Did Daddy ride *his* bike to work?)	6/6
26. Look at the dog on TV	6
27. He walking up the stairs (He *is* walking up the stairs)	6/7
28. Oh, probably to see him friend (Oh, probably to see *his* friend)	6/6

Utterance	Morphemes
29. He gonna play with him friend (*He's* gonna play with *his* friend)	6/7
30 Yep Buttons is my doggie	5
31. And him in the backyard (And *he is* in the backyard)	5/6
32. Buttons like to play with him ball (Buttons *likes* to play with *his* ball)	7/7
33. and drink lots of water	5
34. He splash water all over on the floor (He *splashes* water all over on the floor)	8/8
35. Mommy get mad at all the water (Mommy *gets* mad at all the water)	7/7
36. It all over and sometime I slips and falled (It *is* all over and *sometimes* I *slip* and *fall*)	9/9
37. Wipe it up, yeah.	4
38. Can I have a drink Mommy?	6
39. Grape juice please.	3
40. My sippy cup in the sink (My sippy cup *is* in the sink)	6/7
41. I dranked some at breakfast (I *drank* some at breakfast)	5/5
42. And I have Cheerios. (And I *had* Cheerios)	4/4
43. Daddy have Cheerios too and toast (Daddy *had* Cheerios too and toast)	6/6
44. Put all the animals in the barn	8
45. OK I go first	4
46. Go to the barn horsey	5
47. He up here for a nap (He *is* up here for a nap)	6/7
48. Night-night horsey	2
49. Him sleepy mommy (*He is* sleepy, mommy)	3/4
50. This horsey bed. (This is *the horsey's* bed)	3/6
51. No sheep mommy	3
52. Sheep go outside over here (Sheep *goes* outside over here)	5/6
53. Yeah it go sleep here (Yeah it *goes to* sleep here)	5/6
54. Night-night sheep	2
55. This chicken can sleep with the other chickens	9
56. Where the cows go to sleep? (Where *do* the cows go to sleep?)	7/8
57. I put one here and one here	7
58. It time for breakfast! (It *is* time for breakfast!)	4/5
59. Get up animals	4

Utterance	Morphemes
60. Time for your breakfast	4
61. Come out to the table	5
62. You make breakfast mommy	4
63. Get my kitchen mommy	4
64. We make pancakes for all the animals (We *will* make pancakes for all the animals)	9/10
65. Yeah I want to eat pancakes	7
66. Here pancakes for cows and sheeps (Here *are* pancakes for cows and *sheep*)	8/9
67. Horsey eat pancakes (gobble noises) (Horsey *is eating* pancakes)	4/6
68. Pancake him eat (Pancake *he eats*)	3/3
69. No more pancakes horsey	5
70. Him no drink water (*He does not* drink water)	4/5
71. Why there no water in the bucket? (Why *is* there no water in the bucket?)	7/8
72. Let's go to the sink and get some	9
73. Let's go get some water	5
74. Help me get water mommy	5
75. No that silly mommy (No that *is* silly mommy)	4/5
76. They drink water not juice	5
Total Number of Morphemes Used:	369
Total Number of Morphemes Obligated:	400
Total Number of Utterances:	76
Mean Length of Utterance:	4.86

Grammatical Errors:
Omission of present tense "to be" verb copula *is*,
Omission of article *the*
Omission of possessive *s*
Omission of regular third person singular verb *s*
Omission of infinitive
Omission of *do* in a question
Omission of future tense modal verb
Omission of present tense "to be" verb copula *are*
Omission of present progressive "to be" verb *is* + *ing*
Incorrect use of subjective pronoun *he*

Appendix D

Language Sample Transcription and Grammar Analysis

Child utterances numbered and grammatical errors identified.

1. I want to build too
2. Let me do it
3. That a red block (That *is* a red block)
   omission of copula "to be" verb
4. Here, let me show you how
5. My birthday blocks?
6. Uh hum
7. My mommy and daddy gave them for my birthday
8. Oh look at my tower
9. It big (laughs) (It *is* big)
   omission of copula "to be" verb
10. Me too, mommy!
11. What this? (What *is* this)
    omission of copula "to be" verb
12. That not a block (That *is* not a block)
    omission of copula "to be" verb
13. Where it go? (Where *does* it go?)
    omission of future tense do
14. Where my Kitty puzzle? (Where *is*, my Kitty puzzle?)
    omission of copula "to be" verb
15. I go find it, mommy (I *will* go find it, mommy)
    omission of model verb
16. Maybe it in my room (Maybe it *is*, in my room)
    omission of copula "to be" verb
17. My dolly!
18. Look mommy
19. Her have a pretty dress (*She has* a pretty dress)
    error on subjective pronoun
20. Yeah, green, blue, yellow
21. Red
22. Mommy you like red? (Mommy, *do* you like red?)
    omission of do
23. Daddy like green (Daddy *likes* green)
    error singular verb
24. His bike green (His bike *is* green)
    omission of copula "to be" verb

25. Daddy ride him bike to work? (Did Daddy ride *his* bike to work?)
    error on possessive pronoun
26. Look at the dog on TV
27. He walking up the stairs (He *is* walking up the stairs)
    omission of auxiliary "to be" verb
28. Oh, probably to see him friend (Oh, probably to see *his* friend)
    error on possessive pronoun
29. He gonna play with him friend (*He's* gonna play with *his* friend)
    omission of auxiliary "to be" verb
30. Yep, Buttons is my doggie
31. And him in the backyard (And *he is* in the backyard)
    error on subjective pronoun
    omission of copula "to be" verb
32. Uhm, Buttons like to play with him ball (Buttons *likes* to play with *his* ball)
    error singular verb
    error on possessive pronoun
33. and drink lots of water
34. He splash water all over on the floor (He *splashes* water all over on the floor)
    error on singular verb
35. Mommy get mad at all the water (Mommy *gets*, mad at all the water)
    error on singular verb
36. It all over and sometime I slips and falled (It *is* all over and *sometimes* I *slip* and *fall*)
    omission of copula "to be" verb
    error on singular verb
    error on irregular past tense verb
37. Wipe it up, yeah.
38. Can I have a drink, Mommy?
39. Grape juice, please.
40. My sippy cup in the sink (My sippy cup *is* in the sink)
    omission of copula "to be" verb
41. I dranked some at breakfast (I *drank*, some at breakfast)
    error on irregular past tense verb
42. And I have Cheerios. (And I *had*, Cheerios)
43. Daddy have Cheerios too and toast (Daddy *had* Cheerios too and toast)
    error on past tense verb
44. Put all the animals in the barn
45. OK, I go first
46. Go to the barn horsey
47. He up here for a nap (He *is*, up here for a nap)
    omission of copula "to be" verb
48. Night-night horsey
49. Him sleepy, mommy (*He is,s* sleepy, mommy)
    error on subjective pronoun

50. This horsey bed. (This is *the horsey's* bed)
    omission of copula "to be" verb
    omission of article
    omission of possessive *'s*
51. No sheep, mommy
52. Sheep go outside over here
53. Yeah it go sleep here (Yeah it *goes to* sleep here)
    error on singular verb
    omission of infinitive to
54. Night-night sheep
55. This chicken can sleep with the other chickens
56. Where the cows go to sleep? (Where *do*, the cows go to sleep?)
    omission of do
57. I put one here and one here
58. It time for breakfast! (It *is*, time for breakfast!)
    omission of copula "to be" verb
59. Get up animals
60. Time for your breakfast
61. Come out to the table
62. You make breakfast, mommy
63. Get my kitchen, mommy
64. We make pancakes for all the animals (We *will* make pancakes for all the animals)
    omission of model auxiliary
65. Yeah, I want to eat pancakes
66. Here pancakes for cows and sheeps (Here *are*, pancakes for cows and *sheep*)
    omission of copula "to be" verb
67. Horsey eat pancakes (gobble noises) (Horsey *is eating* pancakes
    omission of present progressive form of "to be" verb
68. Pancake him eat (Pancake *he eats*,)
    error subjective pronoun
69. No more pancakes horsey
70. Him no drink water (*He does not* drink water)
    error subjective pronoun
    error on do + negative
71. Why there no water in the bucket? (Why *is* there no water in the bucket?)
    omission of copula "to be" verb
72. Let's go to the sink and get some
73. Let's go get some water
74. Help me get water, mommy
75. No, that silly, mommy
76. They drink water, not juice

Appendix E

Sample Language Transcription Form—Eric

Child's Name: Eric

Participant's Name: Natalie Collins (N), mother; Kelsey Collins (K), sister

Participant-Observer: Anna Andrews (A), speech-language pathologist

Date: March 9

Location: Child's home

Context	Adult	Child
Playing in family room with child's favorite toys	A: Let's see what we have to play with. A: OK. You look in the bag.	Me look in there Ha-ha a turtle in there Hi turtle Go fast
	A: I think turtles go slow.	No slow Go turtle go
	A: He's a funny turtle. Does he have a friend in there?	Yep Him friend baby bear! What that?
	A: Oh that is the cap to the baby bottle. It came loose. A: Let's look together. A: Do you see it? N: Hey here is the book you got from Grandma. N: Yes it is about the caterpillar. N: Yes, she did. She knew you would like it. N: What? N: Oh, under the table? It looks like a cracker. We should call Buttons over to eat it.	Baby bottle? Me want to see OK me look in there Yeah My book from nana? Nana got book for me What's that? What's that here mommy?
The dog enters the room.	N: Here is Buttons. Good boy. N: Tell Miss Anna about giving Buttons a bath. A: That sounds like fun. Did you get all wet too? N: It sure did. We had to mop it up.	Buttons come eat cracker Here boy eat cracker (giggle) Lick my hand Buttons all wet and he shake all over! Yeah all wet too Splash all over floor huh mommy

Eric directs attention back to the bag	A: It looks like it got caught in this string. What is the string? Oh it is part of the pull toy—a bug I think. A: But now you have that block. What are you going to do with it?	That block stuck Help me get it Pull it out Get it out There it goes Oh boy it got stuck Hm, me need more blocks Build bridge for cars
	A: That sounds like a good idea. Let's gather all the blocks so we can build the bridge.	Let me do that Wow all blocks here Right here by me Let me get that green one Green and red blocks
Big sister comes into the room	A: Here is the green one. Do you want some other colors? A: Can I make a bridge too? A: Great. I think my bridge will be blue and yellow. That will be a pretty bridge.	Sure you got blocks Hi Kelsey Wanna play with me?
	(K) Hi Eric. I can play for a few minutes but I have homework. What are you doing? (K) Looking good. Can I make a tower? (K) I want to make it really tall and then you can knock it down, OK?	Me and mommy and Miss Anna play-ing blocks My bridge is green and red Sure you have mommy's blocks
	(K) You are very good at knocking down towers (K) OK here it is seven blocks tall (K) OK thanks. See you later (N) How about a snack Tiger?	Yeah knock it down Bam, bam, bam Yep very good Wind up and bam knock it down! OK bye Yeah
Mother brings food items into the room	(N) We have some juice and banana and peanut butter.	Me thirsty and hungry
	(N) OK. Do you want some juice? (N) That's a good choice. I 'll get some.	Peanut butter and bananas please No juice mommy Me want water Miss Anna want juice?
	A: That is nice of you, Eric. I think water sounds good for me too. (N) Are you ready for your snack?	Let me see that baby bear. Ok bear play on a bridge Jump down baby bear

| Cell phone rings and mother answers it. | (N) It's OK to have it right here on the floor.
A: Tell me about your snack.
A: Oh I see that you spread it on there.

(N) You are right about that, Eric. Remember when you had some in your hair?
(N) Yes because you had a lot of peanut butter in your hair.

(N) It is daddy and he is bringing home some chicken for dinner.
(N) We'll see if he brings some.
(N) Let's get these toys picked up now, OK? | (giggle) He like jumping down
Fall down baby bear!
Oh he not falling down
Yeah but me playing
OK, me have it here
Right here
Put peanut butter on banana like this
Yeah and it sticky

We wash it out
Wash my hair with soap and water

Who is that?
Some one calling mommy
Maybe daddy calling
Chicken is good
Me want French fries
French fries and ketchup for dinner
My blocks go in my bag
Here's the book |

6

The Saga Continues: Language Development Through the Preschool Years

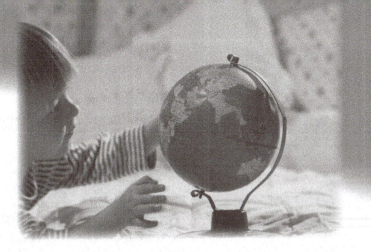

LEARNING OUTCOMES

After completion of this chapter, you will be able to:

- Describe the gains children make in grammar during MLU stages 2 and 3 conversations.
- Discuss how children refine meaning during MLU stages 2 and 3.
- Trace the elaboration of sentences through the use of phrases, clauses, and continued advances in language use during MLU stages 4 and 5.
- Explain the role that comprehension plays in relation to production of concepts, literacy, and later developing forms.
- Explain the similarities and differences in learning two languages simultaneously and successively.

Welcome to the wild and wonderful preschool years, a time of inexhaustible energy, limitless curiosity, and explosive communication development. In this chapter, we examine the phenomenal changes in a child's communication abilities as she runs, jumps, and shrieks through four more stages of language development. At the close of the preceding chapter, the child was just beginning to combine words. By the close of this chapter, she will be an enthusiastic and reasonably competent conversationalist. She will also begin to show evidence of a communication skill we have not seen to this point. She will begin to tell stories, a skill commonly referred to as *narration*. She will also discover that language has regular patterns that can be quite entertaining during participation in songs and games, and that drawing and book-sharing activities are additional and creative ways to interact with others.

Some children will also have the good fortune of learning more than one language at the same time or sometime during their language development journey.

The "Two's" may be terrible for parents trying to keep track of their increasingly active children, but the Two's, the Three's, and the remainder of the preschool years are wonderful and exciting from a language development point of view. As children exit stage 1, they are already talking, but over the next few years they will experience unbelievable gains in language ability. In this chapter, we trace those changes through four more stages of language development. You will notice that virtually all of these changes are elaborations of abilities that emerged in stage 1.

Mean Length of Utterances in Stages 2 and 3: Elaborating Structure

In this section, we will trace the development of grammatical morphemes, pronouns, verbs, phrases, negative forms and question forms, requests and demands, pragmatics, conversations, and metalinguistics across stages 2 and 3. Stage 2 occurs from about 27 months to 30 months and stage 3 follows from 31 to 34 months. Of course these age ranges assume that development is typical, and variations may occur for any particular child.

During stage 2 the MLU is 2.0 to 2.5 morphemes and in stage 3 it is 2.5 to 3.0. Brown (1973) suggests that the greatest change occurring during stage 2 is what he calls the, "**modulations of meaning**" in simple sentences, which are accomplished by the use of grammatical morphemes. To modulate is to modify or regulate, and both of these synonyms are helpful in understanding what occurs when grammatical morphemes are added to base words. For example, by adding *ed* to a verb such as *show*, we can modify the tense from present to past. We use grammatical morphemes to regulate or govern forms of words so that we create the precise meaning we want to express.

Most of the terms used to describe grammatical morphemes will be familiar from our chapter about language sampling and the chapter about the first two years of development, but a few explanations of terminology may be useful. The term **inflection** is used to refer to a change in a word created by adding a grammatical morpheme. Thus, we inflect nouns by making them **plural** (house becomes *houses*) or **possessive** (*Daddy's* shoe). Verbs that discuss actions taking place right now are **present progressive** (*walking*), whereas actions that happened in the past are **regular** (*looked*) or **irregular** (*sat*). The verb *to be* presents some special problems of its own. This verb can be a **copula verb**, or main verb, as in, "He *is* my dog." The verb *to be* can also be used as a helping or **auxiliary verb**, as in, "He *is* running." The child must also sort out when it is appropriate to reduce the pronoun and verb to a **contracted** form, such as, "He's my dog" and, "He's running." He must learn that it is not acceptable to contract "I was running."

Although some grammatical morphemes begin to emerge in the latter part of stage 1, their primary development begins in stage 2 and continues across all the stages. Several studies have focused on 14 grammatical morphemes. Brown (1973) and James and Khan (1982) examined the development of these morphemes in longitudinal studies (children are studied over a period of time), and de Villiers and de Villiers (1973) looked at them in a cross-sectional study (children from each age group are compared to infer developmental trends). Although there are some differences among the three studies, especially with regard to the acquisition of irregular past tense, regular past tense, and the contractible copula, the results summarized in Table 6.1 suggest the order of acquisition for the 14 morphemes.

In all three studies, mastery was determined when 90% of children used each morpheme correctly in *obligatory contexts.* That is, when an utterance *requires* the use of a given grammatical morpheme, the child uses it. If, for example, the child watches his mother jump rope, and the mother says, "What is Mommy doing?" a correct response from the child would include the present progressive form of *jump.* If the child says, "Mommy jumping" or, "Mommy jumping rope," or even if the child says "hopping" or "bouncing" or "running," he has produced the correct grammatical morpheme (*-ing*) for that context.

Although researchers have identified age ranges for the mastery of each of these morphemes, it may be more helpful to emphasize what we know about acquisition in general than to focus attention on specific ages. It is important to note that all of these morphemes begin to emerge during the later months of stage 1 and throughout stage 2. We see mastery of the earliest grammatical morpheme, present progressive, in some children as young as 19 months.

Table 6.1 Acquisition of 14 Grammatical Morphemes

Grammatical Morpheme	Example	Age Range of Mastery (Months)
Present progressive	She run*ning*.	19–28
In (preposition)	Milk *in* cup.	27–30
On (preposition)	Doggie *on* bed.	27–30
Regular plural	Girl*s* playing.	27–33
Irregular past tense	Mommy *went* work.	25–46
Possessive	Billy*'s* ball.	26–40
Uncontractible copula	Billy *was* bad.	27–39
Articles (*the, a*)	Daddy eating *the* cookie.	28–46
Regular past tense	Mommy look*ed*.	26–48
Regular third person singular	She eat*s*.	26–46
Irregular third person singular	Daddy *has* cookie.	28–50
Uncontractible auxiliary	I *was* eating.	29–48
Contractible copula	Billy*'s* bad.	29–49
Contractible auxiliary	He*'s* running.	30–50

Source: Based on Brown (1973) and Miller (1981).

Emergence of the latest of these selected grammatical morphemes, including irregular third-person forms of verbs and the correct sorting of contractible and uncontractible copula and auxiliary verb forms, does not occur until about 28 to 30 months. Although all of these morphemes appear in stage 2, some children do not master them until stage 5 and beyond.

As children begin to master grammatical morphemes, they overextend or overgeneralize their use. When the child begins to make nouns plural by adding *s* to *cat* to make *cats* or the sound *z* to *dog* to make *dogs*, he logically concludes that this rule for plural should work on all nouns. His plural form of *man* is *mans* and his plural form of *child* is *childs*. At some point in his language development, he is likely to overextend the past tense to produce forms such as *goed*, *runned*, *throwed*, and *eated*. Imagine his confusion when he has to learn that the plural of *deer* is *deer* and the plural of *moose* is *moose* or when he learns that the past tense of *burst* is *burst*. Because these productions are unusual and because they catch our attention, we may conclude that they are commonplace in the speech of children at this age. But they occur in only about 5% of utterances (Chapman et al., 1992). In the process of comparing his productions with the productions of those models in his environment who have greater language competence than he does, the child will eventually determine how to apply conventional rules for the use of morphemes.

Pronouns: Words Used to Represent Nouns

Adults use pronouns so easily that we probably do not consider how difficult these words are for children acquiring language. The traditional definition of *pronoun* in English grammar textbooks is something like this: "A **pronoun** is a word used in place of a noun." Actually, there is much more involved than this, and it is the "much more" that should help you understand why children begin to use pronouns in stage 1 or 2 but may not master the use of some pronouns until stage 5 and beyond. In fact, it is not uncommon for adults to struggle with some pronoun forms, and some of us never get them right!

Consider all the language information conveyed by pronouns. Pronouns convey information about gender or the lack of gender (he, him, she, her, it) and about the number of referents (I, we, you, he, she, they). Before the child even enters stage 2, he probably uses a few pronouns including *I, it, this,* and *that*. During stage 2 he will add *my, mine, me,* and *you*. Be aware that the child might not use these pronouns correctly in all situations. He might say, "My ball" at one time and, "Mine ball" at another time. He might use *me* correctly as an objective pronoun when he says, "Kiss me, Mommy," but he might also use *me* as a subjective pronoun when he says, "Me kiss Mommy." It takes time to get all this, that, and the other sorted out. During stage 3, the child will be more consistent in the use of personal pronouns, such as *your, yours, she, he,* and *we* (Owens, 2005) and the demonstrative pronouns *this, that, these,* and *those*.

Children must also learn that pronouns differ, depending on whether they are used as subjects or objects in sentences. The pronouns *I, she, he,* and *they*, for example, are **subjective pronouns**, and their **objective** counterparts are *me, her, him,* and *them*. The child must be able to put the right pronoun in the right part of the sentence. This is not an easy task, and it takes the child some time before he gets it right. According to Wells (1985), most subjective and objective pronouns are not mastered until about 36 months, which places the child in stage 4. Here are examples of how pronouns can be used in the subjective and objective roles in sentences:

Subjective Pronouns	Objective Pronouns
He gave John the tractor.	Dad gave *me* the tractor.
It goes in the toy box.	Mommy put *it* in my toy box.
She has the Peter Pan book.	Jim should give *her* the book.

In addition to knowing where subjective and objective pronouns belong in the structures of sentences, a child must learn that the number represented by the pronoun determines the verb form to be used. She must say, "He is" and, "She is" but, "They are" and, "I am." She must learn the possessive forms of pronouns such as *hers, his, mine, their*, and *your* and when and when not to use reflexive pronouns such as *yourself, himself*, and *herself*.

Because pronouns take the place of nouns, children must learn to establish the topic noun in a preceding sentence so that the listener knows the context. For example, in order for a listener to properly decode the meaning of the pronoun *it*, as in the sentence, "John bought it," he must have heard the previous sentence, "John loved that sweater." This type of reference, in which a pronoun is used to refer to something in a preceding utterance, is called an **anaphoric reference.** It is a very important element in conversations and narratives as it serves as a cohesive strategy to tie ideas together.

Fortunately, there is some order to the potential pronoun chaos. As with all dimensions of language, the child acquires pronouns in a progressive and fairly predictable manner, and we will follow this progress as we move through the remaining stages. In general, you will notice that children acquire subjective pronouns such as *she* and *he* before acquiring objective pronouns such as *her* and *him*. They will then acquire pronouns indicating possession such as *his, hers, their*, and *our*, and, finally, they will use reflexive pronouns such as *myself, yourself*, and *themselves*.

You were introduced to Patrick in Chapter 4 as a one-year-old. In this chapter, some samples of his language during his second and third years show the remarkable journey he makes in the short time from toddler to preschooler. A portion of Patrick's transcript at two years, two weeks of age is analyzed in Table 6.2. His full

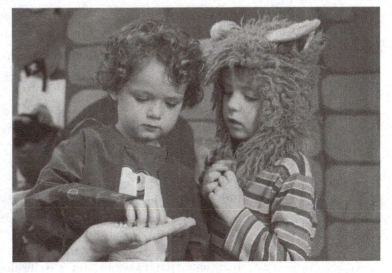

Patrick loves to dress up for his fall preschool party.

Source: Jules Selmes/ Pearson Education, Inc.

Table 6.2   Patrick's Language Sample at 2 Years: Grammatical Morphemes and Other Early Forms (MLU = 2.37; Range = 1.0 to 6.0)

Utterance	Morphemes	Grammatical Form
What's that?	3	contracted copula
What's that, baby.	4	contracted copula
Ah-oh choo-choos	3	regular plural
Choo-choos	2	regular plural
There he is	2	uncontracted copula
Playing	2	present progressive
Building tracks	4	present progressive and regular plural
My chair	2	possessive pronoun
Red engine	2	adjective
Ah there it is!	4	uncontracted copula and pronoun
Right there	2	qualifier
There it is!	3	uncontracted copula and pronoun
Here he goes	4	regular third person singular and pronoun
Where did he go?	4	auxiliary verb and pronoun
Where'd he go?	4	auxiliary verb and pronoun
Take this	2	demonstrative pronoun
There goes	2	regular third person singular
What's that?	3	contracted copula
There he goes	4	regular third person singular
What's this?	3	contracted copula
What's that?	3	contracted copula
More please	2	qualifier
What is that?	3	uncontracted copula
An on where'd he go?	6	preposition
Oh what is that?	4	uncontracted copula
I'll get it	4	pronoun; auxiliary verb and pronoun

transcript revealed an MLU of 2.37 with a range of 1.0 to 6.0 morphemes. Utterances are included that show his emerging grammatical morphemes. You'll notice that he is more advanced than some children, because most children do not enter stage 2 until they are two years, three months old. But, as we have reminded you in the last several chapters, there is much room for individual variation. As we discuss the emergence of grammar and meaning, refer to Patrick's language sample. You will see that he has many of the targeted grammatical morphemes.

Let's look at Patrick's sample to see what pronouns he uses at just two years. It appears that his pronoun use is developing with impressive speed. The variety shows his knowledge of how to use pronouns in place of nouns that are of joint reference to those in the conversation.

What's *that?*	Here *he* goes.
Take *this.*	*I'll* get *it.*
My chair	Where'd *he* go?
There *it* is.	*Mine.*

Auxiliary Verbs

As mentioned earlier, an auxiliary verb is a helping verb. There are **primary auxiliary verbs** such as *have* and *do,* and there are secondary auxiliary verbs such as *can, shall, may,* and *will,* which are also called **modals**. During stage 2, the child begins to use the verbs *have* and *do* as main verbs and as auxiliary verbs. She also produces what are considered semi-auxiliary verb forms such as *hafta, gonna,* and *wanna* as in, "I hafta go potty" and, "I wanna go bye-bye."

As with many language forms, children begin to use auxiliary verbs within a wide range of ages (Wells, 1985). So variable are the ages of acquisition that Wells identified the ages at which only 50% of the children studied were producing selected forms, so that we can see when early emergence occurs. The earliest forms to be used were *do* and *have,* at about 27 months. *Can, be,* and *will* were being produced at about 30 months, and the last two forms to be used by these children were *shall* at 39 months and *could* at 42 months, ages that extend beyond stage 2. The stage 3 child uses these verbs more consistently and adds the verb *to be* as an auxiliary and copula form. The child may not use them correctly to indicate person or number, as in the sentences *They is running, She am my Mommy,* and *We is here.* As we look at Patrick's sample (Table 6.2), we see that he begins to use auxiliary verbs, but not very often. Here are three examples.

Where *did* he go? *Where'd* he go? *I'll* get it.

Phrases

Children in stages 2 and 3 produce combinations of words that are more recognizable as sentences. To do this, the child must develop an understanding of the basic parts or components of sentences. We call these components *phrases.*

A **phrase** is a combination of words that are related to one another, and the combination serves a grammatical purpose, but a phrase does not contain both a subject and a predicate. There are two kinds of phrases: noun phrases and verb phrases. As the name suggests, a **noun phrase** contains a noun and words that describe or modify the noun. There are four kinds of modifiers in noun phrases: determiners, adjectivals, initiators, and postmodifiers (see Table 6.3).

- A **determiner** is the first unit in a noun phrase and is an article (*a, the*), a possessive pronoun (*my, his, he*), a demonstrative pronoun (*this, that, these, those*), or a qualifier (*some, most, any*).

Table 6.3 Possible Constituents of a Noun Phrase

Initiator	Determiner	Ordinal	Quantifier	Adjective	Noun	Postmodifiers
Includes words such as *only*, *nearly*, *almost*, *all*	Includes words such as *the*, *a*, *this*, *that*, *my*, *his*	Includes words such as *first*, *last*, *final*	Includes words such as *one*, *two*, *fifteen*	Includes words such as *big*, *blue*, *little*	Includes words such as *boy*, *girl*, *dog*	Includes prepositional phrases such as *in the middle*, *on the chair*
Example: Only	the	last	six	little	dogs	on the chair

Note: Additional adjectives could be incorporated into the noun phrase to make it even longer.

- An **adjectival** modifies a noun and can be an adjective (*pretty, tall*), an ordinal (*second, last*), or a quantifier (*one, couple, few*).
- An **initiator** comes before a determiner and places a limit on the noun (*only, all, both, just*).
- A **postmodifier** is a modifier that comes after the noun. A postmodifier might be a prepositional phrase, as in "The fish *in the little tank* is Fred," or a clause, as in "The man *who called last night* is my uncle."

Although children produce noun phrases in stage 2, they tend to use only determiners and adjectivals as modifiers in these phrases. Not until the end of stage 4 will he consistently use initiators and postmodifiers (Bernstein, 1989). Patrick uses some elements of the noun phrase (Table 6.2), although they are used sparingly at this point in the following utterances:

> *my* chair (possessive pronoun)
> *more*, please; *right* there (qualifier)
> *red* engine (adjective).

A **verb phrase** contains a verb, and it might contain some other supporting or qualifying words (see Table 6.4). In the sentence "The boy is running," the verb phrase *is running* contains the main verb *run* and the present progressive form supported by *is*. A verb phrase might also contain a modal, which is a word indicating the "attitude" of the verb. Common modals are *can, will, must, shall*, and *may*. Notice the difference in the attitudes of the verb phrases in these sentences when we just change the modal: (1) "John *will* go to the party;" and (2) "John *may* go to the party." The only verb phrase elaboration to be mastered in stage 2 is the present progressive form, but the child does produce primitive infinitive verb forms such as "wanna" and "gonna" (Miller, 1981), and by the end of stage 2, the child typically creates the negative versions of these forms when she produces those sentences we all love to hear: "I can't" or "I won't."

Verb phrases in stage 3 include auxiliary verbs such as *can, do, will*, and the auxiliary form of the verb *to be*. As noted earlier, the verb *to be* may not correctly indicate person and number, and it may not be properly marked for tense. The child might say, "I *is*," or he might say, "She *is*" when he really means, "She was." He is also likely to overextend the regular past tense when he uses irregular verbs to produce, "She *runned* away" or, "I *falled* down" (Miller, 1981).

Table 6.4   Possible Constituents of a Verb Phrase

Other than tense, number, and a verb, the remaining elements of a verb phrase are optional in a simple, grammatically acceptable sentence. Optional elements have been placed in parentheses.

Tense and Number	(Modals)	(Perfect Aspect)	(Progressive)	Main Verb	(Noun Phrase)
All sentences are either present or past in form.	*Can, may, must, shall, will, could, might, should, would*	*have + en* "have forgotten"	Auxiliary verb *to be + ing.* as in "is running." *Is, are, was, were,* or *am + ing*	*Run, kick, play*	The noun phrase can be a prepositional phrase, noun phrase, noun complement, or adverbial phrase.

Note: In the example sentence below, the verb is in the past tense and all of the optional constituents identified above are used. The production of this sentence is based on Chomsky's transformational generative grammar. To generate the example sentence, a rule called the affix or hopping rule enables the speaker to move constituents that can be moved. According to the rule, the speaker can move or affix these members to the stationary member on the right.

In the example sentence, the movable members are tense, the participle ending *en* that accompanies perfect aspect, and the progressive ending *ing* that is the progressive aspect.

After the affix rule is applied, we end up with the sentence "*The boy might have been running in the field.*"

As the child learns to produce and elaborate phrases and clauses, she produces sentences that are more and more complete syntactically and semantically. Although the most dramatic changes in sentences will not occur until stage 3 and beyond, the child in stage 2 produces sentences that contain three, four, and more words. Keep in mind that the upper end of the MLU range in stage 2 is 2.5. The child still produces single-word utterances, with fewer of these short utterances and more multiple-word utterances. Her sentences become longer because she expands her noun phrases and verb phrases. Her noun phrases include personal pronouns such as *my* and *mine*, demonstrative pronouns such as *this* and *that*, and the articles *a* and *the*. Her verb phrases include the present progressive form marked by *ing* as well as semiauxiliary verb forms such as *gonna* and *wanna*. But in stage 3, the MLU increases to 3.0, with more elaboration of the noun and verb phrases.

Negation

Children begin to express negation by late stage 1 and develop its proper use in the early part of stage 4. Klima and Bellugi-Klima (1971) identified three periods that roughly correspond to the stages described by Brown (1973):

- Late Stage 1–Early Stage 2 (MLU 1.5–2.5); "*No* kick that."
- Late Stage 2–Early Stage 3 (MLU 2.25–2.75); "I *no* like that."
- Late Stage 3–Early Stage 4 (MLU 2.75–3.5); "Daddy is *not* going to work."

Notice how the child uses the negative term first at the beginning of the utterance, and then he learns to place it between the subject noun and the verb, finally inserting it between the auxiliary and the action verb. Would it be correct to assume that the child has mastered syntactic negation by the time he reaches stage 4? Not hardly! The child is probably going to be beyond his preschool years before he starts using questions that contain negative forms, such as in the sentence, "Why doesn't Sam like pie?" (Owens, 2016).

Bloom (1970) described three variations of the negative theme during stage 2. The child can express *nonexistence* of something, as when he says, "Cookie allgone," *rejection*, as in the exclamation. "No night-night," and *denial* to express disagreement with another child ("No horsie") who identifies a cow as a horse. In stage 2 the child does not differentiate between *no* and *not*; thus, some interpretation of the child's meaning is necessary in some situations. By late stage 2, *no, not, can't*, and *don't* are used in an undifferentiated manner, but there is progress in locating the negative form between the subject and the predicate. You should note that even though *can't* and *don't* are being used, the child does not use the positive forms (*can, do*) until later (Brown, Cazden, & Bellugi, 1969).

Sentences in stage 3 become more elaborated with continued advances in the use of the negative form as the child adds *no* or *not* between the subject and the predicate to produce a sentence such as, "Daddy no go bye-bye." The child is also adding auxiliary forms to negative forms, as in, "Doggie don't bark." Notice also the use of the contracted negative form *don't* in this sentence. Because in this stage the child also produces affirmative forms of these verbs (*can, do, will*), we can assume that these contractions are based on the application of a rule and are not simply imitations of whole constructions. Brown (1973) considered the changes children make in the use of the negative form to be one of the most important advances to occur in stage 3. In the following excerpt, look at the way in which Patrick expresses negation as he interacts with his Grandpa about the nectarine in a sample of speech at age two years, nine months with an MLU of 3.23:

P:	I want an apple too.
GRP:	This is not an apple.
K*:	What is it?
GRP:	It's a nectarine.
P:	I want a nectarine.
GRP:	You want lunch?
P:	No want a nectarine.
GRP:	Want a nectarine?
P:	Yeah.
GRP:	Okay. I'll cut the nectarine up.
K:	He's gonna give you some nectarine.
P:	[unintelligible] . . . cut the nectarine up.
K:	I don't think you can cut it up. Grandpa has to cut it up.
P:	I don't want cut up.
GRP:	He doesn't want any?
P:	yeah I don't want it cut up.

K: You want to eat the whole thing?

P: Yeah.

Asking Questions

Before we consider what the stage 2 and stage 3 child is able to do in creating sentences using question forms, we should consider the functions of questions. Speakers can ask questions that elicit *yes* or *no* answers, and they can ask questions beginning with *who, whose, whom, what, where, which, when, why,* or *how.* Questions that begin with *wh-* words or *how,* such as, "What time is it?" require answers that provide information.

We create a *yes/no* question by moving an auxiliary verb in front of the subject and closing the sentence with a rising intonation. The sentence "He was going to the store" is transformed into a *yes/no* question by moving the *was* in front of the *he* to create "Was he going to the store?" If the statement to be transformed does not have an auxiliary verb, the speaker must add the appropriate form of *do,* so that "You have my steak" becomes "Do you have my steak?" or "John plans to come home" becomes "Does John plan to come home?" A *wh-* question is formed by inverting the subject and auxiliary and adding the appropriate *wh-* word or *how* to the beginning of the sentence. "He is sitting" can be transformed into "Where is he sitting?" "How is he sitting?" or "Why is he sitting?"

The stage 2 child is obviously not ready for the sometimes convoluted questions adults ask, such as, "Where is he sitting, with whom, and why?" She does ask questions, however, and some of these questions call for more than *yes* or *no.* Klima and Bellugi-Klima (1971) have identified three periods in the development of interrogative forms.

- Late Stage 1–Early Stage 2 (MLU 1.5–2.5) "Go bye-bye↑"
- Late Stage 2–Early Stage 3 (MLU 2.25–2.75) "What Mommy doing?"
- Late Stage 3–Early Stage 4 (MLU 2.75–3.5) "Why is he eating?"

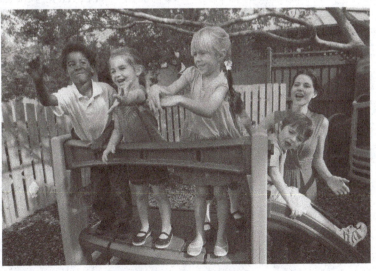

New experiences, new discoveries, and never-ending questions.

Source: Golden Pixels LLC/ Shutterstock

Yes/no questions emerge between the ages of 25 and 28 months, with the child adding rising intonations to simple declarative sentences, the same method she used at the single-word stage of development. In this first phase, she is also asking a few simple *wh-* questions, such as, "What this?" or, "Where Mommy?" *What* and *where* questions are most common, probably because they focus on two of the most prominent semantic categories the child uses at this age, naming and locating. In turn, these may be popular semantic categories because they relate to the child's immediate environment and because caregivers frequently use them to stimulate speech.

During the second period of interrogative development, the child continues to use rising intonation as the primary means by which he expresses *yes/no* questions. In addition to increased use of *what* and *where* questions, he now adds the infamous *why* question, which will become one of his favorite language forms over the next year or so. The child's questions at this point are more elaborate and typically have subjects and predicates, although he still omits auxiliaries. Throughout the first two phases, the child experiences some confusion with *wh-* questions. Until he is about two years old, he interprets most *wh-* questions as *where* questions. After two years, he still responds to some *why* questions as though they are *what* questions. The child, for example, throws his food on the floor. The adult asks, "Why did you do that?" The child responds, "I throwed cookie." In the third phase, the child uses appropriate inverted questions.

Question forms also continue to develop in stage 3. The child is able to use auxiliary verbs and to invert them to ask questions, such as, "Can she go bye-bye?" *Yes/no* questions that include copula verbs are also inverted properly in stage 3, as in, "Am I good boy?" The most frequent *wh-* words used in stage 3 are *what* and *where*, but the child also uses *why, who,* and *how* (Tyack & Ingram, 1977), and most of the child's *wh-* questions are inverted (Klee, 1985), as in, "Where is the cookie?" The following excerpt from Patrick's language sample at two years, nine months shows that questions are certainly on his mind.

> **K*:** Oh boy you are going to swimming lessons today?
> **P:** Want to go with me?
> **K:** I certainly do.
> **P:** Where's grandpa go?
> **K:** He went to get his shorts on.
> **P:** Where?
> **K:** In the bedroom.
> **K:** Where is Patrick? Patrick? Patrick? Oh there you are. Patrick where are you? Boo. Okay. Here comes more!
> **P:** What?
> **K:** Cartoons.
> **P:** What they doing?
> **K:** Looks like they are running in the city! They could be right outside your door! Oh. The cat's running after the mouse!
> **P:** What happened?

Requests and Demands

Because the child has been making requests and demands even before she started to use language, you may wonder when the imperative form of sentences emerges. The child is about 31 months old (early stage 3) before

---

*Kathleen Fahey.

she begins to form true imperative sentences (McCormick, 1990). The imperative form has an implied subject and uses an uninflected verb. If you say, "Turn off the light," it is understood that the subject of the sentence is the person to whom the command is given. The child in stages 1 and 2 certainly uses the imperative function in her communication system. Her body language and prosodic variations are sufficient to make her request, demand, or command obvious to the listener. When the child in the single-word stage says, "Mommy!" with her arms stretched out and urgency in her voice, the imperative message is clear. When the stage 2 child says, "Go bye-bye" while tugging on his mother's shirt and motioning toward the door, the imperative message is also clear.

Check Your Understanding 6.1

Assess your understanding of gains children make in grammar during MLU stages 2 and 3 conversations by completing this brief quiz.

Refining Meaning in Stages 2 and 3: Semantics, Pragmatics, Conversations, and Metalinguistics

When the child begins to put words together, his vocabulary grows rapidly. Carey (1978) estimates that between the ages of 18 months and 6 years, the child adds an average of nine new words every day, and by the age of 6, she may have a comprehension vocabulary that reaches approximately 14,000 words. That becomes impressive when you consider how slowly vocabulary grows when the child creeps into adolescence and adulthood. If you added just one word per day over the next year, you would add 365 words to your vocabulary. I doubt you have had that kind of vocabulary bonanza in more than a few years. The child at 24 months has about 200 to 300 words in her expressive vocabulary. The child in the latter months of stage 2 will probably have a productive vocabulary of about 400 words and at the close of stage 3, about 900.

There are undoubtedly many factors that account for how the child apparently acquires so much information about words so quickly, and it will be many years before we identify all of them. Part of the explanation may be inherent in a process called *fast mapping* (Carey & Bartlett, 1978), described in Chapter 4 on development during the first two years. Recall that the foundation for fast mapping is laid when the child first encounters a new word as he quickly gathers information about the word from the context in which it is introduced. Keep in mind that the child is repeatedly exposed to communicative routines, with caregivers providing him both reviewed and new information (Crais, 1992). As he encounters the same word in different contexts over several days, he gathers additional information that makes his understanding of the word more complete (Childers & Tomasello, 2002).

The increase in word knowledge that occurs during stages 2 and 3 impacts virtually all language components. As was true in stage 1, the stage 2 child talks about people, objects, actions, and events, and multiple-word utterances reflect her understanding of relational meanings. In stages 2 and 3, however, she is using longer and more elaborate sentences, resulting in meanings that are more elaborate and increasingly refined.

One development of note in stage 2 is that the child's cognitive grasp of emotionality is reflected in his language. Some children as young as 18 months begin to talk about emotions (Bretherton, Fritz, Zahn-Waxler, & Ridgeway, 1986), and by 24 months most children are including references to emotion in their language. The stage 2 child identifies emotions, those he is feeling as well as those being experienced by others, and he talks about emotions experienced in the past. As he approaches the end of this stage, he understands that emotions are causative factors in human behavior. If he sees someone crying, for example, he might say, "She sad," reasoning that sadness causes crying.

A child's general understanding of causality is reflected by the appropriate use of the words *because* and *so* as early as 30 months (McCabe & Peterson, 1985). It will be another year before the child is able to provide the language detail consistent with a complete understanding of how a causal factor produces a given circumstance. During stage 2, for example, the child might say, "Milk allgone cause me," whereas in the next stage she might say, "I spilled milk Daddy shirt." Beyond the obvious language differences, we see a more precise understanding of the cause and the effect.

Because it is difficult to isolate the development of understanding within each stage, there is a general discussion of comprehension as it relates to cognitive development and language production at the close of this chapter. This section has provided a preview of the relationships we will examine. That is, as children's understanding of things, people, and events increases, they acquire the vocabulary to name and describe these things, people, and events. As they develop the intellectual capacity to understand concepts, object permanence, causality, and means/ends, they acquire the language by which they can express these understandings. As we established earlier and as we have emphasized throughout this book, it is difficult to separate language and cognitive development. After we complete our examination of stages 2 through 5, we consider this critically important interactive relationship once again,

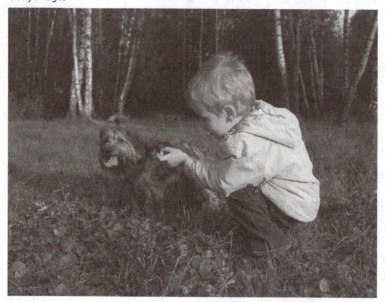

For the stage 2 child, communication is developing rapidly.

Source: Paha_L/ iStock/ Getty Images

this time within the context of children's language abilities as they have developed through the preschool years.

Pragmatics and Conversation

In stage 2, the child uses language to request objects from other people, to request that certain actions be taken, to obtain information by asking questions, and to respond to the questions or comments of others. One interesting development during this stage centers on the word *please*. The child between the ages of 24 and 36 months uses *please* in her requests with some discretion. She is more likely to include *please* if she perceives the listener to be older, more dominant, and less familiar or if the listener has something she really wants (Ervin-Tripp & Gordon, 1986).

Perhaps the most significant change in the child as a conversationalist in this stage is that he simply talks more. There are fewer nonverbal responses. His verbal responses are more frequent, and because of the other changes in his language that we have already noted, his responses are more elaborate (Mueller, Bleier, Krakow, Hegedus, & Cournoyer, 1977). He is also more adept at gaining his listener's attention, and he is able to provide more complete and meaningful responses to his conversational partner's comments and questions (Wellman & Lempers, 1977). In this case, more is better!

In addition to increased verbal output, the child is showing greater skill in introducing new topics into the conversation (Foster, 1986), although he is still not able to sustain a topic for more than a turn or two through stage 3. In addition, even the child in stage 3 has difficulty talking about things or events not in the present, and her comments often catch the listener off guard because they seem out of context (Keenan & Schieffelin, 1976). This, however, is part of the magic of conversations between adults and toddlers. Some adult-to-adult conversations seem to never end. Adult-to-toddler conversations may be confusing and exasperating, but these exchanges have so many beginnings and quasi-endings that they are never boring!

During stages 2 and 3, children have difficulty maintaining a conversational topic. Whereas adults maintain conversation by adding or seeking new information in each turn or by using one comment to prompt a new but related response, the child in stage 2 or 3 is not very adept at using these skills. His primary strategy for maintaining conversation is to repeat. He will repeat part or all of the utterance just produced by his conversational partner. This strategy of exactly matching the topic of one's partner is called **topic collaborating** (Keenan & Schieffelin, 1976).

The child in stage 2 or 3 will also maintain a conversational topic by responding to questions asked by the partner. Adults quickly learn that this is an effective way to keep a young child talking, so the conversational exchange consists of questions from the adult and answers from the child. The limiting factor in this kind of dialogue might be the adult's ability to keep asking questions about a relatively uninvolved topic, such as discussing a chocolate chip cookie.

The child in stage 3 continues to repair her conversational statements by changing words. As we noted earlier, these changes do not always result in more correct statements, but the changes do indicate that the child knows her message was not clear, and she tries to fix it. As her vocabulary grows and understanding of how words are related increases, her repairs will be more effective.

A child in stage 2 or 3 still has much to learn about turn taking and the common courtesies of conversation. Although she is able to participate in conversations with one or two partners, the child does not always allow the speaker to complete his turn before she tries to speak. Ervin-Tripp (1979) has noted that most of these interruptions occur at syntactic junctures or when the speaker's prosody seems to signal a conversational right-of-way. Whereas adults allow about one second between turns, the stage 2 and 3 child allows longer pauses. By the time she reaches her third birthday, however, she learns that these longer pauses can be interpreted to mean that no response will follow, so she shortens her response time to maintain her turn.

One of the skills all conversationalists must learn is **conversational repair**. If you say something to a listener that you believe the listener has not understood, you will revise or repair your message to increase the chances of successful communication. Gallagher (1977) studied conversational repairs in children between the ages of 20 and 30 months, a span that includes stages 1 and 2. During conversations with these children, an adult listener indicated a lack of understanding by saying, "What?" following a child's utterance. More than 75% of the requests for clarifications were followed by revised utterances from the children. Shatz and O'Reilly (1990) found that even though their subjects in this age range tried to repair, only about 38% of their repair attempts were successful. It is important to note that although children throughout this age range regularly try to repair when their listeners do not understand, their approach changes as their language abilities become more sophisticated. According to Gallagher (1977), the younger child is most likely to repair by changing a speech sound. If the child says, "More cookie," and the adult does not understand, the child might say, "More tookie!" The child at 25 or 26 months tends to revise by deleting a word from his original statement. If his original utterance, "That little doggie" is not understood, he might say, "That doggie" or, "Little doggie." By the end of stage 2 or the beginning of stage 3, the child is more likely to repair by changing words. He might revise, "She drink milk" to, "She drink it" or, "Mommy drink milk." It is important to note that a revision or repair is not necessarily more accurate or more correct. In the case of *tookie* for *cookie*, for example, the revision is clearly incorrect. As his vocabulary grows and understanding of how words are related increases, his repairs will be more effective.

It is interesting that even though young children consistently respond to requests for clarification from their listeners, they make few requests for repairs when they listen to adult speakers (Gallagher, 1981). Perhaps these children are so accustomed to understanding only portions of the utterances of adults that they do not feel a need to request clarification, or perhaps, as Gallagher suggests, they are reluctant to imply that adult speakers have not produced clear and effective messages.

Although adults take into account what the child knows in adult/child conversations, the child's presuppositional skills remain relatively undeveloped. As long as the topic is immediately present, the adult will know the child's conversational focus, but the child often uses pronouns when their referents are not identifiable, and he provides little assistance to his listener except for supplying some details about the topic, which might enhance understanding (Owens, 2016).

Along with conversations about what is going on at any given time in households, during trips in the car, and at preschool, there are also opportunities to talk about past and future events as well as hold conversations about stories in books. Parents and other caregivers embed such moments as part of the complex array of talking to their children. They co-construct **narratives** by providing the maximum amount of support necessary to understand the narrative, such as using demonstrations or pictures, as they coax the child's participation. Research also shows that children of mothers who share lengthy interactions concerning past events (topic-extending style) produce longer and more detailed narratives compared to children of mothers who do not elaborate (Hudson, 1990; McCabe & Peterson, 1991). Narratives provide a particular structure to language that assists the child in learning the art of connected discourse, which becomes increasingly important in preschool and beyond. In fact, narrative development plays a significant role in academic success, as it provides a way for children to think about and remember information (Boudreau, 2008).

Thus, in addition to learning the technical skills and artistic nuances of conversation, the child is soon confronted with learning how to tell a story, a common narrative form. Like a conversation, a narrative consists of a series of sentences, not juxtaposed randomly but appearing in an orderly and interconnected sequence. **Narrative discourse** occurs when the speaker produces at least two utterances in a temporal order about an event or experience in the past or future (Beals & Snow, 1994; Boudreau, 2008; Hughes, McGillivray, & Schmidek, 1997). Unlike a conversation in which all participants take turns as speakers and listeners, a narrative requires a monologue whereby the speaker imparts the information. Just as there are rules governing conversations, there are rules for structuring a cohesive and effective narrative.

At this point in language acquisition, the interaction between cognitive attainments and language knowledge and use becomes increasingly important as children build on information about stories. In order to produce narratives, a child must use three aspects of language and cognition: (1) linguistic devices must be used to produce units of discourse including episodes and settings (Peterson & McCabe, 1990); (2) the child must be aware of and responsive to the conversational partner's needs (Hudson & Shapiro, 1991); and (3) she must be able to effectively use working memory and information processing to sequence large amounts of information (Eisenberg, 1985). Nelson (1973) also points out that children need to use their knowledge of the world to construct scripts or schemes about common events, and they need to know how stories are organized.

Children as young as two years old begin to talk about past events, focusing not particularly on the sequence of events, but rather on what interests them (Rathmann, Mann, & Morgan, 2007). In fact, recounts of personal experiences are the most common type of narrative represented in conversations of young children (Hudson & Shapiro, 1991; Peterson, 1990; Preece, 1987). These are statements about what happened in the child's day. Miller and Sperry (1988) refer to early recounts as protonarratives that occur between the ages of 24 and 30 months. The adult who shared the experience often prompts the child to retell the experience. When the child is five or six years old, the adult prompts retelling of stories. A child who spontaneously tells about an experience that occurred without the adult's presence, for example at day care, uses an account.

At stage 3, the child is just starting to use recounts and accounts; thus early narrative development is quite primitive. When the child develops his first narratives, he uses two basic strategies for their organizational structure. Chaining involves ordering events so that one event logically follows the preceding event. Centering involves building a story around a central theme. Each item or action in the narrative is connected to the central theme by an attribute that is related to the theme, however marginal that relationship might seem to the listener. The central themes of early stories tend to focus on unusual, exciting, or upsetting events that have a significant impact on the child's life (Ames, 1966; Sutton-Smith, 1986).

The earliest attempts at narratives between ages two and three consist of unrelated statements connected by a common originating stimulus. Information is simply chained together in an additive fashion without a meaningful sequence, even though you should be able to figure out the association that prompts each succeeding utterance. In these heaps, the meaning would not be altered if the order of the utterances changed in the following example:

Mommy sit here. Baby go "Waa!" Kitty go "meow." Doggie play ball.

We will explore the development of narratives as we discuss the later stages and in the next chapter.

Metalinguistics

Recall from our chapter on development during the first two years that fFamilies engage children in play through rhythmic songs, routines, and games. A child in stage 2 or 3 of language development is not only hard at play, but also captivated by the sights and sounds of these interactions, as well as by television and many variations of electronic media. Because imitation is a very strong skill between 27 and 36 months, it is no wonder that children attempt to sing along, engage in repetitive hand movements, and experiment with verbal routines. For instance, when the child is imitating a song during the holidays, the general melody may be taking shape through vocalizing or humming, and a short phrase may also be repeated. What is more important than the child's ability to say the words in a song or rhyme at this point is the attention he pays to the regularity of the rhythms and phrases. His attention to these features and his ability to imitate them is called metalinguistics. We will see this aspect of language development playing a very important role in future stages in the acquisition of language and literacy.

In stage 3 the child might enjoy a lot of repetition of interactive games, such as Ring-Around-the-Rosy, Itsy-Bitsy Spider, a favorite lullaby, or dancing to Mom and Dad's favorite music. She responds to the predictable patterns involved in each activity, especially when it is a source of fun.

Parents often take advantage of children's high interest and the important foundational skills of oral language by engaging them in **book-sharing activities** (Missall, Carta, McConnell, Walker, & Greenwood, 2008; Snow, Tabors, & Dickinson, 2001). Think for a moment about what happens during book sharing. Imagine a two-year-old child sitting next to her parent on a comfy couch in the living room. What do the parent and child do? Books for toddlers have a lot of pictures and very little print, so the parent might point to the picture first to draw the child's attention and then read the print. Some parents might also point to the print as they read words aloud. These moments are quite important, as they direct the child to focus on particular names of items and actions, but also on the routines involved in book reading, such as holding the book a certain way, talking about the story, pointing to print, and turning each page. Children as young as 1 year of age begin to realize that oral language can be represented by print. This **print interest** serves as a foundation for subsequent development of literacy (Justice & Ezell, 2004; Whitehurst & Lonigan, 2001). We will explore this topic in much more detail later in this chapter and in subsequent chapters. (See Table 6.5 for a summary of stage 2 characteristics and Table 6.6 for a summary of stage 3 characteristics.)

Table 6.5   Stage 2 Highlights

Typical Age Range: 27 to 30 Months
MLU: 2.0 to 2.5 Morphemes

Grammatical Morphemes
- Brown's (1973) 14 specified grammatical morphemes emerge during the later months of stage 1 and throughout stage 2.
- As these morphemes develop, the child overextends his or her use (e.g., *child* → *childs*; *go* → *goed*).

Pronouns
- Enters stage 2 using *I, it, this*, and *that*
- Adds *my, me, mine*, and *you*

Verbs
- Uses *have* and *do* as main verbs and as auxiliary verbs
- Produces semi-infinite forms: *hafta, gonna, wanna*

Noun Phrases
- Uses only determiners and adjectivals as modifiers
- Elaborates in the object position of sentences

Verb Phrases
- Uses present progressive forms of common verbs

(continued)

Table 6.5   Stage 2 Highlights (Continued)

Sentences

- Understands that a sentence contains a noun phrase and a verb phrase
- Produces negation by putting *no* or *not* at the beginning of a sentence
- Produces a *yes/no* question by adding a rising intonation to the end of a sentence
- Asks *what, where*, and *why* questions
- Produces the imperative function but not the imperative form

Pragmatics

- Continues to use language to request, to obtain information, and to respond
- Fewer nonverbal responses than in stage 1
- Sustains topic for one or two turns
- Attempts conversational repairs when the listener does not understand

Metalinguistics

- Tunes in to the regularities of rhymes and songs
- Imitates repetitive phrases in rhymes, songs, and stories

Table 6.6   Stage 3 Highlights

Typical Age Range: 31 to 34 Months
MLU: 2.5 to 3.0 Morphemes

Grammatical Morphemes

- Continues to develop

Pronouns

- More consistent in use of *you, your, yours, she, he, we, this, that, these*, and *those*

Verbs

- Uses the modal verbs *can, will*, and *do* more consistently
- Uses the verb *to be* as both copula and auxiliary, although makes mistakes in terms of person and number

Noun Phrases

- Uses a few quantifiers: *two, some, a lot*
- Elaborates in the subject and object positions of sentences

Verb Phrases

- Elaborates by using modals and the auxiliary forms of *to be*
- Overextends the regular past tense form to irregular verbs (e.g., *"He runned away"*)

Sentences

- Produces negation by putting *no* or *not* between the subject and predicate to create an adult-like form; also uses contracted negative forms: *can't, don't*
- Questions include auxiliary verbs, and the elements are properly inverted (e.g., *"She go bye-bye."* → *"Can she go bye-bye?"*)
- In addition to *what, where*, and *why*, produces questions with *who* and *how*, often properly inverted
- Produces the imperative form of sentences

Pragmatics, Conversation, and Narratives

- Most exchanges are still limited to one or two turns per topic
- Primary strategy for maintaining a topic is repeating part or all of the utterance produced by the conversational partner
- Continues to attempt conversational repairs, usually by using a different word even if it is not a more appropriate word
- Produces early narratives using statements about past events without meaningful sequences

Metalinguistics

- Repetition of phrases in interactive games and rhymes
- Attention and participation during book-sharing activities

Video Example 6.1

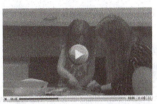

Watch the video of Becca engaged in book sharing with her mother. She is just three years old, so it is likely that she is at the end of stage 3 or in early stage 4. As you watch the video, notice Becca's use of full sentences and her ability to pick out the relevant details from one page to another. Becca's mother uses many strategies to retain her daughter's attention and to connect ideas through the story, such as affirming what Becca says by repeating it, asking *Wh-* questions, and pointing at a picture to elicit comment.

Check Your Understanding 6.2

Assess your understanding of how children refine meaning during MLU stages 2 and 3 by completing this brief quiz.

Mean Length of Utterances in Stages 4 and 5: Elaboration with Phrases and Clauses and Polishing the Act

A child is typically in stage 4 between the ages of 35 and 40 months and has an MLU of 3.0 to 3.75. An increase in MLU from stage 3 to stage 4 indicates that the child continues to elaborate by adding words to his utterances, but in this stage we see elaboration take a new and exciting turn. In stage 3, the child made phrases by adding modifiers or auxiliary verbs. In stage 4, he places a phrase within a clause.

Stage 5 occurs roughly between 3.5 and 4 years (41 through 46 months), a very active and inquisitive time for preschoolers. The child still has much to learn when he completes stage 5, but he has certainly learned all that

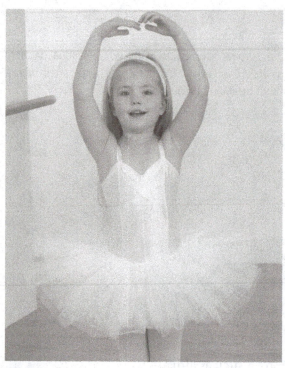

I'm not free, I'm four!

Source: Dave King/DK Images.

can be considered basic in speech and language by the end of this stage. In fact, 9 of the 14 specified grammatical morphemes are mastered by the close of this stage (Brown, 1973; Miller, 1981). During the MLU range of 3.75 to 4.5, the child reaches closure on some language behaviors, elaborates on others, and is still struggling with other aspects of language.

At a local dining establishment on a fall evening, a young family arrived at the counter to be seated. The parents had two children with them. The young boy was around seven years old. The little girl was dressed like a fairy princess, with a lacy pink dress, sparkles on her shoes, tiara on her head, and wand in her hand. She immediately said to the waitress, "It's my birthday." The waitress responded, "Great, that means you are free!" The little girl replied, "I'm not free, I'm four!" This young princess knows a lot about language, but even a child at the end of stage 5 will need time to sort out grammar and meaning!

Morphology, Pronouns, Verbs, Negation, and Questions

Although no dramatic developments in morphology are unique to stage 4, keep in mind that overall growth in vocabulary is rapid throughout the five stages of language development we are describing. The 14 grammatical morphemes we identified as emerging in stage 2 and 3 are continuing to develop. The stage 4 child consistently uses the pronouns *they, us, her, hers, his,* and *them* (Owens, 2016). Personal pronouns (*its, ours, him, their, theirs, myself, yourself*) continue to be refined during stage 5 to convey more precise meanings in sentences such as these:

"The dog has something in its ear."
"Do you have a doggie like ours?"
"I can do it myself."

He also uses modifiers in stage 4, such as *some, something, other, more, one, two,* and *another* (Miller, 1981).

Another attainment in stage 5 and beyond is the emergence of the understanding and production of suffixes. The **comparative** form of adjectives occurs through the addition of the suffix *er,* and the **superlative** form requires the addition of the suffix *est.* The child understands comparative words, such as *taller, colder,* and *faster,* during stage 5, but superlative words, such as *easiest, biggest,* and *smartest,* are not understood until well beyond stage 5. But of course, not all adjectives conform to the application of these suffixes. Two-syllable adjectives usually require the words *more* and *most* instead of the suffixes *er* and *est,* as seen in the example *beautiful/more beautiful/most beautiful.* In addition to these exceptions, absolute adjectives, such as *dead, perfect,* and *pregnant,* do not have comparative or superlative forms.

Children in stage 4 are likely to include some past tense forms of common modals such as *could, should,* and *would* (Chapman, 1978), and he puts *be* and the *ing* form of verbs together to create sentences such as, "He is running" (Chapman, Paul, & Wanska, 1981). As the child acquires more words, he incorporates them into his sentences to make them longer and more elaborate.

By the end of stage 5, the child shows mastery of common irregular verbs such as *sat, went, broke, ate,* and *fell,* but she may continue to have problems with less common verbs such as *hit* and *put* that do not change when they change from present to past tense. She might also try to find regularity where there is none. For example, she might reason that if the past tense of *sing* is *sang,* then the past tense of *bring* must be *brang.* She would, of course, be wrong, but eventually she will figure out most of the exceptions and irregularities.

Another vexing problem for the child in stage 5 is learning the rules for appropriate use of the copula in its contracted form. The child must learn that sometimes it is permissible to contract the copula verb. "He is tall" can be produced as "He's tall." But if the same copula form is in an answer to the question "Is he tall?" the answer "Yes, he is" cannot be contracted. "Yes, he's" is not an acceptable form.

The child has the challenge of learning when the copula is contractible and when it is not, but he also must learn the forms of the copula that reflect person ("I am," "She is"), tense ("I am," "I was"), and the various combinations of these forms, including "They were" and "We will." In like manner, the child is learning the permissible contracted auxiliary forms in combination with negative forms, as in the sentences "He was running away," "He isn't running away," and "They're running away." In Patrick's sample (Figure 6.1), he is appropriately contracting singular subject pronouns with the copula verb ("It's dry," "That's not my mom"), but plural nouns and auxiliary verbs are sometimes not contracted appropriately ("Tom and Jerry's working").

Mastery of the third-person singular verb on the present tense form of regular and irregular verbs is accomplished during stage 5, whereby the child is able to use these forms with ease ("She jumps," "Mary writes," "I do," "He does," "You have," "She has").

Refinement during stage 5 also occurs in the child's use of negative past tense forms of the verb *to be* and common modals, including *wouldn't, couldn't,* and *shouldn't* (Miller, 1981), and in the use of interrogatives where the question form is inverted ("Is he playing baseball?"). The tag question also develops in stage 5 where the speaker adds a *huh* or *okay* to the end of sentence to form a question, such as, "I'm going to leave now, okay?" Beyond stage 5, the child learns a somewhat more difficult form of tag question, where the negative form is not included ("You're going to buy me some ice cream, are you?") to inclusion of the negative form ("You're going to buy me some ice cream, aren't you?").

Another suffix that can be added to words is referred to as the **agentive form.** The *er* is added to a verb in order to change it into a noun. Thus, a

---

Figure 6.1   Patrick's Language Sample at Three Years, Two Months (MLU = 6.1): Playing at Home

---

P When the sun comes out it's dry. (9)

P The rain is not out. (5)

P We don't want the rain to come out. (9)

K* How about Tom and Jerry?

P Tom and Jerry's working. (6)

P You know how to do Tom and Jerry? (8)

P What do we turn on? (5)

P How about Barney? (3)

P How about we play Candy Land! (5)

K Okay, will you go get it?

P My mommy needs to find it. (7)

K Here, let's take this out. Where's the Candy Land?

P Don't take my Light Saber. (5)

K Okay, I won't.

P We have to spread 'em. (5)

K Spread 'em. Spread 'em cowboy.

P That's not my mom. (5)

P That's not anybody. (4)

K That's Grandma silly goose.

P Flip the cards over with Winnie the Pooh on top. (9)

K Can you put these on there?

P Oh oh, I don't know how to do it. (9)

P I don't know how to stack them up. (9)

P You have to stack them up and put them on there. (11)

P Only these two. (3)

P You have to put them on there with those. (9)

P But I can't. (4)

P Let's take a little rest. (6)

---

*Kathleen Fahey.

person who runs can be called a runner, and a person who teaches is a teacher. What might complicate a child's understanding and production of this suffix is the fact that we call a person who puts out fires a fireman and one who delivers mail the mailman. No wonder it takes most children until their fifth year to figure out the nuances of our language! With each stage comes more refinement of the grammatical aspects of language. In stage 5, the child's sentences are a bit longer than in the preceding stage, yet the noun and verb phrases are much the same as in stage 4, where only one pronoun or adjective is in front of the noun. The child continues to have challenges in matching the number of the subject and verb ("The doggies is eating my sandwich."). He must sort out subject and verb agreement, depending on several rules, as shown in Table 6.9, which will take both time and patience.

Phrases Within Clauses

Patrick's sample at two years, nine months (MLU 3.7) in the following excerpt shows the beginnings of elaboration with prepositional phrases and infinitives. Recall that Patrick is about two months advanced in grammar as he heads into stage 4. Let's focus our attention on a few specific examples of elaboration as an introduction to the four kinds of phrases that begin to emerge in stage 4. Notice how many morphemes are being used in each utterance, as well as Patrick's use of various prepositional phrases, infinitive phrases, **adverbial** phrases, and a combination of these phrasal types:

Try *to get* some more dirt *out of the sandbox.* (infinitive and prepositional phrase)

Would you play *with this?* (prepositional phrase)

Oh, go *to the outside,* Grandpa. (adverbial phrase)

He had *to go to the other.* (infinitive and adverbial phrase)

There's cherries *for you.* (prepositional phrase)

You want *to eat* them? (infinitive)

He wanted *to go in there.* (infinitive and adverbial phrase)

Now let's look more closely at common phrase types: (1) prepositional phrases; (2) participial phrases; (3) infinitive phrases; and (4) gerunds. You should not assume that when the child exits stage 4, she produces all of these phrases as embedded forms. Phrasal and clausal embedding are complex processes that develop over a long period of time. The child begins to develop prepositional phrases by using words such as *in* and *on* as early as stage 2, but she does not produce true infinitive forms until stage 5 and beyond (Bloom, Tackeff, & Lahey, 1984; Miller, 1981) and gerund phrases tend to emerge later than infinitives. According to Paul (1981), when her subjects had MLUs about 4.5 (stage 5), more than 90% produced simple infinitive forms, but only about 50% produced sentences that included gerunds. Table 6.7 provides an overview of each phrase type, its definition, and an example.

A complex sentence is created when a speaker embeds one clause in another. A compound sentence is created when the speaker joins or conjoins two independent clauses. Even though the order might seem to violate common sense, the child engages in serious clausal embedding before she becomes proficient in clausal conjoining. There is evidence of some clausal conjoining in stage 4, but Brown (1973) identifies clausal conjoining primarily with stage 5.

According to Brown (1973), there are three types of embedded clauses: (1) the object complement clause; (2) the *wh-*question clause; and (3) the relative clause. In a sentence with an object complement clause, there is an independent clause containing a verb such as *think, hope, know, guess, mean,* or *need,* followed by a noun phrase that functions as an object. In the sentence, "I think you know what I mean," the subordinate clause (*you know what I mean*) functions as the object of the verb *think.* The object complement clause emerges during stage 4.

Table 6.7   Types of Phrases

Phrase Type	Definition	Examples
Prepositional Phrase	Preposition with its object, modifiers, and articles, such as *in, on, under, over, past,* and *with*.	Would you play *with this*? Put the shoes *under the bed*. The car *in the garage* is an antique.
Participial Phrase	Verb form ending in *ing, ed, en,* or *t* that functions as adjective	The women *calling my name* is Aunt Bertha. *Fallen leaves* create a beautiful fall carpet. We listened to the *babbling brook*.
Infinitives and Semiauxiliaries	Verb form introduced with *to* or *in order to*	Noun: Daddy wanted *to go* to the store. Adjective: I have energy *to devote to my hobbies*. Adverb: My father exercises *to increase his physical fitness*. Semiauxiliary: I *wanna* play.
Gerund	Verb form ending in *ing* functions as a subject or object noun	Mary dislikes *walking*. *Diving* is a dangerous sport. *Compulsive eating* is not healthy.

The embedded *wh-* clause also emerges during stage 4, and these clauses also function as objects. Consider the following examples:

"I know what you did."
"He showed me where to get one."
"You probably know when he'll come back."

Because the child learns to use these words in question sentences, it is not surprising that he sometimes produces sentences that seem to mix the inverted structure of the interrogative form and the embedded *wh-* clause. He might say, for example, "Show me where can I get one" instead of the more proper construction, "Show me where I can get one."

A relative clause is introduced by *who, whom, whoever, whomever, whose, which,* or *that* and modifies the preceding noun. A problem for many speakers, including adults, is determining which relative pronoun should be used in a given sentence. Identifying and discussing the rules for selecting the proper pronoun is beyond the scope of this book, but a few examples may help you understand some of what children must learn about pronoun usage:

"He is the man who helped me last week."
"He's the boy whose finger was broken when he was hit in the nose."
"The ball that broke the window was thrown from a passing car."

Although we are introducing the concept of relative clauses as part of our explanation of clausal embedding, be aware that children do not begin to use relative clauses until stage 5 and beyond.

As one might guess, the first conjunction used to link two or more independent clauses is *and*. By the time the child is 25- to 27-months-old, she is using *and* correctly to join words (Bloom, Lahey, Hood, Lifter, & Fiess, 1980). Even though she begins to conjoin clauses in stage 4, the child does not consistently conjoin clauses with *and* and other conjunctions until late in stage 5 (Miller, 1981). It is interesting, though not surprising, that even after the child has acquired many conjunctions and is beyond her fifth birthday, she continues to favor *and* (Bennett-Kaster, 1986).

Embedding and Conjoining Sentences

Prior to stage 5, the child is able to embed phrases within simple sentences. During stage 5, she begins to embed subordinate clauses in the object position of sentences. This means that she is using a complete sentence and adding a clause that also contains a verb to it. The child's earliest relative clauses are used to describe unspecific nouns such as *thing* or *one*. The sentence, "That's the thing that I broke" is an example of a relative clause. Adults often delete the relative pronoun *that* because it is implied, but preschool children may include it to preserve the meaning of the sentence (Menyuk, 1977).

Children tend to use the relative pronoun *that* early on, but they gradually learn to use *who, which,* and *what* to construct relative clauses. Of course, during acquisition, mistakes in their use are common, resulting in a sentence such as, "The glass is the thing what spilled."

Patrick is showing steady progress at 38 months in the development of elaborated sentences through embedding, as seen in the following examples:

> No, I don't think (that) *I go to the pink one.*
> I'll have your(s) *cuz you got mine.*
> I'll see *what we got in there.*
> You know *how to do* Tom and Jerry?
> Oh oh, I don't know *how to do it.*
> I don't know *how to stack them up.*

By the close of stage 5, the child is producing multiple embeddings (Miller, 1981). She might produce a sentence that embeds an infinitive in a subordinate clause that serves as the object of the sentence: "I think I want to eat all the cake." The clause "I want to eat all the cake" is the object of the verb *think.* The infinitive *to eat* is embedded in this clause, so we have a sentence that contains an embedded subordinate clause that, in turn, contains an embedded infinitive. This is only the beginning of the possibilities. As the child moves into the school years, she produces sentences with even more elaborate embeddings, and she learns to embed and conjoin at the same time. That sounds illegal, doesn't it?

Although the child uses the conjunction *and* as early as the end of stage 1 and adds other conjunctions such as *but, so, if,* and *or* in stage 3, he does not conjoin clauses until stage 4 and he does not really get serious about clausal conjoining until stage 5 (Brown, 1973). The child's favorite conjunction is *and*, and he continues to favor it in combining clauses well beyond stage 5 (Bennett-Kaster, 1986).

According to Bloom and colleagues (1980), the semantic relations conveyed in conjoined sentences emerge in an identifiable sequence. In the beginning, a child uses *and* to express all of these semantic relations. The first conjunctive relation to emerge is **additive**, a relation we are most likely to associate with *and*. In an additive sentence, the child combines two clauses that are independent of each other. She might say, "I went to Billy's house, and I'm a big girl." In this sentence, the combined meaning is the same as the added meanings of the separate clauses. The children in Bloom's study also used *and* to connect a clause that described or elaborated on the subject of the preceding clause. The child might say, "I got a baseball bat, and you play baseball with it." The authors called this semantic relation **object specification**. They conclude that the child is using *and* to link subjects and objects appropriately in a listing sense by the end of stage 1 or the beginning of stage 2. The child then uses *and* to express **temporal** relations. In the sentence "I went to Billy's house, and I played with his toys," the child is talking about one event that follows another in time. The child then expresses the **causal relation**. One clause expresses an action or state of being, and the other clause provides a reason or describes the effect. The child might say, "I ate all the cake, and my tummy is full." The combined meaning in this sentence is clearly greater than the sum of the meanings of the separate clauses. The child then expresses the **adversative** relation in her conjoined sentences. In this case, the two parts of the sentence represent a contrast. The child says, "This doggie big, and this one little."

As already noted, some children conjoin clauses with *and* as early as stage 4, but we usually do not see clausal conjoining until the end of stage 5 (Miller, 1981). Although the dominant conjunction continues to be *and* for some time, the child is using *if* to conjoin clauses by the close of stage 5. Other conjunctions, including *because, but, so,* and *when,* do not emerge until after stage 5 when the child's MLU is about 5.0 (Owens, 2005).

To appreciate the sophistication of this stage, compare Patrick's earlier samples with an excerpt of his stage 5 sample at three years, two months (see Figure 6.1). His growth in sentence length, as shown by the number of morphemes in each sentence, and his ability to use language to convey meaning and get things done is quite impressive!

Pragmatics, Conversations, and Narratives

Recall that children in stage 3 do not always recognize that a pause in speech often signals the end of a conversational turn. But by early stage 4, at about three years, the child recognizes that a pause greater than one second means that the conversational partner is probably not going to respond (Craig & Gallagher, 1983). Short pauses, those less than one second in duration, mean that exchanges on this topic will continue. As adults, we are so sensitive to this time factor that long pauses in conversations, especially with people we do not know well, are very uncomfortable. In fact, as we become skilled conversationalists, we learn to overlap our responses so that there are no pauses.

By the end of stage 4 or the beginning of stage 5, at about 42 months, the child is able to maintain a topic for more than two turns (Bloom, Rocissano, & Hood, 1976). Not surprisingly based on everything we know about children, the child is more likely to maintain a topic for several turns if the conversation centers on something in her immediate environment and if the topic interests her. Most adults respond in a similar way. Part of the art of conversation, therefore, is finding a topic that interests your partner, and a good conversationalist is not necessarily someone who has a great deal to say, but rather someone who knows how to get others to talk about what interests them. The lesson to be emphasized at this point, with the stage 4 child, is that the adult, by choosing topics that interest or fail to interest the child, usually determines how long child/adult conversations will last.

The stage 5 child not only continues to be sensitive to pauses during conversational exchanges, as noted in stage 4, but perhaps of even greater significance, he takes into consideration what is likely to be included in the next turn. That is, he shows an awareness of what is being discussed in the present turn, and he anticipates how this topic will be completed in succeeding turns (McTear, 1985). He is sensitive to problems his partner may have in finishing her turn, and when he senses that his partner is having difficulty, he will attempt to help by completing what he perceives to be his partner's thought. In addition, he is developing sensitivity to the problems created by simultaneous talking. When he senses that information will be lost when he and his partner are talking at the same time, he is willing to give up his turn to preserve the conversational topic. By the time the child is ready for school, he has developed considerable turn-taking skills, but conversational inadequacies remain.

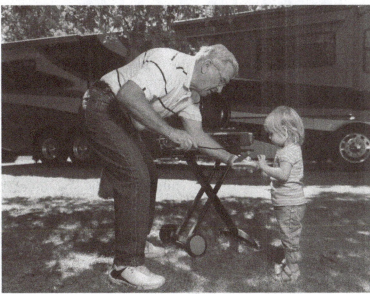

Learning the art of conversation.
Source: Iofoto/Fotolia.

Some preschool children are able to handle conversations involving two partners but struggle with three-party conversations (Ervin-Tripp, 1979). Interruptions remain a problem for young communicators for some time. Remember that interruptions are sometimes necessary to capture one's turn in a conversation. The child must learn how and when to interrupt according to the rules of conversational etiquette. Sachs (1982) found that the preschool child typically does not use polite verbal or nonverbal strategies for gaining the attention of her listener. That is, she does not say, "Excuse me," or does not gently tap her listener's shoulder or lean forward or gesture in a manner that suggests she wants to say something. She simply yells at her listener. Only 36% of the utterances produced by Sachs's subjects, who ranged from 40 to 66 months, were at a conversational loudness level. If you have spent much time around children in this age range, you are probably saying, "Yep, that just about captures it!" Not surprisingly, only the oldest subjects in this study were sensitive to their proximity to their listeners, initiating conversation only when they were within an appropriate range.

Over the course of the preschool years, the child improves his ability to initiate and sustain a conversation. As we have mentioned, the child does not maintain a topic for more than two turns until he is about 42 months old, which marks the beginning of stage 5 (Bloom et al., 1976). By the time the child is 5 years old and well beyond stage 5, he maintains a topic for an average of 5 turns compared to the 11 turns on average by adult speakers (Brinton & Fujiki, 1984). Yet, when the preschool child is maintaining a topic through three or four turns, he is not contributing much new information. He maintains the conversation primarily through repeating part of what his partner has already said or by asking questions about his partner's comments. Even when the child is in the early elementary school years, he seldom adds significant information to a conversation (Brinton & Fujiki, 1984). In this sense, he remains a conversational follower.

We see no radical changes in conversational repairs during stage 5, although as the child's overall language skills improve, she is better able to respond to requests for clarification. As early as stage 1 or 2, the child has shown an awareness of the need for conversational repairs. Throughout the five stages of language development, she tries, within the limits of her intellectual and linguistic abilities, to provide the information her conversational partner finds lacking or confused. Even as stage 5 closes, however, she sometimes has difficulty identifying the part of the message that needs to be repaired (Brinton & Fujiki, 1989), and she still responds readily to requests for repairs more than she makes requests for repairs from her conversational partners.

Before the child's third birthday, his presuppositional skills have been limited. Unless the topic of conversation is immediate, the adult often has difficulty following shifts in the conversation because the child does not provide the information the listener needs to keep abreast of the changes. During stage 4, following his third birthday, the child begins to make some meaningful and helpful presuppositions in his conversations. The stage 4 child understands what the listener needs to know about the topic, and he can determine how much information he needs to provide (Shatz, Wellman, & Silber, 1983; Wellman & Estes, 1987).

The child adjusts the amount of information she provides, depending on whether the listener can directly observe the topic of conversation and depending on what the child assumes the listener knows or understands about the topic. That is, if the listener looks at the object of the conversation or the child believes the listener already knows what he needs to know about the object, the child knows that little additional information is needed. If, however, the child talks about something that is not present or she believes the listener lacks the information he needs to make sense of the communication, the child provides more information. As the child moves past her third birthday, she becomes increasingly proficient in making these presuppositional decisions. Several specific skills emerge at about this time, including the use of anaphoric references, deixis, and grammatical ellipsis.

Recall that anaphoric reference allows a speaker to refer to something through the use of a pronoun that has already been named in the preceding utterance. Consider a simple example. A young boy says, "I played baseball with my new mitt. It is just like the one Sammy Sosa uses." He uses "it" to refer to the mitt, knowing that the listener will make this connection. Children begin to use this presuppositional skill in their third year.

A common thread woven through maturing suppositional skills is the ability to process information from the perspective of another person. We see this thread very clearly in **deixis**. The word *deixis* comes from the Greek word *deiknunai*, which means "to show." In the context of presuppositional skills, a child uses deixis when she demonstrates an understanding that certain words are interpreted differently, depending upon who speaks them. It is easiest to understand deixis if we identify what are called **deictic word pairs**. Examples include *here/there, this/that,* and *I/you*. Imagine conversational partners seated across from each other at an ice cream parlor. One person says, "I bet *this* ice cream tastes better than *that* ice cream." Depending on which speaker makes this statement, *this* and *that* refer to different bowls of ice cream. Let's throw in another deictic word pair to make the point even clearer. Assume that the two speakers are *you* and *I*, and you are eating vanilla ice cream, and I am eating chocolate ice cream. If you are speaking, *this* is vanilla ice cream and *that* is chocolate ice cream, but if I am speaking, *this* is chocolate ice cream and *that* is vanilla. As is obvious to anyone who has watched a child progress though language development, she does not master the complexities of deixis in one neat step. In fact, she appears to move through three phases in learning that deictic word pairs have opposing meanings (Clark & Sengul, 1978). In the first phase, the child uses the members of a deictic pair as though they are synonyms. For example, she will use *this* and *that* as though they mean the same thing whether she is pointing to something in her grasp or something someone sitting 10 feet away is holding. Please note that she understands the basic meaning of *deixis*, which is *to show* or *to point to*. What she is not getting is the speaker's perspective that dictates which word is appropriate in a given context. In the second phase, the child will use one of the two words more often that the other, so that she uses it correctly in some cases but incorrectly in others. In the third phase, she learns when to use each word, depending on who the speaker is and depending on the context in which the word is used. Not surprisingly, the child masters deictic pairs that are more absolute in nature, such as *I/you* and *my/your*, before she masters those that are spatial or more relative, such as *here/there* and *this/that*. The child does well with the absolute deictic pronoun pairs by the time she is 30 months old (Owens, 2005, p. 271), but she may not master the spatial or relative pairs until she is in her early elementary school years.

A language behavior that directly reflects this developing understanding is **grammatical ellipsis**. When a speaker uses grammatical ellipsis, he deletes information when he assumes that the listener already possesses it. He might use this device if he believes the information has been established in prior communicative exchanges, or if he believes the information is obvious because of the nonverbal context in which the communication is taking place. Consider the following scenario: A couple is taking a trip. They stop to eat lunch at a fast-food restaurant. Within minutes after leaving the restaurant, the wife says, "Where's my purse?" The husband says, "Probably in the restaurant." He does not need to provide additional language detail because the context provides all the supporting information the wife needs to make sense of his response. Grammatical ellipsis is not as simple, however, as this example might make it seem. As this skill matures, speakers develop a clearer and more complete understanding about what can be omitted in a communicative exchange and how the number and nature of omissions might need to be amended, depending on who the listener is (Bloom & Lahey, 1978). The evidence suggests that grammatical ellipsis emerges slowly after a child is three years old and is gradually mastered during the school years (Bloom, Miller, & Hood, 1975; Owens, 2005, p. 264).

Keep in mind that presuppositional skills depend not only on the speaker's sensitivity to what the listener may need to know but also on the speaker's cognitive and linguistic abilities to convey information the listener needs. Although the stage 4 child's presuppositional skills have improved, she is still limited in these skills by what she knows and what she is able to express. If the child has a firm cognitive grasp of the topic and if she has the vocabulary and language ability to talk about the topic, she is likely to provide the information necessary. If the topic is beyond her understanding and language abilities, she will have trouble providing the information the listener needs.

We noted that the child's presuppositional skills in stage 4 depend on his knowledge of the topic and his language skills. Nothing has changed in this regard as he moves into stage 5. Naturally, his presuppositional skills improve as he moves toward his fourth birthday, but the limitations are the same. When he talks about things he knows about and understands, he is much more adept at providing the information his listener needs.

▶ Video Reflection 6.1: Parent Prompts Information with 4-Year-Old Son

Watch the video of a parent and her four-year-old son, Ben, discuss an art project he completed just 30 minutes prior to the conversation. Notice Ben's use of presupposition, then answer the question.

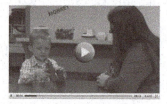

As mentioned earlier, *pragmatics* is concerned with using language to get things done. Adult speakers are often very direct in making requests or demands, such as saying, "Close the door." But requests can be made indirectly to convey a more polite or softer manner or even to use a sarcastic edge: "Can you close the door?" "There seems to be a breeze in here." "Were you raised in a barn?!"

Prior to stage 4, children convey requests first through nonverbal means and then through direct requests (Ervin-Tripp, 1977; Ervin-Tripp, O'Connor, & Rosenberg, 1987). But by stage 4, they are using modals to make requests that are a bit more subtle as compared to direct, thus, they are called **indirect requests,** such as, "Could you give me a cookie?" (rather than "Give me a cookie") or, "Can you pick me up?" These more polite requests are likely to be more warmly received by adults, and they demonstrate how small changes in pragmatic skills make a positive difference in interactions between children and caregivers.

The stage 5 child continues to increase her use of indirect requests, although indirect requests are still far less frequent than direct requests. Between 42 and 52 months, less than 10% of children's requests are indirect, but we see a dramatic increase in use of the indirect form beyond stage 5 at about 54 months (James & Seebach, 1982; Wilkinson, Calculator, & Dollaghan, 1982). The child makes requests such as, "Don't forget to get my cookie" or, "Why don't you get me some candy?" These are clearly requests, but they are subtle and more polite than, "Give me a cookie," or, "Get me some candy." When the child increases her use of indirect requests, she will also include rationalizations for her requests. She might say, for example, "I ate all my peas . . . . Don't forget to get my cookie," a polite and indirect way of saying that she has been a good girl, has fulfilled the obligations of her dinner-eating contract, and now wants a reward.

As early as four years, the child's requests are shaped by his sensitivity to the roles and viewpoints of his listeners and the need to be polite (Gordon & Ervin-Tripp, 1984), and he responds appropriately to indirect requests made to him (Carrell, 1981). He has been using *please* since he was 24 to 36 months old, but in the beginning, he uses it mostly with people who are older or more dominant (Ervin-Tripp & Gordon, 1986). By the time he is four years old, *please* has become the magic word that can be used with almost anyone to get almost anything, and over the next few years, he will learn to use the magic word even more effectively.

In stage 4 we discussed the child's use of early narrative forms. As children transition from age three years to four years, narrative development advances from unrelated chaining (heaps) of ideas to narratives containing **logical sequences.** The most common sequence in the narratives of children raised in Western culture is stories that have a beginning and an end. This temporal organization allows the child to convey ideas in the order in which they happened. Even though it is tempting to characterize sequences as being more organized, the main accomplishment is that the central theme is more developed. There is no plot or causality yet, as demonstrated in the following narrative:

"Mommy took me to the zoo. There was a lion. He made noise. There was a monkey. And I got some popcorn. An we drived home."

What is happening in stage 5 regarding narrative development? Recall that in stages 3 and 4, children tell simple stories that have some beginnings of sequenced ideas but no plot or causality. In stage 5 they expand on these stories by adding more complex grammatical forms, including third-person pronouns, past tense verbs, and conjunctions, that signal temporal concepts in the sequences. We should keep in mind that children who hear storybook narratives have an advantage over children who don't, because hearing the structure of stories repeatedly makes the structural components clearly evident. You can almost hear a four-year-old child ask her parent, "What happens next?"

Video Example 6.2

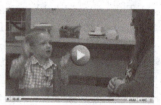

Watch the video to see Ben use sophisticated grammar, but immature verb forms (e.g., "blowed the house down.") Observe Ben's characters as they talk and how he uses some beginnings of episodes and temporal relationships. With some encouragement to continue his story, Ben expands on his interpretation of what the pigs and the wolf do. However, his story remains at a simple level.

The child's narratives will not typically include causality organization until he is five years old (Owens, 2016). When he adds this dimension to his stories, his narratives will change dramatically. We will consider these changes and the continued maturation of the child's narrative skills in Chapter 7.

Metalinguistics and Emergent Literacy

We know that many preschool-age children are exposed to books and other print media within their households, day-care facilities, and educational settings. Newspapers, magazines, books, textbooks belonging to siblings, computerized information, the daily mail, and the creation of shopping lists provide an environment filled with reading and writing activities. As soon as toddlers show interest in books, family members and caregivers are eager to promote and expand upon this interest. There are several very useful activities that serve not only to expand the child's vocabulary, but also to focus his attention on the special attributes of books: pictures; printed words; models for reading, such as the appropriate way to hold and use books; and the narrative structure of simple stories. Books for young children often contain repetitive sentences and the use of rhyming, which serves to heighten the child's focus on words.

The use of storybooks provides a way to interact socially with preschool-age children and to continue to build foundations for literacy. In stage 3 the child's interest may be somewhat fleeting during shared-book time, but by the end of stage 3 and through stage 4, she is much more able and willing to attend to books, pictures, and print. **Print referencing** is one technique that adults use to direct a child's attention to the forms, features, and functions of written language (Justice & Ezell, 2004). The child may respond to nonverbal pointing to printed words or may track words visually as the adult points to words as she reads aloud. She may respond when the adult asks questions or makes requests about print, as in the question, "Where is the letter *B* in that word?" or, "Show me your name." The adult may provide comments about print, such as "That word is in all big letters because it is a loud word, *BANG!* The end result of print-referencing techniques is to heighten the metalinguistic focus of book sharing so that children gain knowledge about print functions, the organization of print through conventions, and the part-to-whole relationships of letters, words, and sentences. More specifically, print referencing has been shown to facilitate print concepts, word concepts, and alphabet knowledge (Ezell, Justice, & Parsons, 2000; Justice & Ezell, 2000, 2002). Of course, children at different levels of language development will need various degrees of scaffolding during book-sharing activities. This is where adults must gauge their interactions to provide concepts slightly beyond a child's current independent capabilities, known as the zone of proximal development, based on Vygotskian theory (see Chapter 2).

▶ **Video Reflection 6.2: Parent Scaffolds to Promote Literacy**

Watch the video of a parent using scaffolding to promote print referencing, then answer the question.

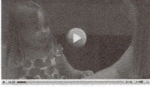

Book sharing during stage 5 continues to promote the regularities of language including rhymes; sound effects of common objects and actions; repetitive phrases in songs, games, and stories; routines involved in book reading; and story structure. Children show emerging **print-concept knowledge**, which is knowledge of the rule-governed organizational properties of print, including being able to show the front of the book, the title, the difference between pictures and print, left-to-right and top-to-bottom directionality for reading, and the concepts of letter and first letter in a word (Justice & Ezell, 2001). In addition to print-concept knowledge, preschool children acquire *alphabetic knowledge*, which includes knowledge of the distinctive features and names of individual alphabet letters (Justice, Bowles, & Skibbe, 2006).

Another aspect of metalinguistic development that emerges in this stage is **phonological awareness**, the child's ability to focus on the sound structure of his language. The child first hears large structures such as sentences. He learns to segment sentences into words, multisyllabic words into syllables, and syllables into sounds. These skills develop gradually across the first four or five years. Awareness of other regularities continues to develop, such that he can detect and produce rhymes, blend the onset of a syllable with its final consonant (*cu-p = cup*), and recognize that several words begin with the same sound (Pence & Justice, 2008). Developmental literature on children's early reading success shows that print-concept knowledge and phonological awareness are the best predictors (Lonigan, 2004). Thus, it is critical that caregivers provide ongoing opportunities to preschoolers during book-sharing activities to focus on both spoken and written words.

For a review of the highlights involved in stage 4, refer to Table 6.8. Table 6.9 shows examples of noun-verb relationships.

Table 6.8   Stage 4 Highlights

Typical Age Range: 35 to 40 Months
MLU: 3.0 to 3.75 Morphemes

Grammatical Morphemes
- Still developing, slowly but surely

Pronouns
- More consistent in use of *they, us, his, her, hers*, and *them*

Verbs
- Uses past tense of common modals: *could, should, would*

Noun Phrases
- Continues to elaborate by adding only one element in front of the noun

Verb Phrase
- Elaborates by including *do* in negative and question forms and by including modals such as *could, would, might*, and *must*
- Continues to overextend the regular past tense form to irregular verbs

Sentences
- Adds the following contractions in productions of negative sentences: *didn't, doesn't, isn't*, and *aren't*
- More consistent in use of *why, who*, and *how* questions; also asks *when* questions

Pragmatics
- Learns that short pauses mean that exchanges will continue; long pauses mean that responses are not forthcoming
- By the end of stage 4, is able to sustain conversation for more than two turns
- Developing primitive presuppositional skills (i.e., understanding what the listener needs to know and providing appropriate information)
- Beginning to make indirect requests (e.g., "Can you pick me up?")

Pragmatics, Conversation, and Narratives
- Produces recounts and heaps to convey topics of importance
- Sequences ideas in simple stories

Metalinguistics and Emergent Literacy
- Learns concepts about literacy through print referencing

Table 6.9   Noun–Verb Agreement Rules

Noun–Verb Relationship	Rule and Examples
Conjoined subject	Singular or plural verb depends on use.
	The *pitcher* and *catcher* are important team members.
	The *director and star* of the movie is Clint Eastwood.
Use of *or* and *nor*	Verb is always singular.
	Rain or shine, the picnic is Saturday.
	Neither *George nor Ralph* needs the job.
Gerund with plural noun as the subject	Verb is always singular.
	Collecting baseball cards is my favorite hobby.
	Washing dogs requires a lot of work.
Plural noun with singular meaning	Verb is always singular.
	Politics is a dirty business.
	Four months is plenty of time to paint the house.
Use of indefinite pronouns	Singular or plural depends on use.
	A few of these are spoiled.
	A few is all he could eat.

For a review of the highlights involved in stage 5, refer to Table 6.10, and refer to Tables 6.11 and 6.12 for summaries of negation and question forms, respectively, in Brown's five stages.

Table 6.10   Stage 5 Highlights

Typical Age Range: 41 to 46 Months
MLU: 3.75 to 4.5 Morphemes

Grammatical Morphemes
- 9 of the 14 specified morphemes are mastered by the close of stage 5.
- The remaining five morphemes (irregular past tense, contractible copula, uncontractible auxiliary, regular third person, and irregular third person) are mastered by 50 months.

Pronouns
- More consistent in use of *its, our, ours, him, their, theirs, myself, yourself*

Adjectives
- Understands the superlative forms of common adjectives but does not understand comparative forms until about 5 years of age

Noun Phrases
- Continues to elaborate by adding only one element in front of the noun

Verb Phrases
- Continues to have difficulty matching the number of the subject and the verb
- Verb phrases become more adult-like as the child masters verb-related grammatical morphemes

(continued)

Table 6.10 Stage 5 Highlights (Continued)

Sentences
- Uses negative past tense forms of *to be* (e.g., *weren't, wasn't*)
- Occasionally uses negative past tense modals (e.g., *wouldn't, couldn't*)
- More consistent in creating questions by properly inverting words (e.g., "He is playing baseball." → "Is he playing baseball?")
- Produces primitive tag questions (e.g., "I'm going now, *okay?*")
- Embeds relative clauses into the object position of sentences (e.g., "That's the plate *that I broke.*")
- Conjoins clauses, usually with *and*

Pragmatics, Conversation, and Narratives
- Conversational skills improve as a direct result of more sophisticated language
- Increases use of indirect requests, although direct requests are still far more common
- Sequences ideas in simple stories

Metalinguistics and Emergent Literacy
- Uses print reference to increase knowledge of print concepts
- Demonstrates phonological awareness of words

Table 6.11 The Development of Negation in Brown's Five Stages

Brown's Stages	Development of Negation	Examples
Early stage 1 12–22 months	Uses single words such as *"No!" "Gone!" "Allgone!"* to express rejection, denial, nonexistence, and disappearance	"Allgone!" to indicate that he ate all of his spinach
Late stage 1 22–26 months	Uses either *no* or *not* as the first element in constructing a simple sentence	"Not cookie!" "No milk."
Early stage 2 27–28 months	No changes	
Late stage 2 28–30 months	Uses *no, not, don't, can't*, and may place the negative element between the subject and predicate	"Daddy can't go."
Early stage 3 31–32 months	More likely to use *no, not, don't*, and *can't* between subject and predicate	"I can't play." "Baby not cry."
Late stage 3 33–34 months	Uses the contraction *won't*	"Mommy won't play."
Early stage 4 35–37 months	Begins using negation with auxiliary verbs	"He will not run away." "Daddy is not playing."
Late stage 4 38–40 months	Begins using *isn't, doesn't, aren't*, and *didn't*	"That isn't my bike." "The boy didn't run."
Stage 5 41–46 months and beyond	Begins using *wouldn't, couldn't, wasn't/*, and *shouldn't*	"The boy wouldn't help me." "The doggie wasn't there."

Table 6.12   **The Development of Question Forms in Brown's Five Stages**

Brown's Stages	Yes/No Questions	Examples	Wh- Questions	Examples
Early stage 1 MLU = 1–1.5 Age = 12–22 Months	Uses a single word with a rising intonation	"Doggie?"	Uses what and where with a rising intonation. What and where are not likely to be complete adult phonological forms.	"What?" "Where?"
Last stage 1 MLU = 1.5–2.0 Age = 22–26 months	Combines two words by putting that + "X" with a rising intonation	"That doggie?"		"What that?" "Where doggie?"
Early stage 2 MLU = 2.0–2.25 Age = 27–28 months			Continues to use what and where to produce the following combinations: What + NP?Where + NP? What + NP + (doing)? Where + NP + (go or going)? (go or going)?	"What kitty doing?" "Where mommy go?"
Late stage 2 MLU = 2.25–2.5 Age = 28–30 months	Continues combining words with a rising intonation	"Doggie go home?"	Produces What and Where + NP + verb?	"What Daddy kick?"
			Produces What or Where + NP + copula (such as "is")?	"Where doggie is?"
			May ask "Why?" as a single word	"Why?"
Early stage 3 MLU = 2.5–2.75 Age = 31–32 months			Toward the end of early stage 3, inverts copula to form comparable to adult	"Where is doggie?"
Late stage 3 MLU = 2.75–3.0 Age = 33–34 months	Auxiliary verb forms such as can and do begin to be incorporated with proper inversion of subject and verb. Rising intonation may still be used without inverting the auxiliary verb.	"Can kitty meow?" "Does kitty like Mommy?" "What is kitty eating?" "Kitty can go bye-bye?"	May add who to productions	"Who is that man?"
Early stage 4 MLU = 3.0–3.5 Age = 35–37 months			May add how to productions	"How did she run?"

(continued)

Table 6.12   **The Development of Question Forms in Brown's Five Stages** (continued)

Brown's Stages	Yes/No Questions	Examples	Wh- Questions	Examples
Late stage 4 MLU = 3.5–3.75 Age = 38–40 months	Continuation of above; more consistent inverting of auxiliary verbs.		Now uses *how* and *when* in productions	"When is he going?"
Stage 5 and beyond MLU = 3.75–4.5 and above Age = 41–46 months and beyond	Auxiliary inversion is consistent; more modals such as *may* and *must* are added.	"Are they going away?" "May I have that?"	*Why* questions now appear in combination with other words; may use some tag questions.	"Why is he doing that?" "I want to go outside, OK?"

Check Your Understanding 6.3

Assess your understanding of the elaboration of sentences through the use of phrases, clauses, and continued advances in language use during MLU Stages 4 and 5 by completing this brief quiz.

The Role of Comprehension and Production in Language Development

Concepts Underlying Words

As you know, it is not possible to separate intellectual growth from language development, and it is not possible to separate comprehension from the production of language. These processes are inextricably connected, and they have interactive relationships. What we say often reflects what we understand about things, people, and events, and it is generally true that clear thinking results in clear speaking and writing. Thus, during the first five years, children are busy learning, understanding, and producing language to reflect what they know and continuing to learn through language.

Many language forms develop by the end of stage 5, whereas others require more time and experience. In fact, language development continues throughout the school-age years, as we will see in the next chapter. The reason for such protracted development leads us back to the relationship between cognition and language. Children must gain understandings of concepts in order to learn to use some forms of grammar and meaning effectively.

Relational words, as the name suggests, identify relationships among people, objects, and events. These words reflect knowledge about space, time, amount, dimensions, and kinship. Table 6.13 shows the various types of relational terms, with examples of the words we use to convey the relationships and information about the typical ages at which these words are understood and used accurately.

Table 6.13 **Comprehension and Production of Relational Words**

Relational Concept	Order and Age of Development	
Spatial terms	*in, on*	2 years
	under	3 years
	beside, next to, in front of	4 to 5 years
Temporal terms	*before, after*	5 years
	since, until, while, during	> 5 years
Quantity terms	*more, less*	> 5 years
	couple, few	> 5 years
Dimensional terms	*big/little, tall/short*	5 years
	thick/thin, deep/shallow	> 5 years
Kinship terms	*mom, dad, brother, sister, grandma, grandpa, aunt, uncle, cousin*	3 years 3 years 4 to 5 years

In all cases, the child must experience these words in many contexts to develop complete understanding of them and rely on caregivers to help her use each of the words appropriately.

The words used in *wh-* questions emerge in the following order: *what, where, who,* and then *when, how,* and *why.* What does this order suggest to you about the order of acquisition of concepts that underlie these words? Why are words such as *when, how,* and *why* acquired later? These last three words relate to the concepts of time and causality, and these concepts are acquired relatively late in cognitive development (Piaget, 1926). Very simply, the child must understand *time* before he can understand or produce *when* questions, and he must understand *cause/effect* before he can comprehend or produce *how* or *why* questions. Before the child has these later *wh-* words, he often responds to *when, how,* and *why* questions as though they are *what, where,* or *who* questions. Tyack and Ingram (1977) suggest that the child with a limited understanding of *wh-* terms uses two strategies in answering *wh-* questions: (1) answer the question as though the *wh-* word is one he already knows; or (2) answer the question in a manner consistent with his understanding of the verb. Using the first strategy in responding to the question, "When did Susie eat?" the child might assume it is a *what* question and respond, "Cracker." Using the second strategy, he might respond in the same way because he associates *cracker* with the verb *eat.*

Piaget (1966) suggested that the child understands the sequencing of events before she understands duration. This too is reflected in his understanding and use of language. The child understands and produces words such as *before* and *after,* indicating *order,* before she uses words such as *until* or *since,* indicating *duration.*

These are just a few examples of the obvious connections between what a child understands about the world at a cognitive level and what he is able to understand and produce in language. Look for the cognitive/language connections in the examples that follow. Some are obvious and others are subtle, but it may be impossible to find any aspect of receptive or expressive language development that is not directly or indirectly tied to a corresponding development in cognition.

Active and Passive Sentences

Consider the problems the child encounters as she tries to sort out active and passive sentences. An active sentence is considered reversible if either noun can be either the agent or the object. For example, we can say, "The dog chased the cat," or, "The cat chased the dog." These are reversible active sentences. To interpret an active sentence, the child must learn that the first noun is the agent and the second noun is the object. The child understands the reversible active sentence in stage 1 or 2 (Chapman & Miller, 1975).

A passive sentence has an entirely different word order. In the passive sentence "The flower was watered by the girl," the first noun (*flower*) is the object of the verb *watered* and the second noun (*girl*) is the agent. Some passive sentences are reversible ("the cat was chased by the dog") and some are not reversible, as is true of the flower example. The child has trouble interpreting reversible passive sentences until she is beyond stage 5. Why is this a problem?

The child in stage 1 or 2 interprets passive sentences in the same way she interprets active sentences. That is, she interprets the first noun as the subject and the second noun as the object. The child does not correctly interpret reversible passive sentences until she is beyond stage 5. During the child's early struggles with passive forms, between the ages of three and four years, she understands passive sentences that include animate objects better than sentences including inanimate objects (Lempert, 1990). Even at 5, the child is more likely to correctly interpret reversible passive sentences containing active verbs than those that contain non-active verbs. That is, "The boy was bitten by the girl" would be interpreted more easily than, "The boy was loved by the girl." The child will probably not sort out passive sentences completely until she is in elementary school.

Our knowledge about children's understanding of passive sentences is based on research, so we must look at the techniques researchers used. Some studies required children to act out their understanding of the sentences they heard, while other studies required children to watch videos: one showing the agent/object relationship reflected in the sentence and the other showing the opposite agent/object relationship (Golinkoff, Hirsh-Pasek, Cauley, & Gordon, 1987). Because acting out sentences is a more intense exercise requiring greater cooperation from the child, it may appear that children gain an understanding of passive and active sentences later than they really do. The video approach, which requires little effort, may eventually demonstrate that this understanding is acquired earlier.

Experts in language acquisition held the belief that comprehension of English forms precedes production of the forms. But Chapman and Miller (1975) studied the comprehension and production of reversible active sentences in stages 1, 2, and 3 children. In the comprehension task, the children were instructed to act out sentences produced by an adult. In the production task, the children were instructed to describe an action produced by an adult. The children in all three stages performed better in the production task than in the comprehension task, leading the authors to conclude that for word order at least, production precedes comprehension. Their conclusions were supported by later research (Gleitman & Wanner, 1982). How can this be?

Notice that in the Chapman and Miller (1975) exercise, the child is instructed to act out a sentence, but she is given no other information. She must rely on linguistic information alone. It may be, therefore, that the child first comprehends linguistic messages within situational and nonverbal contexts, then produces language, and then understands language without the supporting situational and non-verbal contexts. It may be that the kinds of responses required of children in some of these studies obscure what they really know and what they can really do. Acting out sentences and interpreting sentences being acted out may add levels of complexity that mask the child's true receptive and expressive abilities. Techniques that place fewer demands on the child's attention and that require less physical cooperation, such as the video technique developed by Golinkoff and colleagues (1987), may lead us to different conclusions about how and when the child comprehends and produces word order.

Figurative Language

Conversational discourse includes not only relational, spatial, temporal, quantity, and dimensional terms, but also regular occurrences of **figurative language** forms. In fact, these nonliteral forms may occur as often as four times a minute in natural conversational interactions (Pollio & Pollio, 1974; Reid, 2000). Caretakers use a variety of figurative forms including idioms, similes, metaphors, and irony. Very young children must rely on cues such as facial expression and the caregiver's tone of voice to deal with figurative forms. Some children show degrees of understanding during the preschool years, but full understanding emerges in later years. Table 6.14 shows some figurative expressions we might use with young children.

This discussion has not included all that is now known about the development of comprehension during the preschool years. We have provided examples of concepts, words, and structures that must be understood, and

Table 6.14   Types of Figurative Expressions Used by Adults in Interactions with Children

Figurative Form		Meaning
Idiom	Pick up your room.	Pick up these toys on the floor.
	Give me a break.	Let me have some leeway.
Simile	You are like a puppy.	You are soft and cuddly.
	The plane is like a bird.	The plane flies just like a bird flies.
Metaphor	Daddy is Superman!	Daddy is very strong.
	You're a turtle today.	You are moving slowly.
Irony	That's just what I need.	It's not what I needed at all.
	Oh, that's just great!	It is not even good.

we have tried to emphasize the complex relationships that exist among cognitive development, the comprehension of language, and the production of language. Much is still unknown about the interactions of cognition, language comprehension, and language production, but certainly the simplistic notion that comprehension always precedes production is not valid. The relationship of thinking, understanding language, and the production of language cannot be represented on a linear graph with three colored lines. These three phenomena intersect and interact to such an extent that the lines that seem to separate them are blurred and rendered meaningless. Even as an adult thinker and speaker, you must surely sense that these processes do not work independently. Sometimes in talking aloud about a difficult concept, you suddenly understand the meaning of your own words, and your cognitive grasp of the concept is enhanced. In this case, you have actually operated in a manner that appears backward. The production of language facilitates the comprehension of language, which facilitates cognitive understanding.

Check Your Understanding 6.4

Assess your understanding of the role that comprehension plays in relation to production of concepts, literacy, and later developing forms by completing this brief quiz.

Learning More Than One Language

Bilingualism

Let us turn our attention specifically to the rewards and challenges of learning two or more languages. As you have surely discovered by this point in our journey together, nothing in the area of language is ever easy. Terms that seem self-explanatory somehow defy simple definitions. The term *bilingual*, on the surface, seems to mean *two* (bi) *languages* (lingual). The fundamental obstacle to a simple definition can be summed up in a single word, *proficiency*: That is, how competent must a person be in two languages to be considered bilingual? Most of us know snippets of other languages, and many of us routinely use words from other languages. If, as an English-speaking person, I[†] know a few French words, does that make me bilingual? How much French would I need to know before I would be considered bilingual? Good question. Tough answer.

Deciding whether a person is bilingual is further complicated when a child is in the language acquisition period of development and is only partially competent in the language that will be her dominant one. How skilled in a second language must she be before she is considered bilingual?

In the ideal model of bilingualism, a speaker—adult or child—functions well in both languages. The speaker is comfortable and competent speaking English with his English-speaking friends, for example, but when his Spanish-speaking

_____
[†]Lloyd Hulit.

grandmother comes into the room, he transitions easily and smoothly into Spanish. In the *ideal* model of bilingualism, there is no dominant language, as the speaker owns both languages equally. In the vast majority of cases, however, there is a dominant language. A child, for example, might speak Spanish exclusively at home and with his Hispanic friends, but at school he speaks English in the classroom and to his English-speaking friends—but even at school, he speaks Spanish to his Hispanic friends, so even though he is competent in English, he is a more accomplished speaker of Spanish.

Dopke (1992) suggests that we should distinguish between individuals who are *productive* bilinguals and those who are *receptive* bilinguals. The productive bilingual is truly competent in both languages even if one is more dominant than the other. The receptive bilingual clearly has a dominant language and can understand a second language, perhaps even read a second language, but is not a proficient speaker in that language.

If the child's proficiency is essentially equal in two languages, and if she meets whatever standards are established for *language competence* in those languages, she is bilingual, and her bilingualism is considered *balanced*. In most cases, she will be more proficient in one language than in the other, but even in the nondominant language, she is minimally competent. A child meeting this standard is also bilingual, but the stronger of the two languages is *dominant* (Kohnert, 2004). When children learn to speak their languages has a bearing on the development of the languages. We will explore the relationship of timing and learning language first with a discussion of simultaneous acquisition followed by a discussion of sequential acquisition.

Simultaneous Language Acquisition

Simply stated, if children learn two languages at the same time, it is **simultaneous acquisition.** Experts disagree about the age factor in determining if acquisition is truly simultaneous. Some writers have argued that the term *simultaneous acquisition* should be used only if children acquire both languages before their third birthday (McLaughlin, 1978). Some writers apply an even stricter standard—from birth (Padilla & Lindholm, 1984). De Houwer (1995) also asserts that the cutoff age for determining simultaneous bilingualism is three years, and she uses different terminology to make the acquisition difference clearer. She says that a child who acquires two languages from birth experiences **bilingual first language acquisition,** a term which implies that the child becomes competent in both languages, presumably at an equal rate. De Houwer uses the term **bilingual second language acquisition** to describe the child who begins the process of acquiring one language before exposure to the second language. Exposure to the second language, in order to fit de Houwer's understanding of the term, comes at least one month after birth but before the child's second birthday.

Whatever age we use to distinguish between a bilingual child who has been exposed to two languages from the beginning of his life and a bilingual child who learns one language and then another, there is general agreement among those who have studied the development of children who learn two languages very early in their lives that they encounter special challenges. We will examine some of these issues in more detail later in this chapter, but at this point, we need to establish that at the beginning, there are confusions between the two languages, some mixing of the vocabularies and rules. Over time, the child separates the two languages as he becomes increasingly aware of the differences between them. If, however, one language is dominant, as is usually the case, its vocabulary and grammatical rules may continue to have undue influence on the nondominant language. This would mean, for example, that if a person's dominant language were Spanish and the nondominant language were English, his English would always sound like English spoken by a Spanish-speaking person, even if he were quite facile in English.

How dominant a language is for a bilingual speaker depends, in large part, on the nature of inputs she receives while she is learning two or more languages and on how thoroughly she is immersed in the communities in her environment that use each language. All of the variables—home, community, mass media, school—should give you the idea that bilingualism exists on a continuum ranging from two languages used equally to one language as clearly dominant.

Two Languages or a Hybrid?

Because, in simultaneous bilingualism, the child is presumably acquiring two languages at the same time, there is debate about whether the child, in the beginning, is actually acquiring two separate languages or a rather convoluted single language hybrid that includes elements of both languages. The **unitary language system hypothesis**, postulated by Volterra and Taeschner (1978), suggests that the child who is exposed, more or less equally, to two languages from birth, in the first phase of language development, actually functions with a single language that is a hybrid of two distinctly different languages, a hybrid that includes vocabulary and grammatical rules from both languages. As development continues into a second phase, the child differentiates the vocabularies of the two languages but continues to rely on the hybrid grammatical system he developed in the first stage. In the third and final phase, the child differentiates the grammatical systems of the two languages, resulting in a kind of surgical separation of the two languages. The evolution from unitary to separate is not unlike what happens with conjoined twins who, prior to surgery, share organ systems and, after successful separation surgery, function independently. Genesee (1989) offers an opposing view in what he calls the **dual language system hypothesis**. In this case, the name accurately describes the argument. That is, a child who is exposed to two languages from birth uses two separate language systems from the very beginning. The child, according to this hypothesis, does not go through phases in which a conjoined language system is gradually differentiated into two language systems.

Research provides more support for the dual language system hypothesis than for the unitary language system hypothesis. Although simultaneous bilingual children will occasionally mix vocabulary, and although they might occasionally use rules from one language with vocabulary from the other, they do not produce these confusions frequently or in a consistent manner that would suggest that they are *rule-governed*. Even more telling, there is no evidence that these children produce truly hybrid, or amalgamated, rules of grammar, something we would expect in the first stage of development if the unitary language system were valid.

The Impact of the Community on Simultaneous Bilingualism

If we are to understand bilingualism, we cannot overlook the context in which the two languages are learned. In the case of simultaneous bilingualism, we have to consider which language is more highly *preferred* in a child's home and which language is more highly *valued* in the larger community. We must consider if the child's family encourages him to retain his native language in the face of pressures outside the home to extinguish that language in favor of the language of the majority population.

When children grow up in countries that have traditions of bilingualism, many of the *community issues* are not operative, but these issues certainly are operative in the United States. Hispanics who migrate to the United States, for example, must confront these issues and decide if they will retain Spanish only, if they will teach their children to speak English only, or if they will encourage their children born in the United States to be bilingual by exposing them to both languages from birth. Even if they choose bilingualism, there is still the question of which language will be favored, or if equal value will be ascribed to each. These are not easy decisions because they are embedded in larger questions about culture and heritage.

Even if parents decide that their child is best served by remaining truly bilingual, there are forces beyond the home that might shape the child's ultimate linguistic destiny. When it becomes clear to a Hispanic child, for example, that the educational system strongly values English over Spanish, she might decide that little is to be gained by maintaining Spanish. Portes and Rumbaut (2001) found that adolescent immigrants from Asian and Latin countries quickly developed a preference for English. When they were in junior high school, almost three-fourths of the children they surveyed preferred English to their first language. By the time they graduated from high school, nearly 9 of 10 preferred English. Although some people might look at these numbers and conclude that the death of bilingualism is simply one of the costs of becoming an American, we feel compelled to point out that there are clear downsides to the death of bilingualism in a child. We have already noted in previous chapters that there are cognitive advantages to bilingualism, and there are metalinguistic advantages as well. Furthermore, because language is inextricably connected to culture and heritage, it's difficult to imagine what cogent argument could be made to support the idea that a child is best served by disassociating herself from her origins, especially in a country like the United States, which characterizes itself, with considerable pride, as a nation of immigrants.

Monolingual Versus Simultaneous Bilingual Development

Does simultaneous bilingualism cause developmental differences? The easy answer to this question is no. Children who are exposed to two languages from birth follow the same overall developmental patterns and hit developmental milestones at the same ages as children who are exposed to just one language

(Genesee, Paradis, & Crago, 2004). Bilingual children experience the same challenges in language development as monolingual children and make the same kinds of mistakes in grammar and phonology. If a bilingual child does make a unique mistake, it is most likely the product of the unique influences one of his languages exerts on the other. We should also note that we see the same variability in rate of language development among simultaneous bilingual children as we see in monolingual children (Genesee et al., 2004).

Into this simple depiction of developmental harmony, we must inject an important qualification. That is, even though in simultaneous bilingualism a child is exposed to two languages from birth, it is highly unlikely that the exposure will be exactly equal, which means that one language is *dominant* and the other is *non-dominant*. If, during the developmental period, the child is exposed more often and more deliberately to one language than to the other, there is no reason to believe that the development of both languages will be exactly equal. The dominant language will, of course, be accelerated in development in comparison to the nondominant language, but over time, if exposure to both languages remains reasonably strong and consistent, the developmental differences will diminish. Even when the differences are most pronounced, however, one should not conclude that the child is proficient in the dominant language and incompetent or semicompetent in the nondominant language (Genesee et al., 2004). Competence or proficiency is always relative, and there is something else to consider. The dominant language at 3 or 4 years might be the child's nondominant language by the time he is 18.

In a less enlightened time, researchers believed that exposure to two languages retarded development. The evidence they often cited was smaller vocabulary size in bilingual children. Although that may appear to be true, especially if it's the vocabulary of the nondominant language that is measured, when the vocabularies of both languages are combined and when we account for the conceptual bases of the words included in both languages, the size of the vocabularies of simultaneous bilingual children are the same as those of monolingual children during the developmental period (Pearson, 1998; Pearson, Fernandez, & Oller, 1993).

Code Mixing

To argue that the child exposed to two languages from birth *never* confuses the two languages would be silly and not conformant to facts or common observations. My* youngest sister, Jinny, was exposed to Korean and to English at birth, and the exposures were fairly equal during the earliest stages of her language development. She often used Korean words in otherwise English sentences, and she used English words in Korean constructions. She also confused grammatical rules. Code mixing is the norm for bilingual children and adults (Genesee et al., 2004). The fact that most of the bilingual child's code-mixing issues are grammatical means that she is mastering the syntactic systems of the two languages. She could not mix elements of the two grammars unless she were mastering both of them and drawing from one grammar to insert one of its rules into the other grammar. A fact of linguistic life for the bilingual code mixer is that she mixes less and less as language development proceeds.

---

*Lloyd Hulit.

Genesee and his colleagues (2004) state that code mixing is a *communicative resource.* That is, the child draws on his greatest competencies in each language to create a communicative effort that is more complete than it would be if either language were used alone. We should also consider that code mixing, like every other dimension of bilingualism, is a product of the child's familial, community, and cultural experiences. In other words, code mixing is not just a language phenomenon. What is mixed and how it is mixed may well be influenced by factors in the child's life that go beyond the boundaries of language.

Stages of Development in Simultaneous Bilingualism

There are three stages in bilingual development during the infant and preschool years. In stage 1 (Owens, 2005), the child has two different language systems and chooses one system over the other, depending on the communicative context or the communicative purpose in any given circumstance. She might use one system with adults who speak one language and the other system with adults who speak the other language. In the beginning, the child combines the sound systems (phonologies) of the two languages into a single system, but she begins to ascribe the correct phonology to the correct language by 24 to 30 months, and she has them well separated by the time she is 3 years old, at least well enough that she knows the phonology of her native language.

By the time the child enters stage 2, he has two separate vocabularies for his two languages, but he uses one grammatical system in both languages. The words he adds to his vocabularies are drawn from specific contexts, and if he acquires a word in one language, he typically does not learn its equivalent in the other language right away. He tends to learn grammatical constructions that are applicable in both languages before he learns the constructions that are unique to each language, and as common sense would suggest, he learns simple constructions earlier than more complex constructions. If the construction for a given syntactic rule is easier in one language than in the other, he will learn the simpler version first.

In stage 3, the child is fairly consistent in keeping the vocabularies and syntactic systems of the two languages separate. The interference that remains occurs primarily in syntax, when the child applies a rule from one language in producing a construction in the other language. There are very few instances of code mixing in the child's productions by the time she is three or four years old, and some of those mixes seem to occur when the child attends to code mixing in the speech of adults with whom she interacts. In other words, the child seems to learn what her caregivers model for her, mixes and all.

Successive Bilingual Language Development

To appreciate *successive bilingualism* in its most usual form, consider a Hispanic child who lives with parents and members of his extended family who speak only Spanish. He is immersed in this environment for the first three or four years of his life, with few excursions into English-speaking segments of the culture. By the time he is ready for preschool, he is clearly a monolingual Spanish speaker, even though he might know a few words of English. Beginning in preschool, he is exposed to English on a daily basis. If he is not exposed to English until he is five years old, he will understand English before he is able to speak it, and he is not likely to achieve significant strength in his bilingual language system until he is in the sixth or seventh grade (Kohnert & Bates, 2002). Note in this example that he will be 11 or 12 years old. If the child is thoroughly acculturated in his school community and in his peer community, English will become his dominant language, but if he maintains stronger ties to his Hispanic community and culture than to the mainstream English-speaking culture, Spanish will remain his dominant language.

Recall that dual language usage is considered successive or sequential bilingualism if one language is established before the speaker—child or adult—is exposed to a second language. The second exposure could occur when the child is three years old and moving into the latter stages of language development, or it could occur when she is taking language classes in high school or as an adult.

Depending on when the exposure occurs, the challenges involved in acquiring the second language will differ. Early exposure prior to age three may yield more initial confusion than exposure during the adult years, but proficiency will likely be greater if exposure to both languages remains consistent and rich.

Transfer from First to Second Language

In the early stages of a child's exposure to the second language, his productions in that language are influenced by his first-language expertise. When the child applies something from his first language to the second language, we call that *transfer*, a process that may be reflected in grammar, vocabulary, and phonology. The casual observer might notice transfer most easily in his pronunciations. For example, if the speaker's second language contains sounds that do not occur in his first language, he might adjust his production of words containing those unfamiliar sounds to conform to the phonology he knows best, resulting in quaint pronunciations. At one time, transfer was viewed negatively, as an impediment to effectively learning the second language. We now understand that when the child transfers something he knows from his first language to his second language, he is using his first language as a kind of linguistic resource to advance his acquisition of the second language (Genesee et al., 2004). Some transfers, like pronunciations shaped by his greater comfort level with the phonology of his first language, might remain, especially if the second language exposure comes later in life, but most transfers will fade away as the process of separating the two languages moves to completion.

Influence of the Second Language on the First

The child probably uses proficiency in her first language to help her learn a second language, as evidenced by transfer. In many cases, the dominant first language fades, and the second language becomes dominant. This process is called **attrition** (Genesee et al., 2004). In attrition, the first language might simply become the child's nondominant language, or it might fade away entirely so that the formerly bilingual child becomes essentially monolingual. Attrition occurs when the second language becomes required, such as in a school where only English is spoken, or when the child's peer group speaks English.

The journey from dual language to single language by means of attrition is not inexorable, and most experts with interests in language or child development would argue that it is not desirable. No matter what a child brings to life from the genetic pools that merge into his conception, he is also a product of his environment. That environment includes his language, culture, immediate and extended family, and social community.

Stages of Development in Successive Bilingualism

We must, of course, keep in mind that acquiring a second language will not be the same experience or occur at the same rate for all children, any more than learning the piano or learning soccer will be the same experience for all children, even if the amount of exposure to the language, the piano, or soccer is exactly the same. Every child is unique and is influenced by factors, such as the quantity and quality of exposure, motivation, and personality (Wong Fillmore, 1983), and although it's difficult to quantify, some people simply have a greater aptitude for language learning than others (Carroll, 1981). The rate of acquisition is highly variable, and what can be said with a reasonable degree of confidence is that some children are proficient in the second language within one year and most are proficient within two, three, or four years (Genesee et al., 2004).

Generally speaking, a young child has a learning advantage and is likely to become proficient, especially if she has a strong need for that language, is highly motivated, and has a positive attitude, and if she identifies with the community in which that language is dominant. To these generalizations, one more needs to be added. Because this group is exponentially heterogeneous, any stage concept applied to this group must be vague enough to be sufficiently ubiquitous to include the developmental experiences of most, if not all, of its members.

In describing the stages of development for successive bilingualism, Owens (2016) excludes the acquisition of a second language as the result of formal classes. With that in mind, here are some characteristics within each of the three stages:

Stage 1—Social Observer
- Establishing personal and social relationships with speakers of the language
- Using basic vocabulary, standard phrases, social expressions, and gestures
- Listening for repeated linguistic patterns, watching gestures to aid comprehension, and analyses the language forms spoken by others
- Using private speech to practice constructions

Stage 2—Messenger
- Communicating in the second language despite morphological, grammatical, and semantic errors
- Using **interlanguage** that combines rules from the dominant language with rules from the second language to bridge the gap between the two languages

Stage 3—Speaker

- applying the rules of the second language to gradually expand competency in comprehension and production
- using the metalinguistic awareness nurtured in his first language to analyze, understand, and master the second language
- elaborating simple constructions to create complex forms

You should recognize the progression outlined in these three stages, because this is exactly what we observe in the monolingual child. The monolingual child uses single words before he uses phrases. He uses simple phrases before he uses complex ones, and he uses simple sentence forms before he embeds and conjoins.

Others have proposed stages of second language acquisition that offer a similar perspective. Tabors (1997) concluded that there are four stages in second language acquisition, based on a study she conducted with preschool children who were acquiring English as their second language. Tabors noted, as we have repeatedly emphasized, that there was a great deal of variation among these children. The variation in development was so great, in fact, that some children seemed to skip a stage, whereas others seemed to remain in that stage much longer than one would expect. Tabors's stages should be viewed as general descriptions of what a mythical, prototypical child is likely to experience in the step-by-step process of acquiring a second language. There is no suggestion in her conclusions that all second language children will progress through these stages in the same way or according to the same timetable.

Stage 1—Home Language User
- using the first or native language in settings where only that language is spoken

Stage 2—Non-verbal User of Second Language
- depending heavily on nonverbal communication to convey messages to develop relationships and social interactions

Stage 3—Telegraphic and Formulaic User of Second Language
- using imitation of words and phrases to produce direct replications of constructions formulated by others
- creating some original constructions

Stage 4—Speaker of Second Language

- creating original utterances using the basics of the language rules
- retaining the accent and dialectal attributes of the first language in production of the second language
- making grammatical and morphological errors consistent with learning language

Of course, language development does not end with fluency in the second language. Some teachers of English as a second language expect basic fluency in social situations, known as basic interpersonal communication skills (BICS), to be evident within six months to two years of learning a second language. Language skills for academic learning, also known as cognitive language academic proficiency (CALP), usually takes from five to seven years to reach full development (Cummins, 1999). This is important for practitioners in educational settings because they provide support for students. It is not enough for educators to assume that time and practice speaking English is enough for student success. Programming designed specifically to teach the language of the classroom, metalinguistics, vocabulary and concepts, and literacy skills will help students learning English as a second language make the transitions they need for academic learning. Refer to Chapter 7 for a discussion of each of these areas.

The Optimal Age of Second Language Learning

Is there an optimal age for learning a second language? Is there a kind of "acquisition window," an age span during which a second language can be mastered, and once that window closes, it's difficult or impossible to learn a second language? Let's begin with something we know for sure. We know that adults, even adults who are considered *senior citizens* or *elderly*, can and do master second languages, some with relative ease. We also know that some people seem to have a facility for mastering languages, and others seem to struggle in the process.

The question, then, is not *can* someone learn a second language later in life, because that is a simple question with a simple answer—yes, although some clearly do better than others in becoming bilingual. The more important question is whether there is a period of time in a person's life that is optimal for acquiring a second language. The answer to that question is not so simple.

Research does not point to a clear age demarcation, an age before which acquiring a second language is easy and after which acquiring a second language is difficult. Some experts believe that adolescents and adults might actually have an advantage over very young children in learning a second language, in the early stages at least, because older learners bring stronger cognitive abilities and well-developed metalinguistic skills to the process. Collier (1987/1988) asserted that children between 8 and 12 years are the most proficient second language learners. Adults who learn a second language are not as adept as younger learners in acquiring the grammar and the phonology of a second language, and the difficulties in these areas tend to increase as adults age. Furthermore, as one would guess, when a person learns a second language as an adult, she tends to rely heavily on the rules of her first language to understand and formulate in the second language (Sanders, Neville, & Woldorff, 2002). There is, however, no evidence that age, in itself, is an impediment to acquiring a second language.

As with all aspects of bilingualism, we must be cautious when we focus on a single factor, such as age, because no factor operates in a vacuum. Cultural differences may be greater for some immigrants than for other immigrants, as an example. Learning English also depends on supportive opportunities to learn it and use it in both social and academic contexts. Social experiences, language experiences, and cognitive experiences must be recognized as contributors to the language acquisition process. What is remarkable is that in spite of these differences, monolingual and bilingual children acquire language in very much the same way and according to the same general schedule (Bialystok, 2001). In returning to the never-ending argument about nature versus nurture, we reasonably conclude that we retain the biological ability to learn language as long as we live with healthy brains, intact sensory mechanisms, and functional speech mechanisms. We must also recognize that learning is a factor in language acquisition, whether it's one language or two or three, regardless of the age of the learner. We may assume that, for adults, the experience of acquiring a second language is extremely learning-intensive, and it may be for some adults, but for others, learning a second, third, or fourth language is more a process of exposure and social practice than study and drill. We should also not ignore the fact that learning is important in linguistic development for the very young child if the child is learning one language or two. The capacity for language may be innate, but the conventions of the child's language or languages are learned (Bialystok, 2001).

✓ Check Your Understanding 6.5

Assess your understanding of the similarities and differences in learning two languages simultaneously and successively by completing this brief quiz.

SUMMARY

In this chapter we explored the explosion of language in children from 27 months to 46 months. The period between two and four years is truly remarkable, as children quickly expand from single-word utterances and two-word combinations to speaking in sentences that allow them to do all these things: converse with others with increasing complexity using a variety of grammatical forms and with appropriate function and style; attend to and be aware of the predictability of language forms, including the development of print awareness and phonological awareness; listen to and tell simple stories; and understand that language is both literal and figurative. We also discussed learning two languages simultaneously and learning the first language and then the second language.

And That's Not All, Folks!

The child has been a busy language activist during her preschool years, but she still has more work to do. As she moves into her elementary school years, into adolescence, and even into adulthood, her vocabulary will continue to grow, she will refine and elaborate the language structures she has acquired, and she will become a more sophisticated conversationalist. These changes do not occur as quickly as in previous years, and they are not as dramatic, but they are important changes that will make her a more effective language receiver and producer. In the next chapter, we trace language development beyond stage 5.

▯▷ Surfing the Web

If you are interested in exploring topics discussed in this chapter in more detail, search for one or more of the following relevant terms online.

language development stages	development of conversations
development of grammar	narrative development
development of phrases and sentences	emergent literacy skills
development of vocabulary	bilingualism
development of figurative language	simultaneous language acquisition
	successive language acquisition

✓ Chapter Review 6.1

Recall what you learned in this chapter by completing the Chapter Review.

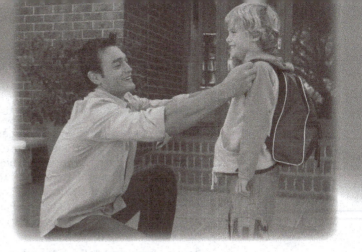

7

Taking Language from Home to School

LEARNING OUTCOMES

After completion of this chapter, you will be able to:

- Describe the challenges that students and teachers face when students are learning English as a second language.
- Discuss the characteristics of the forms of language expected in classrooms as students communicate with teachers and one another.
- List the gains students make in the development of learning about words.
- Describe the changes school-age children make in syntax and morphology.
- Trace the art of conversations and narratives.
- Outline the development of metalinguistic skills and learning to read and write.

Although much of language acquisition occurs from birth through the preschool years, development continues throughout the school years, especially during the primary grades. It is also true that people continue to add to their language knowledge and their communication competencies into their adult years, perhaps all their lives. In this chapter, we consider the continuation of language acquisition as children enter school, including the interactive growth of vocabulary and cognition, and developmental changes in syntax, morphology, and pragmatics. We examine the emergence of gender differences in communication, metalinguistic development, and the application of language knowledge to the learning of reading and writing.

Figure 7.1 reminds us of the exciting experiences that youngsters have as they develop friendships and explore the world outside the home. They have all the language foundation they need to communicate with others and to use information to continue their learning. The five-year-old child brings all of the language skills included in Figure 7.2 to be able to converse with other children and adults, to express his ideas and satisfy his needs, and to embark on learning in the classroom.

Figure 7.1   Experience Leads to Language at School

Paul can't wait to get to his kindergarten classroom on Monday. He just returned from a great day at his friend Joey's house, where they made kites and tried them out in the field. He helped cut out the kite from the pattern that Joey's dad made, and he used bright blue, white, and green paint to make a swirl design across the kite. He made a long tail from an old pillowcase. The wind was just right to make the kite soar high above the field. Show-and-tell for Paul will be his chance to tell all his classmates about kites. He plans to bring in his kite so that they can see it, and his mom even has a picture of him flying it.

Paul's Show-and-Tell on Monday:

Here is my kite. I had fun making it 'cuz we had to paint it and everything. And it drieded in the garage at Joey's house. Joey's dad, he didn't have a car in there. Ah, one time the kite was so high and then it came down, crash! And it didn't break. We had a really long string, so we had to wind it around a ball. I put my name on it, so I can keep it at Joey's house. I hope we go to the field again today. Oh, here is me in this picture.

Figure 7.2   Profile of a 5-Year-Old Communicator

Uses well-developed receptive and expressive vocabulary

Speaks with an almost intact speech sound system

Formulates complete, well-formed sentences, including question and negative forms

Produces declarative and imperative sentences

Understands and uses active sentences with emerging success of passive sentences

Understands and uses indirect requests

Talks about present, past, and future events

Participates in singing, rhyming, and speech-related games

Recognizes written language in books and other print media

Differentiates between writing and drawing

Engages in print-related activities, including emergent reading and writing

---

We must keep in mind that a five-year-old reared in Dallas, Texas, will not sound like a five-year-old in Boston, Massachusetts, and neither of these children will sound like a five-year-old from Tokyo, Japan. The child who grows up in a home full of talkative older siblings and adults who constantly engage the child in communicative exchanges is likely to talk more, and perhaps be more interested in language, than the child who is reared by taciturn parents who make little effort to facilitate speech and language production. The child who is exposed to vulgar words will use vulgar words. The child who is exposed to complete, correct models of language is more likely to use complete, correct sentences than the child who is exposed to models that are syntactically deficient. We must be careful not to extend this too far, because few children are exposed to only inadequate speech and language models, but as a general rule, we would not expect a child's speech and language abilities to be better than the models to which she is predominantly exposed.

The Classroom and Language: New Demands in Diverse Settings

The child learns most of his language in the comfort of his own home, in interaction with the most caring people in his world. The child acquiring language at home has the advantage of knowing the routine of his family life and knowing the nuances of the nonverbal communicative assists provided by his caregivers. If he does not understand all that is said to him, he can fill in the missing information by taking the familiar non-verbal context into account. Most of his conversations at home are one on one, so if there is a breakdown and a repair is needed, his partner will usually recognize the need immediately. If not, he is comfortable enough with his partner to ask for help. Home is a safe and comfortable place for learning and using language, but what happens when the child begins school?

The child soon discovers that the language environment at school differs radically from the language environment at home. To a large extent, the difference reflects the overall purpose served by school. To the casual eye, the classroom for the child just beginning school is a fairly benign place where children color, play, sing songs, learn the alphabet, and learn to count, but those are only the by-products of a much more serious purpose served by our schools. Wilhelm (1994) suggests that schools are the dominant force in the socialization of children, that it is in the schools that students and teachers engage in a kind of "social negotiation," systematically sharing an understanding about the attitudes, values, and knowledge that underlie the major institutions of their society. That's pretty weighty stuff for five- and six-year-old children, but it is an accurate portrayal of what we expect from schools in the new century. Many people talk about getting schools back to the basics of reading, writing, and arithmetic, but that nostalgic view of *school* does not fit the reality of our present world. Teachers should not be expected to be surrogate parents, and they should not be solely responsible for imparting lessons about morality and ethics, but these expectations exist. The language of the classroom is very different from the language of home because it must be. We will explore the challenges that students and educators face to embrace cultural diversity and then focus our attention on the ways in which language is used in classrooms.

Cultural Diversity in the Classroom

Of the total population of the United States, 8% of people have limited English proficiency, including about 5 million children who attend public schools (Camera, 2015). That number is predicted to increase to 6 million by 2020. One of the classroom issues to which we must be especially sensitive in this 21st century is cultural diversity. With dramatic demographic shifts occurring in the United States, no one should be surprised that the language a child uses at home may be quite different from the language she is expected to use in school.

When children are learning English as a second language during their school years, they face challenges as they participate in the language of school.

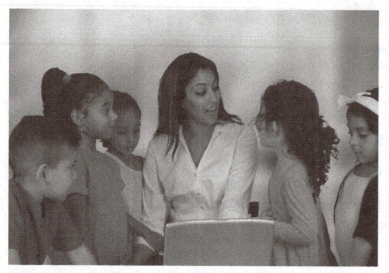

Children learning English as a second language in school.

Recall that they are also working to master their native language with all the challenges of learning grammatical structures, meanings of words and how words are related to each other, and literacy. Now add to that having to learn English, sometimes without support from their families who speak their native language at home, in the context of a busy classroom where only English is spoken. They have the difficult job of learning English while being required to learn the content of the curriculum in English at the same time. It takes several years, as many as seven, for these students to have proficiency in English to use it effectively for learning academic content.

Of course oral language differences are accompanied by disparities in literacy proficiency that further add to the challenges students face in school. A report by Short and Fitzsimmons (2006) summarized literacy statistics from the National Center for Educational Statistics regarding middle and high school students. Of all secondary students, only 30% read with proficiency, whereas 70% fell below proficiency. But the proportion of students of color who do not read proficiently is as high as 89% and the dropout rate is almost 50%, as compared to 10% of white English-speaking high school students. When middle and high school students are learning English as a second language, the picture is even more telling. In 2004, students who reported difficulty with speaking English had an 80% likelihood of dropping out of high school. It is evident that the educational system faces many challenges in meeting the needs of these students.

Literacy development for students learning English as a second language is essential for academic success. It is also quite challenging, particularly for students who enter the American educational system in the later grades. These students have fewer years to master English; less involvement in high-level course content without the contextual supports available in early grades; little formal literacy instruction, common from first through third grade; underdeveloped literacy in the native language; and teachers who are not trained to teach basic literacy skills to adolescents. Students also have varying degrees of success and motivation to learn to read, especially regarding academic subjects. Understanding these factors is necessary for policy makers, preservice teacher preparation programs, school administrators, and teachers as they determine resources and educational efforts to assist students in American classrooms.

At the same time that we value diversity, we also recognize that understanding and speaking English is essential for social and vocational opportunities. There seems little question that our children must be given the opportunity and encouraged to learn English. They must also be given the opportunity to learn those varieties of English that will give them the best chance of succeeding as students and as adults, while at the same time retaining and even strengthening the languages, cultures, and values of their native heritage.

Teacher Preparation, Classroom Environment, and Curricular Approaches

While we acknowledge that students learning English as a second language during the school-age years face a long process complicated by the demands of the curriculum, teachers also must use best teaching practices to assist students to achieve success. However, there is currently a shortage of bilingual teachers, especially those who also have understanding of the sociocultural backgrounds of their students (Camera, 2015). Teachers of U.S. children historically tend to be white, monolingual, English-speaking women from middle-class backgrounds (Boyd & Brock, 2004). Their ways of thinking and knowing are based on their background, experiences, language, and all the factors associated with culture. Diversity in the teaching profession has increased, but according to the U.S. Department of Education (2016), by 2024, 56% will be students of color, whereas 82% of public school teachers identify as white, with that number remaining stable over the past 15 years. However well intentioned, teachers likely have limited cultural competence, especially when their students come from diverse communities. The result is underpreparation for the challenges of teaching diverse learners. Current preservice education for teachers has improved, with courses and experiences in cultural and linguistic differences, resulting in educational practices that are differentiated and evidence based. For example, primary language instruction is one of the most effective ways to increase learning in school for bilingual children (Cummins, 1989), and the inclusion of interactions that mirror the home language environment provides strong messages to children that their home language is valued and respected (Langdon & Cheng, 1992). In addition, an increase in teachers in the workforce with diverse backgrounds will have positive effects for students (U.S. Department of Education, 2016):

- Demonstrating positive role models to change and prevent stereotypes
- Preparing students to live and work in a diverse society
- Implementing and modeling culturally sensitive teaching practices
- Improving the experience of schooling for all students
- Improving academic outcomes to close the achievement gap
- Creating high expectations for all learners
- Advocating for student needs
- Developing trusting relationships with students

Any program designed to help 21ˢᵗ-century teachers prepare for culturally diverse student bodies must include three components: awareness, knowledge, and skills (Sue, Arredondo, & McDavis, 1992). Teachers must become *aware* of their own beliefs, values, and biases, and they must understand how they view their own students. A teacher who lacks appropriate awareness and sensitivity is likely to bring her personal biases into the classroom, biases that will be recognized by her students and will influence how they respond to the teacher and to the learning process. If a teacher acquires *knowledge* about other cultures, she will be able to integrate that knowledge into class material. Her awareness and knowledge will enhance teaching *skills*. She will shape her teaching style to take into account the cultural differences in her classroom. Her interpersonal skills will be improved to the extent that she learns that one communicative style will not be effective with all students, that the way people talk to one another is influenced by their cultural experiences.

It is also true that teachers often refer children from diverse cultures for correction of suspected language and learning disabilities (Langdon & Cheng, 1992; Roseberry-McKibben, Brice, & O'Hanlon, 2005). Referrals can result in over-identification of these students when, in actuality, it is language differences, not disabilities, that are causing academic challenges. Conversely, under-identification of disabilities may occur when teachers assume that language differences, rather than disability, are impacting educational achievements. We should expect that children from diverse backgrounds will have language problems similar to those of children from the majority culture, but we must also realize that there are variations due to the influence of poverty and environmental factors, such as access to health care and education. Limited prenatal care, inadequate treatment for childhood illnesses, inadequate nutrition, and low educational levels are just some of the factors that lead to language and learning difficulties (Roseberry-McKibben, 2007). Knowledge about second language learning and cultural and linguistic differences is important for teachers in order for them to make appropriate referrals when students are having difficulty in academic and social development beyond what would be expected as a second language learner.

 Video Reflection 7.1: Issues in Schools for Students Learning English as a Second Language

Watch the video to gain perspective from a professor in bilingual education and English as a second language regarding language diversity, then answer the question.

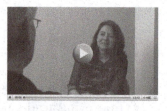

The challenges presented by teaching children who are racially, culturally, ethnically, and religiously diverse are daunting. They are forcing U.S. educators to develop an instructional strategy that takes diversity into account—a comprehensive multicultural education system (Manning & Baruth, 1996). **Multicultural education** asserts, "that all students regardless of the groups to which they belong, such as those related to gender, race, culture, social class, religion, or exceptionality should experience educational equality in the school" (Banks & Banks, 1997, p. 4). If we accept this or some similar concept of what multicultural education means, we will understand how profoundly the U.S. education system must change. To meet the needs of a culturally diverse student population, we must change teacher preparation, teaching practices, the curriculum, and the way we organize the educational process.

Changes in curricula will occur by attention to cultural considerations, including socioeconomic levels, family lifestyles, religions, languages, and learning styles (Manning & Baruth, 1996). Educators will be particularly careful to make their curricula *antibiased*. To create an antibiased curriculum means that it generates, "construction of a knowledgeable, confident self-identity, comfortable, empathetic interaction with people from diverse backgrounds, critical thinking about bias, and the ability to stand up for oneself and for others in the face of bias" (Hohensee & Derman-Sparks, 1992, p. 1). To create this kind of curriculum, educators must identify the cultural features in their school policies that prevent students from achieving their potential. Once identified, these features must be eliminated or modified so that the curriculum and the school environment are culturally inclusive.

Developing a multicultural curriculum is possible only if educators operate in an intentional and systematic manner. Banks and Banks (1997) describe four approaches educators can use to create a truly multicultural curriculum. The strategy that requires the least effort and the fewest changes to the existing curriculum is called the **contributions approach**. Teachers include information on selected heroes and holidays from a range of cultures, and they focus on a few specific characteristics of these cultures.

The second strategy is called the **additive approach**. As with the first strategy, the old curriculum is not discarded. Teachers add to the existing curriculum to take cultures other than the dominant culture into account. They expand content, of course, but they also introduce culturally related concepts, themes, and perspectives without altering the basic structure of the curriculum.

When educators use the **transformation approach** (also referred to as structural reform), the structure of the curriculum is fundamentally changed. It is redesigned to allow students to understand, appreciate, and value concepts, issues, events, and themes from the perspectives of a representative range of ethnic and cultural groups. The students may engage in activities where they experience aspects of the culture through participation in events, demonstrations, and hearing or reading multiple perspectives about a topic. For example, American History would include Women's History, Asian American History, and Latino American History (Gorski, 2015).

Finally, educators may choose the **social action approach**, a strategy that must be used in combination with one or more of the previously identified strategies, most likely the transformation approach. As the name suggests, the social action approach leads students, through their increased understanding of cultural diversity, to make decisions about how best to address social issues affected by cultural differences. Going further, students actually take action to solve problems that are created by cultural differences. They assume responsibility for the problems shared by people who come from widely diverse backgrounds but who are committed to living together as people whose common bonds are stronger than their differences. Ideally, of course, all four of these strategies will be used to develop a curriculum that is relevant to all students, a curriculum that facilitates understanding and respect for all people and all cultures.

Although schools in the 21st century will rely far less on books than schools in the 20th century, textbooks and other printed instructional materials will still be used. Teachers who will be teaching an increasingly diverse student population must take care to use materials that are as bias-free as possible. Gollnick and Chin (1991) suggest that teachers should be aware of at least six forms of bias that can be found in textbooks and other printed instructional materials: (1) invisibility; (2) stereotyping; (3) selectivity and imbalance; (4) unreality; (5) fragmentation and isolation; and (6) language bias. Escamilla (1993) suggests that textbooks should not use sidebars to include information about multicultural issues because sidebars suggest that this information is less important than the information in the body of the text. Textbooks should also avoid a "superhero" approach that suggests that only a few selected individuals from a particular ethnic group have made contributions. Instead, the overall contributions of an ethnic group should be emphasized with reference to some of the major players in these contributions. Finally, Escamilla asserts that textbooks should not be written in a "one size fits all" manner. That is, authors should not write about Hispanic contributions as though they come from a single source. There is no single African culture or single Asian culture. Native Americans and African Americans can trace their cultural backgrounds to many different groups of people. The contributions of each group must be recognized and valued, no matter how convenient it might be to envision that all Africans come from the same place, that all Asians hold the same values, and that all Hispanic people maintain the same beliefs.

Carger (1997) asserts that efforts to create an educational experience that is truly multicultural must include more than just cosmetic adjustments to our current system. Even if we make the kinds of curricular changes the experts recommend to address cultural diversity, and even if teacher training programs include courses and experiences designed to make teachers more sensitive to their culturally diverse students, more needs to be accomplished if we are to ensure that all students achieve the degree of academic, social, and vocational success we believe they deserve. Carger suggests that educating multicultural students does not happen through a *recipe* approach. Teachers must help students experience, "an individualized, lifelong process of learning, discovery, accepting and trying—a little like developing gourmet cuisine versus ordering fast food" (p. 39). This means that a teacher who is serious about being an effective multicultural teacher will immerse students in multicultural literature, art, and music. She will invite guests from widely varying cultural backgrounds into her classroom to share their life stories. She will find ways to give students learning experiences that will expose them to cultural perspectives that differ from their own, perhaps through field trips. Most important, the teacher will lead students to think about, reflect on, and embrace the cultural differences among people rather than allowing them to reject reflexively what they do not understand or what does not fit neatly into their own life experiences.

Check Your Understanding 7.1

Assess your understanding of challenges faced by students and teachers in diverse classrooms by completing this brief quiz.

The Language Forms and Curricula of the Classroom

According to Cazden (1988), children entering school encounter three new forms of language. Each serves a different purpose, each is important, and each must be learned if children are to succeed in school. These language forms are: (1) the language of academic subjects or curriculum; (2) the language of behavior management; and (3) the language by which personal identity is expressed. That these three forms of language are used in the classroom is not a problem. The problem is that they are not clearly identified for children. Their purposes are typically not explained and their rules are usually not delineated or discussed. All three language forms are used during the first day of school and during every day over the next 13 years, but in most American classrooms children are expected to figure them out for themselves. It is not surprising that children are occasionally unsure about how to make these language forms work together in the learning process. It is even less surprising that children who enter school with language skills that fall below age level, who have perceptual deficits, whose intellectual capacities are at the low end of normal or lower, who have sensory problems, who have learning disabilities, and who have emotional problems become terribly frustrated and discouraged. Unfortunately, some of these children drown in the tidal wave of confusion created by these often competing language forms, and they give up.

Most of us, if asked to describe the language of the school, would describe something akin to the first language form identified by Cazden (1988)—the **language of academic subjects or curriculum**. Some children have a head start on this language form because they have heard it at home. They will know words such as *book, arithmetic, map, alphabet,* and *sound* because these and comparable words have been used by their caregivers during their preschool years. They will know how to respond to academic questions, and they will know how to formulate these questions because they have been subsumed within their communication culture at home. Unfortunately, not all children have these experiences before entering school. Still others bring their pencils and crayons to school like all the other children, but they also bring hearing losses, learning disabilities, attention deficits, visual problems, and the like. Still others speak a dialect that does not match the teacher's dialect or that of the majority of children in the classroom. Nelson (1985) describes the **cultural curriculum as the knowledge students must learn regarding the world—knowledge that is shared at particular grade levels, regardless of cultural backgrounds of individual students**. Some students with unique backgrounds will have more to learn than students who have previous exposure to mainstream culture. All of these children must work especially hard to learn the academic subjects language form, or they will quickly fall behind (Bashir & Scavuzzo, 1992).

Teacher/Student Dialogues: Basic Variations

Students are expected to learn the language of academics, including the forms of teacher/student dialogues in an implicit fashion. Westby (2006) described this learning process through experience as "learning to do school." Of course, children learn the rules about who talks to whom and when these interactions should occur over several years. This is sometimes referred to as the **school or classroom curriculum.** They also learn about the attitudes and values of teachers regarding the expectations of how to use language in the classroom (Nelson, 2010).

If you were asked to describe the basic format of instruction in a typical elementary or junior high school classroom, we suspect you would describe what Mehan (1979) calls the **IRE model.** In this version of teacher/student dialogue, the teacher *initiates* (I) a question. The student provides a *response* (R), which the teacher *evaluates* (E). The teacher then asks another question, and the sequence continues until the lesson is completed. Heath (1982b) notes that the kind of question most often asked in this model is the *known-information* question, a self-explanatory term. For example, the students are asked to read specific material and instructed to memorize specific information. The teacher uses the IRE model to determine whether the material was read, memorized, and understood. Obviously, the IRE model is teacher directed. Student/student interactions are usually not encouraged in this format.

Sometimes, of course, instruction occurs in the context of classroom discussions during which students talk to one another as well as to the teacher. This format is known as **revoicing.** In this format, the teacher presents a problem and asks the class to consider possible solutions. One student offers a solution, which another student criticizes as inadequate. Another student suggests that the proposed solution might work if it is amended in specified ways. Yet another student supports the solution as amended but suggests an additional adjustment. The teacher intervenes when she detects that the process has become stagnant or when she notices a lapse of logic that has not been identified by the other students, but she keeps the responsibility for learning in the students' hands by offering questions that nudge the process forward rather than offering a discussion-ending solution of her own. The teacher listens to what the student says, acknowledges it, and asks a question that prompts a response from the original speaker or from other students in the class. The teacher *revoices* the topic as necessary and clarifies as necessary, but she is not the unquestioned dispenser of information. She is a learning facilitator in this format.

When a teacher works with small groups of students, he might use an instructional format called **instructional conversation.** Except for attending more carefully to a designated topic, this format can be almost as informal as regular conversation. At the other end of the formality continuum, instructional conversation might be conducted within the confines of predetermined rules and procedures that keep the participants on topic and that require each participant, including the teacher, to fill the *teacher* role as well as the *student* role. This more formal version of instructional conversation serves the purpose of teaching students lessons about behavior management as well as meeting the learning goals established by the teacher.

We might find it amusing as adults to remember times when we were faced with the **language of behavior management** in school, but we might also remember the embarrassment and pain associated with learning the rules of this language form. Teachers traditionally use this language form to establish who is allowed to talk, what one is allowed to say, and how one is allowed to say it. It is clearly a language of *control.* There is no question that this language form is necessary in the classroom; otherwise, chaos would be the order of the day and nothing would be learned by anyone. Nelson (1985) refers to the expectations teachers have for student behavior as the **hidden curriculum**. Consider, however, that many children are not exposed to this language form, or at least aspects of it, until they come to school. All children are exposed to basic expressions in this language, such as these:

> "Wait until it's your turn to talk."
> "Be quiet and let your sister talk."
> "You listen when I'm talking to you."

Other expressions may be less familiar to the child who is just beginning school:

> "What you said is interesting. Is there anything you want to add?"
> "Your answer is mostly correct, but what seems to be missing?"
> "What you said is confusing. Could you explain it more clearly?"

The third language form employed in the classroom is used to express personal identity. This **language of personal identity** might seem to be a minor player in the educational process until you remember how important it was to you when you were in kindergarten or first grade to find just the right item for show-and-tell, or how it made you feel when you were able to share something about your life with a teacher you adored. Cazden (1988) points out that it is only during these sharing experiences that the child can decide for himself what he wants to say and how he will say it. It may be his only opportunity to talk about himself and to hold the communicative stage for several uninterrupted minutes. We often note that it is during the school years that the child is becoming his own person, establishing his own identity. Part of the process of becoming one's own person is learning to use the language necessary for telling others about yourself. Children viewed as assertive, self-confident, or self-assured are children who are adept at using this language form. Children must also develop and use appropriate styles of language for interactions with peers, also known as the **underground curriculum**. Sadly, notes Michaels (1990), the children who need the most practice in using personal identity language are often denied the opportunity because teachers become impatient when they listen to the personal stories of students who struggle with language due to their disabilities or because they speak a dialect other than the teachers' dialect. If this kind of student does not feel valued when trying to use this language form, he is likely to withdraw from all communicative experiences in the classroom and in social interactions and, as a consequence, fall even farther behind his peers academically and in social relationships.

Check Your Understanding 7.2

Assess your knowledge of the language of school by completing this brief quiz.

Semantic Development

Now we will turn our attention to the strides that school-age children make in their knowledge of words and the relationships words have to each other to enhance meaning.

Throughout the school years, the child makes impressive gains in her knowledge and use of words. Consider the amount of talking that occurs in typical classrooms as teachers and students discuss topics. The language-rich environment of classrooms allows students not only to learn new words but also to learn to use vocabulary in new ways. We will explore several factors that influence vocabulary acquisition, how children use strategies for organizing and retrieving words, the development of word definitions, and the understanding and use of figurative forms. Of course, all of this expansion of language occurs in tandem with maturation of the cognitive shift from concrete to more abstract levels of thinking (Emerson & Gekoski, 1976).

Video Example 7.1

Preschool is a popular choice for families who are able to arrange it, and state-funded programs provide this option for children whose families are in lower income brackets and for children with disabilities. Children who are between the ages of three and six enjoy learning opportunities that provide foundations in word 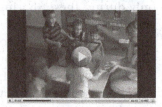 knowledge, concept development, experiences in listening and speaking, literacy, and socialization skills. Children also learn the rules of the classroom during their preschool experience. Watch the video of a preschool classroom that brings to life the concrete and redundant language contexts these students need to discuss the ideas about the tadpole and frog.

Factors Influencing Vocabulary Acquisition

Recall from Chapter 4 that the amount of parent talk is highly correlated with the amount of child talk, and that more talkative children tend to do better academically (Gilkerson & Richards, 2008; Hart & Risley, 1995). Thus, the primary influence on language development generally and vocabulary growth specifically during the early years is spoken language. When the child is about six or seven years old, however, another powerful influence emerges—written language. Research evidence suggests that children 9 or 10 years old who are highly motivated to read, who read often and read well, acquire significantly larger vocabularies than children who are less interested in reading and whose reading skills are not as well developed (Miller & Gildea, 1987; Nagy, Herman, & Anderson, 1985).

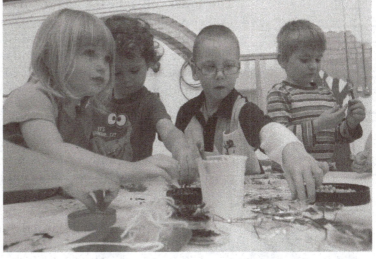

Using language to help solve problems and get things done.

Source: Jules Selmes/ Pearson Education, Inc.

The influence of the written word on vocabulary growth is evidenced in another way. As the child moves through the school years, she acquires words that are increasingly less common than base vocabulary words. These words tend to be more abstract and are used to express more complex concepts than earlier words, which is in line with the child's ability to think abstractly. Not coincidentally, these words are found far more often in written language than in mundane conversation (Nagy, Diakidoy, & Anderson, 1993).

As to how older children and young adults acquire new words and learn their meanings, at least three primary influences seem to be involved: (1) direct teaching from adult models and resources; (2) the use of clues embedded in the context surrounding unfamiliar words; and (3) the ability to use existing morphological knowledge, such as prefixes and suffixes, to figure out the meanings of unknown words (Nippold, 1998).

Adult Models

Home and school environments provide daily opportunities for the introduction of new words and their meanings. A teacher, parent, or some other language model presents a new word and provides its definition or application (Nagy et al., 1985). We all recognize this influence because we have been on both ends of it. When we teach a course in which this book is used, we present words that many students have not used before: *morpheme, phoneme, syntax,* and so forth. We present the word. We define it. We show how it is applied. That is the direct teaching of a word.

In today's world, when a child asks the meaning of a word, he might be sent to his computer for a definition search. The child typically begins to use a dictionary when he is about seven or eight years old and in the second grade (Miller & Gildea, 1987). We should not assume, however, that just because the child looks up the definition of a word, he will understand the definition, especially if the definition is abstract, and we should not assume he is able to appropriately use the word. Miller and Gildea (1987, p. 2) found, for example, that when children 10 to 12 years old were asked to find words in the dictionary and then write sentences using those words, they wrote some interesting sentences. One of the words was *erode*, which means, "to eat out," as in, "My car was eroded by rust." In what we hope was a clear misinterpretation of the definition, one child wrote, "Our family *erodes* (eats out) a lot." Word learning requires much practice for students to be able to apply new words to a variety of situations.

Contextual Cues

The use of context is a skill learned during the elementary years and is refined during adolescence and adulthood (Nagy et al., 1985; Sternberg, 1987). This strategy is encouraged by teachers throughout the school years (Bennett, 1981; Duffy & Roehler, 1981) with many opportunities for a child to use context to expand her understanding of words as she listens to her parents talk and her teachers teach, when she watches movies and television programs, and when she reads books and magazines recreationally. If she is a typical child with a typical curiosity to know, she will use the words she knows to figure out those she does not know. That is, she learns words and their meanings by using *contextual cues*.

Morphological Knowledge

Children also use their understanding of the morphemes that are added to base words to figure out what words mean (Anglin, 1993; Nagy et al., 1993). When a speaker or reader—again, regardless of age—approaches a word he does not know, he identifies the parts of the word he does know to try to determine what the whole word means. If, for example, he is confronted with the word *wholeheartedly*, he might grasp that the word *heart* means something like "spirit." He knows what *whole* means, and he knows that *-ly* is used to indicate an *adverb*. He puts all the pieces together to understand that this word means that the agent is doing something *enthusiastically, with his entire spirit, with his whole heart*. According to White, Power, and White (1989), this strategy is a powerful influence in the vocabulary acquisition of students when they read. Children successfully employ this strategy as young as six years of age (Anglin, 1993), but it obviously becomes a more powerful influence in the acquisition of words and their meanings as children get older.

During our discussion of the preschool years, we explained that fast mapping of words allows the child to gain initial and contextually based meanings of new words, but that through experience with words in many different contexts, she will employ a slow-mapping strategy to expand word meanings. The horizontal expansion of words involves adding semantic features to her definitions. That is, the child will be able to expand her understanding and use of the word in common situations with greater differentiation of it from other words

(McNeil, 1970). Thus, a cup may also be called a glass (even when it is plastic), and a sippy cup is very different from a mug. Words also develop **vertically** when the child understands their deeper meanings, such as understanding that glass is a product found in windows, vases, lamps, and even marbles. Of course, some words occur very often in the language of the home and classroom, whereas other words occur less frequently. Word frequency plays a role in how well the child will know the meanings of words (Marinellie & Chan, 2006).

Storing, Organizing, and Retrieving Vocabulary

Vocabulary acquisition involves more than adding items to one's lexical list. It also involves sorting words into categories. The process of placing words into categories based on their *semantic relationships* is called **chunking**. The child has a cognitive category for animals, for example, and he also has a vocabulary category for animal words, which include *horse, dog, fish*, and *elephant*. As he matures, he chunks in a more differentiated manner. He retains a category for animals but he develops subcategories, so that "farm animals" includes words such as *horse, cow, chicken*, and *pig*, and "jungle animals" includes words such as *elephant, monkey*, and *lion*. These vocabulary chunks facilitate remembering. There is evidence that chunking is a more commonly used strategy for recalling words by seventh-grade children than by children in the first grade (Vanevery & Rosenberg, 1970), a change in vocabulary categorization that is consistent with changes Piaget (1963) identified in cognitive development.

An example of how language knowledge shapes thinking can be observed in a child's efforts to cope with ambiguities among words in her vocabulary. How does the child differentiate among words that sound the same, such as *dear/dear, bye/by/buy, not/knot*, and *right/write*? Perfetti and Goodman (1970) suggest that she addresses the potential ambiguities among these words by sorting them according to their *semantic functions*. That is, *dear* functions as a modifier, and *deer* functions as a noun. *Not* is a negative element, and *knot* is a noun. As the child develops knowledge about the semantic functions of words, therefore, she is able to use this language knowledge to sort and categorize words and their referents cognitively according to the semantic roles they fill.

Another change we see in the child's processing and organization of words occurs in what is called the **syntagmatic-paradigmatic shift** (Ervin, 1961). In a word-association task, the preschool child is likely to respond to a word according to its syntactic role. In responding to "Mommy," for example, he might say, "Kiss." He processes and organizes the stimulus word according to the word that is likely to follow it in a sentence. As he changes his cognitive processing strategies (Emerson & Gekoski, 1976), he responds to words in a paradigmatic manner, based on the semantic features of the word he hears. If he hears "Mommy," he says, "Girl," "Woman," or perhaps, "Daddy" as the opposite of "Mommy." The shift from syntagmatic to paradigmatic processing occurs slowly, but the most rapid change is observed between five and nine years (Muma & Zwycewicz-Emory, 1979), and the shift is not complete until adulthood. Reorganization is a way for the child to keep track of an expanding number of words in his lexicon and the relationships that words have to each other.

These and other changes in cognitive processing account for the growth in vocabulary we observe during the school years and beyond, and they account for the changes we observe in the meanings of the child's words. We are most likely to notice that the child's vocabulary is growing in size, but she also understands words differently as she matures.

As should be abundantly clear by this point in our journey, language cannot be separated from cognition. We see this connection clearly when we consider how vocabulary information is organized, stored, and retrieved. As with every other part of the complex of human behavior we call *oral communication*, the organizational, storage, and retrieval part is very much developmental. The toddler's abilities in this area are primitive. The preschool child's abilities are developing but incomplete. As he moves from childhood to adolescence to adulthood, he becomes increasingly skilled in using basic strategies for pulling words from his memory (Kail, 1984; Kobasigawa, 1974; Kobasigawa & Mason, 1982). At least three strategies are used in retrieval: (1) using semantic categorical information; (2) using externally provided auditory cues including the phonological structure of words; and (3) using visual cues. These strategies are useful because the demands for retrieval of words increase as students move through grade levels.

Semantic Categorization

We have already considered how children use the process of chunking to place words into categories based on their semantic relationships. Chunking actually serves two purposes. It is used to *organize* words according to their semantic features, as we have already established, and it is also used to *retrieve* words from memory when words are stored in categories based on their semantic features. The demands on the ability to retrieve words increase dramatically as the child's vocabulary grows exponentially over the course of language development. When her vocabulary is limited to 50 words, her word-finding choices are limited and the semantic categories in which the words are stored are limited. In fact, the words and categories are so limited that she will often retrieve the same word from two or more categories to represent several semantic relationships. When an adult retrieves words from a vocabulary of 80,000 or more words, the task is considerably more complicated. She needs to find just the right word to express just the right meaning. All children and all adults use chunking in word retrieval, but the chunks change as language matures and vocabulary grows.

Auditory Cues

We would certainly expect retrieval to be a much easier process when hints are provided, and that is correct. Halperin (1974) found that when children in three age groups (6, 9, and 12 years) were asked to recall words organized into several semantic categories that were read aloud to them, they were able to recall more of the words when they were first cued for the category. One of the semantic categories, for example, was *tools*. When the children in all three age groups were asked, "Can you tell me all the tools?" they retrieved more of the tool-related words than when they were not provided the semantic category. It is interesting and important to note that the 9-year-olds and the 12-year-olds retrieved more words than the youngest children even when they were not cued for semantic category, which might suggest that they were better able than the younger children to recognize and use the semantic categories to organize and store words as they were hearing them.

Children are able to retrieve words effectively and efficiently due to a process known as **phonological encoding** (Swank, 1994). This involves the human ability to rapidly process speech and to impose a phonemic (sound) identity to incoming speech sounds. Humans analyze sounds, determine the structure of words, and then store a code for each word, along with its meaning, in long-term, semantic memory. When children want to recall a word, they retrieve the whole word directly, such as when they use a category to rapidly name objects, or they access the speech sound system to use the sounds to access the word, such as for reading and spelling. Have you ever forgotten someone's name? One way to trigger memory is to work through the letters/sounds in the alphabet as you think of the person. Bingo—out pops the person's name!

Visual Cues

What happens when we add visual cues to the retrieval task? Kobasigawa (1974) asked children in three age groups (6, 8, and 11 years) to recall 24 words represented in pictures. Eight semantic categories were represented, with three words in each category. In addition to the 24 pictured words, there were 8 pictures depicting the semantic categories. For example, categories such as food, animals, and tools may have been represented. As the three pictures in each semantic category were shown and named aloud, the children looked at the semantic category picture and were told that those words were associated with that category. After presenting all 24 words, the examiner gave the children the category cue pictures and indicated that they could be used, if the children wanted to use them, to assist in remembering the words. Only one-third of the youngest children used the category pictures to help them retrieve the words, but three-fourths of the 8-year-old children and more than 90% of the oldest children used the category cue pictures. Not surprisingly, the children who used the category cue pictures recalled more words than the children who did not use them. The older children who used the picture cues retrieved more words per category than the younger children who used the cues, indicating that the older children used this retrieval strategy more effectively than their younger counterparts.

We can conclude from all this that finding words once stored is really a two-part process. Successful word finding depends first on successful **word storage**. If we do not store words in an efficient manner and a meaningful manner in readily recognizable categories and with accurate phonological codes, we will have trouble recalling them when we need them. The second and most obvious part of word finding is **word retrieval**. Successful retrieval depends on the efficiency of our storage, but it also depends on our ability to effectively utilize the kinds of retrieval strategies we have identified here—chunking, using auditory cues including phonological codes, and using visual cues. We should note that other factors are involved, of course. We will be able to retrieve a word more easily if it is a word we use often. If we are retrieving a word from memory, we will have less difficulty if we have not stored many other words that have the same or similar meaning. Depending on our understanding of the word, we might more readily retrieve a word we have recently learned, especially if we have a particular fondness for it.

Learning to Define Words

Most of us understand the word *define* to mean, "to determine the boundaries of, to state the meaning of," or words similar to these. When we define a word, we identify its meaning, but we also limit its meaning so that it cannot be confused with a word that is similar but different in some important respect.

We need to appreciate that there is no single way to define a word. Table 7.1 shows us that we may use several different types of word definitions. We are all familiar with *dictionary* definition, or what is sometimes called the *Aristotelian* definition. In this kind of definition, the general category of the thing to be defined is established, and the characteristics that differentiate it from other things in the general category are identified. We might say, for example, that an *apple* is a fruit (general category) that is typically red, yellow, or green and grows on apple trees (differentiating characteristics). This type of definition is the most universal type, but it is also the most abstract and it is **decontextualized**. That is, the defined word is devoid of situation or context.

It is important to emphasize at this point that defining words is not only a semantic exercise. It is also a metalinguistic phenomenon. The semantic part of defining a word involves establishing the general category and identifying the differentiating characteristics—the basic components of a dictionary definition. The metalinguistic part of defining words is the pervasive language awareness that comes with age, maturation, knowledge, developing cognitive skills, and increasingly refined perceptual skills. The more the child knows about life, and the more she knows about language, the more skillfully and completely she will identify the components of the dictionary definition. The metalinguistic influence is clear in the evolution of the child's definitions. We know, for example, that the preschool child's definitions and the early

Table 7.1   Word Definitions

Type	Description	Example
Operational/Functional	Using words to determine an item's presence or properties; describing what an item does	A bat is like a mouse with wings. A dog barks.
Descriptive	Listing attributes	A dog has four legs and a tail.
Categorical	Putting the item into a semantic category	A dog is an animal.
Dictionary	Stating the category and the item characteristics	An apple is a fruit that is red, yellow, or green and grows on trees.

elementary school child's definitions are concrete and personal (Snow, 1990). As he proceeds through the elementary school years and gains more experience with life and language, the child's definitions become more conceptual, more abstract (Swartz & Hall, 1972).

Early definitions tend to be *operational and functional.* For example, to say that a hitter *executed properly* means that he moved the runner. We might define by *comparing,* as in, "A bat is like a mouse with wings." A definition might be based on *negation;* for example, a person might say, "When I say that she is a *strong* person, I don't mean that she's stubborn" (Makau, 1990). At about five years of age, a child's functional definitions allude to something an object does rather than what the object is. If he is asked what a *dog* is, he is likely to say something like, "A dog barks."

Early definitions are also *descriptive.* That is, the child talks about the characteristics of objects ("A dog has four legs and a tail") when asked the meaning of *dog* (Benelli, Arcuri, & Marchesini, 1988; Snow, 1990). By the time the child is 10 years old, more of his definitions will be *categorical,* which is a big step toward *dictionary* definitions. That is, when asked to define *dog,* this child will say, "A dog is an animal" (Al-Issa, 1969).

Johnson and Anglin (1995) found that when defining words, children tend to include correct semantic information before they can put their definitions into correct syntactic form. During the early school years, the child's definitions progress from personal, experience-based understandings to more socially shared understandings, and from single words to sentences with appropriate detail and explanation around age seven (Litowitz, 1977; Wehren, DeLisi, & Arnold, 1981). In addition, as one would expect, children define root words more accurately and completely than they define derived words that contain morphological beginnings and endings.

The ability to effectively combine grammar, word meaning, and metalinguistic knowledge to create definitions is no easy task. The developing child needs formal instruction through school to learn the correct structure and content of definitions (Snow, 1990). The instruction may occur through models from teachers, but incidental instruction occurs as the child encounters definitions in textbooks. In fact, reading and writing provide opportunities for exposure to and practice of definitions (Benelli, Belacchi, Gini, & Lucangeli, 2006; Sinclair, 1986; Snow, 1990).

Research tells us that the understanding and expression of definitions change with maturation, as we might expect. The frequency with which a child encounters words is related to the quality of word definitions, with high-frequency nouns and verbs being defined more completely than low-frequency nouns and verbs (Marinellie & Chan, 2006). We must also keep in mind that the advances in constructing and using definitions are related not only to increasing age and word frequency but also to differing educational levels. Benelli and her colleagues (2006) showed that Italian adults with a lower educational level expressed more primitive definitions than did 11-year-old participants. These authors suggest that actual practice with definitions in school may be necessary to sustain high-level use.

Having Fun with Words: Literal to Figurative Forms

It might seem reasonable to assume that preschool children use language only in literal ways, an assumption that is not true. Recall that adults use figurative language quite frequently in their interactions with children during the preschool years, so they have ample exposure to many types of figurative expressions. As discussed in the previous chapter, preschool-age children often use language creatively, but their creativity is usually not intentional. The cute and unusual expressions of a preschool child are often the products of incomplete language knowledge. That is, the child will use the language he has to describe things, people, and events in the absence of more appropriate language he has not yet acquired. When my* oldest daughter was about three years old, she ran out of our apartment without benefit of clothing. When I called for her to return, she yelled, "Look, Daddy, my bottom is barefootin'!" She understood that a foot without a shoe is a "barefoot," so she applied this language to other parts of her anatomy, including her naked tush! This was not, strictly speaking, figurative language. It was my daughter's honest and direct attempt to describe her public nudity, using the language available to her. (There were no arrests.)

We discussed several figurative forms that adults use in everyday language with children in the previous chapter, but we know that although children are able to understand some figurative language at age five (Nippold & Sullivan, 1987), preschool-age children do not have the language knowledge to use these forms (Hakes, 1982). Refer to Table 6.14 for examples of idioms, similes, metaphors, and irony.

Although idioms are the most common form of figurative language used in conversational and classroom contexts (Kerbel & Grunwell, 1997; Lazar, Warr-Leeper, Nicholson, & Johnson, 1989), they are acquired very gradually as the preschool and early elementary child learns to understand them, first using a literal interpretation and then moving to the figurative interpretation in his later elementary years, teenage years, and into adulthood (Chan & Marinellie, 2008; Nippold & Duthie, 2003). Idioms are quite difficult for nonnative speakers because they require both knowledge of the vocabulary and the meaning of the figurative use of the words in the context of the social use within the culture. Keeping in mind that Piaget (1963) describes the child's thinking as "concrete" throughout the elementary school years, we would not expect her to produce and process metaphors and similes frequently and effectively until she moves into the formal operations stage of cognitive development, which takes her from the sixth grade through her sophomore year in high school. That is, during the preschool and elementary school years, the child thinks and talks about what is real and immediate. As she moves into her junior high and high school years, she begins to think and talk more abstractly.

Consider the problems one might have trying to interpret literally the following American English **idioms** in simple sentences:

He was beating around the bush.	It takes two to tango.
I beat you to the punch.	I lost my shirt in that deal.

---

*Lloyd Hulit.

I'll fix your wagon.	Just keep your pants on.
I put my foot in my mouth.	Did the cat get your tongue?
The cat's out of the bag.	She'll have to face the music.

The child learning English as his native language does not encounter the problems associated with translating idioms from English into another language, which creates extraordinary and sometimes humorous confusion, but he must still learn how to use and understand idioms.

Research on the acquisition of idioms suggests that these forms are learned and stored as single lexical units. These "giant words" cannot be understood or explained by the meanings of the individual words; their meaning must be associated with the entire sentence (Swinney & Cutler, 1979). Our earlier discussion of word definitions relates here to a child's ability to understand and express the meaning of idioms. It is no wonder that she will have considerable difficulty defining idioms in the elementary school years, with gradual improvement in her definitions as her linguistic, metalinguistic, and cognitive abilities increase in middle school, in high school, and into adulthood. As is true for word definitions, increased familiarity and practice in defining idioms may allow the child opportunities to acquire the critical elements necessary for accurate and complete definitions (Chan & Marinellie, 2008).

There is evidence that idioms are learned more quickly by children who have superior reading and comprehension skills (Nippold, Moran, & Schwartz, 2001), and that certainly makes sense. The more immersed a child is in language and in the processing of language, the more familiar he will be with the figurative nuances that add the layers of meaning characteristic of idioms.

Another figurative form that is evident in everyday communication is **irony**. This form occurs in 8% of conversational turns when adults talk among friends (Gibbs, 2000). The ability to understand and produce irony reflects the social competence of speakers. But, as we have seen with other language forms, irony is perhaps more complex than we might think.

One form of irony is the **ironic criticism**. Here, the statement is positive but the intent of the statement is negative, as when you say, "You are so graceful," when you really mean that tripping on the sidewalk is clumsy. The second form of irony is the **ironic compliment**, in which a negative statement calls for a positive interpretation. The statement, "He is just such a bore" suggests that the person is fascinating. Of course, when we use statements such as these, we typically use prosody and facial cues to enhance our meanings. These cues help us to convey our meanings, especially when we converse with children.

For children to be successful in interpreting irony, they must detect whether the speaker is using literal or figurative language and they must judge the speaker's intended meaning of the remark through inference. Ackerman (1983) found that children had the most difficulty with inference. Pexman and Glenwright (2007) studied 6- to 10-year-old children's understanding of ironic remarks. The ability to understand irony develops with age and children understand ironic criticisms more easily than ironic compliments, perhaps due to the frequency differences with which these forms are used. They also found that children were able to detect teasing in both forms according to a developmental progression.

A **proverb,** (also known as an adage, or maxim) is a commonplace, wise saying or a precise statement of truth. Proverbs often provide commonsense advice or cautions. See whether you can interpret the meanings of the following proverbs:

> You can lead a horse to water, but you can't make him drink.
> An ounce of prevention is worth a pound of cure.
> A penny saved is a penny earned.
> A rolling stone gathers no moss.
> The grass is always greener on the other side of the fence.

Now try to imagine how the preschool child would interpret these statements. As with idioms, the young child initially interprets proverbs literally. Proverbs are more difficult for the child to understand than other forms of figurative language, including idioms and metaphors. There are some fairly logical reasons for this difficulty. The syntactic structures of proverbs are often unusual. They sometimes contain unfamiliar words or familiar words used in unfamiliar ways and the concepts that underlie proverbs are often difficult for the young child to comprehend. Even if you can help the preschool child unravel the language meaning of, "There is none so blind as he who will not see," you will probably find it difficult to teach her the proverb's lesson. Truth and wisdom, no matter how precisely or eloquently stated, are difficult matters for mature adults. We should not expect the child to easily grasp the truths in proverbs or understand the language in which they are packaged. Although a child may understand some common proverbs during the early elementary school years, she will typically not understand proverbs until she is an adolescent (Billow, 1975).

Figurative language plays an important role in humor, and we see the same growth in the child's understanding of the language of humor that we see in his understanding of metaphors, idioms, and proverbs. A joke can be a physical prank, but we normally think of a joke as a brief humorous narrative, a funny language form. Humans typically laugh at actions or words that are unexpected or incongruous. Consider the following common riddle: "What is it that a man does standing up, a woman does sitting down, and a dog does with one leg in the air? Shake hands." Sometimes the humor in language is not by design, especially when children are involved, but the humor is still evoked because what is said is unexpected. When a Sunday school teacher asked a child about the "epistles," he said, "The epistles were the wives of the apostles." Another child in talking about Mount Vesuvius said, "Vesuvius is a volcano. You can see the creator smoking there day and night." A nine-year-old girl, came home from school on the Monday before Easter. She was terribly excited as she told her mother that this was going to be the last week of school. Her mother, knowing that school would be in session for several more months, told her daughter that she must be mistaken. The little girl said, "But, Mommy, it's true. The teacher sent home a note about it. It says that all Brownsburg schools will be closed for Good Friday."

To appreciate the humor in each of these examples, one must understand the incongruities. As we have already established, preschool children tend to interpret language literally, and because they do not understand multiple meanings of words or appreciate that some words that sound alike have different meanings, they are likely to miss the humor in common jokes. Research (Lund & Duchan, 1988; Schultz & Horibe, 1974) indicates that as a child matures and comes to appreciate and understand figurative language, she responds to progressively more sophisticated forms of humor. Prior to her sixth birthday, for example, the child will laugh at slapstick actions, the physical pratfalls and pie-in-the-face antics of circus clowns, but she will not understand language-based jokes. Between the ages of six and nine years, she will laugh at jokes based on words that are *phonologically similar* to other words she knows, as in this example provided by Lund and Duchan:

> A diner says, "What is this?"
> The waiter responds, "It's bean soup."
> The diner says, "I don't care what it's been. What is it now?"

Between the ages of 9 and 12 years, the child appreciates the humor in jokes that rely on words with *multiple meanings*. You may remember this oldie from your own childhood: "What's big and white, has four wheels, and flies? A garbage truck." When the child passes his 12th birthday, he understands humor based on two or more possible meanings within a single sentence, as in this classroom classic:

> A teacher asks, "Where was the Declaration of Independence signed?"
> The student answers, "At the bottom."

Most jokes adults find funny are based on words with multiple meanings or on *sentence structures* that can be interpreted in two or more ways. What makes them funny is that the listener anticipates the most obvious meaning and is caught off guard by a different meaning or by an unexpected twist in the way a word is used.

It should be easy to understand, therefore, that the child will understand language-based jokes only to the extent that he knows and understands all the possible meanings of the words contained in these jokes and only to the extent that he understands that a single sentence might have two or more possible underlying meanings. These understandings develop throughout the school years and even into adulthood. We all know a few adults we think of as naive, innocent, or gullible because they do not seem to know all the possible meanings of the words in punch lines, especially unsavory or potentially offensive meanings.

Check Your Understanding 7.3

Assess your knowledge of semantic development by completing this brief quiz.

Syntax and Morphology

There is so much to understand about the pieces of language and about how to put the pieces together in grammatically acceptable ways that the business of acquiring syntax and morphology is never really complete. One of the fascinations of language is that it is a creative process—there are always innovations and new adaptations of old productions. This is true in art and music, and in a very real sense, it is true of language. From birth through the preschool years, the child has learned the rudiments of language. During the school years, she improves her language skills by expanding the forms she has already acquired, by increasing her language knowledge, and by learning how to use language creatively.

In this section we will describe the following changes school-age children make: figuring out passive sentences; interpreting sentences that violate the principle of minimal distance; learning to use complex conjunctions to conjoin and embed clauses; expanding noun and verb phrases; and understanding and using morphological modifications.

Figuring Out Passive Sentences

In the preceding chapter, we described active sentences, where the first noun is the agent and the second noun is the object. In passive sentences, the order changes, and this apparently causes the child to be confused. The preschool child understands the active sentence, "The dog chased the cat," but has trouble interpreting the passive sentence, "The cat was chased by the dog." Passive sentences remain troublesome throughout most of the child's elementary school years.

The 4-year-old child begins to use reversible passive sentences, where the agent and the object can be interchanged ("The girl was chased by the dog." "The dog was chased by the girl."), but it isn't until age 11 that he also uses the nonreversible form ("The candy was eaten by the boy"; Horgan, 1978). Even at age five, children understand passive sentences including action verbs, such as *hit* or *eat*, but they produce very few passive forms. In fact, it is not until 8 years or even as late as 11 years that they will produce full passive sentences (Baldie, 1976; Horgan, 1978).

The Principle of Minimal Distance

As noted by Slobin (1978) and others who study the development of language, a young child goes out of his way to avoid exceptions. He learns general rules first, and then over time he gradually sorts out and masters the exceptions to the rules.

One intriguing example of learning an exception was studied by Carol Chomsky (1969), who analyzed the problems children have in interpreting sentences that violate the **principle of minimal distance**. She was specifically interested in sentences containing the verbs *ask*, *tell*, and *promise*. According to the principle of minimal distance, the preceding noun closest to the verb is treated as the subject of the sentence (Subject Noun–Verb–Object Noun), such as, "The boy hit the ball" or, "Mom picks me up after school."

In each of these sentences and in countless others that we all produce every day, the subject immediately precedes the verb. When there is a separation, it is typically only one word, as in, "Mom *always* picks me up after school." Chomsky found that the principle of minimal distance, and exceptions to the principle, are demonstrated in sentences that include the verbs *ask*, *tell*, and *promise*. If the verb *tell* is used, the principle of minimal distance can be consistently applied in sentences such as, "Tanya told Joe to cook dinner." In this sentence, *Tanya* and *Joe* precede the infinitive verb *to cook*, but *Joe* is closer to the infinitive verb, and according to the principle of minimal distance, it is the subject of this verb. In this sentence the principle works because Tanya is the one doing the telling and Joe is the one doing the cooking.

Consider what happens, however, when we use a verb that violates the principle of minimal distance, as in the sentence, "Tanya promised Joe to cook dinner." Even though the surface structure of this sentence is the same as in the earlier example, the principle of minimal distance cannot be used in the interpretation. In this sentence Tanya is doing the promising, but she is also the one who will be doing the cooking, even though *Joe* is closer to the infinitive verb *to cook*.

The verb *tell* consistently adheres to the principle of minimal distance, and the verb *promise* consistently violates the principle. The verb *ask* is especially troublesome because it sometimes adheres to the principle and sometimes violates it. If we say, "Tanya asked Joe to cook dinner," application of the principle of minimal distance will result in a correct interpretation; but if we say, "Tanya asked Joe what to cook for dinner," the principle will not work. In the first case, Joe will be doing the cooking, but in the second case, Tanya will be doing the cooking. What really matters here, of course, is that someone will be cooking dinner, because Tanya and Joe are getting hungry!

A child uses the principle of minimal distance by the time she is about five years old, but learning the exceptions takes time. In reference to the verbs in Chomsky's (1969) study, she will have little trouble with *tell* because it adheres consistently to the principle. She will have only somewhat more trouble with *promise* because, although it violates the principle of minimal distance, it violates the principle consistently. Chomsky found that the child correctly interprets *tell* and *promise* by the time she is 9 years old, but she does not master her interpretation of the pesky, inconsistent *ask* until she is about 10.

Conjoining and Embedding: Becoming More Complex

Making language constructions more complex does not occur by simply pasting words onto the ends of sentences. Increased complexity is the product of combining constructions and by placing new strings of words within already existing constructions. You may recognize these as the processes of **conjoining** and **embedding**.

Complex Conjunctions

Over the course of the school years, the child increases the complexity of his sentences by using more embedded and conjoined forms. He begins to conjoin clauses during the preschool years, usually with the conjunction *and*. During the school years, when his narrative skills are improving, he continues to favor *and* over other conjunctions. In fact, as many as 80% of the sentences in the narratives produced by the school-age child begin with *and*. As the child grows older, he relies less on this conjunction. By the time he is an early teenager, *and* initiates about 20% of his narrative sentences; when he writes narratives at this age, the percentage drops to about 5% (Scott, 1987).

The school-age child not only conjoins more often but also uses a wider range of conjunctions expressing more complex relationships among the clauses of his sentences. Through the later elementary school years, he commonly uses *because* and *when*, and *if* and *in order* are produced, but are used less frequently (Scott, 1987). Menyuk (1969) identified the categories of conjunctions the child will eventually acquire to express the more complex clausal relationships he is expressing: *conditional* (*if*), *causal* (*so, because, therefore*), *disjunctive* (*but, or, therefore*), and *temporal* (*before, after, when, then*). There is evidence that the child may use some of these conjunctions before he fully understands them (Hood & Bloom, 1979). Among other concepts, he must understand time and the subtleties of truth as expressed in language before he can understand and use all of these conjunctions meaningfully. Nevertheless, by the time he completes his elementary school years, that understanding is emerging, and he is using most conjunctions appropriately most of the time. However, some thorny issues with some conjunctions persist for a time.

The conjunction *because* is troublesome because the child must understand the underlying cause/effect relationship expressed in the conjoined clauses and the temporal relationship between the events described. In the normal thought process, a cause is identified before its effect is considered. For example, if we stand in the rain (cause), we will get wet (effect). The preschool child understands cause/effect relationships and can express them in conjoined sentences such as, "I fell down the stairs, and I hurt my knee." Notice the difference, however, between this sentence and a version using the conjunction *because*: "I hurt my knee because I fell down the stairs." The cause and effect are now reversed. "I hurt my knee" is the *effect*, but it is mentioned before the *cause* ("I fell down the stairs"). The child who is accustomed to interpreting cause/effect on the basis of **order of mention** is likely to be confused. Prior to her seventh birthday, the child will use *because, and*, and *then* as though they mean the same thing (Corrigan, 1975). She might say, for example, "I fell down the stairs, *and* I hurt my knee," but she might also say, "I fell down the stairs *because* I hurt my knee." Apparently, the child has less difficulty when she is describing two events that are occurring simultaneously or that overlap in time than when she is describing related but distinctly successive events. That is, she can produce and understand sentences such as, "I'm eating ice cream because it tastes good" (simultaneous events) and, "I throw the ball because we're playing baseball" (overlapping events), but she has trouble interpreting sentences such as, "I have to stay in my room because I told a lie" (distinctly successive events). Not until she is about 10 or 11 years old does she fully and consistently comprehend the ordering and causal meanings of *because* (Emerson, 1979).

Other conjunctions pose similar problems for the child. He must understand *contrast* before he can use *but* correctly. He must understand *consequence* before he can use *therefore* appropriately and *condition* before he can use *if* properly. Wing and Scholnick (1981) have noted that the child at 10 years may still have problems with the conjunction *unless* because he does not fully understand disbelief and uncertainty. Conjunctions may seem to be simple words, but the concepts and relationships they denote are clearly not simple. The child must have a cognitive understanding of the concepts underlying conjunctions before he is able to comprehend and produce conjoined sentences that include these conjunctions. As the child moves through his school-age years, his understanding of the concepts and his ability to apply this knowledge to language interpretation and production improve steadily.

Embedding

The same persistent, if occasionally stumbling, improvements we observe in conjoining are observed in embedding during the school years. The preschool child produces relatively few embedded sentences, and when she does, she embeds infinitive phrases, object complements, and relative clauses modifying noun phrases in the object position but not in the subject position. Over the course of the elementary school years, the percentage of sentences with embedded elements grows to about 30% (Scott, 1984). Her repertoire of relative pronouns grows to include *whose, whom,* and *in which* (Scott, 1988a). After she passes her seventh birthday, the child will produce sentences in which the relative pronoun is deleted but understood, as in "I just saw a movie [that] you would really enjoy," and she will embed in the subject position or center of a sentence, as in "The man *who bought our car* is a teacher" (Menyuk, 1971). As the child matures, she produces more multiple embeddings as well. This is quite noticeable in the narratives of school-age children. The first- or second-grade child seldom includes multiple embeddings in her narratives, whereas they are common in the narratives of the fifth- and sixth-grade child.

Sentences involving the subject position or center embedding are initially difficult for the child to interpret because they violate the expected subject-verb-object order. If the child hears "The dog that bit the cat ran away" and applies the subject-verb-object rule, he may conclude that the cat ran away. He may understand the sentence correctly if he relies on his understanding of semantic roles. That is, in the world most children understand, dogs are aggressive toward cats, not the reverse. If that is the child's understanding, he will interpret the sentence correctly even if the subject-verb-object rule is violated. Confusion in center embedding may be avoided if the object of the center embedding is inanimate (Maratsos, 1974). For example, if the child hears, "The dog that chewed the shoe ran away," he will correctly conclude that the dog ran away, not the shoe. If the child cannot depend on his understanding of semantic roles to figure out center embeddings, he may have trouble interpreting these structures because of limitations on his auditory memory (Lewis, 1996). As he grows older and his auditory memory retains more information for longer periods of time, he is able to sort out the possible ambiguities presented by these embeddings. By the time the child is about 12 years old, he will correctly interpret embedded sentences no matter where the embeddings occur, and he will base his interpretations on his grammatical knowledge, not simply on word order or semantic roles (Abrahamsen & Rigrodsky, 1984).

Noun and Verb Phrases: Still Expanding

Do you remember the first time a teacher asked you to write a 500-word essay? You may remember thinking that it must be almost impossible to write 500 words about any topic. If you didn't write enough words, you may rarely have considered elaborating your thoughts. Your first instinct may have been simply to add words to the sentences you had already created. Surely you remember how this works:

The man walked. (3 words)
The man walked across the street. (6 words)

The haggard, gray-bearded man, whose last meal must have been consumed about three weeks before the birth of the New World, walked with short, labored, arthritic steps across the windswept, deserted street to the dark and desolate hole in the wall that 20 years ago was the most exquisite restaurant in the city. (53 words . . . only 447 to go!)

As this example suggests, a sentence can be made longer by adding adjectives and adverbs, and by embedding prepositional phrases and subordinate clauses in the original sentence, which consisted of a basic noun phrase (*The man*) and a simple verb phrase (*walked*). The child has been elaborating these phrases throughout the preschool years. As she moves through the school years, she produces longer and more elaborate noun and verb phrases. She refines forms she has been producing. She adds new forms. She learns which language forms must be retained and which forms can be eliminated because they are redundant.

When the child is about five to seven years old, he may still be omitting articles (*a, an, the*) even though he adds other redundant information, such as the infamous double negative. The child might say, for example, "I don't got [the] ball no more." This same child is likely to have problems with using some prepositions, with marking verbs appropriately for tense, and with marking plurality (Menyuk, 1971). As one would expect, cases of plurality and tense changes that violate the regular rules are the most troublesome for school-age children. As the child moves through elementary school, he addresses each of these problems. He learns to retain function words, including the articles. He eliminates redundant negative terms, and he gradually learns the exceptions for verb tense, plurality, and other language forms.

A child also completes her sorting of pronouns. She learns to separate subject pronouns (*I, we, he, she, they*) from object pronouns (*me, us, him, her, them*), and she learns to use reflexive pronouns such as *myself, herself,* and *themselves.*

The school-age child learns to recognize the antecedents of pronouns even when the nouns and pronouns are in different sentences, as in the following example: "Joe's brother was badly hurt in an automobile accident. He [Joe] goes to see him [Joe's brother] in the hospital every day."

As demonstrated in the example in the opening of this section, one of the ways to elaborate noun phrases is to add adjectives. When the child begins to string adjectives together, he must learn the rules for ordering adjectives. Each adjective in a sequence refers to a specific attribute of the noun being modified or described. There are rules for how adjectives are ordered (Whorf, 1956), although we do not have a complete understanding of these rules. We do know, however, that "three hyperactive preschool children" *sounds* right, whereas "hyperactive preschool three children" does not sound remotely correct. We also know that children as young as three years demonstrate some of the same sequencing rules used by adults (Richards, 1980). During the school years, the child will develop a more complete understanding of the attributes reflected in adjectives and a more complete understanding of how these attributes are related to one another. As these understandings mature, she will learn the remaining rules for sequencing adjectives, even if she is never able to express the rules.

You are probably familiar with the differentiation between a *common noun*, which refers to a general class of people, places, or things, and a *proper noun*, which refers to a specific member of a class. Nouns are also classified as *concrete* (names of real, tangible objects), *abstract* (names of ideas, emotions, concepts), *collective* (names of groups of people or things), *count* (nouns that can be counted or tallied), and *mass* (names of homogeneous, aggregate substances). The child learning language must understand all these categories of nouns, of course, but the distinction between count and mass nouns is especially difficult. The child gradually comprehends the difference between these categories and learns which quantifying adjectives can be used with each category (Gathercole, 1985).

English speakers modify count nouns by numbers, of course, but adjectives such as *many* and *few* can be used as in the following examples:

There are *few* students in class today.
Miguel keeps *many* pencils in his desk.

Mass nouns require different modifiers, such as *little* and *much*, as in the following examples:

There was *little* meat left on his plate.
You put too *much* sugar in my coffee.

Now mix these adjectives by using *few* for *little*, *many* for *much*, and vice versa. You will quickly discover that you know which adjectives should be used with count nouns and which should be used with mass nouns. A child has usually mastered this understanding by the time he approaches adolescence, although he might still use *much* when *many* is appropriate, as in, "Can you believe how much girls were at that party?" While he is trying to figure out which adjectives should be used with which category of nouns, he might use *lots of* in reference to both categories. In fact, if you listen carefully to the speech of adults, you may hear sentences such as the following:

Miguel keeps *lots of* pencils in his desk. (count)
You put *lots of* sugar in my coffee. (mass)

Because one can get lots of mileage out of *lots of*, one may tend to use *lots of* lots of the time!

School-age children learn what adverbs mean and how to use them. As with other categories of words, some adverbs are easier to understand than others. Adverbs of likelihood such as *definitely, probably,* and *possibly* are especially difficult because, although they can be used in the same contexts, they express varying degrees of likelihood. The differences may seem small or nonexistent to the young child, but they are critical. Assume that you are standing with your back to a friend, who tells you to fall straight backward. You ask, "Will you catch me?" You will listen very carefully to the adverb of likelihood in your friend's answer because you know there is a bodily risk difference between "I will *probably* catch you" and "I will *definitely* catch you." During the preschool years, the child does not understand the subtle but vital differences among adverbs of likelihood, but she has a fairly good grasp of the differences by the time she is in the fourth grade. She does not learn these adverbs at the same time, and, as you might guess, she tends to understand *definitely* before she understands *probably* and *possibly* (Hoffner, Cantor, & Badzinski, 1990).

Morphological Modifications

Vocabulary expansion occurs by *morphing*, or reshaping, root words. These modifications are clearly the products of the child's growing understanding of how words are formed and how the constituent parts of words can be manipulated to change their meanings or to affect how they are used in relation to other words. He uses inflectional suffixes to indicate things such as plurality and possession, and changes in verb tense mature, but the most dramatic improvement comes in his use of inflectional prefixes, such as adding *non* to *sense* to create the word *nonsense* or adding *dis* to *respect* to create the word *disrespect*. In both of these examples, the inflected words are opposite the root words in meaning. We also see improvement in his use of derivational suffixes, such as adding *-ly* to *slow*, changing the word from an adjective to an adverb, or *ness* to *sad*, changing the word from an adjective to a noun (Nagy, Diakidoy, & Anderson, 1991).

Morphophonemic Alterations

One of the more interesting developments in morphology that occurs during the school years is something called **morphophonemic alteration.** If we analyze the parts of this term, we will understand what it means. *Morph* refers to morpheme, which refers to the smallest unit of meaning in language. *Phonemic* refers to *phoneme*, which refers to speech sound. *Alteration* means change. A morphophonemic alteration, then, refers to a speech sound change that occurs when the shape of the base morpheme is changed. For example, the final sound in the word *public* is the *k* sound, but when *public* becomes *publicity*, that *k* becomes an *s* sound. That is a morphophonemic alteration. In the word *sign*, the letter *g* is silent, but notice what happens when *sign* is morphed into *signature*—the *g* is now pronounced. The child learns to make many of these changes during the elementary school years.

By the time a child is in the first grade, she understands a very basic morphophonemic alteration related to plurality. She knows that when a noun ends with a voiceless consonant, she adds the sound *s* to make it plural (*c a t* → *c a t s*), but when it ends with a voiced consonant, she adds the sound *z* to make it plural (*d o g* → *d o g s* [z]). Within another year or two, she will know that some words require vowel + *z* to make a plural (*d i t c h* → *d i t c h e s* [z]).

Yet another type of morphophonemic alteration, vowel shifting, is not mastered until the child is at the end of the school years, when he is perhaps 17 or 18. When the shapes of certain words are changed, their vowels change. For example, in the word *finite*, the first vowel is a long vowel, but when the word is morphed into *infinity*, the corresponding vowel is short. In the word *profound*, the *ou* is produced like "ow," but when the word is changed to the noun form, *profundity*, the spelling changes, as does the pronunciation of the corresponding vowel—it is now produced like "uh." Some adults struggle with these changes because they do not always follow the rules of common sense.

Gerunds

Early in the elementary school years, at about age seven, children understand how to produce gerunds. A gerund, you may recall from earlier discussions, is a noun created by adding *-ing* to the verb and then using the word as a noun. *Running* is the gerund form of *run* in the sentence, "Running is a sport," for example, and *fishing* is the gerund form of *fish*. The seven-year-old child also understands the agentive forms of common verbs (Carrow, 1973). The agentive form identifies the person who performs the action of a verb. Someone who *runs*, for example, is a *runner*, and someone who *sings* is a *singer*, but as with other language forms, there are many exceptions. Someone who *cooks* is a *cook*, not a *cooker*, although *cooker* refers to a certain kind of cooking pot. Someone who fishes is a *fisherman*, not a fisher. A person who *types* is a *typist*, not a *typer*, but a person who sets type is a *typesetter*.

Adverb Forms

When the child is seven years old, she also understands and is able to produce the adverb forms of common adjectives by adding the bound morpheme *-ly*. By adding this morpheme, the adjective *slow* becomes the adverb *slowly*. The adjective and adverb forms of *slow* are included in the following sentence: "The train moved *slowly* [adverb] down the tracks on a *slow* [adjective] day in August." We can create many adverbs by adding *-ly*, including *quickly*, *rapidly*, and *swiftly*, but notice that the child must learn exceptions here, too. The adjective *fast*, for example, does not have an adverbial form, *fastly*. The adverb form of *fast* is *fast*, and sometimes nouns can function as adverbs, as in the following examples:

After watching the movie, Tony went *home*.
Nora moved *yesterday*.

In the first sentence, *home* modifies the verb *went* by specifying *where* Tony went. In the second sentence, *yesterday* specifies *when* Nora moved. Still other adverbs, which always function as adverbs, do not end in *-ly*, such as *again*, *often*, *now*, and *never*.

Check Your Understanding 7.4

Assess your knowledge of grammatical development by completing this brief quiz.

Conversations and Narratives

The most dramatic changes in language development during the school years are in how the student uses language to relate to others. Improvements in conversation involve using language to manipulate the behaviors, feelings, and attitudes of other people. The student learns how to manipulate people so indirectly with his words that they scarcely know they are being manipulated. He learns how to adjust his vocabulary and modify his language style to accommodate listeners of varying ages and backgrounds and both genders. He learns the art of narration, or the telling of stories.

In this section we explore what changes occur in conversations, including topic maintenance, honing pre-suppositional skills, making conversational repairs, using indirect requests, and using adverbial conjuncts and disjuncts. We also describe the development of narration as the student engages in story telling.

Topic Maintenance and Presupposition

Gradual changes occur as the child becomes more capable of maintaining a conversational topic, moving from one topic to a related topic, and introducing new topics, but this progress is slow. She becomes increasingly sensitive to the issue of relevance, which guides the conversations of adults. That is, the more pertinent, useful, or timely a topic is, the more likely the older conversationalist is to sustain that topic.

With conversational experience, the school-age child learns how to shade conversations by moving from one topic to a different but related topic. In adult conversations, shading occurs so subtly that it is often difficult to determine, based on the final topic, how the conversational partners got there. Recall that a young child talks about concrete things, people and events in the here and the now. By the time the child is 11 or 12 years old, he is able to discuss abstract topics and ideas.

How a topic is maintained changes as the child develops. The elementary school child maintains a conversation by adding new information to the established topic, whereas adolescent and adult speakers maintain their conversations not only by adding information during their turns but also by shading one topic into another.

The child also provides more specific information to his conversational partner when the listener does not have the details (Krauss & Glucksberg, 1977), understands when information can be left out because the listener shares the information (presupposition), and understands the importance of organizing and sequencing information for his conversational partner. For example, he is able to explain how a game is played. He first describes the purpose of the game and clarifies what is required to win. He then delineates the rules and explains the mechanics of playing the game, step by step. He also is able to use repair strategies when his message is not being understood. Repetition is used primarily until about age nine, but thereafter he is able to determine the breakdown in the interaction and specifies and defines his terms, fills in missing background, and talks about the repair (Brinton, Fujiki, Loeb, & Winkler, 1986).

As you can see, during the school-age years, the student becomes very adept at conversational exchanges with flexibility to move within and between topics with skill. Teachers and parents increase the conversational demands to suit these expanding abilities. Some students learn the art of debate during their high school years and even compete in forensic competitions.

Indirect Requests

Requests are made very directly in early childhood, as you know, and the child has difficulty understanding indirect requests (Ervin-Tripp, 1977); the difficulty relates to the terms used within the request and whether the request is declarative or interrogative. For example, he will understand declarative terms such as *you should, you shouldn't,* or *you must* more easily than he will understand their interrogative versions, *should you? shouldn't you?* and *must you?* He will understand positive forms more easily than negative forms (Carrell, 1981; Leonard, Wilcox, Fulmer, & Davis, 1978).

The seven-year-old child is fairly proficient in producing indirect requests (Grimm, 1975) and she becomes increasingly adept at using non-standard or creative forms of indirect request using brevity and a non-demanding manner (Ervin-Tripp & Gordon, 1986). This allows her to use indirect requests to shape the manipulative behaviors that bring joy and delight to the lives of all who know and love her through her school years. Even at the tender age of eight years, the child understands the importance of being more polite to adults than to her peers and to people whose favor she is trying to win than to people whose favor she already possesses (Corsaro, 1979; Parsons, 1980). After the age of eight years, the child's indirect requests are more likely to be influenced by her sensitivity to her listener's situation (Ervin-Tripp & Gordon, 1986). She will no longer assume that a request will be filled but will ask in a manner that suggests that the listener has a right to exercise a real option. Whereas a younger child might say, "Take me home," or, "Can you take me home?" the older child might say, "If it's not too much trouble or too far out of your way, could you take me home?" She recognizes the need to be polite in making requests increases when she is interrupting her listener or when she is asking the listener to do something that is difficult or inconvenient (Mitchell-Kernan & Kernan, 1977).

There is a difference, you see, between, "Would you mind opening that door for me?" and, "Excuse me, I know you're busy, but when you finish painting your house, you wouldn't mind painting mine . . . would you . . . perchance?"

By adolescence, the student responds to indirect requests as well as adults do, although even adults become confused by negative and interrogative forms of indirect requests (Clark & Chase, 1972). It should be evident that the ability to understand and create indirect requests spans from early children through adulthood.

Conjuncts and Disjuncts

Logic and reasoning are directly applied to language constructions in the form of what are called **adverbial conjuncts** and **adverbial disjuncts**. To appreciate these language forms, however, we need to understand the forms of logic they express.

Most people who have studied logic even superficially associate basic forms of logic, called *syllogisms*, with Aristotle, the ancient Greek philosopher (384–322 B.C.E.). According to Freeley (1993), there are three major types of syllogisms: *conditional, categorical,* and *disjunctive.* Sternberg (1979) addresses a fourth that is relevant to our discussion: *conjunctive.* Each type is defined and presented with examples in Table 7.2.

As the child is learning the nuances of conversation, she learns to use language forms that express the types of logical conclusions that are subsumed in these examples. In the process of linking her utterances together, she also learns to use words designed to make her attitude about what she is saying clear to the listener. Speakers use *adverbial disjuncts*, for example, to provide a kind of buffer between their attitudes about what they are saying and the actual

Table 7.2   **Types of Syllogisms**

Type	Definition	Example
Conditional	The if/then logical statement	If you tickle Peyton's belly, he will laugh. Nina tickled Peyton's belly. He laughed.
Categorical	A general major premise of fact or truth is exemplified with a minor premise	All mammals are warm-blooded animals. A bear is warm-blooded. A bear, therefore, is a mammal.
Disjunctive	A general statement includes options and leads to one of the options	We can either drive my car or walk to the restaurant. The restaurant is an easy walk, perhaps three blocks. Because it is so close, let's walk.
Conjunctive	A statement made about two conditions that coexist	In football, some players are permitted to go downfield on pass plays, and other players must stay behind the line of scrimmage. Only running backs, receivers, and the quarterback may go downfield. Therefore, linemen must stay at the line of scrimmage on pass plays.

content of their messages. When a person says, "To be quite honest with you, you're making a mistake," he is disjoining or separating his attitude of honesty from the surface message of his utterance that might be intended to soften the message or perhaps to focus attention on the speaker's purpose, apart from or in addition to the communication.

An *adverbial conjunct* is a device that connects, but it can be either concordant or dissonant. If a person says, "He ran around with the wrong crowd. Consequently, he has been in constant trouble with the law," there is concordance, or harmony, between the two statements. The word *consequently* is an example of a concordant adverbial conjunct. If someone says, "Catherine has always studied hard and earned good grades. Jane, in contrast, spends almost no time studying and she is just scraping by," there is dissonance between the two statements, as reflected in the words *in contrast.*

Conjuncts emerge in the child's conversational applications gradually over the course of the school years and into adulthood. As with every other aspect of communication, the ability to understand conjuncts outpaces their actual use (Nippold, Schwarz, & Undlin, 1992). By the time the child is six years old, he is using some adverbial conjuncts, including *now, though, so,* and *then,* but he uses very few disjuncts. By the time he is 12 years old, he has expanded his repertoire of conjuncts to include words such as *however, therefore,* and *anyway,* and he is using the disjuncts *probably* and *really.* The gap between children and adults in their use of these devices is substantial. Scott (1988b) found that adults use conjuncts at three times the rate used by 12-year-olds.

Gender Differences in Conversations

There are differences in the way men and women talk, and these differences reflect both biological and environment influences such as maturation rates, neurological development, role models, and experiences during their childhood and into adulthood (Bornstein, Hahn, & Haynes, 2004). We see gender differences in language acquisition as early as the toddler years. For instance, girls begin talking earlier than boys do, producing vocabulary and two-word combinations faster in their second year (Fenson et al., 2000; Huttenlocher, Haight, Bryk, Seltzer, & Lyons, 1991). In addition, boys have a higher prevalence of language impairments, estimated at 2 or 3 to 1 as compared with girls (Dale, Price, Bishop, & Plomin, 2003).

By the time a child is in first grade, she is able to determine the gender of a speaker based on the vocabulary used in emotional expressions (Edelsky, 1977), and she is able to vary her conversational style depending on her conversational partner. When speaking to a girl or woman, the child uses a more open and complimentary style, such as, "That box is heavy, isn't it? Let me help you," whereas a more directive style would be used when she is speaking to a boy or man, as in, "Here, give me that."

According to Tannen (1990), the difficulties men and women sometimes have in communicating to each other can be traced to the way boys and girls grow up; however, again we are speaking in generalities. Boys tend to play in large groups, and their play is activity oriented. Their games have winners and losers, and there are elaborate rules about which participants frequently argue. Boys also brag about their skills and compete for first place. Speech is used in the context of play to achieve status and establish a hierarchy of superiority. They tell stories and jokes, and they interrupt and challenge one another to determine who is the quickest or wittiest. Boys with high status give orders to those with lower status. Sometimes speech is used as a tool of aggression, not only to establish one's status but also to defend one's position when verbally attacked.

Girls, according to Tannen (1990), play and communicate in small groups or pairs. Many of their activities do not have winners and losers. In fact, taking turns and sharing experiences are emphasized. They tend not to boast about their skills because they seek acceptance. Rather than giving orders, girls are more inclined to try to manipulate the behaviors of others by offering suggestions or indicating their preferences. Speech is used as a means for interacting with other people and for sharing thoughts and feelings.

As children grow older, they are influenced less by their caregivers and more by their peers. This shift of influence is apparent in the way children interact with one another and talk to one another. During the school years, children tend to segregate themselves by gender, so that same-gender influences are more profound than influences across gender lines. Not surprisingly, we see the same gender-based differences in children that we see in adults. During the school years, girls seek relationships, whereas boys try to establish authority and independence (Gilligan, 1982; Maltz & Borker, 1982). When school-age girls interact with other girls, conversation is a focal point, and they are much more likely than boys at this age to talk about their feelings (Aukett, Ritchie, & Mill, 1988; Barth & Kinder, 1988). As they mature to around 11 years, they also become adept at using verbal language, such as gossip, as an indirect form of aggression to exclude a peer from a clique (Bjorkqvist, Lagerspetz, & Kaukiainen, 1992). School-age boys are more likely than girls to use coarse language, including profanity (Jay, 1992; Martin, 1997) and use language for abusing and accusing, shouting, and name calling as a direct form of aggression (Bjorkqvist et al., 1992).

The developmental trends just described lead to the interactional styles of men and women, of course. Women tend to communicate to establish and maintain relationships with others and they seek collaboration, cooperation, mutual agreement, and approval from peers. They concern themselves with shared problems and seek understanding through empathy and sympathy as they express and read emotions. Men tend to be independent and relate to other men as partners or rivals and they are goal oriented. They are more private in their thoughts and feelings, but they offer advice and like to solve problems.

Research showed that women tended to use more tentative and polite words, while men were less polite and used language to establish dominance and to gain tangible outcomes (Leaper, 1991; Mulac, Bradac, & Gibbons, 2001). When men and women relate to each other in a competing manner, and when men or women talk to men, they tend to decrease the use of imprecise and noncommittal language forms (e.g., *sort of, possibly, perhaps*) and increase the use of direct forms (Dixon & Foster, 1997). Men and women also differ in their use of nonverbal and verbal language in conversations.

Although we do not know the full importance of these findings, research has demonstrated that parents talk differently to their sons and daughters. Both parents, but particularly fathers, influence the development of genderlects (the differences in the way males and females communicate) in their children (Perlmann & Berko-Gleason, 1994). Mothers imitate their preschool daughters more often than their sons, and they spend more time talking to their daughters (Cherry & Lewis, 1976). Fathers attach nicknames such as *nutcake* and *ding-a-ling* to their sons, but they call their daughters *sweetheart* and *honey* (Berko-Gleason & Greif, 1983). Consistent with gender differences noted among adults, fathers interrupt their daughters more often than their sons (Warren-Leubecker, 1982).

Gender differences in language are fascinating, not so much because of what they tell us about language as because of what they tell us about the differences between the genders. Figure 7.3 lists some comparative observations reported in the literature (Swacher, 1975; Tannen, 1994b; Willis & Williams, 1976). Keep in mind that these are only trends and do not describe particular individuals.

Gender differences in interests and in language emerge early.

Source: Philipus/Fotolia.

Figure 7.3   Gender Differences in Communication

Women face their conversation partners, whereas men are more distant.

Women make eye contact more often than men.

Women converse more thoroughly about topics, whereas men change topics frequently.

Women use fillers to indicate their attention to the speaker more often than men.

Women introduce new topics more frequently than men.

Women sustain a topic infrequently (36%), whereas men frequently sustain topics (96%).

Women talk less than men, and conversations are longer when men talk to other men or when men talk to women.

Women interrupt less than men, and men are more likely to interrupt women than they are to interrupt men.

Women are more likely to surrender their conversational turns than are men.

Women tend to talk openly about their relationships and feelings, whereas men prefer to talk about impersonal subjects.

Narratives

In Chapter 6, we introduced the concept of personal narratives as a means by which children share their experiences. We use personal narratives to share our experience throughout our lifetimes, primarily in social situations. These narratives develop in complexity and style over time and with experience. Recall the last time that you told a story about one of your experiences. Often, a personal narrative leads to several other people telling similar stories.

 Video Reflection 7.2:   Personal Narratives of 6-Year-Old and 9-Year-Old Students

Watch the video to observe the personal narratives of a six-year-old and a nine-year-old, then answer the question.

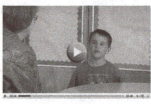

 Video Reflection 7.3:   Fictional Narratives of 6-Year-Old and 9-Year-Old Students

Watch the video to focus on the content of two fictional narratives, then answer the questions.

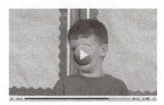

Recall that children in the preschool years are also listening to stories told by family, caregivers, and educators. Some children are fortunate to have a high frequency and amount of story exposure. Not only is this exposure valuable for increasing vocabulary and exposure to complex grammatical structures, but it is also the way in which children develop the knowledge about **story grammar**. In all cultures, storytelling is an important tradition. Story structure varies culturally, but stories have structure nevertheless. Mainstream Western culture has a typical structure that children learn first through listening to lots of stories, and then through constructing their own narratives. You will no doubt recognize the typical story structure (Stein, 1982; Stein & Glenn, 1979): setting; initiating event; internal response; attempt; consequence; reaction. Each of these elements can be simple or highly elaborated and duplicated as narratives become more complex through children's maturation and experience.

Teachers use this structure to guide children in speaking, comprehending, and writing personal and fictional narratives.

In Chapter 6, we saw the emergence of early narratives consisting of unrelated statements called *heaps*. These early recounts and accounts do not have a story grammar. They are a collection of unrelated ideas. Gradually, with prompting from parents and others, the child adds a beginning and a middle to these accounts and recounts, or **event sequences**, with a central character or topic, but the stories lack plot, organization, additional characters, cause/effect relationships, and endings (Kemper & Edwards, 1986). Approaching the fourth year, children talk about events, the central character or topic, and cause/effect relationships in **primitive narratives**. Logical sequencing of events emerges in **focused chains** at around five years, but plot is still not present as children this age do not have understanding of motivations and goals of characters. Most 6- and seven-year-old children have developed causal relationships in **true narratives** including motivations for actions of characters and plots begin to emerge. It isn't until children are eight years old that their stories have plots including a problem, internal responses by the characters, a plan of action for solving the problem, and the results of the action leading to a definite resolution of the central problem (Peterson & McCabe, 1983). Storytelling reaches its peak in the middle grades, with fully formed narratives, perhaps because fictional narratives are prominent in the school curriculum during these years. These narratives include greater detail and more information on the relationship of the characters, moods, motivations, and circumstances. The storyteller ties information together and may specify the significance of an event.

Recent research (Ukrainetz et al., 2005) shows that the art of **expressive elaboration** in fictional narratives develops incrementally from 5 to 12 years of age, with increases in narrative length and more sophisticated use of expressive elaborations including opening appendages (introductory information), orientation (background information), and evaluations (emphasis and meaning). Thus, children do not simply increase the length of their stories. They use many different ways to construct and convey artful and creative stories.

Although narratives tend to have the same components, compelling evidence indicates that the way children and adults relate personal narratives is dependent on the cultures in which they live (McCabe, 1996; Roseberry-McKibben, 2007). For example, the narratives of children who are Hispanic center far more on interpersonal relationships, especially family relationships, than on the events in their stories (Rodino, Gimbert, Perez, & McCabe, 1991). They tend to favor descriptions over sequences of events (McCabe, 1997; Mahecha, 2003). Children who are Japanese construct their narratives in a manner reminiscent of haiku, a popular literary form in their culture (Minami & McCabe, 1995). A haiku is a very disciplined literary form based on the principles of minimalism and immediacy. It is the principle of immediacy that is particularly noticeable in the narratives of these children. They connect events by theme rather than presenting them in temporal order so that the aggregate of events is presented at once.

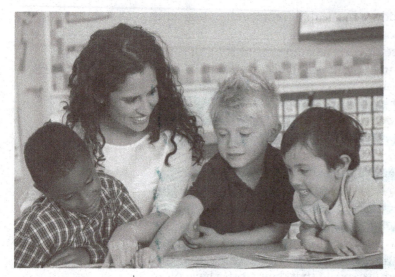

Narrative styles vary with cultural experiences.

How narratives are constructed is also affected by more narrowly defined cultures. American-born children who are white and from the middle SES, for example, tend to generate narratives that are topic-based. Their narratives center on single characters or on single events that have clearly defined chronologies. Girls who are African American from working-class families generate very different narratives. Their stories are topic-associating (Michaels, 1991), which means that they connect two, three, or more different events that share a common theme. Each episode in the narrative might have different characters, and the stories might occur in different places and times. Speakers who tell topic-associated stories also presuppose shared knowledge between them and their listeners, which results in lack of detail. Champion and Mainess (2003) found that students who are African American tell lengthy stories that contain figurative forms and exaggeration.

The contrast presented here between the narrative styles of American children who are white of both genders and girls who are African American should give us pause about what might happen in school. If a classroom teacher knows only the narrative style of one group, she might not respond appropriately to the narratives generated by other children in her classroom, placing greater value on the style she knows (Michaels, 1991). From the teacher's perspective, the topic-associating style might be viewed as *scattered* or *not sufficiently focused* or *undisciplined*. It is, of course, none of these. This style used by girls who are African American is the strategy used to make sense of their life experiences, just as the topic-based style is the strategy children who are white use to make sense of their life experiences. Neither is inferior to the other. Each is *right* within the cultural experiences of the children who use it. Our previous discussion about the diversity of children in our schools should remind us that a teacher's knowledge, appreciation, acceptance, and encouragement of cultural differences is applicable here.

Check Your Understanding 7.5

Assess your understanding of conversations and narratives by completing this brief quiz.

Metalinguistics and the Development of Reading and Writing

The most noticeable and dramatic increase in metalinguistic awareness occurs between the ages of five and eight years (Bernstein, 1989, p. 145). Beginning at this time but continuing even into adulthood, the child notices and develops an understanding of each of the basic components of language, including phonology, semantics, syntax, and pragmatics. Not surprisingly, the development of metalinguistic awareness is related to cognitive development, intellectual capacity, scholastic achievement, reading skills, and environmental factors, including the child's play experiences and the kind of stimulation he receives from adults (Saywitz & Cherry-Wilkinson, 1982). Although most discussions of metalinguistics generally focus on the relationship between words in verbal exchanges, metalinguistic awareness also plays an important role in reading comprehension (Zipke, 2007).

The typical adult may not have a sophisticated understanding of the components of language, but every adult has an awareness of each component and has at least a rudimentary understanding of the rules that govern the various dimensions of language. It is a speaker's metalinguistic ability that allows her to make judgments about whether a sentence sounds grammatical or about which marker for tense or plurality sounds correct. When a speaker produces language, she does so automatically, with little or no conscious attention to the rules she is applying, but when she is asked to make a judgment about a language form, she must consciously attend to the form and apply her knowledge of the rules to determine whether the form is correct. The production of language is a linguistic function. The evaluation of language is a metalinguistic function.

Awareness of Speech Sounds

The ability to realize and reflect upon the sounds and syllables that make up words is called **phonological awareness**. It is the child's conscious awareness and ability to manipulate the smaller linguistic units within words. Phonological awareness has received a lot of attention in recent years, because studies have shown a direct link between its development and vocabulary size and speech perception (Rvachew, 2006), and with theory of mind (Farrar, Ashwell, & Maag, 2005; Rvachew, 2006), as well as with the acquisition of reading and spelling (Rvachew, 2006; Stanovich, 2000). Numerous studies have shown that phonological awareness in preschool and kindergarten predicts reading ability in later elementary and high school grades (Bryant, MacLean, Bradley, & Crossland, 1990; Fawcett & Nicolson, 1995; Wagner et al., 1997).

Phonological awareness skills develop over time. The child responds first to rhymes in stories and activities. Thus, books that contain rhyming words and games that promote rhymes are favorites in preschool and kindergarten. In addition to rhyming, segmentation of words into syllables allows the child to focus on the structure of words. A child in the five- to seven-year range will be able to segment sentences into words and words into sounds. The ability to segment words into sounds allows for the spelling of simple words. The child is also able to recognize and generate alliteration (Gilbertson & Bramlett, 1998). The early elementary school child can identify words that begin with a certain sound and end with a certain sound (Yopp, 1992; 2000). As students gain phonological awareness, tasks require more manipulation of words. The tasks listed below represent an order of acquisition of phonological awareness (Paul, 2007; van Kleeck, 1990):

- Rhyming words
- Counting sounds and segmenting sounds in words
- Counting sounds and segmenting sounds in longer and more complex words
- Determining letter and sound correspondence in words (phonics)
- Segmenting words into onset and rhyme components (*c-at, r-un*)
- Segmenting words that represent a variety of syllable shapes
- Manipulating sounds in words to omit the first or last sound or to redistribute sounds in words
- Using knowledge of sounds to spell words

Awareness of Semantics

A child's awareness of word meanings evolves as he encounters words in various contexts. The child's awareness of word meanings can be evaluated by asking him to judge words as hard or easy or as big or little. If the child is asked, for example, whether the word *whale* is big or little, he might say it is big because he is not able to separate the meaning from the word. The child who is aware of semantics at the word level understands that the connections between words and the things they represent are arbitrary. Sometimes a little word represents a little thing (e.g., *ant*), but sometimes a big word represents a little thing (e.g., *microorganism*), and sometimes a little word represents a big thing (e.g., *ship*).

The fact that words are arbitrary labels might also mean that one word can have two or more very different meanings. A child comes to this realization, for example, with the word *down*; it is most commonly understood to mean *in a lower position*, but the word *down* also refers to soft, fluffy feathers. Researchers have used riddles to determine whether children understand the multiple meanings of key words. Consider the following riddle: "Why did the man throw his clock out the window? Because he wanted to see time fly." To understand this riddle, the child must understand that the word *fly* has at least two possible meanings: (1) to move through the air; and (2) to pass quickly. By the time a child is six or seven years old, she is able to separate words from their referents, as evidenced by her ability to understand multiple meanings of words and to recognize the arbitrary connection between words and the things they represent. Even though the child will understand many of these expressions during the elementary years, she will be in junior high school before she will be able to explain to someone else the reason for their meaningfulness (Westby, 1994).

As one might suspect, practice makes a difference in developing definitional skills. Snow (1990) found that the ability of elementary school children to create correct formal definitions was associated with their experience with language, and specifically with their experience in using language to talk about what words mean. That is, definitional skills depend on the opportunity to practice definitions. In this case, practice does not necessarily make perfect, but practice does make better.

Researchers have evaluated awareness of sentence meaning by asking children to evaluate the acceptability of sentences based on their semantic appropriateness. A child who is aware of the rules governing sentence meaning will be able to judge whether a sentence makes sense. For example, he will recognize that the sentence, "The dog ate the cookie" is meaningful, whereas the sentence, "The paper ate the cookie" is not meaningful. The child can typically make judgments about the semantic appropriateness of sentences as early as five years of age, and he can often point out the problem. In the example cited, he might say, "'The paper ate the cookie' is wrong because paper can't eat."

Awareness of Morphology and Syntax

Children gain in their knowledge of morphemes as a direct result of learning to read and spell (Numes, Bryant, & Bindman, 2006). The awareness that comes with learning to decode words which have inflectional and derivational morphemes and learning to add morphemes when spelling words provides increased knowledge about these structures. Thus, teaching children about morphemes has a positive effect on their spelling ability, and teaching spelling has a positive effect on morphological awareness.

We determine metalinguistic awareness of syntax when we ask a child to decide whether sentences are grammatically correct or incorrect. To ensure that the child is making a judgment about a sentence based on a grammatical error, we can ask her to correct the mistake. If she is able to make the grammatical correction, we may assume she has developed syntactic awareness. At about age six, she is able to determine that the sentence, "The dog chased the cat tree up the" is incorrect, and she is able to produce the correction.

A somewhat more difficult judgment involves the identification of syntactic ambiguities in sentences. For example, "Visiting relatives can be a pain" can be interpreted in two ways: (1) going to visit relatives can be a pain; or (2) having relatives visit can be a pain. The child may be 11 or 12 years old before he has enough metalinguistic awareness to recognize this kind of ambiguity.

Awareness of Pragmatics

Less attention has been given to the development of pragmatic awareness than to other metalinguistic skills. We do know that by the time the child is five or six, she is able to make judgments about whether enough information is contained in a message, such as whether instructions are adequate. At about this same age, the child recognizes glaring contradictions or inconsistencies. For example, a character in a story cannot be the hero and the villain at the same time. She understands that a man saying, "When I was a little girl . . . "

does not make sense even if the sentence is correct according to all the rules of syntax.

If there is a communicative failure that requires repair, preschool children usually fault the listener for the failure, not the speaker, but by age eight, the children understand that the speaker is sometimes responsible for the failure (Robinson, 1981). In another interesting preschool-to-school-age comparison, preschool children tend to answer strange, nonsensical questions without asking for additional information or clarification. For example, in a study by Hughes and Grieve (1980), children were asked questions such as, "Is orange taller than purple?" and, "Is dirt higher than sand?" The five-year-old children in the study answered these questions as though they were valid. The seven-year-old children indicated in their responses that they did not understand the speaker's communicative intent.

By the time the child reaches adolescence, she has fairly well-developed pragmatic skills, at least as they are applied in the most common social experiences she is likely to face (Berko-Gleason, Hay, & Cain, 1988), and she purposely violates the pragmatic skills we would categorize as common rules of courtesy. She might purposely snub someone, knowing that this is so inappropriate that it will be noticed and that it has the potential to offend. She might consciously avoid saying, "Thank you," or, "You're welcome," as a way of sending a message of defiance or, if we wish to be gracious in our assessment of her intention, an expression of independence. Figure 7.4 summarizes metalinguistic awareness and abilities in school-age children.

Figure 7.4   An Overview of Metalinguistic Awareness and Abilities in School-Age Children

School-age children:

- Differentiate basic units of language—i.E., Sounds, syllables, words, and sentences
- Attach correct inflections to unfamiliar words
- Recognize when words are used incorrectly in sentences, and know when word order is incorrect
- Understand how it is possible to construct varying sentence types, and convey understanding to other people
- Understand the possible meanings framed within sentence types
- Know when utterances are acceptable based on who the listener is and/or the setting in which the communication is taking place
- Know how to define words in a manner that makes their meanings clear to others
- Demonstrate an understanding of the language forms used in creating humorous constructions, such as puns and riddles

---

Note: It is well established that preschool children have some metalinguistic awareness, but their metalinguistic awareness and abilities are not complete until they are about seven or eight years old.

Learning to Read and Write

There is convincing evidence that human beings are born to speak. But are they genetically predisposed to read and write? The answer to this question lies, to some extent, in two basic facts about human beings as communicators. Anthropologists have never discovered a group of people, no matter how primitive their lifestyle, without a highly developed spoken language. They have found, however, groups of people whose languages have no written forms. In addition, there are many people who speak languages that do have written forms but who are unable to read and write. It is reasonable to conclude, therefore, that a more powerful biological drive exists for humans to speak than to read and write. Although humans are innately endowed with the sensory, perceptual, and cognitive abilities to learn to read and write, environmental factors are more crucial in the emergence of these language capabilities than in the emergence of speech.

Extensive language research conducted over the past several decades has changed our views about how language is acquired, even if this research has not answered all the questions we have posed about how the acquisition process occurs. At the same time that language researchers have tried to understand how children acquire language, other researchers have tried to understand their learning of reading and writing. They have used their findings to suggest more effective strategies for facilitating literacy development in children, both in their homes and in their schools.

The Components of Reading and Reading Instruction

In Chapter 6, we discussed the importance of emergent literacy activities to build awareness of all the aspects of oral language and to develop experiences in using books as a focal point for interactions and sharing stories. Knowledge about books and print lays the foundation for reading and writing.

The school-age child will certainly continue to enjoy listening to stories and continue to use his knowledge to understand rhymes, alliteration, word meanings, and story structure, but the attention in the curriculum shifts to teaching him specifically to read and write. How should reading and writing be taught? Systematic analysis of research on reading instruction by the National Reading Panel provides guidance on the components that lead to successful learning (National Institute of Child Health and Human Development, 2000). The International Reading Association's Division of Research and Policy (2002) summarized the panel's conclusions about the skills that are necessary for effective reading instruction.

Phonological awareness skills offer the child an understanding that spoken words have sound segments. The child is able to isolate the beginning sound in a word and to recognize the same sound occurring in different words, that sounds blend together, and that it is possible to add, change, or delete sounds in words. This awareness about the makeup of words is valuable as the child prepares to read and spell.

When printed language is used, the child is now exposed to the relationship between the printed word and the spoken word. **Phonics** allows the child to link sounds to letter symbols and combine them to make words. Phonics skills include decoding regularly spelled words, reading nonsense words, using the sound-symbol relationships to decode words and then speak or write the words, learning the orthographic patterns of words, and beginning to read orally and silently with comprehension of the text. All of these skills require direct teaching and this occurs between kindergarten and third grade.

Reading fluency is an important literacy achievement, because it reflects the child's ability to read with accuracy, speed, and comprehension. There are many different avenues teachers can use to facilitate reading fluency, such as guided and repeated oral reading. Silent reading strategies are also important where students can focus on comprehension as the primary goal.

The goal of reading instruction is to increase the child's ability to derive meaning from reading text. While there is much attention to increasing decoding skills in the early elementary school years, decoding for word recognition is the way in which readers gain access to the meanings embedded in what they read. One critical outcome, then, is to gain meaning from the words and the words within the context of phrases, sentences, and paragraphs. **Vocabulary instruction** is enhanced through printed materials. Teachers can make children aware of root words and their prefixes, suffixes, and other morphological attributes, word definitions, new words and their associated meanings, and expansions of word understandings in sentences and paragraphs.

Teachers should also focus on strategies that increase **text comprehension**. That is, they can guide the child to greater understandings of meanings through the use of cognitive strategies, such as teaching the child to generate questions, and asking the child to answer questions about the meaning of texts, to engage in summarizing what was read, to transfer information to new situations, and to understand increasingly longer and more complex reading materials. Students benefit from teaching strategies that help them think about what they are reading, share their understandings with others, organize information, and be able to offer key ideas.

Historically, reading instruction has been dominated by distinct philosophies that favored only parts of the areas just described. Some instructional approaches focused on decoding strategies at the expense of reading comprehension strategies; other approaches stressed reading comprehension and ignored or only lightly emphasized decoding and reading fluency. These differences in instructional practices result from opposing views about how we learn to read. One view suggests that reading is taught through systematic and direct instruction (transmission model). The other view suggests that reading develops as part of the child's natural language development (transactional model), thus, methods should mirror natural contexts (Weaver, 1994).

Children's Reading Development

We know from watching children who grow up in households where reading and writing occur that they come to school knowing a great deal about literacy. In literate homes, oral and written language are interwoven within everyday interactions as families use books, newspapers, magazines, bedtime stories, and even grocery lists in their interactions (Miller, 1990; van Kleeck & Scheule, 1987; Wallach & Miller, 1988). Children who attend preschool often engage in activities that build phonological awareness, metalinguistic skills, vocabulary, print awareness, experience in hearing and telling narratives, and social routines about reading and writing (Kuykendall & Fahey, 2000). Children who do not have written language exposure in their homes and do not attend preschool are at a disadvantage upon entering school, because they have not had the opportunity to develop these skills.

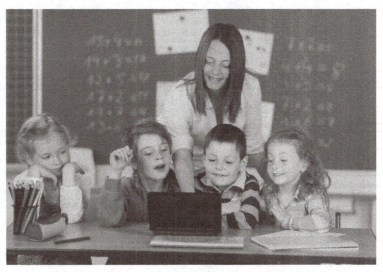

Learning to read and enjoy books.

Source: Contrastwerkstatt/ Fotolia.

Reading development occurs across several years in a continuous, seamless process. We will identify categories of development, but these categories should not be understood as periods of mastery in which one category is completed before the next category begins. The reader will note instead that there is a great deal of overlap as we move from category to category, and the emphasis is always on continuous development. Three broad categories of readers will be identified and described in the following sections: emergent, developing, and independent.

Emergent Readers

Emergent readers are at the beginning of the reading adventure. They have learned that books contain stories, that they can visit these stories as often as they like, that the words will be the same each time they return, and that the pictures accompanying the stories help construct and more fully develop meaning. Emergent readers show progressively more interest in trying to read without assistance from others. They are able to discuss what is happening in a story, and they can predict what is likely to happen next. They are also beginning to recognize certain words in varying contexts. As important as all this is to the development of reading, we need to be very clear about the fact that children at this stage, which typically occurs between 30 and 48 months, are not reading. They are pretending to read (Kaderavek & Sulzby, 2000). We need to remember, however, that pretending is a very good thing in young children because it sets the stage for *representation*, which helps form the very foundation of language—spoken and written. Caregivers should encourage their emergent readers, not just because it is a step toward true reading, but also because there is evidence that children whose caregivers actively promote exposure to reading have greater phonological awareness than children who live in homes that are less reader-friendly (Foy & Mann, 2003).

Jean Chall's (1983, 1996) model links specific aspects of reading development to specific ages and stages. The preparatory stage extends from about six months to six years. During this stage, which corresponds nicely to the emergent reading period, the child is *exposed* to reading in the sense that he looks at books, usually in the company of a caregiver. Early on, he might pretend that he is reading. During the preschool years, he will probably recognize some of the letters of the alphabet and might recognize traffic signs and the names of franchise restaurants. He might know the stop sign more by its color and shape than by the letters in the word *stop*, but he is at least paying attention to the symbols he will soon process in real reading. It is very likely that the preschool child knows McDonald's more by its golden arches than by the letters in the restaurant's name, but again, he is beginning to make a connection between symbols and the act of processing symbols, and that is the basis of reading.

It is important to choose books for emergent readers with their needs and competencies in mind. The books should provide opportunities for these children to enjoy literature even though they cannot yet read independently. The text and illustrations should be clear, the plots simple. Recall that understanding and use of story grammar develop over this time frame, thus, books should be slightly more advanced than the child's own language abilities. The language should be repetitive, rhythmic, and natural. Ideally, the illustrations should assist emergent readers to predict what the text might say and what is going to happen next in the story. Books should possess an invitational tone that encourages children to participate to the extent that they can until they are able to read on their own. Within the context of the transactional model, it is most important that books for emergent readers be designed to guide children toward an understanding of what they are reading rather than focusing on individual words. From the very beginning of literacy development, children should be made aware that the essence of reading, and indeed the essence of language in all its forms, is meaning.

Developing Readers

Developing readers have established the habit of reading for meaning, at least in the sense that they understand that meaning is the bottom line. They use the text, the illustrations, and their own knowledge of print conventions to sample, to predict, and to confirm printed words. These children also use letter/sound associations, within context, to help confirm their predictions about words. Teachers encourage them to:

- Use their own life experiences as context for what they read
- Take interpretative risks
- Make approximations about what words are or what words mean
- Move beyond unfamiliar words to find lexical content they do recognize to help them figure out unfamiliar words
- Reread and self-correct when the process of interpreting meaning has been interrupted or when the printed words do not seem to make sense

You recognize, of course, that these are strategies adult readers use when they have difficulty determining the meaning of printed words. What is important to understand is that these are strategies, according to the transactional model, which should be encouraged from the beginning of reading development.

In Chall's stage 1, the child is six to seven years old and receives *direct instruction* in reading. She learns how letters are connected to sounds. She learns how to *sound out* simple words, typically single-syllable words, and by the end of this stage, she can actually read about 600 words.

In stage 2, she is seven to eight years old. Instruction is still direct and she learns to read simple stories. She becomes increasingly adept in using her decoding skills and she learns more about the connections between words and meanings, and by the end of the stage, she can read about 3,000 words.

Reading instruction for students in the developing reading stage often focuses on phonological awareness and decoding strategies in order to teach reading accuracy for words and sentences. Students learn to recite the alphabet, recognize and name letters, retrieve sound/symbol relationships, sound out words, compare words for beginning and ending sounds, and identify words with certain vowels (Adams, 1990). They encounter regular patterns for spelling words, and they discover that irregular forms also exist. Well-balanced reading programs include many different strategies to focus students on comprehension, including the variety of purposes for reading, the meaning of words and text, using knowledge of spoken syntax and semantics as cues for decoding and creating meaning, story structure, and comprehension monitoring techniques. The inclusion of all five components produces readers who have efficient and effective reading ability and complete comprehension of the information.

In comparison to books chosen for emergent readers, books chosen for developing readers draw on a wider range of life experiences, and they expand readers' horizons to a significantly enlarged world, complete with more elaborate, mature understandings about how the world works. The vocabulary bases of these books match the rapidly growing vocabularies of the children reading them. They are designed, in fact, to increase readers' vocabularies and to introduce them to more complex and varied language structures. These books, in comparison to the books used by emergent readers, employ a wider variety of cues to help children sample, predict, and monitor what they are reading, and to construct and maintain meaning.

Independent Readers

Independent readers read on their own and when they are alone. These children are confident and competent readers who integrate into the process of reading all the cueing systems available in language. They pay little conscious attention to the details of printed words because their focus is on constructing and maintaining meaning. For independent readers, the printed details are not ends, but means to understanding and interpreting meaning. Independent readers are able to read increasingly longer and more structurally complex sentences with meaning and they process a wide variety of prose and poetry. They learn to adjust their reading rate to accommodate the purposes for which they are reading. One of the most obvious characteristics of independent readers is variety, not just in what they read but also in the databases on which they draw to make sense of what they read. To a much greater extent than developing readers, independent readers use knowledge gained from their personal experiences in their homes, schools, and communities, as well as knowledge gleaned from previously read books, movies, and television, to understand what they are reading right now. As their reading choices expand, they encounter books that are increasingly challenging in terms of content, format, and style. They read stories about people and places far removed from their own lives in time and space in nonfiction as well as fiction. They read essays, poems, novels, plays, and, dare we acknowledge it, even textbooks. As their language becomes more complete and their reading experiences become more varied, these children experience a knowledge explosion that cannot be fathomed by people who cannot read. The true miracle in this experience is that it all happens inside readers' minds, bounded only by the limits of their imaginations, and all this can take place in the family room or the classroom. The power of books in the hands of readers is truly amazing. As their reading experiences increase in frequency and variety, independent readers learn to enjoy reading. As they learn to enjoy reading, they risk becoming what are called *voracious* readers. You know these people. They are knowledgeable, interesting, creative, and productive.

Once students advance to the independent reading stage, reading instruction is often not directly the focus of the curriculum; rather, students use their reading ability to engage in high-level thinking for learning new information and for solving problems. They not only read at the literal and inspectual levels of younger children, but also expand their reading to the analytic and comparative levels to comprehend academic subjects (Kamhi, 1997). The **literal level** allows the student to focus on word meanings and the relationships between ideas conveyed in the paragraph. The **inspectual level** allows the student to quickly scan reading materials to determine the main ideas. The **analytic level** activates the student's deep processing of the information, and the **comparative level** involves his use of all the other levels to reflect on information from multiple sources in order to compare meanings (Craik & Lockhart, 1972).

The independent reader is in Chall's stage 3 from 9 to 14 years of age. He now uses reading as a primary vehicle by which he learns independently. Reading provides the background for class discussions, and he is learning to dissect words more thoroughly to understand the breadth and depth of their meanings.

Stage 4 according to Chall's scheme extends from about 15 to 17 years. This stage is essentially an extension of stage 3 during which the emerging young adult becomes more expert in his reading skills and expands his application of these skills to an increasingly large array of topics.

At 18 years and beyond, the reader is in stage 5—the stage in which he remains during his adult years. The stage 5 reader continues to expand his reading vistas. If he was not a self-motivated reader earlier, he is now becoming one, especially when he finishes school and is no longer motivated by the threat of a failing grade that might be the consequence for not reading assigned material. In or out of school, he reads to understand more fully knowledge he has already attained and to acquire new knowledge.

Throughout our discussion of language development, we have emphasized that children do not proceed through development at the same pace. We conclude with the same emphasis here. Although the general development of reading competencies will be the same for all children, they do not all achieve these competencies at the same ages. Rather than becoming unduly concerned about whether a child is on schedule in terms of literacy development, we should be concerned about doing whatever we can to facilitate development. What we can do is fairly simple. We can support and encourage children who are learning to read and write. We can trust that their natural language abilities, in combination with teaching/learning paradigms that foster natural, language-based reading instruction, will ultimately produce effective and efficient adult readers.

Components of Writing and Its Development

Even the casual observer will understand that reading and writing are closely related processes, sharing language as a common bond. Butler and Turbill (1987) note that reading and writing are also functional cousins in that each is an act of composing. More specifically, they observe, "Readers, using their background of knowledge and experience, compose meaning from text; writers, using their background of knowledge and experience, compose meaning into text" (p. 11).

In a very real sense, then, reading and writing are different facets of a single process. In the development of reading and writing, the knowledge of each process is enhanced by the knowledge gained in the other. This means that the more a person reads, the more she will know about writing, and the more she writes, the more she will know about reading (Fields & Spangler, 1995). From the point of view of Butler and Turbill, the tie that binds reading and writing together is meaning. As the reader processes the printed symbols on the page, she constructs meaning, not by paying attention to every detail, but by sampling only those details she needs for meaning closure. You know from your own experience that if you are reading material with which you are not familiar, you process many more details of the printed symbols than if you are reading material you know well. The reader's knowledge and experience help her gauge how many details are enough in a given reading situation. Alas, sometimes the reader exhausts all the available details and, for want of more, never achieves meaning closure. We have all been there, too.

Writing offers a different challenge. A writer begins with ideas, morsels of meaning, and must decide which symbols in which combination will best represent those ideas. If the writer understands the nuances of this kind of communication, he will also take into account the audience to whom he is directing his packaged morsels of meaning, and he will select the literary style he believes is most appropriate for conveying his message. This proactive and self-directed process is sometimes referred to as **self-regulated writing** (Bashir & Singer, 2006). Consider the differences in symbols and literary styles that might be reflected in the following: writing a diary entry, writing a letter to a lover, writing a letter of inquiry about a job, and writing an essay for a philosophy professor on the relative dangers of optimism and pessimism in humankind's efforts to save the planet.

We should step back for a moment and consider what has been discussed about writing to this point. The opening paragraphs in this section have been devoted to what might be called *real writing*, in contrast to the act of copying letters or words a teacher has written on the chalkboard. It needs to be emphasized that *real writing* is not the same thing as *handwriting practice*. For many years, teachers assumed they were teaching writing when they taught their students how to print their letters and then produce them in cursive, the physical skills included in *penmanship*.

Today, teachers recognize that although the physical skills involved in forming letters are important, the process of real writing is far more important. They value writing as a powerful communication tool and believe their students have the potential to become authors, that they can actually transform meaning into text (Fields & Spangler, 1995). Writing is, as writing experts today remind us, about meaning, and it is about language. The developing child who processes meaning in the speech of others, and who learns how to create meaning in her own oral expressions, eventually extends these meaning/language skills to the processes of reading and writing. Just as she can express meaning in what she says, she can express meaning in what she writes.

Even though, as we have noted, there is a more powerful biological drive in human beings for the production of speech than for the production of language in written form, there can be little doubt that children have a natural inclination to write. They show evidence of a strong desire to write even before they enter school. Preschoolers are infamous for marking up walls, sidewalks, and newspapers with crayons, chalk, pencils, and pens (Graves, 1983). If speech begins in cooing and babbling, writing begins in the preschool child's scratches and scrawls.

The physical process of moving the fingers and hands to put letters on paper is closely related to drawing in that writing and drawing are both processes of symbolization (Dyson, 1983). Writing and drawing, however, are not the same thing. The child demonstrates that writing and drawing are differentiated processes when he is about three years old (Gibson & Levin, 1975). As soon as the child can hold and manipulate a pencil or crayon and is given an opportunity to experiment with these instruments of expression, he will begin to make marks on any surface that is available. These early marking and scribbling exercises form the foundations of writing. Figures 7.5 and 7.6 offer two views of scribbling from a 32-month-old and 36-month-old. Especially if the young child has been exposed to printed language in books and magazines, he will try to make forms that resemble letters of the alphabet. These early attempts are crude approximations at best. At this point, the child does not know the names of the letters he is trying to form, nor does he understand that printed words represent spoken words, but he is beginning the journey that leads inexorably to written language (Sulzby, 1981).

Figure 7.5   Scribbling at Two Years, Eight Months

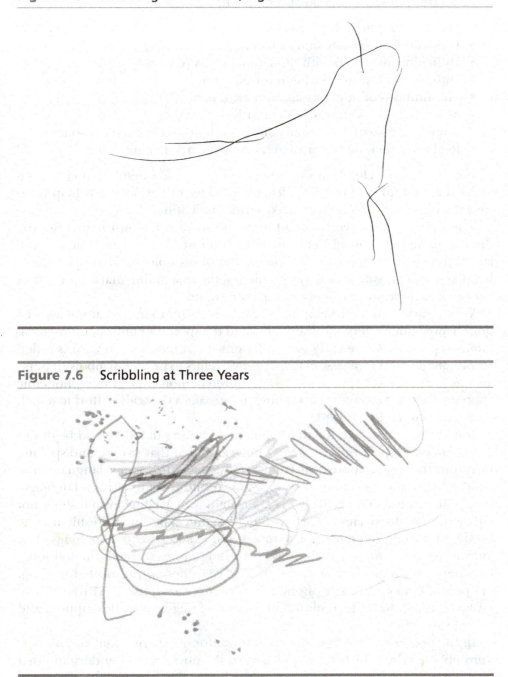

Figure 7.6   Scribbling at Three Years

By the end of kindergarten, teachers expect children to be able to write their full name, write both upper and lowercase alphabet letters, and use invented and conventional spellings of several words (Snow, Burns, & Griffin, 1998). Richey (2008) studied the writing and spelling skills of children in kindergarten. She found that by the end of kindergarten, children demonstrate a variety of skills in steady progression:

- Writing many alphabet letters
- Difficulty with visually similar letters (e.g., *b–d, u–v*)
- Difficulty with letters with directional shifts (e.g., *z–s*)
- Difficulty with words having less frequently occurring letters (e.g., *q, w*)
- Substitutions of upper and lowercase letters
- More difficulty with vowels than with consonants
- More success with the initial consonant followed by final consonants
- Real-word spelling better than nonsense-word spelling

Let's look more closely at the process children use when learning to spell and write. As with oral language learning, stages of development help us to view the ways in which children make strides in writing.

The first word the typical child learns to write is his own name. Shortly thereafter, he will probably learn to write other words with which he is familiar, including *Mommy, Daddy,* and the names of his siblings. These personally familiar words provide the child with his first understanding that a connection exists between printed symbols and spoken sounds.

Very early in writing development, children begin to make natural associations between the letters of the alphabet and the speech sounds they most commonly represent. These early sound/letter associations lead to what is called **graphophonemic awareness,** in which *grapho* refers to printed symbols (letters) and *phonemic* refers to speech sounds. Children demonstrate graphophonemic awareness when, in a contextual setting, they make a conscious effort to match letters to sounds (Read, 1981).

It is at this juncture in the development of writing that the child begins to sense a need to spell; thus we need to be reminded that writing and spelling fit within the larger context of language. Just as with spoken language, the child must risk, experiment, develop, and refine rules in written language. In fact, the typical child is likely to experiment with spelling even if she is not encouraged to do so. Her earliest spelling risks and experiments result in some pretty interesting sequences of letters, often called **invented spellings.** The journey from invented to conventional spelling moves through the following four stages, each of which involves progressively more sophisticated spelling: (1) prephonemic; (2) early phonemic; (3) letter/name; and (4) transitional (Weaver, 1994). Refer to Table 7.3 to view these stages, their description, and some examples.

In the **prephonemic stage,** the child is wantonly experimental and blithely uninhibited. When she tries to spell a word she does seem to understand that longer words require more letters, and she knows that when letters are strung together, they "say" something, but she does not yet understand that there are specific, if not always consistent, relationships between the letters of the alphabet and the sounds of speech.

The changes in the **early phonemic stage** are not dramatic, but they are important because they reflect more sophisticated understanding about

Table 7.3   Spelling Development in Elementary School

Stage	Description	Age Range	Examples
Prephonemic	Letters strung together without regard to letter/sound correspondence	3 to 4 years	T C L M K V
Early Phonemic	First letter used alone; first letter matches the first sound in the word; no vowels appear	4 to 6 years Kindergarten/early first grade	D (Daddy) D B M S (Daddy) B T S
Letter Name	Both consonants and vowels are used and letters match their names	5 to 6 years End of first grade	J A S N X R A
Transitional	Recall of some printed words Application of some rules with over-generalization Letter–name spelling	5 to 8 years Second grade	Teeth, Fine Lefe (Leaf) Shuger (sugar)

spelling and sounds. In this stage, the child often attends only to the first letter of a word that represents the entire word even if other letters are included. The other letters typically have no correspondence to the remaining segments of the target word. As he gains more experience and knowledge, he may also include the letter that represents the last sound of the word. The middle of the word is a kind of mystery spelling package in the sense that no one, including the child, knows what letters might be included from one spelling attempt to the next on the same word. Early phonemic spellings include consonants and exclude vowels. As the child gains more experience with letters and the sounds they represent, phonemic spellings begin to shade into spellings that more obviously reflect letter/sound relationships.

In the **letter–name stage**, the child represents vowels as well as consonants with letters whose names sound like the speech sounds they purportedly represent, such as *P, D,* and *O* in the words *peach, Dean,* and *opal.* Because she has been nurtured in a risk-free environment, this understanding that there are relationships between printed symbols and speech sounds, or graphophonemic awareness, enables the child to move to the transitional stage of spelling.

In the **transitional stage**, the child will try a number of spelling strategies. He might use a particular spelling because he *remembers* seeing the word spelled that way in print. He might try to apply rules for spelling he has observed in his own reading. Perhaps he observed that when a word contains a double vowel (e.g., *teeth*), the vowel sound is long, or when a word ends with *e* (e.g., *fine*), the preceding vowel is long. In his attempts to apply these rules, he makes errors that show he is using generalization strategies. He might also continue to rely on letter–name spellings and the use of sounding-out strategies to spell words.

A writing sample of a child in the transitional stage of spelling might include productions based on several different spelling strategies, including the examples provided here and others. The typical child is still experimenting. In fact, the development of spelling is facilitated by successful use of an expanding range of spelling strategies (Wilde, 1992). After all, a strategy that works well in one spelling challenge may be of absolutely no help in another.

Given the inconsistencies between the way words are spelled and the way words are spoken, the child who aspires to a competent speller must have a plethora of spelling strategy options at her disposal. The truth is, many of the strategies used in the transitional stage are used by adult spellers as well. The child learns much of what she will ever know about spelling patterns during the elementary school years, but most people continue to learn how to spell throughout their adult years, and we all rely to a certain extent on our computers to spell-check when we are writing.

Obviously, much more is involved in writing than in forming letters and spelling. Even as these foundational processes continue to develop, the child is learning to express himself through writing, and he is learning the rules of grammar, capitalization, and punctuation that make writing "correct." Whatever limitations others may see in the young child's writing abilities, he is typically unabashed about expressing himself on paper, and the products of these early attempts are often delightful. In the following essay written by a seven-year-old boy, you will notice spelling, punctuation, and capitalization errors but also the simple elegance of the written message:

> spider live in hot dezerd.
> but not oll of them. sum live here.
> sum cude hurt you. they are deadles.
> I saw one before it was not deadles.
> It was a dade-long-legs he was on
> me. they are not fast
> they are not good jumpers at all
> THE END
> of the spiter story

Just as spelling proceeds through stages of development, so does writing. Kroll (1981) suggests that there are four stages or phases in the development of writing: preparation, consolidation, differentiation, and integration. Refer to Table 7.4 for a summary of these writing attainments during the elementary school years. The child is typically a preschooler during the **preparation phase**. He is learning the ground floor basics of writing—how to form letters. His caregivers and teachers provide models that he imitates. It is a painstaking, but absolutely necessary, phase in writing development that usually continues through kindergarten and first grade.

When the child is about seven years old and in the second grade, he enters the **consolidation phase**. He now writes strings of words, using the same vocabulary and rules of grammar he uses in his speech. In Figure 7.7, the seven-year-old writer and artist shows his use of complete sentences, capitalization, and

Table 7.4   Writing Development in Pre- and Elementary School

Stage	Description	Age/Grade Range	Examples
Preparation	Child copies letters from a model and practices letters and words.	3 to 6 years	S S S S S S A M
Consolidation	Child writes strings of words using spoken vocabulary and grammar.	7 to 10 years	I'm Sam and my doggy is Shaggy.
Differentiation	Writing is more sophisticated than the spoken grammar.	10 to 11 years	My name is Sam. I have a dog and I named him Shaggy.
Integration	Child expresses mood, attitude, and personal style and creativity.	Beyond 11 years	It is fair to say that my dog, Sam is the smartest dog on the planet.

punctuation, and the ability to stay on the topic. Jacob is a reluctant writer and was prompted to continue his story about a field trip after the first sentence and to write an ending. He finds spelling challenging, asking how to spell *animals, skulls, aquatic,* and *insects.*

When a student is in the fifth grade, or about 10 years old, she enters the **differentiation phase**. During this phase, the way she writes becomes

Figure 7.7   Writing in the Consolidation Phase at Seven Years

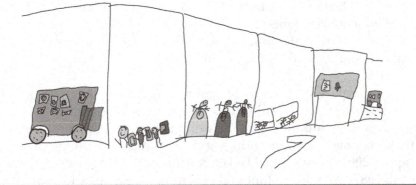

differentiated from the way she talks through the use of more sophisticated grammar in writing than in speaking, a trend that continues for many people throughout their lives. All writers proceed through the first three phases.

Not all children will enter the final phase, **integration**. In this phase, a writer develops a *style* that reflects his own personality, makes him unique, and allows him to express varying moods and attitudes in his writing. Less sophisticated writers are fairly regimented in the way they write. They may obey the rules of grammar and their writing may be clear, but it lacks personal expression. The difference between a writer in the integration phase and one who never enters this phase is comparable to the difference between a concert-level musician and one whose playing is competent but mechanical. Both musicians play all the right notes, but the concert-level musician plays in a manner that is creative and personally expressive. The integration phase writer uses standard words and conventional rules of language, but he uses written language creatively and expressively.

Development in writing has been described at the most mechanical, grammatical level (Perera, 1986). As the child matures, for example, she uses more passive sentences in her writing. At the age of 13, she is producing three times as many passive sentences in her writing as she produced at 8 years. The length of her clauses, calculated on a *words-per-clause* basis, increases systematically. The mean length of a written clause at eight years is six-and-a-half words. That number increases to 8.6 at 17 years; by adulthood, the writer is creating clauses that average 11.5 words in length. Writers increase the length of their clauses by adding modifiers and by including more words to signal adjustments such as tense changes and modality.

Many of these changes in writing, particularly those associated with developing one's own *style*, continue to evolve on the journey through adulthood. Many professional writers will look back on their earlier work as being less mature, less expressive than their present work. Just as *life is a journey and not a destination*, so is learning to be an effective writer.

As students advance through elementary school and enter middle and high school, writing takes on more formal purposes. Students write in expository style to create reports about what they read, essays about what they think and to persuade others, and term papers to integrate ideas about topics. Writing is no longer a private matter, but is intended for other audiences as a way to share information (Maxwell & Meisser, 1997; Nippold, Ward-Lonergan, & Fanning, 2005). High school students are expected to be skilled in independently accessing information from the library, the Internet, and other sources and using the information to read and write for many academic purposes (Tunmer & Cole, 1991).

Teachers expect students to engage in revision processes before, during, and after writing. But learning to revise written text is difficult because it places heavy demands on cognition, working memory, linguistic and metalinguistic knowledge, self-monitoring, and social understandings (Alamargot & Chanquoy, 2001; Butterfield, Hacker, & Albertson, 1996; Kellogg, 1994; Pea & Kurland, 1987). Myhill and Jones (2007) studied a group of 13- and 15-year-old students to observe their use of revisions during writing and to discover their beliefs and reflections about their revision behaviors. Most of the students did engage in some form of revision during writing. Their reflections about their writings revealed several interesting themes:

- Reread as a revision strategy
- Revise for accuracy of spelling, punctuation, and sentence and paragraph structure
- Revise for coherence of meaning and making sense
- Revise to add to the text in order to provide more detail and to clarify or expand the information
- Revise to avoid repetition
- Revise to achieve general improvement in the writing

The authors point out that the students did use many types of revision during writing, and they were able to think about and talk about these revision activities, suggesting that they have metacognitive awareness of revision behaviors. However, most students in the early-teen years were not able to identify precise problems with their writing, and they struggled to implement effective strategies to solve writing problems.

Another advance in writing during adolescence and through adulthood is the persuasive essay. Nippold et al. (2005) found that 11-, 17-, and 24-year-old students make gradual improvements across all language domains in their persuasive essays. They also showed greater flexibility of thought consistent with formal operations reasoning with increased age, allowing for the inclusion of a greater number of reasons to convince their audience of their point of view, as well as being able to acknowledge differing points of view in their essays.

Check Your Understanding 7.6

Assess your knowledge of the development of literacy by completing this brief quiz.

And the Beat Goes On . . .

What a magnificent adventure this has been! Children, by virtue of their genetic background, are born to talk, but acquiring language and the abilities to express language through speech and writing is not as simple as acquiring freckles. Language acquisition depends on social and environmental opportunities and on the child's interactions with the important people in his life. It depends on motor, sensory, perceptual, and cognitive development. It is a complex process that begins before birth, accelerates through the child's first five or six years of life, and continues, only slightly abated, through the remainder of his school years. Even then the learning does not end. As adults, we learn new words. We understand syntactic rules more completely and we learn the multiple meanings of words and the differences between the denotations and connotations of words, which allow us to use words more effectively to convey the exact messages we intend. Language is indeed a wondrous and exciting phenomenon, and we continue to experience the wonder of language as long as we live and speak and listen and read and write.

This marks the end of our journey through the joys and travails of speech and language development, but more chapters remain. Throughout our discussion of language development, we have mentioned the sound system of speech but we have not specifically traced its development. In Chapter 8, we take a closer look at phonology, the acquisition of speech sounds, and how phonology and morphology are influenced by accent and dialects of English. Finally, we review some of the common disorders of speech and language in chapter 9.

SUMMARY

Children who enter school should have a solid foundation in their native language, but they still have a lot to learn, practice, and refine during the elementary years and beyond. In this chapter we considered the complex nature of school and we explored the strategies children use in learning the meanings and the uses of thousands of words. We discovered that the complexity of grammar continues to develop, especially in the ability to use passive and complex sentences. School-age children are able to use sophisticated repair strategies as they refine their meanings and they become skilled in telling stories. The classroom environment requires children to learn new forms of language and the development of literacy skills allows children to read and write for enjoyment and as a vehicle for learning academic information. Language is truly a multi-layered ability that provides the way and means for continued learning and interactions with others.

Surfing the Web

If you are interested in exploring topics discussed in this chapter in more detail, search for one or more of the following relevant terms online.

- communication development in the school years
- cultural curriculum
- classroom curriculum
- IRE model of instruction
- cultural diversity in the classroom
- slow mapping for vocabulary development
- strategies for vocabulary organization and storage
- strategies for learning word meanings
- figurative language development
- narrative structure
- narrative development in children
- gender differences in communication
- metalinguistic development in children
- development of reading
- development of writing

Chapter Review 7.1

Recall what you learned in this chapter by completing the Chapter Review.

8

Development of Speech Sounds and Cultural Variation in Speech and Language Production

LEARNING OUTCOMES

After completion of this chapter, you will be able to:

- Describe speech sounds using phonetics and distinctive features.
- Explain the emergence of speech sounds during the prelinguistic and one-word stage.
- Discuss the development of speech sounds in two-word utterances and beyond.
- Define phonological processes and give examples of the major types used during early childhood.
- Summarize trends in language dialects for Spanish English, Asian English, and Native American English.
- Compare the characteristics of regional dialects.

The preceding chapters have focused primarily on language development, but we have made frequent references to speech, and we have made occasional references to speech sounds. We want to emphasize that for the child with normal hearing and typical development, the speech sound system does not exist apart from language. The child acquires it and learns its underlying rules at the same time that she acquires language.

You must be reminded, however, as we noted in the opening chapter, that *speech* is not a synonym for *language* and that speech can exist apart from language, as it does when a mynah bird "talks," and language can surely exist apart from speech, as it does when the person who is deaf communicates through sign language. Because speech is related to language but in some ways is separate from language, and because the speech sound system is mastered according to a different developmental schedule than language, we have chosen to devote this chapter to the speech component of the larger communication system.

When I[*] was in high school, I lived in Egypt for two years. Although I had some extraordinary experiences during that time and saw many remnants of a remarkable ancient civilization, nothing impressed me as much as the great pyramids outside Cairo. From a distance, the surfaces of the pyramids appear relatively smooth, almost seamless. A closer view reveals structures of enormous size consisting of many huge blocks piled on top of one another in precise patterns. In the years since my visit to the pyramids, I have looked at modern buildings, especially brick buildings, with an eye not only to the total structure, but to the bricks that together make the building complete.

We can think about human speech in much the same way. As senders and receivers of speech, we pay attention to the message, but even a simple sentence is actually a structure consisting of many small pieces. A sentence is a string of words, of course, but the words themselves are strings of speech sounds or phonemes, which are the building blocks of speech. And when someone speaks, there are no markers at the beginnings and endings of words. An utterance consists of a long, uninterrupted string of sounds. Only our knowledge of the language being spoken and our perceptual abilities allow us to know which segments of the string are words.

In a practical sense, we have little reason to pay attention to the sounds of speech any more than we should pay attention to individual bricks in a building. Individual bricks become important only when they fall out or break, threatening the structural integrity of a wall. In much the same way, we usually pay attention to specific sounds of speech only when they are missing or misarticulated in ways that affect our ability to understand the words of which they are members.

One cannot fully appreciate human speech, however, unless one understands the sound system from which specific phonemes are drawn to make up spoken words. We call the study of speech sounds and the rules that determine how sounds can be sequenced into syllables and words phonology. In this chapter, we take a look at how speech sounds are described and classified and how sounds interact with one another when they are joined to form syllables, words, and phrases, and we consider some of the major theories that attempt to explain how a child acquires his sound system as language is emerging.

Some of you reading this chapter are studying in the area of communication disorders in preparation for a career as a speech-language pathologist or audiologist. You will need this introductory information about speech sounds and much more detailed information later as you work with children and adults who have quite a variety of disorders affecting the speech sound system. Other students focusing on general education and special education are learning about children and adults as they face challenges in learning language, literacy, and academics, especially in schools but also in the home and community. Your knowledge about speech sounds is important as you make connections for children about their awareness of the sounds of speech in spoken language (metalinguistics and phonological awareness) and of the

---

[*]Lloyd Hulit.

sound/symbol correspondence in learning the alphabet principle for reading and spelling (phonics), it will also help you determine which children appear behind in speech development, requiring a referral to the speech-language pathologist, or to an audiologist if hearing loss is suspected. Early childhood educators also need information about the development of speech sounds, as referral for early diagnosis and intervention of speech sound system disorders is of high importance. Dare I say that any adult who shares responsibility for the development of children will be able to apply knowledge of the sound system to his or her work? Even professionals working with adults to learn English as a second language will find the information about the characteristics of English sounds useful for teaching it.

Describing Speech Sounds

We begin by distinguishing between sound differences that matter and those that do not matter. A phoneme is often described as a distinctive speech sound. That is, a phoneme is a speech sound that is recognized as a specific sound and is distinctly different from all other speech sounds. Consider the words *seat* and *seed*. These two words, when spoken, are exactly the same except for one small, but important, difference. Each word consists of three sounds. The first sound in each word is *s*. The second sound in each word is the long vowel, *e*. Now notice the last sound in each word. Say each of these sounds aloud and feel what is happening in your speech mechanism during each production. Both the *t* and the *d* are produced with the front portion of the tongue pressed against the alveolar ridge, and in both productions, the tongue is quickly released to complete the sound. The only difference between *t* and *d* and, in the example used, the only difference between *seat* and *seed*, is that when the *d* is produced, the vocal folds vibrate and when the *t* is produced, the vocal folds do not vibrate. The difference between vocal fold vibration and no vibration, therefore, is a difference that makes a difference. It is a difference that can differentiate one phoneme from another.

Not all differences matter, however. In American English, for example, it does not matter if you produce the word *cat*, with a release of air following the *t*, known as **aspiration**, or with no released air. The listener will hear both productions as *cat* and will perceive the final sound as *t*. Although aspiration is a distinctive sound difference in some languages, it is a nondistinctive speech sound difference in English. That is, it is a difference that does not make a difference. A non-distinctive speech sound change is called an **allophone**. In the *cat* example, the aspirated *t* and the unaspirated *t* are allophones of the *t* phoneme. Think of the phoneme as a sound family. Allophones are members of the family. Each allophone is a little different from every other allophone, but allophones are so similar to one another in all important respects that they are recognized as members of the same family. All of this information is preliminary to a brief overview of phonological acquisition and a summary of major theoretical views about how the sound system of language emerges.

Traditional Phonetics

The International Phonetic Alphabet (IPA) uses symbols that differ from our English letters for some sounds, so that the alphabet can be used to describe many neighboring languages. Consonant symbols that differ from English letters include the voiced and voiceless *th* sounds, as in the words *thanks* ([θænks]) and *those* ([ðoz], the *sh* sound in *shoe* ([ʃu]), the final sound in the word *beige* ([beʒ]), the *ch* sound in *chop* ([tʃap]), and the *ng* sound in *sing* ([sɪŋ]). As you can see in Table 8.1, the vowel symbols also differ.

Table 8.1   Characteristics of English Phonemes

Voicing/Manner	Sound in Word		Place
Voiced Stop	b	boat	Bilabial
	d	dog	Lingual-alveolar
	g	girl	Lingual-velar
Voiceless Stop	p	pan	Bilabial
	t	toy	Lingual-alveolar
	k	key	Lingual-velar
Voiced Fricative	v	velvet	Labial-dental
	ð	there	Lingual-interdental
	z	zoo	Lingual-alveolar
	ʒ	beige (end sound)	Lingual-palatal
Voiceless Fricative	f	five	Labial-dental
	θ	thanks	Lingual-interdental
	s	sun	Lingual-alveolar
	ʃ	shoe	Lingual-palatal
	h	ham	Glottal
Voiced Affricate	d ʒ	jungle	Lingual-palatal
Voiceless Affricate	t ʃ	chew	Lingual-palatal
Voiced Nasals	m	mitten	Bilabial
	n	never	Lingual-alveolar
	ŋ	sing (end sound)	Lingual-palatal
Voiced Glide	w	wish	Bilabial
	j	yes	Lingual-palatal
Voiced Liquid	r	racoon	Lingual-palatal
	l	lucky	Lingual-alveolar
Vowel	i	bean	High-front, tense
	ɪ	bin	High-front, lax
	e	bait	Mid-front, tense
	ε	bet	Mid-front, lax
	æ	bat	Low-front, lax

Table 8.1 Characteristics of English Phonemes (Continued)

Voicing/Manner	Sound in Word		Place
	ə	button	Mid-central unstressed, lax
	ʌ	button	Mid-central stressed, tense
	ɚ	butter	Mid-central unstressed, lax
	ɝ	Bert	Mid-central stressed, tense
	ʌ	butler	Low-central stressed, tense
	u	boot	High-back, tense
	ʊ	bush	High-back, lax
	o	boat	Mid-back, tense
	ɔ	bought	Mid-back, lax
	ɑ	bother	Low-Back, lax
Diphthong	a ɪ	bite	Low-front to High-front
	a ʊ	about	Low-front to High-back
	ɔɪ	boy	Mid-back to High-front

The most basic approach for describing consonant speech sounds is the threefold classification system used in traditional phonetics. Each consonant is identified according to place of articulation, manner of articulation, and voicing. **Place of articulation** identifies where in the oral cavity the essential articulatory contact or movement is being made. There are several major places of articulation. The articulators interact in various combinations and the tongue (lingual) is a key player in the production of many sounds.

Lips and teeth: /b, p, m, w, f, v, θ, ð /
Alveolar ridge: /t, d, n, s, z, l/
Hard palate: / ʃ, ʒ, tʃ, dʒ, j, r/
Soft palate: /k, g, ŋ/
Glottis: /h/

Manner of articulation describes how a consonant sound is produced. The term *stop* is used to describe a consonant produced by stopping the flow of air out of the mouth and then suddenly releasing it. It may be helpful to remember that a stop sound is produced in a somewhat explosive manner. The stop sounds in English are /p/, /b/, /t/, /d/, /k/, and /g/.

The production of a *fricative* sound requires forcing air through a narrow constriction, producing a friction-like sound. The following sounds are fricatives: /f/, /v/, /s/, /z/, /θ/, /ð/, /ʃ/, and /ʒ/.

The *h* is also considered a fricative in traditional phonetics, even though one would be hard-pressed to identify where the constriction is since this sound is made as air is released through the space between the vocal cords.

An *affricate* is a unique sound that combines stop and fricative qualities. There are two affricates in English, /tʃ/ and /dʒ/. The /tʃ/ sound is actually a /t/ and a / ∫ / pushed together into a single sound that retains qualities of both original sounds. In the same way, /dʒ/ combines /d/ and /ʒ/.

A *nasal* consonant is produced with nasal resonance. The only consonants in English that should be produced with nasal resonance are /m/, /n/ and /ŋ/. All others should be produced with oral resonance only.

A consonant is considered liquid when the tongue is near a point of contact but it does not obstruct or constrict the flow of air to create turbulence. The unique speech sounds are determined by the position of the tongue to channel the flow of air. A *lateral* production involves directing the flow of air out of the mouth along the sides of the tongue. There is only one lateral consonant in English, and it is easy to remember because it is the first and last sound in *lateral*, the /l/ sound. The other liquid consonant is not lateral and it requires the flow of air to be close to the roof of the mouth for the production of /r/.

The *glides*, /w/ and /j/, are also called *semivowels*, and both names are helpful in understanding how they are produced. They are called *glides* because their productions involve movement. They are called *semivowels* because they are somewhat vowel-like in the sense that they involve a relatively free and continuous flow of air through the oral cavity, unlike other consonants, which involve varying degrees of constriction or closure.

Voicing is simple. A consonant either involves vocal fold vibration or it does not. The majority of consonants are *voiced.* Those consonants that are *voiceless* are partners with voiced consonants. We call these voiced and voiceless partners *cognate pairs*. A cognate pair consists of two consonants produced in the same place and in the same manner but differing in voicing. For example, /p/ and /b/ are both produced with the two lips and both are produced in an explosive manner (also called a stop or plosive consonant), but /p/ is voiceless and /b/ is voiced. They are a cognate pair. Cognate pairs account for 16 of the 24 consonants we use in English. The eight consonants that are not members of cognate pairs are all voiced—except for /h/, which is voiceless.

Classifying vowels in traditional phonetics is more difficult than classifying consonants, primarily because vowels are so variable in their production. Consider the vowel /i/, as in the word *bee*. The /i/ is classified as a high-front vowel. That is, the tongue is positioned at the front of the mouth in a relatively high position, but with very little effort, you will discover that you can produce the /i/ with the tongue in almost any position. In fact, with a little dexterity, you can produce an /i/ with your tongue protruding from your mouth. How and where vowels are produced depends on the sounds that precede and follow them, and vowels can adapt to virtually any phonetic environment. The traditional phonetics classification for vowels, therefore, is a general guide based on the production of these sounds in isolation.

A three-fold classification is also used to classify vowels: height of tongue (i.e., high and low), location of primary resonance (i.e., front, central, and back), and tension of the tongue (i.e., tense or lax). High vowels have narrow resonating spaces, whereas low vowels have wider resonating spaces. You can test these tongue height positions for yourself by producing the high vowel in the word *root* and the low vowel in the word *rot*. Vowels are also produced in the front, middle, and back of the oral cavity. The front vowel in the word *day* ([de]) is contrasted easily with the back vowel in the word *doe* ([do]). Finally, vowels are either tense, as in the word *beet* ([bit]), or lax, as in the word *bit* ([bIt]). Tension refers to the duration of the vowel and the degree of muscle activity required for its production.

Throughout this discussion of the description of speech sounds using traditional phonetics, you may have noticed that the classification of speech sounds is based on certain basic contrasts. For example, in cognate pairs we contrast voiced and voiceless sounds. We contrast nasal sounds with all other consonants that are oral. Stops are contrasted with fricatives on the basis of how they are produced, plosives by stopping the airstream completely before release, and fricatives by forcing air through a narrow constriction. With the vowels, we contrast high and low, front and back, tense and lax. The idea of classifying speech sounds by contrast eventually led to a more elaborate system of describing speech sounds known as the **distinctive feature approach**.

Distinctive Features

Distinctive feature theories view speech sounds as consisting of several constituents that make them different from each other. We discussed the most prominent of these earlier in the place, manner, and voicing of speech sounds. According to these theories, features are considered to be universal properties of speech segments. That is, each spoken language has sounds that can be described using distinctive features. Several distinctive feature systems have been created, but all of them distinguish each feature through a binary (+, −) approach in which the feature is either present or absent (Chomsky & Halle, 1968; Jakobson, 1949; Jakobson, Fant, & Halle, 1952; Ladefoged, 1971; Singh & Polen, 1972). An important difference between traditional phonetics, which focuses only on the production of sounds via the speech mechanism, and distinctive features is that the distinctive feature approach emphasizes the entire system of attributes involved in sounds across languages. Distinctive feature theory allows us not only to view each sound as being distinct from other sounds, but also to group sounds that share features according to classes by their manner (Sloat, Taylor, & Hoard, 1978). In English, these classes are: stops, nasals, liquids, glides, fricatives, and affricates. We can also group sounds into voiced versus voiceless sounds or sounds made according to a particular place in the oral cavity, such as bilabial or lingual-dental sounds.

Feature differences help us to contrast sounds from one another. Some examples of contrasts include the following:

- Consonantal (consonants) versus vocalic (vowels)
- Continuant (constricted sounds with gradual release of air, such as /f, s, θ, ʃ/) versus non-continuant (limited constriction with sudden release of air, such as stop consonants)
- Coronal (front portion of the tongue for /s, t, l, n/) versus non-coronal (/k, g/)
- Strident (fricatives with a primary and secondary constriction, such as /s, z, ʃ, ʒ/ non-strident fricatives (/f, v, θ/).
- Rounded vowels (/u, ʊ, o, ɔ/) versus unrounded vowels (e.g., (i, e, I, æ/)

Distinctive features also are useful for considering the characteristics of **natural sounds** and **marked sounds**. Natural sounds are common to all languages and emerge first in a child's speech development, whereas marked sounds are found less frequently in languages and develop later because they are more difficult to produce. It is noteworthy that a child who is slow to develop her sound systems will have more difficulty learning the marked sounds, whereas the natural sounds are typically learned more easily (Ingram, 1989). Research studies on development of the sound system show that preschool children master the nasal, grave (front and back sounds), voiced, diffuse (front sounds), continuent, and strident features (Menyuk, 1968), and these features develop gradually from 1 to 30 months (Singh, 1976).

It should be evident from the descriptions of the speech sounds that we know a great deal about their characteristics. Linguists have mapped out the characteristics for all or most of the languages of the world. Regarding English, we all know accurate speech when we hear it, and when the speech of an individual isn't produced accurately, we are able to use our knowledge of sounds to determine what has gone awry. We now can use this information to discover how children acquire this complex system.

 ### Check Your Understanding 8.1

Assess your knowledge of the sound system of English by completing this brief quiz.

Development of Speech Sounds in the Prelinguistic and One-Word Stages

Researchers used the traditional phonetic view and the distinctive feature view of speech sounds to study children's acquisition of speech sounds, especially when they begin to use words. Prior to first words, however, the developmental course of speech sounds is typically described in a few stages, although we again caution that development should be viewed as a continuum of changes across time.

As we have seen in previous chapters, infants very quickly learn to communicate with caregivers. The journey from an infant's cries, coughs, gurgles, and hiccups as reflexive responses to her physical condition and environment, to using speech sounds, to talking about her wants and needs is remarkably fast and predictable. Researchers have divided the course of this development into several age-related periods. Although these periods may differ slightly, it is clear that during the first year we see growth patterns that prepare the infant for speech production.

During the first two months, reflexive fussing, crying, grunt-like sounds, and vegetative sounds occur. These **quasi-resonant nuclei** sounds have a low pitch and a muffled resonance quality (Oller, 2000; Stark, Bernstein, & Demorest, 1983).

The child demonstrates comfort between two and four months through the production of vowel-like and consonant-like sounds that together literally sound like cooing. It is at the end of this period that the vowels begin to become **fully resonant nuclei**, with a full range of frequencies and resonant characteristics. To the delight of his parents and siblings, the child at four months old is able to laugh.

The period between four and six months is very exciting as the child experiments with her voice to produce extremes of loudness and pitch. This **vocal play** includes noises, such as squeals, grunts, screams, and growls, and the always popular "raspberries." Some children seem to fixate on one particular kind of noise for a few days before moving on to another noise, and then sometimes return to an old favorite for a time. **Marginal babbling** consists of single consonants and vowels that are made in a row, such as "a, a, a," and "da, da, da."

The *babbling* period takes center stage between 5 and 10 months as the child interacts more directly and intentionally with his family and environment. Consonants and vowels are combined into CV syllables and even some CVCV syllable combinations. Note that during this period the number of consonants the child has is quite limited. Many syllable combinations are reduplicated ([baba]), but some syllables show nonreduplicated forms ([badu]; Nathani, Ertmer, & Stark, 2006). The sounds the child is producing do not have the consistency of adult phonemes, but they most closely resemble a few stops, nasals, glides, and liquids in combination with the lax vowels. The child also incorporates patterns from his native language, including intonation, rhythm, and pausing, into his babbling (Crystal, 1986). These long strings, known as *jargon*, sound quite similar to sentences, but it will be another couple of months before the child uses his first words. Refer to the third video in Chapter 4 for an example of babbling and jargon.

Although there is considerable disagreement about how phonology develops in a general sense, as we will see when we sample common theories of phonological development, experts generally agree that what happens during the first year of phonological development is largely the result of physical maturation in combination with the human instinct to talk. The best evidence of this is that children from widely varying language and cultural backgrounds sound remarkably similar during this first stage of phonological development.

Before we leave this first stage of phonological development, we should briefly address a central controversy regarding the relationship between *babbling* and *true speech*. The controversy was sparked by two very different interpretations of this relationship. The first view, *babbling drift*, is probably most closely associated with Mowrer (1952). According to this view, caregivers selectively reinforce child vocalizations, so that children's emerging phonological system is gradually shaped to fit the phonological system of their caregivers' language. That is, children's babblings *drift* into adult speech.

Opposing this view is the *discontinuity theory* most closely associated with Jakobson (1968). According to Jakobson, babbling and true speech are two entirely separate stages of development. Whatever relationship they might have to one another is almost coincidental. During babbling, the child produces a wide variety of natural sounds common to many of the world's languages. When the child begins to produce meaningful speech, she stops babbling. She might even experience a period of silence before she begins to acquire the true sounds of her native language. The acquisition of true speech sounds, according to this view, is a slow and deliberate process.

Both of these views have problems. If the babbling drift theory were correct, we would expect that children from varying language backgrounds would sound different from one another by the end of the first year because their babblings would be differentially reinforced. That is, a Japanese child's Japanese-like sounds would be reinforced and a Russian child's Russian-like sounds would be reinforced. Because of the phonological differences among these languages, these children would sound different. But, they do not. If the discontinuity theory were true, we would expect that there would be dramatic differences between the sounds we hear in babbling and the sounds we hear in early speech productions, and we would expect that babbling would have a definite ending and true speech a clearly defined beginning. Neither of these expectations is supported by research. Most children continue to babble for several months after they produce their first true words, and the sounds we hear in true words are remarkably similar to the sounds we hear in babbling.

If neither view is correct, what do we conclude? We conclude that even if we do not fully understand the purposes served by babbling relative to the emergence of speech, the facts of development speak for themselves. That is, the child does not stop babbling one day and begin to produce true words the next. For several months covering the end of the first year and the beginning of the second, babbling and true speech co-occur. To make matters even more interesting, as noted in an earlier chapter of this book, the child will produce what are called vocables (also known as quasi-words, protowords, and phonetically consistent forms) during the transition period between babbling and true speech. A vocable is a production that it is used consistently with clear communicative intent. It does have phonemic and semantic consistency, but it is not an adult word, and it may not even be an attempt at an adult word. The child may call his high chair a *baki*, for example. If he uses this production consistently in reference to the same object, it is a protoword, and it is just as meaningful as *high chair*. The transition, then, from babbling to true speech is just that, a transition. Perhaps the most important conclusion we can reach about babbling itself is that, based on the evidence we have gathered and examined so far, phonological development begins during babbling, before the child begins to produce his first true words (Lowe, 1994; Storkel & Morrisette, 2002).

Not only do we have evidence that babbling and early speech development are continuous developmental processes in typical children, but we also know that children with hearing impairments exhibit different babbling patterns. They babble later and with less frequency than children who hear, and their syllable combinations are not as diverse, especially after about eight months (Oller & Eilers, 1988; Stoel-Gammon & Otomo, 1986). Keep in mind that parents provide lots of contingent social feedback to their infants and the infants look at their faces, thereby gaining feedback and information about how sounds are made. It is also true that parents who are deaf use their hands to babble in a manual way to their children who are deaf and infants respond in like manner (Petitto, Holowka, Sergio, & Ostry, 2001).

At around the time of the child's first birthday, we see a combination of babbling, protowords, and the emergence of **first words**. The first words differ from the earlier forms in that the child conveys meaning in a purposive, consistent, and specific way. Of course, the addition of first words is a very important step in becoming a verbal communicator, but the child is still constrained by his development thus far. It is also true that the timing of first words and the individual words that children choose to say are quite variable from child to child (Grunwell, 1981; Vihman, Ferguson, & Elbert, 1986; Vihman & Greenlee, 1987).

When we examined first words from a language point of view, we suggested that the child often chooses her first words based on the personal importance of their referents, as well as their semantic properties and grammatical functions. To this list of selective factors we can also add phonological characteristics. That is, if the language and personal factors are equal, the child will select words that contain phonological segments that are included in her speech sound system, and she will avoid words that contain phonological information she does not yet possess. This means that given a choice between the targets *dog* and *miniature Schnauzer*, the young child will attempt to say *dog* because its phonological makeup is more consistent with her developing sound system than the phonological makeup of *miniature Schnauzer*. However, it is amazing what children do that seems to defy logic. A child growing up in my extended family was fascinated with the world outside the back door of his home. Construction on new homes captured his attention and his parents were stunned when out of the blue he pointed and said, "bulldozer!" When prompted and bribed with his favorite snack, he was not able to duplicate it. This is a good example of a word that sounds like the adult target but is not used consistently by the child. He understands what a bulldozer is, but he has not mastered its form.

Once the child acquires her first few words, vocabulary development occurs quickly. By the time she is 18 months old, the typical child will have about 50 words in her productive vocabulary, but do not forget the caution about age. It would not be unusual for a child to be using 50 words as early as 13 or 14 months, and it would not be at all unusual for a child to be producing her first 50 words as late as 20 to 24 months.

The title of this chapter reminds us that units of speech are like building blocks for our language, but we also recognize that this analogy is limited. One example of this limitation is the observation that children use **whole-word templates** in the early stages of the acquisition of first words. Vihman and Croft (2007) remind us that children learn language through access to patterns, including verb use, subject-verb-object order, word learning, and phrase learning. Thus, they use whole words or phrases as *frozen* forms as they take in and imitate speech input from the environment and receive social interaction as a result of their attempts. Early frozen forms tend to mirror the consonant and vowel combinations the child has developed thus far and the individual words the child is acquiring. The authors explain that the child will use particular patterns to represent a variety of words, as in the following examples:

Example: palatal nasal used to produce any multisyllabic word containing /n/

Finger—[ne:ne], [ni:ni]

Window—[ne:ne]

Another—[nana]

As we have already seen, children begin to use a few speech sounds in various combinations through the production of their first words at one year of age. Researchers found that between eight months and one year, children used an average of five different consonants in the syllable-initial position (CV) and about three different consonants in the syllable-final position (VC, CVC; Robb & Bleile, 1994). The one-word stage, however, lasts anywhere from 10 months to 18 months, so that by the time the child is 18 to 24 months old, the two-word stage will commence. During this relatively long period of time, there is a good deal of development in the speech sound system. Data collected show that children between one and two years of age use about 11 consonants in the syllable-initial position and 5 consonants in the syllable-final position (Robb & Bleile, 1994). This trend for more consonants emerging first at the beginning of words compared to at the end of words is a consistent finding across many studies (Dyson, 1988; Preisser, Hodson, & Paden, 1988; Stoel-Gammon, 1985).

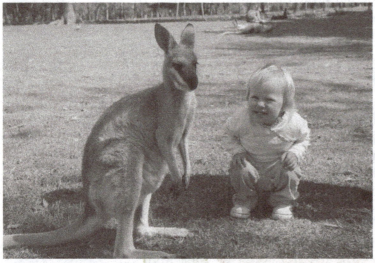

"I'm going to tell my mommy all about this!"

Source: Peter Galbraith/Fotolia.

As mentioned previously, there is much individual variation in the particular sounds children use during the single-word period, but studies show that children acquire sounds from each of the sound classes (stops, nasals, glides, liquids, fricatives, affricates); however, some sounds are not used by most children until later. Stoel-Gammon's (1985) research revealed that at least 50% of her subjects studied longitudinally used the phonemes /h/, /w/, /b/, /t/, /d/, /m/, /n/, /k/, /g/, /f/, and /s/ in the word initial position of words in their spontaneous speech and /p/, /t/, /k/, /n/, /r/, and /s/ in the word final position.

Check Your Understanding 8.2

Assess your understanding of the sound system of English during the prelinguistic and first-word stages by completing this brief quiz.

Development of Speech Sounds in Two-Word Utterances and Beyond

Several systematic studies of English phonemic acquisition in the United States and in Great Britain have been conducted as far back as 1931 and as recently as 2007 (Dodd, Holm, Hua, & Crosbie, 2003; Poole, 1934; Templin, 1957; Vance, Stackhouse, & Wells, 2005; Wellman, Case, Mengert, & Bradbury,1931). These studies were designed to establish norms for phonemic acquisition by assessing the phonemic abilities of large numbers of children within a broad age range. Although the specific methodologies of these studies varied, there was a fairly consistent general design and the outcomes provide information about the range of emergence and mastery of phonemes.

Many studies show that the acquisition of speech sounds is gradual. Some sounds emerge during the babbling, jargon, and first-word stages. Emergence is defined as customary production. This means that about half of children tend to use these sounds in at least two word positions (i.e., first and last sounds in words) before age two. Sounds that emerge prior to age two include /m/, /n/, /p/, /b/, /w/ and /h/. At about two years of age, as children start combining words into two-word combinations, many more sounds appear. These include /ŋ/, /t/, /d/, /k/, and /g/. Notice that the nasals and stops emerge quite early. As you might anticipate, these sounds are also among the earliest to be mastered. Sounds that are considered mastered appear in the speech of 90% of children at a given age. The stops and nasals and glides /w/, /j/ and the liquid /l/ are mastered from three years to four years of age. Note that sound development occurs within a range of time for individual children as it does when comparing children within groups.

▶ Video Reflection 8.1: Two-Year-Old Speech Production

Watch the video to listen to a two-year-old child produce speech: then answer the question.

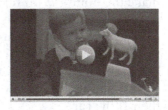

Next in the development journey are the fricatives and affricates. These tend to emerge and become mastered across several years, depending on the particular sound being considered. The /h/, /w/, and /f/ emerge during the first two years, but they are mastered somewhere between ages three and four years. Likewise, the /s/ and /z/ emerge around the third birthday, but can be acquired by some as late as six years.

A group of sounds within the fricative and affricate classes are among the latest sounds to develop. These include the /θ/, /ð/, /ʃ/, /tʃ/, and /dʒ/.

Their emergence occurs during years 3–5 and they are mastered between ages four and seven, with the /θ/ and /ð/ as late as age eight in connected speech.

A sound that presents trouble for some children is the /r/. This sound is sometimes difficult to produce because it requires modification of tongue position when the /r/ follows a vowel. To appreciate the differences, say the following words aloud and hear and feel how the vowel and /r/ interact: *painter* (/ɚ/); *fern* (/ɝ/); *steer* (/ɪr/); *care* (/ɛr/); *tour* (/ʊr/); *more* (/ɔr/); and *dark* (/ar/). Some experts refer to the vowel-r combinations as /r/-colored vowels.

Consonant Clusters

You probably surmise that because the acquisition of single phonemes progresses slowly across many years, the use of consonant clusters is also likely to show this trend. You are correct in this assumption, but you may not know that clusters actually begin to emerge quite early in the speech acquisition process. Going back to the idea that the child interacts with others about the people, objects, and places in his experiences, words that contain clusters are being spoken all the time. So, it should come as no surprise that he will begin to use clusters as early as two years of age (McLeod, van Doorn, & Reed, 2001). We create these **consonant clusters** through using the /l/, /w/, /r/, and /s/ with other consonants. The /l/, /w/, and /r/ follow another consonant (e.g., *play, tweet, truck*), whereas the /s/ precedes them (e.g., *swim, story, split*) or occurs at the end of words (e.g., *skates, dogs, cookies*). Consonant clusters begin to emerge early, but mastery depends on the development of the sounds listed here. Early clusters include the phonemes the child has already acquired, such as /p/, but the phoneme that is paired with it to make the cluster may not yet be developed; thus, the child will create the next best production through substitution. For example, he might point to the sky and exclaim *plane* ([pwen]) using the /w/ as an acceptable replacement for the /l/. Early clusters also help the child add morphemes to the ends of words. For example, in order to make the noun *cup* plural, /s/ will create a final word position cluster /ps/. As is true of phoneme development, cluster development is first focused on those containing stops, with clusters involving fricatives emerging later. In addition to these trends, clusters containing two sounds develop earlier than clusters containing three sounds. Clusters, therefore, are mastered between the ages of four and eight years, with most children using mature productions during their fifth year.

Intelligibility

The best indicator of sound system development is the extent to which others are able to understand the child. Parents and teachers have expectations for how a child should be able to speak at two years of age and how that same child should sound at three, four, and five years of age. We also have data from research that informs us about **intelligibility** expectations. During the child's second year, she should be understood about 50% of the time. During her third year, she is about 75% intelligible and she is completely intelligible at age 4 (Paul, 2007). Researchers and clinicians use a procedure to determine a more precise measure of intelligibility known as the percentage of consonants correct (PCC). From a spontaneous speech sample, the consonants produced incorrectly divided by the correctly produced consonants times 100 yields the estimate of intelligibility. Typically developing children demonstrate 25% to 50% intelligibility during the period between 1.5 and 2 years. Intelligibility increases from 50% to 75% during the second and third years, and during years 4 and 5, children achieve 90% accuracy. Fine-tuning of sounds continues during year 5 and beyond (Hoffman, 1982; Stoel-Gammon, 1987; Watson & Scukanec, 1997). Similar findings for British children show that 3-year-olds are about 82% correct, children 4 to 5.5 years are about 90% correct, and those 5.5 to 7 years are about 96% correct (Dodd, Holm, Hua, & Crosbie, 2003). Of course, English is spoken in many countries around the world; thus, many variations are not only possible, but probable (McLeod, 2007) and English is influenced by the native language of speakers in the U.S. We will consider some of these later in this chapter.

Consider what we can conclude about phonemic acquisition based on the findings of large cross-sectional and longitudinal studies. We can conclude that there is a tendency for some sounds to emerge before others, but we must be careful not to assume that there is a specific order of mastery. As we have already noted, wide individual differences exist among children, which are reflected, to some extent, even in the data provided by researchers. It is also prudent to note that longitudinal or diary data on phonemic acquisition in individual children and the results of studies of small groups of children attest that the individual variability in phonemic acquisition is so great that establishing reliable norms is difficult at best. We should use ages of customary production and mastery, therefore, only as general guidelines for understanding phonemic acquisition and for making determinations about how an individual child is progressing in his own phonemic development. Intelligibility is the most important goal of phoneme acquisition, and the same cautions apply as we consider how individual children are establishing and refining their speech sound system.

Check Your Understanding 8.3

Assess your understanding of the development of the sound system of English during the two-word stage by completing this brief quiz.

Phonological Views of Development

So far, we have focused on the emergence of phonemes as single units of speech, without consideration of their functions within words and longer units of language. The discussion in the literature about phonology began with generative phonology (Chomsky & Halle, 1968). This theory introduced the rule level as part of the representation the learner develops about phonemes as they are combined into larger units. Phonological rules pertain to the regularity that occurs when phonemes are arranged. For example, when a word contains a nasal sound (/m, n/), especially when it comes after the vowel, the vowel becomes nasalized. It is impossible to say the word *hand* without the vowel having some of the nasal feature of the /n/ involved. Thus, a rule might be written stating that a vowel preceding a nasal will be nasalized. There are many rules that explain how phonemes influence other phonemes, depending on their arrangements in words.

Another view of phonology, proposed by Stampe (1979), introduced the concept of phonological processes, which are considered to be "mental operations present at birth that act to restrict a child's speech productions" (Lowe, 1994, p. 9). Essentially, they are simplification strategies that allow a child to produce words even when he does not have mastery of the sounds within the words. Phonological processes are considered to be innate; thus, each child must learn to suppress those that are not appropriate to his native language. Take, for instance, a typical three-year-old child who attempts to the say the word *cup*, but says [tʌp] instead. He must learn to eliminate the process called *fronting* so that he can produce the word accurately. This theory is used quite often in speech-language pathology in order to determine a child's error patterns and to focus on intervention when a phonological disorder exists.

A young child developing speech may simplify words through phonological processes in at least four ways: reduction of syllable structure, substitution of sounds, assimilation of sounds, and changes to vowels. She may decrease the **syllable structure** of words by omitting one or several consonants or by eliminating one or more of the syllables that do not receive primary stress. Table 8.2 shows examples of some typical syllable structure processes. The consonant/vowel combinations seen in the first 50 words include CV, VC, CVCV syllable reduplications, and occasional CVC forms (Ingram, 1974; Stoel-Gammon & Cooper, 1984). As consonant clusters begin to emerge during the second and third years, syllable shapes expand to include single-syllable words containing CVCC and CCVC combinations and two- and three-syllable words with and without clusters (McLeod et al., 2001). The child's task is to gradually eliminate the tendency to reduce clusters in order to produce words containing these complex forms.

Another form of simplification, **substitution processes**, occurs when a child uses phonemes within his developmental level as substitutes for sounds he is not able to use consistently. You will recognize these patterns most often in preschool-age children. Recall that the sounds learned early (natural sounds) will be most likely used as substitutes for later (marked) sounds.

Assimilation processes are rather tricky to identify because they reveal the influence that sounds and syllables have on each other in words. Sounds that occur at the beginning of words can influence what the child produces at the end of the words (*progressive assimilation*), and sounds at the end of words can have a bearing on what the child produces at the beginning of the words (*regressive assimilation*). In either case, the tendency is for one sound to take on the

Table 8.2   Four Types of Phonological Processes

Syllable Structure	Word	Child's Production	Transcription
Weak syllable deletion	alligator	*gator*	[getor]
	telephone	*tel phone*	[tɛlfon]
Consonant cluster reduction/simplification	spoon	*poon*	[pun]
	cream	*weam*	[wim]
Final consonant deletion	boat	*boa*	[bo]
	house	*hou*	[haʊ]
Substitution	Word	Child's Production	Transcription
Stopping	shoe	*to*	[tu]
	valentine	*balentine*	[bælɛntaln]
Fronting	cake	*tate*	[tet]
	go	*do*	[do]
Gliding	lake	*yake*	[jek]
	rose	*wose*	[woz]
Assimilation	Word	Child's Production	Transcription
Velar	dog	*gog*	[gɔg]
	goat	*goak*	[gok]
Alveolar	bunny	*nunny*	[nʌnl]
	party	*darty*	[darl]
Labial	guppy	*puppy*	[pʌpl]
	bottle	*babo*	[babo]
Vowels	Word	Child's Production	Transcription
Centralization	paper	*papa*	[papa]
	bacon	*button*	[bʌtən]
Lowering	rain	*ran*	ræn

identity (or some of the characteristics) of another sound. Refer to Table 8.2 to appreciate a few types of assimilation. Notice that you must look across the entire word to see what is happening when the child simplifies it.

Vowel processes are not as common as processes affecting consonants, but they are important nonetheless. Generally, the child will produce vowels in the center of the oral cavity, making it neither high/low nor front/back. Changes in either of these dimensions will result in vowels that are either too high or low or made too far in front or back of the intended target. Vowel simplification is common in children with hearing loss.

As you might imagine, this pattern approach is quite efficient and effective in allowing the child to convey many ideas with only a few forms. A big drawback to this strategy, however, is that many words sound the same (homonyms), so there is much potential for misunderstanding. These patterns are used with less frequency as the child adds phonemes to her repertoire.

The processes included here are only examples. Hodson and Paden (1991) describe nearly 40 processes, not including idiosyncratic rules that are unique to individual children. We will probably never have a complete list of processes precisely because children are very inventive in their phonological strategies. Just when we think we have heard them all, we will find a child who uses a rule we have never heard before.

With all three phonological descriptions in mind, consider how each would be used to describe what a child does when she makes "errors" on speech sounds. Using the traditional phonetics point of view, if the child says *bu* for *bus*, we simply say that she has an /s/ problem. A distinctive features specialist might speculate that the /s/ is deleted because the child has not yet mastered the strident feature. The phonological processes specialist, taking into account other productions in which final consonants are deleted, might conclude that the problem has nothing to do with /s/ specifically or even with the strident feature. The child says *bu* for *bus* because she applies final consonant deletion to all words that end with consonants.

Each of these approaches to describing phonological productions leads to a somewhat different interpretation about how phonology develops. The traditional phonetic view suggests that phonemes develop as whole entities. The distinctive features view suggests that the child masters features. When he has all the features for which the /s/ sound is marked, for example, he will produce /s/. The phonological processes view suggests that the child masters the adult phonological system by gradually suppressing his rules or processes in favor of adult rules. The two-year-old, for example, applies the final consonant deletion rule to all words ending in consonants, but by the time he is four or five years old, he has suppressed that rule in favor of the adult rule that says that some words do, in fact, end in consonants.

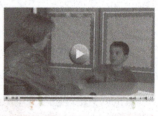 **Video Reflection 8.2:   6-Year-Old Speech Production**

Watch the video to listen to a six-year-old child's speech production, then answer the questions.

Coarticulation and Suprasegmental Aspects of Speech Production

If you had never experienced speech, you might assume that a child learns individual speech sounds before she combines them, in much the same way that children learn the alphabet as the foundation for learning to spell, read, and write. However, children who are just beginning to acquire speech do not practice sounds in isolation, and even their earliest utterances involve combinations of sounds involving complicated interactive adjustments of the speech mechanism.

In the opening of this chapter, speech sounds were compared to bricks in a wall. As is true of most analogies, the brick comparison has limitations. It is true that any given word consists of a finite number of sounds just as a wall, no matter how large, consists of a finite number of bricks. In the case of a brick wall, however, each brick retains its individual identity. It looks and feels the same whether it is in the wall or separate from the wall. When speech sounds are joined into words, they lose some of their individual characteristics. They blend together and influence one another so that the final product is something other than the sum of the sounds. We call the influence sounds have on one another in context **coarticulation**.

We know that coarticulation works in a forward and a backward manner. That is, an early-appearing sound sometimes affects how a following sound will be produced, and sometimes a later-appearing sound will affect how an earlier sound is produced. When an early sound affects a later sound, it is called **retentive coarticulation**. In producing the word *new*, you cannot avoid producing the *ew* with nasality because of the influence of /n/. That is, nasality is retained on the *ew*. If you put the nasal sound after a vowel, the same influence will occur in the other direction. When you produce the word *aim*, the vowel is nasalized because you are anticipating the nasal sound /m/. This is called **anticipatory coarticulation**.

Feel what happens to your lips on the production of the two /s/ sounds as you say the word *seesaw*. Now say the sound /s/ in isolation a few times. Repeat *seesaw* a few more times and sense the lip adjustment again. What is happening here? The sounds influencing the /s/ productions are the vowels (/i/) and (/ɔ/). The /i/ is a front vowel produced with the lips slightly spread, so the /s/ in the first syllable is produced with the lips in a slightly spread position. The /ɔ/ is a back vowel produced with lip rounding, so the /s/ in the second syllable is produced with the lips rounded. These are examples of anticipatory coarticulation. What is truly amazing is that you have no idea you are making these adjustments, and if we asked you how you knew to make them, you could not provide an answer.

Consider what happens when you put two or more consonants together in a cluster or blend as in the words *cluster* and *blend*. In both words, you actually begin to produce the /l/ before you release the first sound. Try to produce the beginning of each word in slow motion. In *cluster*, you are using the back of the tongue for /k/ at the same time that you are moving the front of the tongue to the alveolar ridge for /l/. In saying *blend*, you contact the alveolar ridge for the /l/ before you release the bilabial closure for /b/.

We may not be able to explain *how* we coarticulate, but we should be able to understand *why*. Coarticulation allows us to speak in the most efficient manner possible within the limits of our speech mechanisms. Articulation follows the path of least resistance, which means that the speaker is constantly adjusting according to the challenges presented by the sounds combined in a word or phrase. The adjustments sometimes result in compromises. In saying the word *little*, for example, the /t/ is usually produced as a /d/ because every other sound in the word is voiced, and it's too much trouble to turn off voicing for one sound, and the /d/ is produced with lateral emission rather than frontal emission because it is surrounded by /l/ sounds, which are laterals. Because we all coarticulate according to the same rules, these adjustments and compromises have no effect on the ability of people to understand one another. In fact, if we concisely articulated every sound in every word, we would sound a little strange. Speech that sounds too perfect is not normal!

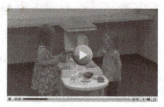

▶ Video Example 8.1

Watch the video of Sophia, who is two years and eight months old, and Becca, who is three years old, engage in parallel play. Listen to each child, focusing on the coarticulation of their utterances. Along with the accuracy of speech sounds, what do you notice about their use of suprasegmental aspects of speech, including the vocalizations of protest from Sophia?

In addition to the constraints on our speech mechanism to coarticulate sounds, languages also conform to particular patterns of stress that influence the degree of emphasis we put on syllables within words and the way syllable stress alters the speech segments. A number of theories help us to account for the variable effects of continuous speech. These include the more general prosodic theory (Waterson, 1971, 1981), the autosegmental theory (Goldsmith, 1990; Hayes, 1988), and the metrical theory (Liberman, 1975; Liberman & Prince, 1977).

Theorists continue to seek explanations for the complexities of speech production. The linear theories described earlier view speech production as a progression of phonemes produced in time in a continuous fashion. One sound and syllable follows another in a "linear string" throughout the speaker's message (Clements & Keyser, 1983). But nonlinear theorists view speech production a bit differently. They seek to account for the effects of the suprasegmental characteristics of speech, particularly syllable stress and the tone of vowels as syllables are combined into words and words are combined into sentences.

Autosegmental theory uses hierarchical tiers to describe the phonological features of sounds as they interact with other sounds and syllable stress. The multilevel tiers provide a way for theorists to view affricates (combinations of stop and fricative sounds), the relationship between sounds within various syllable structures, and the effects of coarticulation as features spread from one sound to another. Feature geometry is a related theory that explains the spreading of some features and the neutralization of other features as sounds are produced in words (Bernhardt & Stemberger, 1988; Clements, 1985; McCarthy, 1988). A detailed journey into these theories is not appropriate here, but awareness that sounds interact within syllables and syllables combine to form words is important for our understanding of the complexities of speech production.

Whatever we might conclude about the value of any of the theories briefly described in this chapter, we can certainly agree that the process of phonological acquisition is far more complex than envisioned by early researchers. We can also agree that we are still searching for a theory that addresses all relevant aspects of development. Such a theory will address the cognitive and perceptual aspects of oral communication as well as the productive aspects. It will account for how developing cognitive and perceptual abilities are related to the neuromuscular requirements for speech. It will certainly attempt to reconcile universal patterns of phonological development with individual variations in acquisition tied to language environment and to children's active role in the process of discovering phonological patterns. Such a theory will address how children formulate hypotheses about how these patterns work and should be applied to newly acquired words, how they test their hypotheses in real-life communication challenges, and how they use their communicative experiences to help build the phonological systems of their languages.

Someone once observed that the more you know, the more you know what you don't know, and that is certainly true in our attempts to understand speech and language, even in an area like phonology, which at one time seemed so simple. Researchers such as Wellman et al. and Poole in the 1930s and Templin in the 1950s thought all we needed to do was count the bricks—the sounds of speech—but the more we have learned about phonology, the more complex we have discovered it to be. It is impossible to separate what the child produces from what she hears. It is impossible to separate what the child performs from what she understands, and it is impossible to separate what she knows and understands from the physical processes that generate speech sounds. Although we are learning more about these intricately interconnected relationships every day, we must accept that a complete understanding of the development of phonology lies somewhere in the future.

Check Your Understanding 8.4

Assess your understanding of phonological development by completing this brief quiz.

Cultural Variations in Speech and Language Production

Throughout our journey to describe the development of the various components of language, we have emphasized the interrelationships between the child's biological system, including physical structures and his emerging perceptual and intellectual abilities, and the role that communication plays in the child's socialization in her community. The home language is a primary contributor in the development of speech sounds and how these sounds are used within the broader context of the production of language. We have focused on the sound system so far in this chapter, but we must include other aspects of language when we discuss the many influences on how we produce our language.

Dialects and Accents

It should be apparent that the issue of language variation is fraught with sensitivities. We must take care to approach this topic with thoughtful and considerate respect, beginning with an understanding of dialect. The term **dialect** is used often, and it is often used with incomplete understanding. Wolfram and Christian (1989) suggest that dialect should be understood in a "technical" sense as well as the "popular" sense. They define dialect as, "any given variety of a language shared by a group of speakers" (p. 1). Taylor (1990) offers a more elaborate version of the same definition: "A dialect is a variety of language that has developed through a complex interplay of historical, social, political, educational, and linguistic forces" (p. 131). All students of dialectology and sociolinguistics would agree that dialect should be understood and treated as a neutral term.

A dialect typically corresponds with other differences among groups of people who happen to be united by culture, social class, or region. That is, people who live in the same region and who share cultural, ethnic, educational, and social values tend to speak the same variety of their national language. The dialect spoken by any given group of people is neither superior nor inferior to the dialect spoken by any other group of people. It must also be understood that every speaker of a given language speaks a dialect of that language. There are dialects of English spoken by many people and dialects spoken by fewer people, but number of speakers does not indicate superiority or correctness. Every dialect of English is linguistically correct within the rules that govern it, and every dialect of English is as valid as any other (Taylor & Leonard, 1999).

A **standard dialect** is considered a variety of a language spoken by people of relatively high status who have economic, political, social, and educational power. Those who speak such a dialect may maintain condescending attitudes toward other dialects and the people who speak them, but one must always keep in mind that standard is relative and there is no absolute Standard English, for example, against which variations are evaluated. The standard dialect of the rich and powerful in Texas is not the same as the standard dialect of the rich and powerful in New York, so that what is standard in one place may be nonstandard in another place.

If we accept that there are some "standard dialects" of English, we must accept that there are nonstandard dialects as well. This is not a problem as long as we remember that nonstandard does not mean inferior. Another term sometimes used for nonstandard dialect is **vernacular dialect**. This may be a better term because it does not connote value. *Vernacular* emphasizes what Wolfram and Christian (1989) refer to as the, "indigenous community dimension of these language varieties" (p. 3).

Whether dialects are standard or vernacular, the differences that separate them occur in grammar, phonology, semantics, vocabulary, pragmatics, and all other dimensions of language. In our discussion of dialects, we consider some of these differences in two major categories of language differences: social/cultural and regional.

Before we continue with our discussion of dialect, we should differentiate between *dialect* and *accent*. These terms are sometimes treated as synonyms by laypersons. Is there a difference, for example, between a southern dialect and a southern accent? The two terms can be separated if one understands **accent** to indicate characteristics of speech or variations in pronunciation and dialect to indicate language differences as well as speech differences (Abercrombie, 1967, p. 19). Understood in this way, *dialect* is the broader term and subsumes *accent*. If a listener perceives only pronunciation differences in the speech of someone else and no language differences, he perceives an accent. If he hears pronunciation and language differences, he hears a dialect that differs from his own.

Social/Cultural Dialects

In introducing the concept of a social/cultural dialect, it is important to reiterate that dialects are not products of biology, but products of culture. In this section, we consider the characteristics of four social/cultural dialects: African American English, Hispanic English, Asian English, and Native American English. All possible variations of English that fit within these broad categories are the products of social, cultural, ethnic, educational, and occupational influences. These dialects are then influenced by regional dialects; thus, African American English in Atlanta, Georgia, differs from African American English in Philadelphia, Pennsylvania, and Hispanic English in New York differs from Hispanic English in Miami, Florida. Keep in mind that we are only highlighting features of four social/cultural dialects. McLeod (2007) provides a comprehensive text that discusses the characteristics of languages across the globe and how the characteristics influence the production of English as a second language.

African American English

Without question, the most studied and most controversial dialect in American English is African American English (AAE), which is also called Black Dialect, Black English Vernacular, and Ebonics (Smitherman, 1994, p. 1; Taylor, 1990, p. 140). The controversy surrounding AAE is the result of misunderstanding, ignorance, and the continuing racial prejudices that tend to divide all black/white issues into "good/correct" and "bad/incorrect." Based on what has been presented in this chapter, you should understand that these evaluative terms have no relevance in any discussion about dialects, because no dialect is inherently superior to any other. Furthermore, it is absolutely unreasonable for any educated person to believe that all African Americans speak AAE. Although there is risk even in the following generalization, it may be relatively safe to say that AAE is the dialect spoken by most working-class African Americans living in working-class African American communities.

Each dialect of a language has its own social and cultural history. AAE has a long, diverse, complex history. According to the creolist theory, AAE is a complicated hybrid derived from several African languages and Portuguese, Dutch,

French, and English (Taylor, 1990). Most of the Africans brought to the United States as slaves came from the west coast of Africa. On the east coast, Swahili was the dominant language, but natives of Africa's west coast spoke hundreds of languages that, although similar in terms of phonology and syntax, had different vocabularies (Taylor, 1972). When speakers of these various languages interacted, they developed common languages so that they could communicate with one another. A common language, called a pidgin, develops as speakers of a non-dominant language accept a few key words, usually related to business or trade, from the dominant language. A pidgin begins as an informal language consisting mostly of nouns and many gestures. As it develops, the pidgin becomes more formal. The vocabulary of the dominant language is absorbed into the non-dominant language, which retains revised versions of its original phonological and grammatical systems. When the pidgin becomes the primary language of a group of people, it is called a creole language. At this point, the original non-dominant language ceases to exist. As the language evolution continues, the creole language becomes increasingly similar to the language of the dominant culture, a process called decreolization (Taylor, 1972, 1990). Part of the development of AAE, then, can be traced to the creolization of the west coast African languages. Elements of these creoles came with the people who were brought to America as slaves.

The influences of European languages on AAE can be traced to the trade initiatives of European countries in Africa. In the early 1500s, Portugal sent ships to West Africa for commercial purposes. Because the Portuguese traders could not learn all the African languages in this area, the Africans learned Portuguese. As one would expect, however, the Portuguese language that became the trading language of West Africa evolved into a creole, the product of Portuguese merged with various African languages. Black Portuguese came to America with the slaves who were brought to Portuguese and Spanish colonies. The Dutch took over Portuguese trading bases in the early 1600s, adding mostly Dutch vocabulary to Black Portuguese. At about this same time, England and France were becoming trading powers in Africa, and their languages were thrown into the mix. The French especially were active in the slave trade, but unlike the Dutch, they did not adopt Black Portuguese as their trade language. Their involvement in the slave markets of Africa, therefore, produced another creole, Black French. The original AAE also came to America by way of the slave trade. Unlike Black Portuguese and Black French, however, AAE became widely and firmly established in the United States because of the constant and intensive contacts between slaves and their English-speaking owners (Taylor, 1972).

Although AAE has changed considerably over the years, mostly as a result of social and educational pressures, it remains a distinct dialect with its own identifiable characteristics and rules. All variations between AAE and Standard American English (SAE) must be understood not as errors but as characteristics of a viable and valid dialect. According to Williams and Wolfram (1977), there are at least 29 linguistic rules of AAE that vary from SAE rules. As should be expected, many of these 29 rules overlap the rules of other dialects of SAE, especially the standard and non-standard dialects of the South. Because African Americans have strong historical connections to the southern states, this overlapping of dialects should be viewed as inevitable.

A complete analysis of AAE would require an entire book. Our purposes will be met by including a summary of selected characteristics of AAE. The selections include some features most of you will readily recognize and features that may be less familiar. Unlike regional dialects that are characterized primarily by vocabulary or lexical differences, AAE differs from

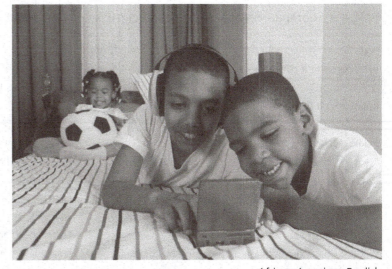

African American English is a valid and valued dialect.

Source: liquidlibrary/Getty Images

SAE in a variety of ways. There are phonological and syntactic differences as well as lexical differences. Examples of some of these differences are included in Table 8.3. As you work through these examples, note the array of differences in how speakers of AAE apply the phonological and grammatical rules of English.

Some of the grammatical differences between AAE and SAE center on whether a rule is obligatory. In SAE, for example, there are obligatory rules for marking plurality and possession. *Dog* is made plural by adding *s* to produce *dogs*. *Dog* is made possessive by adding *'s* to produce *dog's*. In AAE, plurality may be indicated by adding *s*, but it may also be indicated by using words that identify quantity either specifically or generally. This rule results in productions such as *I have two dog* or *I have many dog*. The rule for possession in AAE is similar. That is, possession is understood as long as the possessor is identified, resulting in sentences such as *That's Jim car* or *Mary is John mother*. Refer to Table 8.3 for examples of verb forms.

Some irregular rules in SAE are made regular in AAE. In SAE, for example, the third person singular form of a verb differs from the first and second person forms, resulting in *I hit* (first person), *you hit* (second person), and *she hits* (third person singular). In AAE, the irregularity for third person singular forms is eliminated, resulting in *I hit, you hit, she hit.* Table 8.3 shows examples of regularization of other verb forms, articles, and demonstrative pronouns.

There are at least two differences between SAE and AAE in the production of negation. *Ain't* is a common feature in many dialects of American English as a substitution for *am not, isn't,* and *aren't.* In AAE, *ain't* is substituted for these forms, but it is also used for *haven't, hasn't,* and *didn't* (Taylor, 1990). For example, the sentence *She didn't go to school* becomes *She ain't go to school.* We all learned about double negatives in school, and we were all probably taught that two negatives cancel out into a positive, so that *She don't got no money* means that she does, in fact, have money. Despite the warnings, all children and many

Table 8.3   Comparison of Selected Characteristics of SAE and AAE

SAE	AAE
Final consonant clusters such as /st/ and /sk/.	Tendency to delete second sound of the cluster at the end of words: *rus* for *rust* or *des* for *desk*.
Initial voiced phoneme: *th* /ð/ as in *that, those, them*.	May substitute /d/ in the initial position in a word, as in *dat* for *that*.
Final voiceless phoneme: *th* /θ/ as in *tooth, both*.	May substitute /f/ in the final position in a word, as in *toof* for *tooth* or *bof* for *both*.
Intervocalic phoneme: /r/ as in *carrot*.	May delete /r/, as in *caot* for *carrot*.
Phoneme /l/ in the postvocalic position: may be a final consonant or part of a cluster (e.g., *toll* or *help*).	May delete /l/ in the postvocalic position, as in *toe* for *toll*. May delete /l/ when it precedes /t/, /d/, and /p/, as in *bet* for *belt* or *hep* for *help*.
Plural *s*: obligatory addition of /-s/ to the end of a word, as in *I have two dogs*.	Not obliged to add /s/ if a quantifier is present, as in *I have two dog*.
Possessive *s*: obligatory addition of /-'s/ to the end of a word, as in *That's Jim's car*.	Not obliged to add /'s/ if the possessor is identified in the sentence, as in *That's Jim car*.
Regular past tense: obligatory addition of /-ed/ to the end of a word, as in *She talked to me yesterday*.	Not obliged to add /ed/, resulting in a sentence such as *She talk to me yesterday*.
Copula and auxiliary *to be* verb forms: Obligatory and contractible in certain contexts. Copula: *She is a beautiful woman* or *She's a beautiful woman*. Auxiliary: *They are running fast* or *They're running fast*.	Copula *may* be deleted, as in *She a beautiful woman*. Auxiliary *may* be deleted, as in *They running fast*. See next structure for possible exceptions.
Person and number agreement of copula and auxiliary *to be* verb forms: Copula: *They are beautiful people*. Auxiliary: *They are running*.	If not deleted, inclusion of the *to be* form may result in a lack of subject–verb agreement. Copula: *They is beautiful people*. Auxiliary: *They is running*.
Irregular third-person singular, present tense, as in *She kicks*.	*May* be deleted, as in *She kick* instead of *She kicks*.
Articles *a* and *an*: Obligatory rule says use *a* if the word modified begins with a consonant; use *an* if the word modified begins with a vowel: *a car* versus *an automobile*	General rule is to use *a* whether the sound that follows is a consonant or a vowel: *a car* or *a automobile*
Pronouns *those* and *them*: The pronoun *those* is used as the subject while the pronoun *them* is used as the object. *Those dogs belong to us* (subject). *We washed them yesterday* (object).	Use *them* as both subject and object in sentences, as in *Them dogs belong to us*.
Negation: Substitute *ain't* for *am not, isn't*, and *aren't*, but don't substitute it for *haven't, hasn't*, and *didn't*.	Use *ain't* for all negative forms, as in *she ain't go to school*.

adults of all dialects occasionally use double negatives. In AAE, the rule is that the more negative terms there are, the more negative the sentence, so that *Joe ain't going to no doctor at no time no how!* conveys a fairly powerful message about what Joe intends *not* to do.

One of the most interesting characteristics of AAE is a syntactic device called *aspect* (Warren-Leubecker & Bohannon, 1989). When a speaker wants to convey that an action or state of being is continuing or occurs intermittently, he uses the verb *be*. For example, if the speaker is referring to someone who talks constantly and is now talking, he would say, *He be talking*. If the speaker is referring to someone who seldom talks but is now talking, he would say, *He talking*. In Standard English, both observations would be expressed in the same sentence, *He is talking*. In AAE, *been* is used to describe an action or state of being that occurred a long time ago but no longer exists. To say *Joe been sad* means that Joe was sad a while ago, but he is feeling better now. The SAE equivalent of this sentence is *Joe had been sad*. In AAE, the sentence *I been had this cough* means that this is not a recently developed cough but a cough I have had for a long time. What is most interesting about this feature is that there is no directly comparable version of it in SAE. Labov (1966) has identified this aspect as a feature of several West African languages. It would be reasonable to speculate that this feature of AAE is a remnant of the creole used by the West Africans who were brought to America as part of the slave trade.

One would expect that there would be vocabulary, or lexical, differences between AAE and SAE, and there are. Examples abound (Smitherman, 1994). Unfortunately, the lexical characteristics of AAE change so quickly that any examples provided today could be passé by the time you read this paragraph. Some words used in AAE at the beginning of the 21st century will persist in the dialect for many years. Some will be assimilated into other dialects of American English. Many others will be faddish today and historically quaint a few tomorrows from now. Rather than focusing, then, on an aspect of AAE that evolves faster than our ability to record it, we will turn our attention to the forces that will drive the evolution of the dialect in the future.

Stockman's review (1999) of the semantic development of African American children revealed that semantic knowledge increases with age in AAE, as it does for other speakers of English, but vocabulary is often less developed than that of children who speak SAE. These differences are due to socioeconomic factors, not ethnicity. Keep in mind that the communication system of every person who speaks AAE is also subject to the influences of the regional dialect of English spoken where he or she lives. In addition, as noted by Walker (1999, p. 41), the acquisition of AAE by each child is affected by variables such as family environment, learning strategies, the child's gender and age, the parents' occupations, and the family's socioeconomic level.

Certainly the interactions children have during their developing years will influence not just their language development but their cultural development as well (Taylor & Clarke, 1994). These interactions include but are not limited to the following: child/caregiver, child/family, child/peer, and child/community. If you think about all the variables subsumed within each of these interactions, you will understand that AAE is not now, nor will it ever be, a single dialect. Furthermore, if you consider the power of these interactions to influence the child's development, you will appreciate that the development of AAE will never be static. In fact, the evolution of the dialects of AAE is likely to accelerate during the 21st century because people are, at an ever-accelerating rate, becoming connected globally through the power of mass communication, including the Internet. No matter how much isolationists on all continents might object, we are moving toward a global society. One of the consequences of that movement is that distinctions among dialects, even distinctions among languages, will become increasingly blurred.

Hispanic English

The history of Hispanic English (HE) is not as convoluted as the history of AAE because the historical influences in HE are connected to a single language. This is not to suggest that all forms of Spanish are the same, because that is clearly not true, but AAE is an amalgam of many distinctly different languages spoken by people from widely varying cultures. The evolution of HE followed a much more direct line from one language spoken by people whose cultures had some common denominators.

By the mid-1500s, Spain had a strong presence on the American continent. Spanish explorers moved to the west and the north across what is now Mexico and the southern portion of the United States, taking their language and their culture with them (Ramirez, 1992). Original Spanish settlements established in the 1500s that eventually became major cities in North America include St. Augustine in Florida, Mexico City, San Juan, Santo Domingo, and Havana. In the 1600s, Spanish communities were established in what is now Texas and New Mexico, and between the mid-1700s and the early 1800s, Spanish communities were founded in California. When its territory was largest, New Spain reached from today's Panama to the southwestern boundaries of the United States (Chang-Rodriguez, 1991). New Spain, of course, eventually became Mexico. We see then that the influences of the Spanish culture and the Spanish language began when Columbus arrived in Santo Domingo in 1492 and were firmly entrenched in the Americas by the early 1800s.

A historical factor that affected the Spanish introduced to the Americas was triggered by an event in Spain. When the Moors were driven out of Spain, Queen Isabel decreed that the Castilian dialect should be spoken by all the people of Spain in order that they might become more united. This convergence of events—the defeat of the Moors, the establishment of the Castilian dialect as the national Spanish dialect, and the colonization of the Americas—meant that the Castilian dialect would also be introduced to the Spanish settlements in the Americas.

Even though the Spaniards who settled in the Americas used Spanish, it did not capture the linguistic imagination of Native Americans as Queen Isabel had hoped it would. Especially the settlers who were missionaries found that they could communicate more effectively with Native Americans in their own languages. In some cases, the Spaniards taught Spanish to a few Native Americans and encouraged them to teach the language in their own communities, but many Native Americans resisted, probably for the same reasons people resist having languages imposed on them today. That is, the substitution of a new language for one's native language is tantamount to the abdication of one's culture. It is difficult to imagine any group of people who would not resist this kind of change.

Even though Castilian Spanish was considered the most prestigious Spanish dialect at this time, another dialect emerged as a major influence on what would become HE—Andalusian Spanish. The Spaniards who settled in the islands of the Caribbean and along the coastal areas of the Americas maintained commercial contacts with shipping companies in the southern part of Spain—Andalusia. Spanish spoken in the Caribbean and in the coastal regions of the Americas, therefore, was and continues to be heavily influenced by the Andalusian dialect (Fontanella de Weinberg, 1992).

As the first half of the 19th century concluded, Spanish control in the Americas was waning. Some countries, including Colombia, Peru, Bolivia, Venezuela, and Ecuador, became independent nations (Chang-Rodriguez, 1991). What is now Florida became part of the United States. Mexico, including the territory that is now Texas, gained independence from Spain. Texas then became independent from Mexico and eventually became part of the United States. Other territories that included parts or all of what are now Arizona, California, Colorado, Kansas, Nevada, New Mexico, Oklahoma, and Wyoming were added to the United States, by treaty, in 1848.

As the geography changed, the language influences changed. Changes that occurred in the Spanish spoken in Spain did not occur in the dialects of Spanish spoken in the Americas. The people who lived in those regions that had been under Spanish control but were now under the control of the United States began to use English as their dominant language. Only those communities that were isolated—in the mountains, for example—continued to speak Spanish only. As Spanish-speaking individuals have moved to states such as Texas, Arizona, and California, their Spanish has evolved to become more like the Spanish spoken in Mexico, and more changes in this century are inevitable.

Consider that Spanish is a significantly used language in 21 countries in the Americas (Grimes, 1996). In some countries, it is the first language of almost all citizens. It is the first language of 90% or more of the citizens of Argentina, Chile, Colombia, Costa Rica, Cuba, El Salvador, Honduras, Nicaragua, Uruguay, and Venezuela. Spanish is the first language of 88% of Mexicans. Of the U.S. citizens who speak Spanish as their first language, 10% do not speak English at all, 18.3% do not speak English well, and 71.8% speak it well to very well (Grimes, 1996; U.S. Bureau of the Census, 2007).

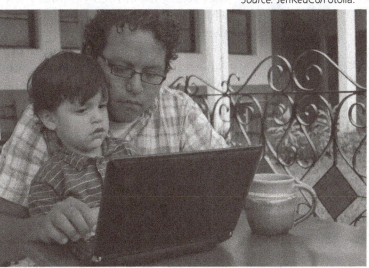

Hispanic English is a widely used dialect in the United States.

Source: JenKedCo/Fotolia.

The reason these numbers are significant can be identified in one word: *immigration*. The influx of Spanish-speaking individuals into the United States has been strong for many years, and it will continue to be strong. There is a factor related to this immigration that cannot be ignored if we are to understand the continuing evolution of HE: not all Spanish-speaking individuals come from the same place. They do not come from a single culture. They do not speak a homogeneous form of Spanish. The most current census figures indicate that among residents of the United States who consider themselves Hispanic, 64% trace their origins to Mexico; 9% to Puerto Rico; 7.6% to Central America and the Caribbean; 3.4% to Cuba; 2.8% to the Dominican Republic; and another 5.5% to South America. More than one-third of these people are first-generation immigrants (U.S. Bureau of the Census, 2007). If we are to understand both the present and the future of HE, we must appreciate what all of these people will bring to HE from their native dialects of Spanish and from their cultures.

Consider, for example, the powerful influence of the family among people who live in Latin America, and we are not talking here about just Mom, Dad, and siblings. In Latin American cultures, children spend considerable time with the extended family, including grandparents, aunts, uncles, and cousins. It is not unusual for a child to be a part of her extended family's daily activities. Godparents are also important players in the child's life. In the United States, being a godparent is largely ceremonial, but that is not true in Latin America. Godparents and members of the extended family are active participants in the child's life. They attend the important events in her life, of course, but they are present for mundane events as well, and they are often consulted when parents are making decisions about the child's life (Bedore, 1999, p. 161).

In Latin American cultures, language, and especially the oral expression of language, is important. A person who has extraordinary speaking talents is held in high esteem. Even when children are very young, they are strongly encouraged to participate in conversations with adults. Storytelling is also highly valued. Children are exposed to narratives early in their lives, and much of what they learn about their culture, their family, and even the towns and cities in which they live is learned through narratives. They listen to these stories, and they learn how to tell them (Bedore, 1999, p. 161).

Even though we can identify factors such as these that seem to tie Latin American cultures together, we should remember that they are only loosely linked because there is considerable diversity among Latin American people, diversity in their cultures and diversity in the variations of Spanish they speak. The lessons in all this are twofold: (1) Those who speak HE are influenced in their language development and their language use, as are people who speak any language, by a multitude of factors; and (2) to appreciate the evolution of HE, we need to be aware of the range of origins from which HE is derived, including Latin America, which presents a variety of cultural, family, and religious influences and its own repertoire of Spanish dialects.

Speakers who have Spanish as their primary and dominant language will find that it differs considerably from English; thus, Standard English reflects these differences. A few examples are provided here, but many more exist. English contains 24 consonants and 12 vowels, whereas Spanish contains 18 consonants and only 5 vowels (Merino, 1992). These differences account for the pronunciation variations of native Spanish speakers as they produce English words. There is no Spanish equivalent for the /t/, /d/, /z/, /tʃ/, /v/, /⁻ð/, / ʃ /, and /dʒ/ phonemes; therefore, English words containing these sounds will be modified to align with the sounds present in Spanish. The five consonants permissible in the final position of words include /l/, /n/, /r/, /s/, and /d/; thus, most syllables consist of the consonant/vowel configuration (Bedore, 1999). The long vowels that predominate in Spanish will take the place of short vowels in English words (Merino, 1992).

Word order is an important aspect of English syntax, but Spanish uses more inflections on words to convey meaning. Thus, questions are made by raising intonation, specific articles show agreement with nouns and pronouns based on number and gender, and verbs are inflected across five distinctions as compared to three in English.

Examples showing the most common ways that Spanish speakers use English grammar include the following (Langdon & Merino, 1992):

Omission of Forms:

The auxiliary verb *is* (*The man eating*/The man is eating)
Pronouns (*Suddenly smiled*/Suddenly she smiled)
Articles (*Dog ate bone*/The dog ate the bone)

Variation in Use of Forms:

Negatives (*He not play*/He doesn't play)
Pronouns (*She is fixing his hair*/She is fixing her hair)
Questions (*How the man feel?*/How does the man feel?)
Noun-verb agreement (*The teacher are coming*/The teachers are coming)

It is also noteworthy that phonological and syntactic forms vary from speaker to speaker, depending on the particular dialect of each speaker. Of course, the dialect of the native language will influence the pronunciation and grammar of English (Taylor & Leonard, 1999).

Children learning to speak Spanish gain vocabulary at rates similar to those of children learning English and other languages (Jackson-Maldonado, Thal, Marchman, Bates, & Gutierrez-Clellan, 1993), but some different strategies appear to be used as they focus on the grammatical cues particular to Spanish (Bedore, 1999).

Asian English

Our focus on AAE and HE in this chapter is certainly justified by the integral role African Americans have played in the cultural history of the United States and by the demographic shifts in our nation that have made the Hispanic population an increasingly influential minority, a minority that continues to grow in numbers, as well as in economic and political influence. At the same time, it is important to recognize that many of those who have immigrated to the United States over the past 40 years have come from Asia, and the projections indicate that the influx of new citizens from Asia will be strong for the foreseeable future. So what can we say about Asian English (AE)? First and foremost, we must emphasize that the cultural and linguistic diversity of those who come from Asia is staggering, so that whatever generalizations we make about AE must be made in the broadest possible strokes, and each generalization will be fraught with the likelihood of exceptions.

To gain more respect for the problems inherent in describing AE, allow yourself a brief lesson in geography and then consider the languages spoken by the people who live in the countries that comprise Asia. When most people think about AE, they think about a form of English spoken by people who come to the United States from Japan, China, Taiwan, Korea, and a few other countries thought of as belonging to the *Far East*. Actually, speakers of AE from the Far East come from, in alphabetical order, Brunei, Cambodia, China, East Timor, Indonesia, Japan, Laos, Malaysia, North Korea, the Philippines, Singapore, South Korea, Taiwan, Thailand, and Vietnam.

But now, look at a map and you will see that Asia is a huge landmass that includes what we typically refer to as the *Middle East*, not just the Far East. The Middle East includes 21 countries: Afghanistan, Bahrain, Cyprus, Iran, Iraq, Israel, Jordan, Kuwait, Kyrgyzstan, Lebanon, Oman, Pakistan, Qatar, Saudi Arabia, Syria, Tajikistan, Turkey, Turkmenistan, the United Arab Emirates, Uzbekistan, and Yemen. Very few of us would think of immigrants from these countries to the United States as speakers of AE. Other countries in the part of Asia that is not considered the Middle East include Bangladesh, Bhutan, Burma, India, Mongolia, and Nepal.

You should be getting a sense here that one of the problems we face in trying to describe AE is that we are dealing with people who come from countries that cover a very large portion of our planet. More importantly, there are not many ties, other than being in the same general geographic neighborhood, that bind all these countries together, but there is an even more significant problem. When we talk about HE, we are at least talking about the interfacing of just two languages, English and Spanish. We have already acknowledged, and we have repeatedly emphasized, that the Spanish spoken by people in Spain is not the same as the Spanish spoken by people who live in Puerto Rico, but at least it is more or less the same language.

What languages are spoken in the Far East that will interface with English when people from that part of the world move to the United States and learn our language? We can say with certainty that the most commonly spoken language is Chinese, but it is far from the only language. People who live in Japan speak Japanese. Those who live in North and South Korea speak Korean. Most people who live in Thailand speak Thai. The official language of Laos is Lao. In most of these countries, however, multiple languages are spoken. In Taiwan, for example, most people speak Chinese, but Japanese and Vietnamese are commonly spoken as well. In Thailand, in addition to Thai, people speak Chinese and Korean. Citizens of Malaysia speak Chinese, Japanese, and Tamil. Without question, the multilanguage champion of the Far East is Singapore.

Citizens of this tiny country, with a total population of about 4.2 million, speak Bengali, Chinese, East Punjabi, English, Hindi, Japanese, Java, Korean, Malay, Sindhi, Teluga, and Thai. According to the Singapore visitors' website, English is their "working language," and it is the most widely spoken language used in that country, but their national anthem is sung in Malay. If you are now sufficiently exhausted by information overload, we can settle comfortably into the point that must be made and understood before you examine Table 8.4. That is, there is clearly no single Asian language that affects the production of English to create what we are calling AE. At most, there are a few common issues that arise when the languages spoken by those who immigrate to the United States from the Far East portion of Asia collide with SAE. We consider some of those English/Asian language characteristics, those we believe are reasonably comparable.

Native American English

There are nearly 2 million individuals in the United States who identify themselves as Native American (U.S. Bureau of the Census, 1990) and they live in every state, especially in the Southwest. But there is nothing homogeneous about Native Americans, just as there is little similarity about any ethnic group living in different parts of the country. In fact, with about 500 distinct tribal entities, each with a separate governing body, language, and culture, it is impossible to discuss Native American English (NAE) as if this includes only one or a

Table 8.4 Comparison of Selected Characteristics of SAE and AE

SAE	AE
Final consonants: Obligatory rule applies.	Omissions of consonants such as /p, t, v, s, z/ are frequent.
Plural /-s/: Obligatory rule applies, as in *He lost two dollars*.	May be omitted, as in *He lost two dollar*. May be added to irregular forms, as in *She saw the mans*.
Possessive /-'s/: Obligatory rule applies, as in *Lane's dog is a wonderful pet*.	May be omitted, as in *Lane dog is a wonderful pet*.
Auxiliary *to be* verbs *is, are, was, were, am* + *ing*: Obligatory rule applies, in that *be* verbs must accompany the use of *ing* on the end of the main verb, as in *The dog is barking loudly*.	May be either omitted or included without marking for person or number, as in *The dog barking loudly* or *They is running*.
Regular past tense /-ed/: Obligatory rule applies, as in *She kicked the ball*.	May be omitted, as in *She kick the ball*.
Articles *the, a*: Obligatory rule applies to specific types of nouns, as in *I have the keys to the car*.	May be omitted, as in *I have keys to car*.

Source: Based on Cheng (1987).

few variations. It is also true, just as with other groups, that geography, lifestyle, and socioeconomic status play a large role in the ways in which Native Americans learn and use English.

We do know that some Native Americans live on the 278 reservations and in the 209 Alaska Native villages located in remote and rural areas (Harris, 1992), and that these isolated areas make accessibility to health care and other services challenging. We also know that rural areas are often challenged in terms of income and educational opportunity (U.S. Bureau of the Census, 2000). There is a very high incidence of otitis media compared to other groups in the United States and across the world (Canterbury, Dixon, & Gish, 1981; Harris, 1992; Toubbeh, 1985), and fetal alcohol syndrome is a major health problem (May, Hymbaugh, Aase, & Samet, 1984).

Native American cultures do share some worldviews, such as those about spirituality, relationships, family structures, and adult–child interactions and child-rearing practices, that differ from those of mainstream American culture. These worldviews influence their interactions with the members of their communities and the wider cultural landscape of the United States. Traditional values and practices have been maintained throughout Native American cultures. Factors summarized by Harris (1992) that determine traditional values and practices include clan affiliation, society membership, formal education, intermarriage, urbanization, and technology.

Like AAE, HE, and AE, NAE is not a unitary variation of SAE. The dialectal variations of English spoken by Native Americans reflect the phonological and syntactic influences of their tribal languages. Several variations of NAE have been described in the literature. Harris (1992) provides a comparison of the phonological and syntactic differences between English and the Navajo language; a few examples of these differences follow:

Phonological System

Six consonants do not occur (/v, f, dʒ, θ, r, η/).
There are limited consonant clusters, and none in the final position of syllables.
Eleven consonants occur in the final position of syllables.
Fifteen sounds do not occur in English.
Simple vowel system with vowel lengthening is used to distinguish meaning.

Grammatical System

There is an intricate verb system for action-oriented language.
There is limited use of plural form on nouns because the number is implied by the verb.
Possession is not marked by a pronoun or suffix but is marked by the noun/possessive pronoun/noun structure (*man his dog*).
Contrasting opposites are made by using the negative (good/not good).
There is no adjective class, but neutral verbs express state, quality, or condition

Our review of the influences of the home language and culture on the development of all aspects of English should cause readers to marvel at the dynamic nature of language in societies. Languages are ever-changing with the complex factors that come to bear on individuals living in their social world. The sociocultural dialects not only are products of the diversity we enjoy in the United States, but also provide diversity to our towns, cities, and states. Another influence on dialect is geography, which we now explore.

Check Your Understanding 8.5

Assess your knowledge of cultural variations of English by completing this brief quiz.

Regional Dialects

For the sake of convenience, we assume greater homogeneity within each identified regional dialect than actually exists. In fact, it is difficult to clearly separate social dialect from regional dialect. Technically, a **regional dialect** refers to a variety of language used by people living in a restricted geographic area, but within that area several social dialects may be spoken by people who are grouped by factors other than geography, including social class, ethnicity, educational level, occupation, and religion. The social dialect is influenced by the regional dialect, however, so that a group of people linked by factors such as those identified here have a different dialect in Houston than in Boston. In other words, regional and social dialects interact, producing variations within dialects of language.

As you might imagine, not all experts agree about the number of regional dialects because they do not all draw lines on dialectal maps in exactly the same places, and regional dialects are defined according to geographic boundaries. Taylor (1987), a specialist in regional U.S. dialects, there are six major regions, which can be divided into many layers and subregions. There are five places along the eastern and southern coasts of the United States from which most regional dialects have evolved: Boston, Philadelphia, tidewater Virginia, Charleston, and New Orleans (Carver, 1987, p. 7). These centers are called **cultural hearths**. In some cases, as in Boston, the original dialectal influences remain strong. In others, the original dialect has been largely lost. In all cases, American dialects constantly evolve as a result of changes in population centers. Because we tend to be increasingly mobile and increasingly connected to one another through a variety of mass media, dialects will continue to evolve, eroding many of the speech and language differences that now exist.

Our discussion of regional dialects includes samples of language differences that have been noted and explained by Carver (1987). This analysis is certainly not complete in breadth or depth, but it provides you with a sense of the dialectal differences that exist in the United States. Regional dialects are characterized by differences in all components of language, including phonology, grammar, and semantics, but the dimension most affected is vocabulary. Certain words that are common to the vocabularies of people living in New England may be unknown to people living in the Midwest. Some words are used and defined differently from region to region. Our discussion focuses on selected examples of these vocabulary differences in just three of the six regions identified by Carver.

The New England and Northeast Region

When many of us think about the speech of people who live in New England, especially in the Boston area, we think about what these people do with the /r/. That is, they drop the /r/ when it should be present in a word, and they sometimes add it where it does not belong. The Bostonian might say *"ca"* for *car*, for example, but he might say *"tuber"* for *tuba*. As with all regional dialects, however, the most notable features of the dialects in this region are in word usage.

The past and present of New England have been powerfully influenced by the sea, and this influence is observed in the language of the people in this area. They use words such as *nor'easter* and *nor'wester* to describe the movements of winds and storms. When the wind calms, they say it is *lulling down*; when the wind increases, they say it is *breezing up*. Some words that were originally nautical terms have developed broader usage. For example, a *bulkhead* refers to a partition between compartments of a ship. The term is now used in New England to refer to the sloping doors of a cellar.

Those who came to this part of the country from England sometimes found new phenomena for which they had no vocabulary, so they adapted words to describe these things. The weather in England, for example, is fairly constant, but the weather in New England changes rapidly and often. Nautical folks in the 18th century referred to a sunny day as an *open* day, so that over time the expression *open-and-shut day* came to mean a day when the clouds come and go. Settlers from England were also unfamiliar with mountain passes, so, using a word known to them, they called this kind of opening between mountains a *notch*.

Many terms in the dialects of this region reflect not influences of the sea but experiences of rural living. *Creepers*, for example, are metal cleats fastened to boots for the purpose of providing sure footing on ice. A bobsled is called a *double runner*, *double ripper*, or *traverse sled*. When

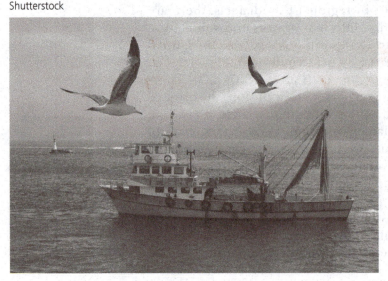

The influence of the sea is apparent in New England dialects.

Source: Martin Lehmann/ Shutterstock

one hauls something, he *carts* or *teams* it. If a horse or cow is uncooperative or mean, it is described as *ugly*, but an *ugly top cow* is a bull, and not necessarily ill-tempered.

This region has produced many unique terms for food items. Some of these terms, such as *Boston brown bread* or simply *brown bread*, refer to recipes unique to the region, but most are terms used to name food items found throughout the country. For example, a submarine sandwich is called a *grinder*, and a soft drink is called a *tonic*. *Hamburger* and *frankfurter* are often shortened to *hamburg* and *frankfurt*. A poached egg is called a *dropped egg*, a term unique to New England dialects.

Many other terms peculiar to this region do not fit the categories already identified. For example, older residents of the region may refer to a funnel as a *tunnel*, and if liquid poured through the funnel comes out slowly, it is coming out in *dribs and drabs*. An apartment building is called a *tenement*, and a veranda or open porch is called a *piazza*. Someone who is especially rigid or fastidious is called a *fusspot* or *fussbudget*. Taking a shortcut is *cutting cross-lots*.

The Northeast region beyond New England includes New York, most of New Jersey, and Pennsylvania (Carver, 1987), but the influences of the dialects in this region extend to the North and West. Since this portion of the region was settled by New Englanders migrating westward, many of the terms used in New England are used by other speakers in the region. Some words, however, are associated with specific areas of this region beyond New England. For example, although the term *cruller*, referring to a doughnut, is widely used in many areas of the country today, it was originally a word unique to speakers from the Hudson Valley. Speakers from New York refer to a freeway or expressway as a *throughway*, to curdled or sour milk as *lobbered milk*, and to a whisk broom as a *brush broom*. Speakers from the greater New York metropolitan area, including northern New Jersey, refer to a particularly large and aggressive mosquito as a *Jersey mosquito* or *Jersey bomber*. Other words are common to speakers throughout the region, including *nightwalker* for night crawler or large earthworm, *soda* for soft drink, *scallion* for small onion, and *grass* for asparagus. There are also slang words or phrases characteristic of the dialects in this region, including *can* in reference to buttocks, *nanna* in reference to one's grandmother, and *get a wiggle on* to mean hurry up!

The Northern and Midwest Region

The boundaries of this area are difficult to define with great precision, but it may be useful to think of this region as spreading from coast to coast, with the Ohio River as a rough dividing line between North and South. Even though this region covers a wide geographic area, the dialects have been primarily influenced by only two cultural and linguistic hearths: New England and southeastern Pennsylvania. As these cultures moved westward across the United States, they mixed and influenced each other, eventually producing a shared dialect. There are variations within this broad dialect, of course, but our focus is primarily on the common features.

Although some dialects, including the New England dialect, still show influences of older English and include words borrowed from other European languages and American Indian languages, the dialects of this region are remarkably free of these influences. A few words such as the German word *fest,* meaning "festival" or "holiday," are retained in the dialects of the Northern/Midwest region, but *fest* is most often included within the words *gabfest* or *talkfest* to refer to an informal conversation or gossip session. Other self-explanatory words have been coined from the morpheme *fest,* including *beerfest, slugfest,* and *funfest.* Another word borrowed from German and used in this region is *gesundheit,* an expression used in response to a sneeze. Some speakers who use this expression may believe it means, "God bless you," but it is actually just a way of saying, "I wish you good health."

A number of slang and colloquial expressions are used throughout the country but are most common in this region. For example, a person who works hard sweats *like a butcher.* A cigar is called a *rope,* and a cigarette is called a *coffin nail.* A common euphemism for regurgitate is *toss one's cookies.*

Speakers in the upper portion of the North region use *squealer* in reference to an informer, *milquetoast* in reference to someone who is shy and timid, *crusty* in reference to someone who is aggressive and nervy, and *souse* to mean a drunk. There are also phrases common to this area, as shown here. The meanings of these phrases should be clear:

> I wouldn't run a marathon *for all the tea in China.*
>
> He's always trying *to get the best of* his friends.
>
> Jim's brother is *meaner than dirt.*
>
> Why, I haven't seen that movie *in a dog's age.*

The Southern Region

We tend to think of the speech of people who live in the southern states as representing a single dialect. In actuality, there are a variety of dialects in the South, but we treat it as one region and provide dialectal examples from throughout the region. The dividing line between North and South extends westward from central Delaware, along the traditional Mason-Dixon Line and the Ohio River to an area west of the Mississippi River, including some or all of Texas, depending on whose version of the region one accepts.

The dialects of this region are characterized by uniquely American words and phrases, including *snake doctor* for dragonfly, *calling the hogs* for snoring, *egg turner* for spatula, and *cooling board* for the slab on which a corpse is laid. Other words are adaptations of common English words, including *puny* to mean not only small and weak but also sickly, *harp* for harmonica, *rogue* for a thief or scoundrel, *spew* for gush, *slouch* for a bungler or clod, and *piddling around* for wasting time.

Because the South is primarily a rural area, a definite rural flavor is evident in the dialects of the region. Words relating to the farm experience include *hand* for farm worker, *overseer* for supervisor, *dusky dark* for twilight, *critters* for animals, *juicing* for milking cows, and *cowlot* for pasture. If a farmer works too hard, he may feel *wore out*, and if he continues to work too hard, he may *take sick* and lose weight or *fall off* a bit.

Other common words and phrases heard in the dialects of the South include *fussing* for fighting, *draw up* for shrink or squeeze, *slosh* for spill or splash, *johnny* or *commode* for toilet, *booger* for child, *sowbelly* for pork, *calaboose* for jail, *ruther* to show preference, *earbob* for earring, *dead cat on the line* for something that is suspicious, and *jump the broomstick* for getting married.

One of the more distinct subregions in the South includes Louisiana and especially the area around New Orleans. The French were among the first to settle this area, and even though settlers came from other parts of the world, including Germany, Spain, and what is now known as Nova Scotia, the French influence has remained strong. It is, in fact, this French influence that gives New Orleans its unique character. The dialect of this region retains a distinct French flavor. Carver refers to this dialect as "Louisiana French" (1987, p. 141). It contains words borrowed directly from French and incorporates other words borrowed from British English, Spanish, and Indian languages. Words common to Louisiana French include *armoire* for a dresser or bureau, *gallery* for porch, *lagniappe* for a modest gift or bonus, *bayou* for a marshy stream or creek, *pirogue* for canoe, *marais* for swamp, and *coulee* for dry creek bed.

Many people associate New Orleans with excellent French food. Louisiana French includes culinary terms such as *praline* (candy made with pecans and brown sugar), *gumbo* (stew containing meat or seafood and vegetables), *jambalaya* (rice with tomatoes and herbs along with chicken, ham, oysters, or shrimp), *brioche* (coffee cake), *bisque* (cream soup), and *pigeonnier* (roast pigeon).

It is rather fun to test your knowledge of words and their pronunciations from various parts of the United States. Several websites have quizzes about vocabulary and accents. Give them a try!

Check Your Understanding 8.6

Assess your understanding of regional dialects by completing this brief quiz.

SUMMARY

We devoted this chapter to the development of speech sounds because it is an important aspect of our language system. We described speech sounds according their characteristics and discussed how speech sounds and speech sound clusters develop during each stage of language, starting with the prelinguistic period and ending with multiword utterances. Children who are learning to speak use simplifications of words as a normal developmental strategy, so we describe the most common types of these phonological processes as examples of how children gradually move from simple forms to more complex forms as they perfect their speaking skills. Speech acquisition is a complex endeavor that requires the interdependence of our biological structures and functions, cognitive abilities, and social interactions.

This chapter also focused on sociocultural dialects and regional influences that produce much variety in the way that English is spoken across the United States. We show some prominent features and examples of the components of language to highlight dialectal trends.

▐▌▶ Surfing the Web

If you are interested in exploring topics discussed in this chapter in more detail, search for one or more of the following relevant terms online.

English phonetics
development of English phonemes in children's speech
phonological development in children

development of consonant clusters
phonological processes in children's speech
coarticulation of speech sounds
suprasegmental aspects of speech
dialects and accents in the U.S.
quizzes to test knowledge of American dialects

Chapter Review 8.1

Recall what you learned in this chapter by completing the Chapter Review.

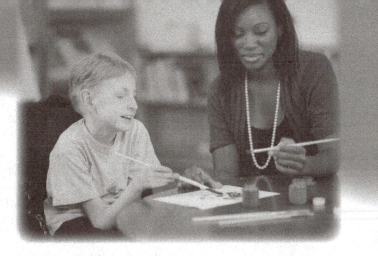

9

Speech and Language Disorders in the Home, School, and Community

LEARNING OUTCOMES

After completion of this chapter, the reader will be able to:

- Differentiate between what is considered normal and disordered speech and language.
- Discuss the interrelationships of speech and language and their impact on learning.
- Describe the causes, contributing factors, and types of communication disorders.
- Discuss the characteristics of several speech disorders.

> "The fitness of the person of the 21st century will be defined, for the most part, in terms of his or her ability to communicate effectively" (Rubin, 2009, p. 9). We live in an age in which we depend on our communication skills far more than in ages past. In fact, Ruben reflected on data from the U.S. labor, that at the end of the 20th century, 62% of employed citizens used communication skills as a primary function of their work, compared to only 20% at the beginning of the century. Additionally, the remaining 37%, who were farmers and blue-collar workers, reported that communication was necessary in their work. Our reliance on effective communication depends on normal development of the many aspects of speech and language that we have addressed in this book.

Defining Communication Disorders

The acquisition of speech and language is so natural that we may not truly appreciate the complexity and power of human oral communication unless or until something goes wrong. In the United States, about 10% of the population have speech, language, or hearing problems. Some may be surprised that this many people have communication disorders. When we consider how much language knowledge the child must acquire, how quickly she acquires it, and the incredible neuromuscular mechanisms that must be coordinated to make speech work, we must be amazed that more people do not have communication problems. In fact, it's a wonder that any of us master the mysterious and magical processes of speech and language.

When speech, language, and hearing problems occur, they pose significant challenges for individuals, their families, and society. Consider the child who is born with a developmental disability leading to lifelong limitations in language, education, social, and employment outcomes. Unemployment rates and low income are associated with individuals with disabilities. The U.S. Department of Labor reported that in May 2013 people age 16 and older without disabilities had a 64% employment rate and an unemployment rate of 6.9%. Conversely, individuals who had a disability were employed at the rate of 18%, with 13% unemployed (U.S. Department of Labor, 2010).

Communication disorders are estimated to affect from 5% to 10% of the population and are among the most common disabilities in the United States. It is difficult, however to derive a true sense of the prevalence of communication disorders because there are many types of disorders and prevalence figures vary depending on the ages one considers. The American Speech-Language-Hearing Association (ASHA) reports on both the incidence and the prevalence of communication disorders. **Prevalence** refers to the number of people in a specified population who have a disorder at a given time. **Incidence** refers to the number of people in a specified population who had, have now, or will develop a disorder during their lifetimes. The incidence of stuttering is 4-5%, which means that from 4% to 5% of the members of a population will develop stuttering at some point during their lifetime, but the prevalence of stuttering, reflecting the number of people in the same population who are stutterers at a given time, is just 1% (Andrews, 1984; ASHA, 2008a; Zebrowski, 2003).

Let us consider some data regarding communication disorders in children from ASHA (2008b) and the National Center for Educational Statistics (2013):

- More than 6 million school-age children were served under the Individuals with Disabilities Education Act (IDEA Part B) in 2012.
- Speech or language disorders as the primary disability account for 21.4% of children served under IDEA Part B.
- A positive family history (parent or sibling) of communication disorders is present in 28-60% of cases.
- Fluency: 4-5% of the population experience stuttering in the second to fourth year and persistent stuttering is more common in boys than in girls. About 1% of the population stutters.
- Voice: Hoarseness is the most common symptom in 6-23% of school-age children and children respond to treatment. Lifetime voice problems occur in 30% of the population.

- Phonological: It is the most commonly treated disorder in prekindergarten (68.8% of caseload;).
- Language: Prevalence of language disorders in preschool children is 2-19% and specific language impairment affects 7% of children.
- Hearing: Genetic hearing loss affects 1-6 per 1000 live births and about half of all cases of infant hearing loss are from genetic causes; children served for hearing impairments under IDEA Part B comprise less than 1% of the total.
- Learning disability: Among school-age children, 43.8% have some form of learning disability with a lifetime prevalence of 3-13%. Learning disabilities account for 4.7% of children served under IDEA Part B.
- Autism: There is wide variation in prevalence reports between professional disciplines, resulting in a range of from .2 to .6 per 10,000 individuals. School-age children served under IDEA Part B (2002) for autism account for 7%.
- Dyslexia: Reading disorders affect 5-20% of the population.

We have emphasized repeatedly in previous chapters that there are predictable patterns in the development and use of each aspect of human communication. We also continue to point out that individuals vary considerably from one to another. Normal differences account for this variability and include intellectual abilities; hearing and visual status; early environmental factors affecting social, emotional, and learning abilities; physical development; and the integration of factors that make us who we are. Given the complexity of human growth and development, it is not difficult to imagine how one or more factors can impact the development and use of speech and language for communication and learning. As we consider communication disorders, you should keep in mind that we often cannot determine a single cause of a problem. In most cases, a combination of factors is responsible. We certainly look for the factors that may contribute to a specific disorder, because some ongoing factors may be amenable to intervention. For example, we can use parent education to increase the number of words and communication exchanges parents have with their young child in order to assist the child in learning many more words, or we can seek medical management of chronic ear infections so that a child will no longer have repeated difficulties hearing everyday language.

You probably have encountered people with communication disorders, and there may be individuals within your own family who have communication challenges. We recognize that at some point, the individual variations diverge too significantly from what we consider normal. It is not always easy to make this determination, because the way a person is able to function depends on the context of the interactions. A child in his home environment will be able to communicate with his parents even when speech and language are significantly impaired, because not only do they share a social and an emotional bond, but they also have the experience of interacting on a daily basis.

 Video Example 9.1

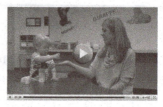

Jackson is 21 months old and uses mostly single words. Although two-word utterances are scarce in his repertoire, they are expected between 20 and 26 months. Watch the video to see Jackson's mother express her concerns about her son's limited expressive vocabulary and two-word combinations. She discusses his medical history as one factor that might relate to his language development and the strategies she is using to increase his language skills.

Some criteria help professionals determine when a communication disorder exists. In 2001, the World Health Organization (WHO) developed the International Classification of Functioning, Disability and Health (ICF). The classification system helps practitioners to assess a person's disability and its effect on other aspects of her life. The first consideration is the body structures and functions. For example, if a person has a cleft lip and palate, the *structure* of the speech mechanism is not normal. When the cleft involves the soft palate (velum), the amount of tissue may not be adequate for the velum to make contact with the wall of the pharynx. This lack of contact will cause exhaled air to leak out the nasal cavity rather than be directed into the oral cavity for production of sounds. Thus the *function* of the mechanism is impaired. During the production of speech, the person with the cleft lip and palate will have too much nasal resonance during speech (hypernasal resonance) and will have difficulty producing sounds that require oral air pressure. Recall from Chapter 8 that stops, fricatives, and affricates are the classes of sounds that require air pressure. When air leaks into the nasal cavity, pressure is lost or is even expelled through the nose upon consonant production. The resulting speech problem may be severe enough to limit the *activities and participation* of the child. Speech may be very difficult to produce and the child may both be delayed and have very poor speech quality. As a result of poor speech, the child may develop a low self-esteem and have difficulty establishing friendships. The *social* consequences due to difficulty communicating must be taken into account when determining the impact of a disability. The use of the ICF is one way to think about the far-reaching effects of communication disorders.

One of the most widely used definitions of disordered speech is offered by Van Riper and Erickson (1996): "Speech is impaired when it deviates so far from the speech of other people that it: (1) calls attention to itself; (2) interferes with communication; or (3) provokes distress in the speaker or the listener" (p. 110). The advantage of this kind of definition is that it focuses our attention on what might be called the keys of communication abnormality. Van Riper and Erickson suggest, in fact, that their definition can be reduced to three key adjectives: *conspicuous, unintelligible,* and *unpleasant.* The disadvantage of this definition, in either the long or short form, is that it is very subjective.

Nevertheless, it provides an appropriate foundation for understanding what is meant by disordered communication.

Most communication disorders, in their most severe forms, are *conspicuous*. You have perhaps observed a person who has a severe stutter whose face becomes distorted as he struggles to get out a single word. Maybe you have listened to a person with a cleft palate who is so excessively nasal that you pay more attention to the quality of his voice than to the content of his words. Whenever speech is so far removed from normal that listeners' attention is drawn more to the manner of speech than to the message being conveyed, it may be considered disordered.

When speech differences reduce *intelligibility*—that is, when they interfere with the ability of listeners to understand what a speaker is saying—there is probably a communication disorder. We have all listened to youngsters who do not have complete sound systems. They leave out so many sounds, or substitute for them, that we understand little of what they are trying to say. When a child is 24 months old, we would not expect her speech to be completely intelligible, and if we could understand only half of what she was trying to say, we would probably not consider her speech disordered; but if the same child at the age of 6 years was still only 50% intelligible, we would undoubtedly agree that her speech was disordered. However, reduced intelligibility might be the consequence of regional or cultural dialects, and, as we established in Chapter 8, dialectal differences are not considered disorders. Some individuals have intellectual and motor challenges that make speech production difficult. It is sometimes necessary for social and academic purposes to teach them to use assistive technology as they are learning to produce speech with acceptable intelligibility.

 Video Example 9.2

Watch the student in this video work with her speech-language pathologist to request objects using her high-technology assistive device. When the student strings picture icons together and presses play, she is able to hear her sentence. Practice creating requests will eventually lead to spontaneous verbal participation through the use of the device in the classroom.

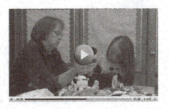

Deciding what is *unpleasant* to a speaker or his listeners might be the most troubling aspect of understanding disordered speech because it is the product of individual perception. The range of tolerance for speech differences is as wide as the range of tolerance for all other human differences. It would probably be fair to say that we would not call speech disordered, on the basis of listeners' perceptions, unless *many* people found the difference unpleasant.

The only single perception that really matters is that of the speaker. If she considers her speech to be unpleasant, it really does not matter whether anyone else agrees, especially if the rest of us cannot persuade her that nothing is wrong with her speech.

We must not forget that speech is only one aspect of communication. Language competence is necessary for effective communication. Thus, normal language at any given age must include the appropriate levels of understanding and expression of all aspects of language we have addressed in earlier chapters. Incomplete development in some or all of these components will result in conspicuous, unintelligible, and maladaptive communication. It is also true that oral speech and language attainments are foundational to the development of literacy. While reading disorders may exist in children without speech and language disorders, children who have these disorders are at high risk for literacy problems. Let us look at the interaction of speech, language, and literacy problems in four cases described in the next section.

Check Your Understanding 9.1

Assess your understanding of the characteristics of communication disorders by completing this brief quiz.

Interrelationships and Impact of Speech and Language Disorders

We have discussed the various aspects of speech and language in previous chapters, especially phonology, morphology, syntax, semantics, and pragmatics. It is fair to say, however, that speech and language problems are rarely confined to these neat categories. Recall that from the beginning of this book, we have stressed the interrelationships and the dynamic and interactional processes of speech and language. In keeping with this philosophy, we describe speech and language problems through the use of four student profiles. As you read about each of these four individuals from an educational standpoint, consider also the impact that their communication disorder likely has on their home life and their interactions within their community. Communication disorders have far-reaching consequences throughout a lifetime for interactions with family members, academic success, social and emotional development, and vocational choice and fulfillment.

Four Students with Speech, Language, and Learning Problems
Jacob is three-and-a-half years old.

He currently attends a literacy-based program for preschoolers where stories form the basis of interactions about language. Jacob's parents note that he was very late to talk, saying his first words at 20 months and putting words together at 36 months. He is gaining vocabulary slowly, and two-word utterances still dominate his expressive utterances. Jacob appears to understand some of what others say to him, but his parents use both gestures and demonstrations to make their meanings clear. He requires a lot of repetition in order to gain understanding and use of words. Although Jacob is quite outgoing, his speech is difficult for others to understand. Children his age like to play with him on the equipment at the neighborhood playground, but they often don't include him in conversation. Children just one year older refer to him as "the baby."

The speech-language pathologist working with Jacob (Ms. Reed) describes him as having a severe language disorder. His phonological development is significantly delayed as evidenced by his production of consonant/vowel constructions that include early-acquired speech sounds in place of sounds consistent with the intended sounds we would expect to hear from a child his age. He is beginning to show frustration by walking away or getting angry when others do not understand him. Jacob is also using noun/verb and verb/noun constructions (e.g., *doggie bark; go daddy*) to communicate his ideas. He is learning many new words during his four hours of intervention each week, yet review and practice of these words are necessary for him to retain them. Ms. Reed noted the following characteristics about Jacob:

- Limited intelligibility of single- and two-word utterances
- Use of CV and VC combinations for words
- Frustration due to his difficulty in using language with others
- Limited receptive and expressive vocabularies
- Poor retention of new vocabulary, with need for repetition
- Expressive language combinations limited to nouns and verbs
- Incomplete comprehension of language

Max is nine years, two months old and in the third grade.

He attended child care during his third, fourth, and fifth years and began kindergarten at age six. His parents decided to wait one year past his fifth birthday to enroll him in kindergarten due to his poor speech development. Max had chronic ear infections (otitis media) from birth through age three. Consistent medical care and the insertion of pressure equalization tubes at age three ended the ear infections and presence of middle ear fluid. Max began talking late, using single words from 15 months to just before his third birthday. When he started to combine words and use simple sentences, his speech was unintelligible to listeners outside of his family. Max received speech-language therapy from ages three to six years. The speech-language pathologist's goals for Max were to increase his development of phonology to improve speech intelligibility, heighten his awareness of the properties of sounds within words (phonological awareness), introduce print awareness, and build his syntactic abilities.

Ms. Moore is Max's third-grade teacher. She notes that Max sounds immature for his age and has residual speech errors, including /r/, /l/, /θ/ and /s/ and blends that contain these sounds. He is also the poorest reader in her class, and his writing is slow and filled with spelling and grammar errors.

Max has not fully mastered the alphabetic principle and he lacks metalinguistic knowledge, including rhyming and segmentation of words by syllable and sound. Ms. Moore describes his classroom difficulties:

- Articulation errors during speaking that affect his social interactions
- Reading fluency problems due to poor word attack skills at the first-grade level
- Recalling and using sound/symbol relationships in decoding words
- Using context to solve decoding problems
- Understanding what he reads due to poor decoding and long delays
- Learning to write short sentences using accurate sentence structure
- Learning to write words and sentences using accurate spelling
- Frustration with language arts class

Megan is fourteen years, three months old.

She attended a half-day preschool at four years and began full-day kindergarten at five years of age. Megan is now in the eighth grade, having repeated the fifth grade. Throughout her schooling, she has remained motivated and hardworking, yet has a high degree of frustration when the outcome of her work does not match her effort. Megan struggles mostly with semantics. She has difficulty learning, retaining, retrieving, and using new concepts and vocabulary; connecting acquired knowledge with new information; and reasoning and problem solving. She appears to have mastered the basic structural aspects of language for articulating clearly and constructing complex sentences, yet she doesn't always fully comprehend complex sentences and multiple directions in the context of classroom instruction. Megan has a small group of friends and appears to be a happy, well-adjusted teenager. She sometimes feels left out at social outings and doesn't understand the use of slang and the subtle humor of jokes and puns. Megan is interested in being a teacher someday, but wonders how she can overcome her language and learning problems to do well in college and function as a teacher in the classroom.

Megan's teacher encounters her frustration on a daily basis. Mr. Bailey is an experienced teacher who believes that all students can succeed. He teaches all of the subjects in Megan's grade except math and science. He encourages Megan to complete her work and rewards the extra time she uses for homework with the help of her parents. Megan is having difficulty with many aspects of the curriculum. Specifically, she struggles with social studies/history, science, English literature, and story problems in mathematics. Mr. Bailey describes her primary difficulties in the classroom:

- Understanding complex oral and written directions for projects and assignments
- Recalling information on exams or during class discussions from lecture or readings
- Using background knowledge to predict outcomes from discussions, debates, narratives, or plays
- Using background knowledge to make inferences during discussions or readings

- Understanding and using multiple meanings of words through contextual cues
- Developing new and expanded definitions for words, as wells as flexibility and variety of word use
- Explaining and understanding metaphors and other figurative forms encountered in readings, discussions, and social interactions

---

 Video Example 9.3

Students having difficulty in the semantic domain of language face challenges in understanding and using a variety of words with flexibility and confidence. Watch the video of a second-grader determining how to use adjectives in sentences.

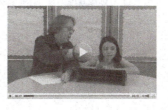

Tory is seventeen years, seven months old.

He was adopted from a Korean orphanage at age three. Tory's early life circumstances are unknown, but his physical condition at the time of his adoption was poor. He was malnourished and had pulmonary tuberculosis, several internal parasites, and delayed motor and language development. He had meningitis at three-and-a-half years of age, however, his recovery was complete, and his hearing was normal. Tory's language development during his preschool years was quite delayed across all areas, and he had great difficulty in social interactions. However, he made rapid progress in speech-language therapy and by age six attended kindergarten. Tory's language structure (articulation, morphology, and syntax) was challenging early on, but he rapidly acquired phonological and syntactic abilities, such that he was completely intelligible and he used compound and basic complex sentences by age seven. His understanding of concepts and vocabulary also blossomed, so that he is now adept at acquiring new information and using past knowledge and experiences to construct new ideas. Tory is an avid reader and enjoys novels, poems, autobiographies, biographies, and expository material. He is especially interested in movie production and aspires to earn a bachelor's degree for work in the film and television industry. Tory's residual language difficulties are in his social use of language (pragmatics). He and his family are concerned that his poor oral communication skills will limit his ability to fulfill his career goals. Tory is also concerned that he doesn't have friends and has problems communicating with others in both social and academic settings.

Mrs. Karrington is Tory's 11th-grade homeroom and English teacher. Tory's primary area of difficulty in high school is using language to interact socially and educationally with others. He is able to construct narratives, but is hampered in his ability to engage in conversation and discussion. In the classroom, his social interaction is limited to asking and answering questions, giving book or other oral reports, and writing. Mrs. Karrington is using literature in her classroom to teach various literary genres, and she employs a discussion-based style. She has concerns about Tory's limited participation in class, which is affecting his grades in her class and in other classes, as well as his social development, self-esteem, and career goals. She describes his primary classroom difficulties:

- Demonstrating and using knowledge of various oral genres, such as persuasion, debate, and storytelling
- Using language to convey opinions, procedural knowledge, directions, and exposition when interaction with others is involved
- Engaging in discussion to share ideas, using turn taking and topic maintenance
- Conversing with others to arrive at a consensus regarding a course of action
- Conversing with others for social interactions
- Using and interpreting figurative and nonverbal language appropriate to situations

These four students, ages 3.5 to 17.5 years, with their strengths and needs in classroom situations, represent a wide range of language-learning problems that teachers encounter in their classrooms. Teachers often understand how each student's language problem directly impacts the tasks that are required within the classroom, sometimes without knowing or recalling the specific causes if known, or the results of language assessments.

It should be evident from these profiles that language problems occur early in a child's life, and they are often detected when parents determine that their child is not gaining the components of language in a timely fashion. This may seem to be a simple matter, but recognizing the point at which a child is not progressing is far from straightforward. It is also true that most communication disorders are not easily remediated, and the way the disorder affects the individual depends on the language task demands of home, school, and community activities. A preschool-age child will have the support of parents and siblings at home, but when the child goes to school, the demands of the curriculum will become increasingly difficult for the child who has a weak language system.

Check Your Understanding 9.2

Assess your understanding of the interrelationships of the components of language by completing this brief quiz.

Causes and Types of Communication Disorders

It is challenging for speech-language pathologists in many cases, such as with the four students discussed previously, to determine the cause of a disorder. This is because speech, language, and literacy disorders are behaviors that do not lead us directly to conclusions about cause. As we have seen, human behavior is complex and results from a myriad of factors. We use case history and interview techniques to explore all aspects of a child's background, including prenatal and birth history, medical history, early developmental history, and educational history, to consider potential factors as to the origin of the communication disorder. However, unless there are obvious connections between a cause, such as a traumatic brain injury, and an effect, such as a language disorder, no one-to-one correspondence can be made. We do our best to describe the communication characteristics of each individual child and the factors that taken together may account for the disorder. In some cases, factors that perpetuate a disorder, such as hearing loss or low parent interaction, can be changed through intervention.

A disorder is considered **functional** if, after using the best diagnostic procedures and technologies available, we fail to identify a pathology of an organ system. Functional influences on the development of the systems involved in communication include reduced environmental stimulation, poor motivation for learning, and emotional issues that suppress learning. Disorders that have no known organic cause include phonological disorders and specific language impairment, for example. As our technology becomes more sophisticated, it may be only a matter of time before we pinpoint organic causes of these disabilities.

An **organic disorder** is one that is caused by a demonstrable pathology of an organ system. Organic influences that result in communication disorders include hearing loss and deafness, genetic syndromes that affect the structure and movement of the oral structures, growths on the vocal folds or paralysis of one or both folds, neurological conditions that result in reduced movement and control of the speech mechanism, and intellectual disability from known causes, such as Down syndrome. Acquired organic conditions include traumatic brain injury, degenerative neurological conditions, and damage to brain-related speech and language functions due to stroke, dementia, and brain tumors.

The important point of considering whether a disorder is functional or organic is to understand the relationship between the environment, biological systems, and the resulting effect on communication development and to determine whether educational interventions and/or referral for medical management is necessary.

Environmental Factors

There are many ways in which the environment plays a role in the prevalence of communication disorders. Consider that each human fetus has the genetic makeup of his or her parents. If that genetic makeup is typical, the child should develop with the potential for normal speech and language development.

If there are prenatal environmental factors that alter the course of development during gestation, the child may already be at a disadvantage for communication disorders, physical abnormalities, and learning. Prenatal care is a critical factor predicting with a degree of confidence that the developing fetus will thrive. The mother must take care of herself with proper nutrition, physical activity, and rest. Any toxins to the fetus, such as nicotine, nonprescribed drugs, and alcohol must be avoided, as these can cause serious physical and developmental consequences (Center on Addiction and Substance Abuse, 2005). Premature (born before 37 weeks' gestation) and low-birth-weight (less than 5.5 pounds) babies have underdeveloped vascular systems, feeding and digestive difficulties, and respiratory problems (Rosetti, 2001). These infants are at risk for communication and learning disabilities.

In addition to prematurity and low birth weight, a small group of children have complications at birth leading to neurological damage. Partial (hypoxia) or total (anoxia) lack of oxygen to the brain causes severe damage to the cerebral cortex. The damage often results in severe communication disorders, motor disorders, impaired cognition, and feeding and swallowing disabilities (Fogel, 2008). Unfortunately, these problems are not reversible, and the challenges to affected individuals are lifelong.

The postnatal environment of the developing child contains a variety of factors that affect communication growth. We know that each child needs a lot of supportive interaction with parents and others in a rich, healthy environment. When there is deprivation of positive social interaction, abuse and/or neglect of the child by parents or others, reduced conversational turns and spoken words, and limited opportunities for learning experiences, the child is at risk for communication disorders. Some prenatal and all postnatal factors are preventable; thus, education of parents and other caregivers and programs that aim to prevent the aforementioned social problems are extremely important.

Sensory Factors

Hearing Loss and Deafness

Hearing loss is unfortunately a common physical condition affecting 1 out of every 22 newborns in the United States, with severe and profound losses occurring in 2 to 3 of every 1,000 live births (Albright & O'Neal, 1998; Barsky-Firsker & Sun, 1997; Mason & Herrmann, 1998). About half of hearing loss at birth is genetic (Morton, 1991). In fact, hearing loss occurs in over 300 genetic syndromes (Gorlin, Toriello, & Cohen, 1995; Van Camp & Smith, 1991). The average age of diagnosis of hearing loss in children occurs from 14 months to 3 years of age and otitis media (middle ear infection) is the most frequent reason for childhood visits to the emergency room (Schappert, 1992). Its prevalence for school-age children who qualify for services as a result of hearing loss is 83 out of 1,000 children. Hearing loss can be caused by heredity, diseases such as chronic ear infections and meningitis, trauma, certain medications, long-term exposure to loud noise, and aging (Fogel, 2008).

There are three types of hearing loss: **conductive**, **sensorineural**, and **mixed**. The degree of loss is determined by the level of loudness of the tones an individual hears. Conductive hearing loss occurs when there is poor transmission of information from the outer or middle ear to the inner ear. The most common cause of conductive hearing loss is fluid in the middle ear, but malformations of the outer ear, impacted cerumen, perforation or inflammation of the tympanic membrane, and poor functioning of the tiny bone of the middle ear (stapes) can also interfere with transmission of sound.

Damage to the auditory nervous system, due to heredity, infection, trauma, exposure to toxins, or repeated exposure to loud noise, results in sensorineural hearing loss. The damage may be located in the cochlea of the inner ear, in the auditory nerve, at various points along the auditory pathway, or in the primary auditory cortex in the temporal lobe of the brain. Mixed hearing loss is a combination of conductive and sensorineural hearing loss.

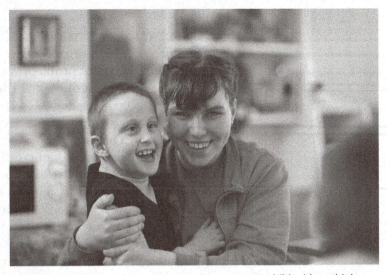

A child with multiple disabilities, including hearing loss, with his teacher.

The degree and type of communication disorder seen in children with hearing loss depend on a variety of factors. Most notably, the age of onset, the age of identification and management, the type of loss, the sound frequencies most affected, and the presence of other handicapping conditions all predict the speech and language outcomes (Hedge & Maul, 2006,; Tye-Murray, 2004). Early detection is critically important. Thus, all professionals who interact with children must be alert to potential hearing problems. Referring parents to hearing screening programs and audiological services when hearing loss is suspected is a necessary and valuable step in early identification and intervention.

The development of normal speech and language requires an adequate hearing system. When hearing loss exists, and especially when the loss is in both ears, speech and language input will be degraded. Because we learn language primarily by hearing, faulty input will impede language learning. All other factors being equal, the greater the hearing loss, the greater the language impairment is likely to be. Children who are deaf or hard of hearing have an impoverished speech and language environment, no matter how much speech is generated at home and regardless of the quality of parents' and siblings' speech and language models. Early identification of hearing loss is critical, because amplification with hearing aids will provide normal or at least near-normal hearing to these individuals. Even individuals who are deaf have a good chance of hearing through cochlear implant technology. When implantation occurs early, hearing is restored to levels that afford the child access to speech and language.

Another avenue for the development of language is through American Sign Language (ASL). Many individuals who are deaf communicate through ASL, and some people combine speech and ASL. This visual mode of communication is sometimes preferred within communities of people who are deaf for social, educational, and vocational interactions. We must keep in mind that communication is a very personal attribute, and the mode one chooses is certainly a person's right.

Low Vision and Blindness

Hearing and visual deficits can result from similar causal factors, such as genetic syndromes and prenatal exposure to substance abuse; thus there is a higher incidence of visual problems in the deaf and hard-of-hearing population (Barraga, 1983). But of course visual problems can also exist as a single sensory deficit at birth or later.

A person with **low vision** (visual acuity 20/70) has some functional use of sight ranging from a moderate to severe impairment. While corrective lenses or surgery may produce some benefit, full restoration is not successful. A person is deemed **legally blind** when visual acuity is 20/200 or less in the better eye, or has a 20-degree visual field (American Foundation for the Blind, 2013).

Children who have low vision or blindness face challenges in language development during the first few years, but with support from others the potential for normal language development is high (Wilton, 2011). Recall that early social interactions require adults and children to engage in mutual gaze, joint attention, and using gestures to convey information about wants, needs, and referencing objects in the environment. These early interactions require being able to see people, objects, and events. Children with low vision or blindness are at a disadvantage in using these early communicative strategies. They also tend to rely on others to initiate language, rather than being directive in their interactions, and they have difficulty interpreting the emotional states of others in the absence of visual information (Landau & Gleitman, 1985). Word learning occurs rapidly in children as they incidentally encounter new objects and experiences. But children with visual impairments preferentially use words to name people, but may be as much as a year delayed in the use of words for requesting objects. Children also may have difficulty learning meanings of verbs, prepositions, and pronouns, because the meanings of these types of words depend on the perspective of the speaker (Nelson, 2010). Just as with children who have normal vision, it is particularly important for parents of children with visual impairments to provide verbal language along with actions and allow them to explore objects as they are described.

Pragmatic communication is an area where children who are blind or have low vision show developmental challenges (Tadic, Pring, & Dale, 2010). The use of facial expressions, gestures, and body language provide important social cues for children. When these cues are not available, children require additional verbal and tactile cues in order to learn social interaction strategies.

As is true for hearing loss, early identification of visual impairments is critical for the well-being and development of young children. It is never too early to bring concerns to the attention of parents and to provide them with resources to secure an evaluation of their child's vision.

Developmental Factors

Developmental Disability

There are many conditions in early childhood that lead to severe chronic physical and/or intellectual disabilities. A child born with cerebral palsy, for example, will face challenges in gross and fine motor skills, including the production of speech. A child born with fetal alcohol syndrome will have physical and intellectual impairments. **Developmental disability** is a broad term used when the disability occurs prior to the age of 22 (American Association on Intellectual and Developmental Disabilities, 2013). Children who have developmental disabilities often have speech and language problems. The specific cause of the disability, known or unknown, does not predict the nature or severity of the speech and language disorder. Rather, the speech and language characteristics depend on many factors regarding the disability, including age of identification, age of interventions, environment, personality, and more.

Intellectual Disability

In the case of intellectual disability, we should begin with the common ground. There is no dispute that a connection exists between intellectual disability and language impairment, and that the severity of language impairment is correlated with the degree of intellectual disability. Please keep in mind, however, that "intellectually disabled language" is a meaningless description because the intellectual disability continuum is fairly broad. Some individuals at the mild end of the continuum use language quite well. Individuals at the severe end are often noncommunicative, and we find a wide range of language abilities between the extremes.

What is **intellectual disability**? The definition most often used today was established by the American Association on Intellectual and Developmental Disabilities (AAIDD). Intellectual disability, according to AAIDD, occurs when a person has significant limitations in intelligence, as determined by an IQ test score below 70, and limitations in adaptive behavior. Adaptive behavior is composed of three main areas that include many sub-areas: conceptual skills, social skills, and activities of daily living. A person exhibits *deficits* in adaptive behavior when she demonstrates an inability to function independently or behaves irresponsibly in common social situations. Another criterion for intellectual disability is that it occurs during the developmental period, before the age of 18 years.

Keeping in mind that wide individual variations exist among individuals with intellectual disability in terms of their speech and language abilities, Kamhi (1981) observes that children with intellectual disabilities experience more language difficulties than normally developing children even when they are matched for mental age. That is, a typical child with an intellectual disability who is six years old, but who has a mental age of three years will have more trouble with language than a normally developing child whose chronological and mental ages are three years. It is also noteworthy that even when children with intellectual disabilities have other developmental problems, including neuromuscular difficulties or social skill deficits, language impairment is usually the most critical problem they face. Language impairment may, in fact, be the single most defining characteristic of this population.

Owens (2004), after thoroughly reviewing the literature, provides an excellent summary of the language behaviors of children with intellectual disabilities. Even though these children exhibit gestures and intentions that are similar to those used by normally developing children, they tend to be submissive conversational partners and are not as effective as their mental age-matched peers in clarifying their messages when misunderstandings occur. Children who have intellectual disabilities acquire morphemes in the same order as other children, and the sequence in which they produce varying types of sentences is similar to that of normal children, but they tend to use shorter and less complex sentences than their mental age-matched peers. Although all children begin with word meanings that are concrete, children with intellectual disabilities do not make the change from concrete to abstract meanings as quickly and easily as other children, and their word meanings remain restrictive. They experience slower vocabulary growth, and they have more trouble with figurative forms of language than their mental age-matched peers. Children with intellectual disabilities tend to use phonological processes that are typical of younger children, and they are slower to suppress these processes than their peers who have normal intellectual abilities. Finally, these children produce more articulation, or motor production, errors than other children.

If we put all these pieces together, we understand that children with intellectual disabilities acquire language forms more slowly but in the same order as normally developing children. In some cases, when we match children with intellectual disabilities and normally developing children for mental age, they perform about the same. In other cases, even when we account for mental age, children with intellectual disabilities are less effective in their use of language and more restricted in their use of the language forms they do have than their mental age-matched peers.

Given the range of abilities and challenges that children with intellectual disabilities show, it is necessary that parents, teachers, and members of a child's special education team meet regularly to establish and maintain understandings of the child's strengths and needs. Many children are effectively included in regular education classrooms, developing social and academic goals with their typical peers. These positive outcomes require conscious planning and implementation of goals based on the principles of family-centered practice. That is, the priorities of the family in collaboration with school-based professionals are used to design age- and grade-appropriate goals, and families participate in the achievement of those goals.

 Video Reflection 9.1: Intervention Planning Meeting - Child Strengths

Watch the video on a child intervention planning meeting focusing on strengths, then answer the question.

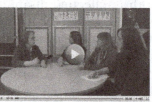

Video Reflection 9.2: Intervention Planning Meeting—Child Needs

Watch the video on a child intervention planning meeting focusing on needs, then answer the question.

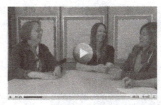

Neurological Factors

Autism Spectrum Disorder

The fifth edition of the Diagnostic and Statistical Manual of Mental Disorders (DSM-5), released in 2013, defines **autism spectrum disorder** (ASD) as having five primary characteristics. For a complete list of subcharacteristics, and for the specific criteria required for the diagnosis, refer to the DSM-5.

1. Social communication and interaction deficits (expressive and/or receptive)
2. Repetitive or restricted patterns of behavior
3. Onset of symptoms in early childhood
4. Significant impairment in functioning in contextual situations
5. Other developmental disorders do not explain the disturbances

In earlier versions of the DSM, autistic disorder, Asperger's disorder, and pervasive developmental disorder not otherwise specified led to inconsistencies in diagnosis. The DSM-5 recommends autism spectrum disorder as the appropriate classification.

In 2012, the Centers for Disease Control and Prevention revealed that the prevalence (number of existing cases in a defined group of people during a specific time period) of ASD was 1 in 88 children in the United States and it was five times more common in boys than in girls. Research has shown that the prevalence of autism has been on the rise. The reason for the increase is not clear, but it has produced great concern. One factor may be increased identification at early ages and identification as a category of disability within the schools (Autism Science Foundation, 2013; Newschaffer, Falb, & Gurney, 2005).

The cause of autism has not been established, but there is speculation that it may be a genetic disorder, that it may result from a degenerative neurological disease, or that it may be an autoimmune disease. The prognosis is uncertain in all cases, but it is considered poor for children with autism who are not talking by the time they are five years old. At this time, there is no single established treatment, but most treatments stress education and behavior modification principles, with emphasis on teaching small segments of information and strictly controlling inappropriate and maladaptive behaviors.

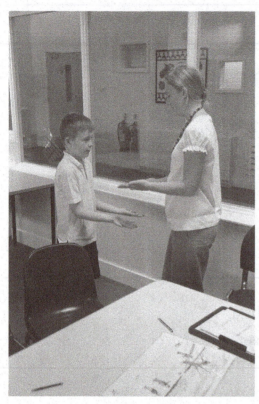

Child with autism spectrum disorder interacting with his teacher.

The primary focus of concern for children with autism, as it is for children with intellectual disability, is severe language impairment. According to Tager-Flusberg (1985), all individuals with autism have impairments that affect their ability both to understand language and to produce language. Paul (1987) notes that half of the population with autism fails to develop functional language and more than a few communication skills of any kind. Beyond this general and not very positive view, we can make a number of generalizations about the language abilities of children with autism.

Children with autism have difficulty establishing the kind of mutual attention that is necessary for communicative exchanges. They have trouble initiating conversation and using language to inform, skills that are basic to social interactions (Wetherby, 1986), in addition to poor conversational turn-taking skills. They also utilize a very limited range of communication functions (Donnellan & Kilman, 1986; Mirenda & Donnellan, 1986). Considering our general description of individuals with autism, it is not surprising that they exhibit difficulty with abstract words; poor word retrieval; and trouble expressing their emotions. Children with autism often refer to themselves with second-person (*you*) and third-person pronouns (*he, she*) and they often construct sentences without regard to underlying meaning (Bartolucci, Pierce, Streiner, & Eppel, 1976). The least-affected component of language is phonology, although phonological problems are common in this population. The sequence of phonological development is the same as for normal children, and development is not distinctly delayed (Fay & Schuler, 1980).

In summary, the language problems of children with autism are diverse because they are members of a diverse population. Some of these children eventually use functional language, but just as many never do. Some of the language problems associated with autism seem to be the result of developmental delay, but other problems go beyond delay. When children with autism are matched for mental age with children who have intellectual disabilities, have specific language impairment (SLI), and are normally developing, the syntactic abilities of the children with autism are equal to those of children with intellectual disability and with SLI. What does this mean? According to Swisher and Demetras (1985), it may mean that children with autism construct sentences differently than normally developing children, that they derive surface structures from incompletely understood deep structures. Taking into account research on the development of all components of language, Swisher and Demetras conclude that there is evidence of delay, but in some cases, there is also evidence that these children follow developmental patterns that are unique. And we will reiterate one more time that, given what we know about the characteristics of autism, it is not surprising that there would be evidence of unusual developmental patterns.

Traumatic Brain Injury

A sudden trauma to the brain that causes injury is called **traumatic brain injury** (TBI). In the United States, there are about 1.5 to 2 million victims of TBI each year, with concussions accounting for about 75% of these injuries. Vehicular accidents are involved in about half of all TBIs and falls are the most common among young children and adults over 75. Other causes of TBI include domestic violence, childhood physical abuse, and nonvehicular accidents. Children and adolescents may experience complete, or nearly complete, recovery from their brain injuries. Sadly, some people will retain significant disabilities for the remainder of their lives.

Children with TBI are members of an extraordinarily heterogeneous group with widely varying behaviors over a wide range of severity for varying periods of time. The severity and location of the injury, the age of the child when the injury occurred, the general health of the person, and the rehabilitative efforts affect the outcomes of TBI (ASHA, 2010). In addition, we must note that the language impairments associated with TBI differ in some respects from the language impairments that have developmental etiologies.

TBI may affect cognition, sensory processing, communication, academic learning, and mental health (ASHA, 2010; Ewing-Cobbs, Fletcher, & Leven, 1985). Depending on the severity of the injury and on the site and extent of the damage, problems in these areas might persist for weeks or months, or they might be permanent. Children with TBI tend to be highly distractible, may perseverate, and may have a low threshold for frustration. Imagine for a moment the combination of these behavioral characteristics and language impairment, academic problems, and the social challenges inherent in interpersonal relationships. To say that TBIs, even those in the mild and moderate categories, can be life altering is an understatement.

As with the other categories of language impairment we have already discussed, we must be careful to acknowledge that whatever generalizations we make about the language impairments of children with (TBI) are just that, generalizations. Here, then, are a few generalizations. These children often make statements during conversations that are not topic focused. They have problems organizing their thoughts into language forms, and they have difficulty expressing complex ideas orally and in written form. Language that is automatic, including the language we use when we greet one another, tends to be unaffected by TBI; but when language is intentional or purposive, and when it is important, communication becomes more difficult. It is not unusual for children with TBIs to experience some problems with language comprehension. They might, for example, have problems affixing meanings to the syntactic structures of sentences, but most of these children will be able to interpret the sentences included in ordinary conversational exchanges.

Body language, nonverbal signals, emotions, and intonations are sometimes not accurately interpreted. Individuals with TBIs often struggle to name things, and they have problems with word retrieval even if their vocabularies are relatively intact. The sentences they produce tend to be long, aimless, fragmented, and inappropriate. Sensory deficits in hearing, smell, taste, or touch may occur. Children with TBI typically do not have phonological problems as a result of their brain injuries, but they might have some articulation difficulties associated with injury-induced dysarthria and/or apraxia.

Brain Damage from Stroke or Disease

Another cause of brain injury is internal. That is, several conditions within the brain itself can be triggered to cause a lack of blood flow and oxygen, such as when an artery is clogged or bursts. A **cerebrovascular accident** (CVA), commonly called a *stroke*, may result in mild to serious motor, speech, and language problems. A stroke can occur prenatally or anytime in a person's life, but generally there is a much higher occurrence in older adults. It is a leading cause of death in the United States and 10% of children who have a stroke will die. Survivors of stroke often experience long-term disabilities including paralysis of limbs on the opposite side, speech and language disorders, higher-level cognitive deficits, seizures, and coma (Mackay & Gordon, 2007).

The incidence of stroke in childhood is 2.5 per 100,000 per year, with strokes more often occurring prior to the second birthday and becoming less common with advancing age (Nicolaides & Appleton, 1996). Strokes in infants, children, and adolescents account for less than 5% of the total incidence of stroke in the general population (Gulati & Kalra, 2003). Risk factors such as congenital heart disease, vascular anomalies, and sickle cell disease increase the potential for strokes in children (Roach, 2000).

Children who sustain brain injury are far more likely to recover language abilities as compared to adults. There is strong support that their favorable speech and language outcomes are due to the neural and behavioral plasticity of the brain. Please note, however, that the number of injuries, the extent and site of injury, and postinjury care of the child are factors in recovery (Bates et al., 2001).

Language-Learning Disabilities

A **learning disability** is a general term that is used to designate difficulties in acquiring spoken language, written language, and mathematical skills. Learning disabilities are not the result of sensory, intellectual, or emotional disorders and they are not due to environmental factors, such as inappropriate instruction or cultural influences (National Committee on Learning Disabilities, 1991). The complete definition of a learning disability is lengthy and has been modified across many decades to reflect characteristics, causes, and factors not considered to be causative. As is true of other disorders, the label does not tell us much about any particular person, as there is much individual variation in the acquisition of skills. Although a specific cause is unknown, learning disabilities are presumed to be due to central nervous system dysfunction and they result in lifelong consequences. Estimates of the prevalence of learning disorders in the general population range from 2% to 10% (Alterac & Saroha, 2007; ASHA, 2008a). In the school-age population (ages 6 through 21 years), there are close to 3 million children receiving special education (U.S. Department of Education, 2005).

Dyslexia

Dyslexia is often considered a specific learning disability with a neurological origin. The term is used when a child has difficulty using phonological components to decode written words (Catts & Kamhi, 2005; Snowling, 2000). Children and adults with dyslexia have persistent difficulties in word recognition; thus, reading comprehension is often poor, and they are poor spellers. Of course, some reading problems lie not with decoding, but with comprehension. The preferred term for this problem is *specific comprehension deficit* (Catts, Kamhi, & Adolf, 2012).

Language Disorders of Unknown Origin

Specific Language Impairment

The complexity of learning language during the toddler and preschool years is remarkable, to say the least. We have introduced the many factors and conditions that can affect an individual's progress toward normal communication, some of which are known early in the child's development through medical diagnosis and severe social interaction difficulties. The existence of language impairments, however, is not always so clear early on.

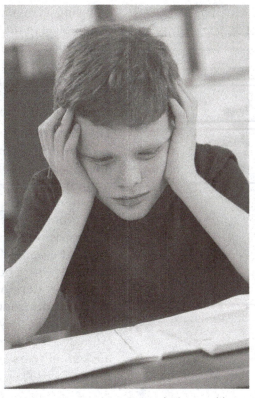

Stressed 10-year-old boy who has a reading disability

Specific language impairment (SLI) is a term used to categorize a language disorder that is *not* accompanied by deficits in hearing, intelligence, neurological functions, or motor function (Leonard, 1998; Shames, Wiig, & Secord, 1998). Children who have SLI have a range of communication problems. Paul (2007) summarized research findings to focus on the relationship of SLI to other abilities. First, the language acquisition of these children follows a typical developmental sequence, but the various components of language are not only delayed but also frequently uneven. Thus, vocabulary may be delayed by two years, but grammar may show a three-year delay (Paul, 2007). Deficits in both short-term and working memory; processing of rapidly changing phonological, morphological, and syntactic information; and nonverbal cognitive abilities have been found through research (Archibald & Gathercole, 2006; Haskill & Tyler, 2007; Kamhi, 1981; Tallal, Stark, & Mellits, 1985) Pragmatic difficulties, if present, are usually in the mild range; however, behavioral and social difficulties may occur (Paul, 2007).

Children who have SLI are likely to be identified as having learning disabilities when their language difficulties interfere with the development of reading and writing, as well as during classroom interactions. The educational impact of having a language disorder highlights the importance of the changing role of language in the child's experiences. Children may function fairly well when they are communicating with family members and friends, but the demands for the use of higher language skills in the classroom and during reading and writing tax the abilities of children with language disorders.

Phonological Disorders

The term **phonological disorder** is used to describe children who not only have speech errors on the surface, but whose errors indicate an underlying disorder in establishing and using the appropriate rules for sounds and their combinations. Children with phonological disorders have difficulty mastering where to use speech sounds in order to make words sound different from each other. For example, when a child leaves off sounds at the end of words, the words sound like other words. Words such as *boat, bone,* and *bowl* will sound the same ([bo]) when the child simplifies them through final consonant deletion. The many phonological processes a particular child might use during her development will diminish her intelligibility. Children with phonological disorders often have difficulty acquiring phonological awareness abilities; thus, they are at risk for problems in the development of literacy. It is estimated that as many as 70% exhibit general academic difficulty throughout the school years (ASHA, 2008b).

Check Your Understanding 9.3

Assess your understanding of the causes, contributing factors, and types of language disorders by completing this brief quiz.

Speech Disorders

The most obvious disorders that adults recognize in children are those that are readily seen and heard. When a child produces speech, the parents expect that sounds will become accurate and intelligibility will improve with maturity. When a child does not speak clearly as compared to others at or near his age, it can be a sign that speech acquisition is delayed. There are many factors that should be considered in determining what causes delay in any particular child.

The speech mechanism itself is of course an important factor. Children must have the structural and functional components, such as lips, tongue, hard palate, and soft palate, in order to create speech sounds using place, manner, and voicing features. Children must also have adequate breath support, vocal tone, and resonance and all these need to be coordinated with the signals from the brain. Some structural problems involve malformations, such as cleft lip and palate or severe dental and occlusion conditions. Functional difficulties include tongue thrust, coordination problems, or limited mobility of the tongue or soft palate. Neurological conditions can greatly diminish the control and speed a person has in order to produce speech in a rapid and accurate manner.

Articulation Disorders

Whether a speech disorder is caused by a known condition or it is present due to unknown factors, the resulting problem is the articulation of speech sounds. When the disorder is in the use of the speech mechanism to form the necessary place, manner, and voicing of sounds, we refer to it as an **articulation disorder**. A child may, for example, have difficulty producing precise /s, f, l, r/ phonemes. We generally call articulation disorders *surface structure problems* because they are present when the child speaks aloud. Thus, the errors are on the surface for all to hear. Articulation disorders can be mild to severe, and intelligibility is the main concern. The errors are described as substitutions of one sound for another, distortions, and omissions of sounds in words. When articulation problems are accompanied by incoordination of the speech mechanism or by rate and prosody issues, intelligibility problems will often increase.

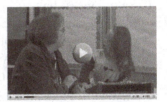

Video Example 9.4

Watch the video of a first-grader practicing speech sounds in syllables with her speech-language pathologist. Down syndrome results in low muscle tone, so precision of articulation is impaired. Children with Down syndrome also have at least some degree of intellectual disability, which has an effect on language development in addition to the acquisition of speech.

Voice Disorders

We convey much about our general health, our emotional state, our personality, and, of course, what we are communicating through our voice. Therefore, when the voice is disordered, individuals find that it affects their lives in significant ways. Surveys conducted by experts in this disorder indicate that 3% of adults and as many as 7% of school-age children have voices that can be considered disordered (Boone, McFarlane, Von Berg, & Zraick, 2010). There are many causes of voice disorders, and experts classify them in various ways. Four categories of voice problems, summarized by Boone and colleagues, include organic voice disorders, neurogenic voice disorders, psychogenic voice disorders, and muscle tension dysphonia. The names of these categories reflect the cause of each of these problems.

The most common cause, **muscle tension dysphonia**, is the result of using too much effort during vocalization. Children and adults who speak in loud voices develop hoarseness and fatigue as they overuse their respiratory, phonotory, and articulatory mechanisms. When this behavior persists over time, actual changes in the vocal fold tissue can result in various growths that require medical management, voice therapy, or both.

Another category that is also related to behavior is called **psychogenic voice disorders**. Because our voices reflect our state of being, severe emotional trauma or conflict can result in hoarseness without a physical cause (functional dysphonia) or complete loss of the voice (conversion aphonia). People who have psychogenic voice disorders find daily social and vocational interactions quite difficult.

There are numerous types of organic voice disorders in which the physical structures involved in phonation and resonation are affected in some way. For example, cancer of the larynx, congenital abnormalities of the laryngeal structures, contact ulcers and cysts of the vocal folds, infectious laryngitis, and chronic gastroesophageal reflux disease represent some of these *organic conditions*. Organic conditions are discovered through medical examination, but their symptoms may be first noticed through the characteristics of the voice.

Vocal characteristics can also tell us when there is something amiss with a person's neurological status. The category that includes a variety of conditions related to muscle control and innervations of the muscles involved in respiration, phonation, resonation, and articulation is called **neurogenic voice disorders**. The nervous system in humans is quite complex, with many pathways responsible for the ability to consciously and unconsciously breathe, produce voice, and articulate speech. Neurological difficulties can occur anywhere in the central and peripheral nervous systems. Recall our brief description of dysarthria earlier in the chapter. Among the characteristics of dysarthric speech is an alteration in voice quality, pitch, and loudness. The several kinds of dysarthria are indicative of where in the system the neurological problem exists. Neurological problems involving cranial nerves can also lead directly to voice disorders. Damage to cranial nerve X, the vagus nerve, for example, leads to vocal fold paralysis.

It is important for educators to be aware of the many ways that children and adults can acquire voice disorders. Prevention of muscle tension dysphonia can be effective by building awareness of healthy vocal practices and discouraging vocal misuse and abuse. Referral to pediatricians and otolaryngologists when the vocal characteristics of a child cause concern is important not only in determining that a disorder exists, but also in making sure that the health of the child is not at risk by ruling out medical problems. These preventive efforts are equally important for adults, especially those who use their voices daily in their work.

Fluency Disorders

When most people, even many speech-language pathologists, talk about fluency disorders, they limit their consideration to **stuttering**. In fact, stuttering is just one of the fluency disorders therapists are called on to treat. Obviously, there are common denominators among fluency disorders, but it is important to differentiate among them because they are not simply variations of the same disorder. They have different etiologies and different symptoms.

Any disorder characterized by hesitation, repetition of speech segments, or prolongation of sounds that impedes the forward flow of speech is a fluency disorder. Beyond this commonality are many differences. Fluency problems often accompany neuropathologies. People with epilepsy or cerebral palsy, or people who have suffered strokes or head injuries, often have fluency problems along with other communication disorders. Whether all of these conditions should be called *stuttering* is the subject of considerable debate (Hulit, 2004).

Developmental Stuttering

For purposes of this discussion, *developmental stutterers,* or simply *stutterers* with no qualifying adjectives, are individuals who are normal neurologically and who do not have serious psychological problems. Consider, however, that even if we limit ourselves to this population, we encounter another problem. All speakers occasionally experience fluency failures. All speakers repeat syllables, words, even phrases. They all stumble, hesitate, revise, add superfluous interjections, and produce all the other behaviors associated with stuttering. It is not as easy to differentiate between stuttering and normal fluency failures as you might imagine. You might be tempted to conclude that the difference is frequency of fluency failure. That is, people who stutter fail more often than people who do not stutter. Although frequency of fluency failure is one factor in the difference, it is not the only difference, and it may not even be the most important difference. Stutterers and nonstutterers actually have more similarities than differences as communicators (Hulit, 2004). They are separated as much by their *perceptions* of speech, speaking situations, sounds, words, and listeners as by the struggle associated with stuttering.

One of the most difficult problems we face in discussing stuttering is defining it (Bloodstein, 1995; Guitar, 1998; Silverman, 1996; Wingate, 1997). Experts over the centuries have argued about what stuttering is, what causes it, why it seems to run in families, why it is more common in males than in females, why some children recover spontaneously from it and others do not, and how to treat it. Suffice it to say that even though much has been written about stuttering, and even though it is among the most thoroughly investigated of all communication disorders, there is still far more we do not know about stuttering than we know.

Developmental stuttering is a disorder that begins in childhood, usually between the ages of two and six years. Many children who begin to stutter spontaneously recover by the time they are about six years old. Some experts, based on empirical research, believe that about 40% of young children who stutterer recover spontaneously; a few place the recovery rate as high as 80%. Stuttering is much more common in males than in females. When children are young, the ratio is about 2:1. By adulthood, the ratio is 4:1 or 5:1.

When stuttering begins, it is relatively simple and uninvolved. The child who stutters repeats single-syllable words or the first syllable of multisyllabic words, and he stutters without struggle, awareness, or concern.

Early stuttering is usually episodic. That is, weeks or months go by when speech is relatively nonfluent, followed by weeks or months when speech is relatively fluent. The episodes of fluent speech and non-fluent speech might continue for several years until the child enters a fluent period and never has another episode of excessive non-fluency. Such a child has *recovered spontaneously*. If stuttering continues, the behaviors increase in number and become more complicated. The child who stutters becomes more aware that he is producing fluency failures, becomes more concerned about his speech, and eventually begins to include *stutterer* as a major component of his self-identity. As severity increases, the child or adult who stutters adds what are called *secondary symptoms* to his repertoire of behaviors. These include facial grimaces, head jerks, and extraneous movements in the limbs that reflect his struggle to fight through moments of stuttering.

Most experts believe that the prognosis for the adult who stutters is not good. She may learn how to control her speech to the extent that she can dramatically improve her ability to communicate, but it is not likely that she will ever again be a "normal" speaker. On those rare occasions when an adult is completely liberated from her disorder, the liberation is typically the product of a life-altering experience.

As noted at the beginning of this section, the term *stuttering* is often applied to disorders that do not fit the profile of developmental stuttering. Some individuals have fluency problems that are clearly and directly connected to neuropathologies. Although these individuals may produce similar behaviors to developmental stutterering, there are differences between developmental stuttering and *neurogenic stuttering*. Other people may have a fluency disorder that is the product of a psychological problem, a disorder called *psychogenic stuttering* or *hysterical stuttering*. Again, some common ground is shared by developmental stuttering and psychogenic stuttering, but important differences are evident as well. Finally, a disorder called *cluttering* differs from stuttering in many respects even though both are fluency disorders.

Neurogenic Stuttering

Stuttering that begins after an individual suffers damage to the central nervous system (CNS) has been described by many authors (Davis, 1993; Hertrich & Ackermann, 1994; Mavlov, 1994; Nagafuchi,1994). In most cases the individuals had no history of stuttering prior to the CNS damage and the onset was sudden.. In other cases, the individual had a history of stuttering that either reappeared or noticeably worsened after the neurological damage. Damage to the CNS can be caused by a cerebral vascular accident (stroke), a blow to the head, the development of a tumor, a reaction to drugs, dementia, or a number of diseases that affect the nervous system. The person whose stuttering is neurogenic is less likely to acquire secondary symptoms (Lundgren, Helm-Estabrooks, & Klein, 2010).

Psychogenic Stuttering

Cases of individuals who stutter as the result of psychological problems, known as psychogenic stuttering, have been reported (Attanasio, 1987; Mahr & Leith, 1992; Roth, Aronson, & Davis, 1989). As with neurogenic stuttering, the onset of psychogenic stuttering tends to be sudden and appears to be associated with a specific, identifiable psychological trauma. In some cases, the trauma is the result of violence the individual has experienced or observed. In other cases, the trauma is associated with a powerful and aversive life-altering experience, such as the sudden, unexpected death of a loved one or an unusually acrimonious divorce. It is also reported that it may occur in people with degenerative conditions, seizure disorders, and closed head injury (Baumgartner & Duffy, 1997). Unlike the individual with developmental stutterering who stutters in response to certain situational and linguistic cues, the person with psychogenic stutterering tends to stutter in all communicative situations. She does not develop secondary behaviors such as facial grimaces and head jerks. She does not avoid words or speaking situations, and she tends to be so completely unconcerned about her stuttering that she is essentially detached from it (Freund, 1966).

Cluttering

Cluttering is as misunderstood a communication disorder as stuttering, and it has received far less attention from U.S. authors than from European authors (St. Louis & Rustin, 1992). Cluttering is as difficult to define as stuttering, but it may best be thought of as a speech and language problem. Cluttering is just one symptom of that problem. Others include delayed speech, developmental phonological disorders, reading and writing disorders, disorders of rhythm and musicality, and even general behavior problems such as restlessness and disorderliness (Weiss, 1964).

Further descriptions by Daly (1993) and Daly and Cantrelle (2006) indicate that cluttering involves both speech and language errors including sound omissions and distortions, irregular rate and lack of pausing, poor awareness and self-monitoring, incomplete phases, and disorganization in the construction and execution of verbal information. Speech intelligibility is reduced due to the interaction of all of these aspects.

Check Your Understanding 9.4

Assess your understanding of speech disorders by completing this brief quiz.

SUMMARY

This chapter on speech and language disorders provided introductory information on the many aspects of communication that may not develop within the typical timeframe or manner. We identified the incidence and prevalence of communication in children to highlight the likelihood that you will work with them in your future career and for you to consider the impact these disorders have on children's social and educational development. We described four school-aged students in detail to show the interrelationships

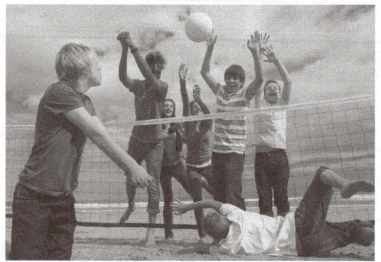

Teens enjoying their time together

of the various aspects of communication on success in the classroom. We provided a brief overview of many contributing factors that put individuals at risk for communication disorders: environmental; sensory; developmental; neurological; and unknown. In addition, we described several speech disorders that are common in school-aged children.

Final Thoughts

We have come to the end of our story. As you have progressed through the pages of this book, we hope you have developed a new appreciation for the miracle of speech and language. We may never fully understand how human beings can think, edit thoughts, pull language from their memory banks, transform language into speech, and combine speech with all the critical aspects of nonverbal communication. We should, however, appreciate that this communicative ability is one of the great gifts humans pass from generation to generation.

Although there is a powerful innate drive to acquire language and to speak in all human children, parents should do all they can to encourage their children during the acquisition period. Parents and teachers are usually the first to notice when a child is having difficulty with speech and language. It is their responsibility to seek professional help from speech-language pathologists who are qualified to diagnose and treat communication problems. If there is any doubt about whether a child has a communication disorder, the child should be evaluated and treated, if necessary. It is far easier to treat communication disorders in their early stages than after inappropriate habits have become established. Children who can talk have one of the most important tools they need to explore and understand the exciting world awaiting them.

▮▷ Surfing the Web

If you are interested in exploring topics discussed in this chapter in more detail, search for one or more of the following relevant terms online.

incidence and prevalence of communication disorders

types and causes of communication disorders

speech and language disorders and diseases

risk factors associated with communication disorders

communication disorders due to hearing loss and deafness

preventing traumatic brain injury

communication disorders after traumatic brain injury

language and learning disabilities

specific language impairment in children

phonological disorders in children

articulation disorders in children and adults

voice disorders

language development in children
with low vision and blindness
communication disorders and
intellectual disability
autism spectrum disorders

fluency disorders
developmental stuttering
neurogenic stuttering
psychogenic stuttering
cluttering

 ## Chapter Review 9.1

Recall what you learned in this chapter by completing the Chapter
Review.

10

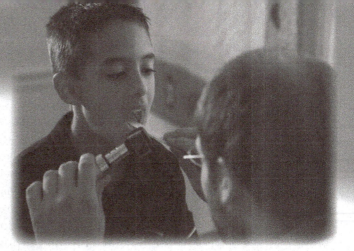

The Anatomical and Physiological Bases of Speech, Language, and Hearing

LEARNING OUTCOMES

After completion of this chapter, the reader will be able to:

■ Describe the four processes of speech production.
■ Discuss how the brain is the control center for speech, language, and hearing.
■ Explain the mechanism of hearing.

It is impossible to understand human speech without examining the anatomical structures and physiological processes that produce speech. Speech is, after all, the direct result of muscle contractions innervated by the nervous system that move structures in ways that force air out of the lungs, vibrate that air, resonate it, and break it up into speech sounds. In this appendix, we look at the structures that together make up what we call the *speech machine*. We also examine the hearing mechanism, which is important to speech in two ways. First, we receive the speech of others through the hearing mechanism. Unless there are ears to hear what is said, we cannot complete the *vocal-auditory channel*, one of the design-features of speech (Hockett, 1960). Second, a speaker depends on the ability to hear himself so that he can monitor the content of his speech as well as things like rate, pitch, stress, rhythm, and articulatory accuracy.

Speech as the Product of Borrowed Structures: Four Processes of Speech

All of the structures involved in producing speech are designed for other, more basic biological purposes. Breathing, for example, is important for speech, but the primary reasons a person breathes are to absorb oxygen into the bloodstream and to release waste in the form of carbon dioxide. The *larynx*, commonly called the *voice box*, is a valve in the throat that prevents the ingestion of foreign substances into the lungs. The tongue, which plays a major role in the production of speech sounds, exists primarily to facilitate eating. Every structure that is a part of the speech machine is, in a sense, borrowed from the body's life maintenance systems. Human beings have adapted certain bodily structures for the purpose of producing speech.

You should not interpret this to mean that speech is the product of an anatomy ill suited for this purpose. On the contrary, every part of the body that plays a role in speech is ideally designed in structure and function for speech, but we should never forget that speech is an activity that is overlaid on biological functions that are more basic to our physical survival than is speech. This is one of the wonders of human oral communication—that we have been able to use structures intended for other purposes to create a communication system that is convenient, efficient, and unmatched in power and sophistication by any other communication system in the animal kingdom. Other primates, for example, have anatomies remarkably similar to ours, but they have not been able to adapt their structures to produce oral communication systems even remotely comparable to speech. The structures themselves, although similar, are not capable of the intricate, controlled adjustments required for speech. The larynx of a chimpanzee, for example, resembles the human larynx, but the vocal folds in the chimpanzee's larynx do not allow the range of length and tension adjustments that are possible in human vocal folds. Although it is true, therefore, that the structures humans use to produce speech have more fundamental vegetative responsibilities, they work so well for speech that they could have been specifically designed for that purpose.

Speech can be most easily understood as the product of four separate but inextricably related processes: respiration, phonation, resonation, and articulation. As indicated in Figure 10.1, each process makes a specific contribution to the end product. *Respiration,* or breathing, provides the power for speech. The speaker inhales to capture air in the lungs and then, in a controlled manner, exhales to force a column of air into the larynx. *Phonation* occurs when the vocal folds of the larynx are drawn together by contraction of specific muscles, and the exhaled air causes the folds to vibrate in a manner that disturbs or vibrates the air column. As the vibrating air column passes through the throat, the mouth, and sometimes the nasal cavities, it undergoes *resonation,* which means that the tone of the noise from the vocal folds is modified according to the size and shape of the resonating cavities. As the vibrating and resonated air column passes through the mouth, the tongue, teeth, and other structures in the mouth break up the airstream into the sounds of speech, a process called *articulation.*

As described here and depicted in Figure 10.1, the reader might get the impression that there is a discrete order from one process to the next, beginning with respiration. It is more accurate to understand speech as the product of the successive and simultaneous interactions of these four processes. In other words, it is true that speech must begin with exhalation, and the airstream must be phonated before it can be resonated, and it is articulated as it

Figure 10.1 The Processes of Speech

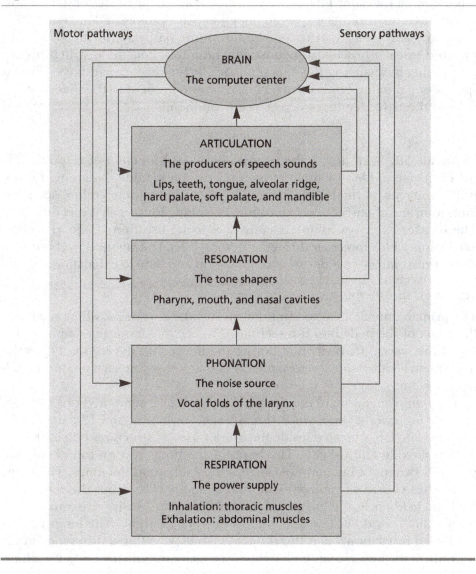

passes out of the mouth, but in continuous speech, all four of these processes are occurring in a precisely integrated and synchronized manner. While one part of the vibrating air column is being articulated, another part of the air column is just beginning the journey from the lungs into the larynx.

For the sake of convenience, we will look at each process as a separate entity, but you should remember that, as in any machine, each part of the speech machine depends on every other part, and the machine functions only when the parts work together. Many man-made machines have become so complicated in their structures and functions that they must be managed by internal computers. The human speech machine is also incredibly complex and also requires an internal computer to make sure that all the parts function in proper synchrony. The speech machine's computer is the brain. It is the brain that coordinates the activities of all the processes of speech and ensures that the product is speech, not gibberish. As indicated in Figure 10.1, the brain sends out instructions along motor pathways to the structures involved in each process and constantly monitors how these structures are responding by analyzing the data sent back by the sensory pathways. Normal speech is maintained only if correct instructions are sent to the speech structures and reliable feedback is received from them.

Respiration

As has already been noted, the primary biological function of respiration is the exchange of life-sustaining oxygen for carbon dioxide. Breathing for life is involuntary and rhythmic. About 50% of each breathing cycle is spent on inhalation and about 50% on exhalation. Breathing for speech is very different. The speaker exercises voluntary control over the breathing cycle, especially exhalation, which forces air through the vocal tract. During speech, about 15% of the breathing cycle is devoted to inhalation and 85% to exhalation.

Structures of *Breathing*

The primary muscle involved in inhalation is the *diaphragm*, which separates the trunk of the body into two sections. The section above the diaphragm is called the *thorax*, the cavity that houses the lungs, and the section below the diaphragm is called the *abdomen*, the cavity that houses internal organs including the kidneys, liver, and intestines.

The bony framework of the thorax (Figure 10.2) is composed of 12 *thoracic vertebrae* posteriorly, the *sternum* (breastbone) anteriorly, and 12 pairs of *ribs*, laterally. The *lungs*, located inside the thorax, are the structures that exchange carbon dioxide and oxygen. The bases of the lungs rest on top of the diaphragm. Two moist membranes called *pleurae* surround the lungs. The lungs themselves consist of spongy tissue that is highly elastic, but there are very few muscle fibers in the lungs, which means they are passive structures. They receive air. They do not suck in air, as some people think. The lungs receive air during inhalation when the thorax expands, creating a difference in air pressure in the lungs compared to the air pressure outside the body. Breathing depends on a very basic principle of physics known as *Boyle's law*.

Basic Physics in *Breathing*: Inhalation and *Exhalation*

According to Boyle's law, "If a gas is kept at a constant temperature, pressure and volume are inversely proportional to one another and have a constant product" (Zemlin, 1988, p. 33). This means that if we have a given number of gas molecules at a constant temperature, we can change the pressure exerted by those molecules by changing the volume of the container. If we double the volume of the container, the pressure is reduced by one-half. If we triple the volume of the container, the pressure is reduced to one-third of the original pressure, and so on. However, if we cut the volume of the container in half, the pressure exerted by the gas molecules doubles, and if we reduce the volume to one-third of the original volume, the pressure triples, and so on.

Figure 10.2 The Thorax: Front and Rear Views

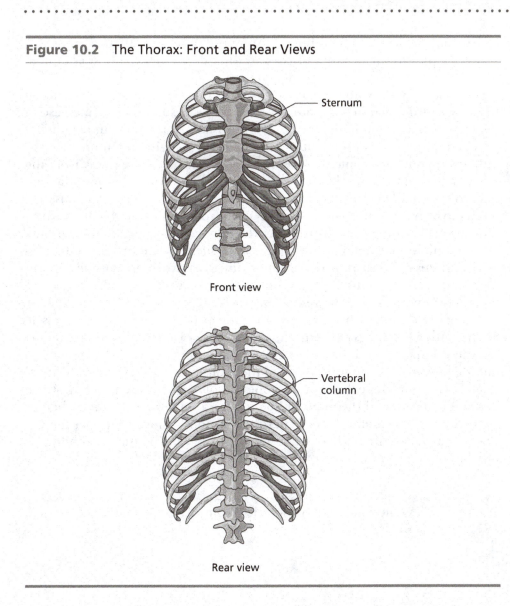

Sternum

Front view

Vertebral column

Rear view

Consider how this law is applied to breathing. The lungs are housed inside the thorax, an airtight cavity connected to the outside air through the *trachea*, or windpipe, and the mouth and nose. If the volume of the thorax is increased, the air pressure inside the lungs decreases proportionately; what will happen if the pressure inside is less than the pressure outside when there is a direct connection between the lungs and the outside air? Air will rush into the lungs to make the pressures equal, of course. Therefore, *inhalation* occurs when the volume of the thorax is increased, creating pressure in the lungs that is less than the outside pressure. In *exhalation*, the volume of the thorax is reduced, creating pressure inside the lungs that is greater than the outside pressure, and what happens? Air rushes out of the lungs until the pressures are equal again. Breathing, then, depends on the very practical application of Boyle's law and the simple principle of equilibrium. What remains to be understood is how the volume of the thorax is increased in inhalation and decreased in exhalation.

During normal quiet breathing, the amount of oxygen inhaled is approximately equal to the volume of carbon dioxide exhaled, and a complete inhalation/exhalation cycle occurs about 12 to 15 times per minute.

The diaphragm is dome-shaped in its resting configuration. Inhalation begins when the diaphragm contracts or flattens, resulting in an increase in the vertical dimension of the thorax (Figure 10.3). At the same time, muscles attached to the ribs contract, lifting the ribs and swinging them upward and outward in much the same way the handle on a bucket moves away from the side of a bucket when it is lifted (Figure 10.4). This action also causes the sternum to be moved up and out. The muscles of inhalation, therefore, cause the thorax to be increased from side to side, from front to back, and in the vertical dimension. The lungs, which are effectively attached to the sides of the thorax by the pleurae that surround them, expand when the thorax expands. This action creates reduced air pressure in the lungs relative to the outside air pressure, and air rushes into the lungs until the pressures are equal, completing the inhalation portion of the respiratory cycle.

Exhalation in quiet breathing is a passive process, not involving muscle activity. After the lungs fill with air, the muscles of inhalation relax, reducing the volume of the thorax and creating another imbalance of inside and outside pressures. Air now flows out of the lungs until the pressures are equal again. This completes exhalation and one complete cycle of respiration. We do this automatically and rhythmically about 12 to 15 times per minute, whether asleep or awake (Zemlin, 1988). There are obviously more cycles per minute when we are active than when we are relaxed, and when we sleep soundly, the number of cycles per minute is further reduced.

Figure 10.3   Vertical Increase in Thoracic Volume as the Diaphragm Contracts

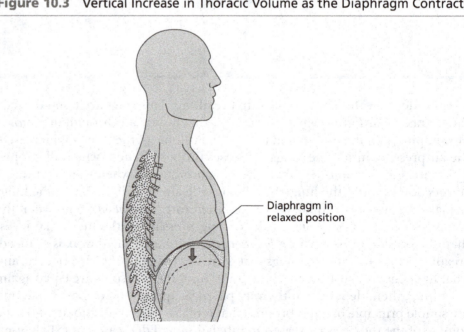

Diaphragm in relaxed position

Figure 10.4   Lateral and Anteroposterior Expansions of the Thorax

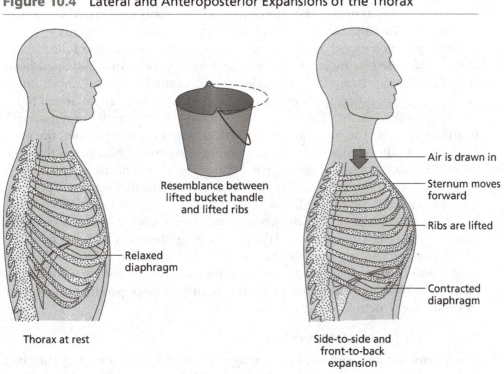

Resemblance between
lifted bucket handle
and lifted ribs

— Relaxed
diaphragm

Thorax at rest

— Air is drawn in

— Sternum moves
forward

— Ribs are lifted

— Contracted
diaphragm

Side-to-side and
front-to-back
expansion

Breathing for *Speech*

Breathing for speech differs radically from breathing for life. As mentioned earlier, speech is a muscular activity requiring the precise synchronization of all four
processes of speech, including respiration. Breathing for speech necessitates
delicate control of each respiratory cycle and particularly the exhalation portion
of the cycle. When we breathe for speech, we extend and control exhalation for
up to 15 seconds. If we were unable to do this, talking time would be restricted
to two-and-a-half-second spurts, the average duration of exhalation during quiet
breathing (Zemlin, 1990). We would be able to produce only a few words at a
time instead of the lengthy sentences that characterize normal speech.

In addition to changing the nature of the respiratory cycle, speech affects
breathing by introducing varying degrees of airflow resistance at a number
of places in the speech mechanism. If the vocal folds are brought together,
for example, and the lips or the tongue are positioned for the production
of certain sounds, the power of exhalation must be great enough to force air
through the constriction points. Instead of just relaxing the muscles of inhalation as we do during quiet breathing, we must partially contract these muscles
and actively contract muscles of exhalation to maintain sufficient airflow force
and control for speech production. Breathing for speech, therefore, requires
a complex balance of the muscle activities involved in inhalation and exhalation, a balance that allows us to sustain exhalation for periods up to six times
longer than exhalation during quiet breathing. The air we exhale for speech
moves into the larynx, the tone-producing structure in the speech machine.

Phonation

The *larynx* is a structure in the anterior neck commonly known as the *voice box*. The *vocal folds* are the components in the larynx responsible for generating the noise upon which speech is superimposed. The larynx sits on top of the trachea and is suspended by means of muscles and ligaments from a U-shaped bone called the *hyoid*. Although the hyoid is not part of the larynx, it is important to laryngeal function because a number of laryngeal muscles are attached to it.

As mentioned earlier, the larynx acts as a valve to prevent foreign materials from entering the trachea and lungs. If something threatens to enter, the vocal folds close while exhalation continues until the force of the air below the folds literally blows them open. You may recognize this action as the cough.

The secondary function of the larynx is sound production, a purpose for which it is ideally constructed. The vocal folds are relatively long and are capable of the wide range of adjustments in length and tension that are essential for voice production. During normal quiet breathing, the vocal folds are relatively wide open, but during speech, they are drawn together to obstruct the flow of air from the lungs, setting up the conditions necessary for vocal fold vibration. We will take a closer look at the mechanics of voice production after we examine the structure of the larynx.

The Parts of the Voice *Generator*

The larynx is composed of nine cartilages (Figure 10.5) bound together by a complex network of membranes. The inside of the larynx is lined with a membrane that is continuous with the membrane lining the trachea below and the pharynx above. There are three single cartilages in the larynx and three pairs of smaller cartilages. We are concerned with only the most important of these cartilages: thyroid, cricoid, epiglottis, and arytenoids.

The *thyroid* is the largest of the laryngeal cartilages. It is the part of the larynx that tends to protrude in the neck and is often referred to as the *Adam's apple*. This unpaired cartilage is made up of two plates joined in front in a V-shape whose open portion faces toward the back. Each plate has two projections called *horns*. The *superior horn* extends upward toward the hyoid bone, and the *inferior horn* extends downward to connect with the cricoid cartilage. This pivotal connection allows the thyroid cartilage to be tilted downward and forward, an action that lengthens the vocal folds.

The lowermost portion of the larynx is the *cricoid* cartilage, which sits on top of the trachea. The cricoid is in the shape of a ring, with a plate on the posterior side and a narrower band forming the front and sides.

Attached to the angle of the thyroid is the third single cartilage, called the *epiglottis*, which is shaped something like a narrow leaf. It is attached at its top margin to the hyoid bone by a ligament. Even though the epiglottis is an interesting-looking structure, it makes little, if any, contribution to speech.

The only paired cartilages that are important to laryngeal function are the roughly pyramid-shaped *arytenoids* (Figure 10.6), which are situated on top of the posterior plate of the cricoid. Each arytenoid has a *vocal process* and a *lateral* or *muscular* process. The vocal processes extend anteriorly and have the vocal

Figure 10.5 The Cartilages of the Larynx: Front and Rear Views

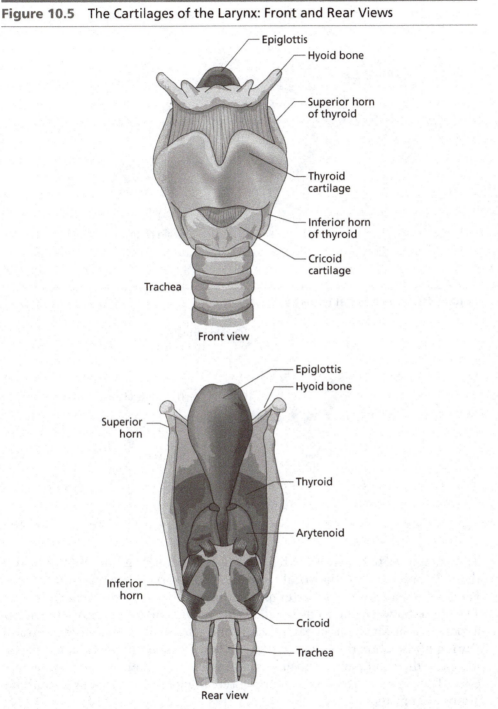

Epiglottis

Hyoid bone

Superior horn
of thyroid

Thyroid
cartilage

Inferior horn
of thyroid

Cricoid
cartilage

Trachea

Front view

Epiglottis

Hyoid bone

Superior
horn

Thyroid

Arytenoid

Inferior
horn

Cricoid

Trachea

Rear view

folds attached to them. The lateral processes have muscles attached to them
that act to move the vocal folds together or apart.

As has already been mentioned, the vocal folds (Figure 10.7) are the vibrating elements of the larynx and consist of muscles and ligaments. They originate

Figure 10.6   The Arytenoid Cartilages and Related Structures

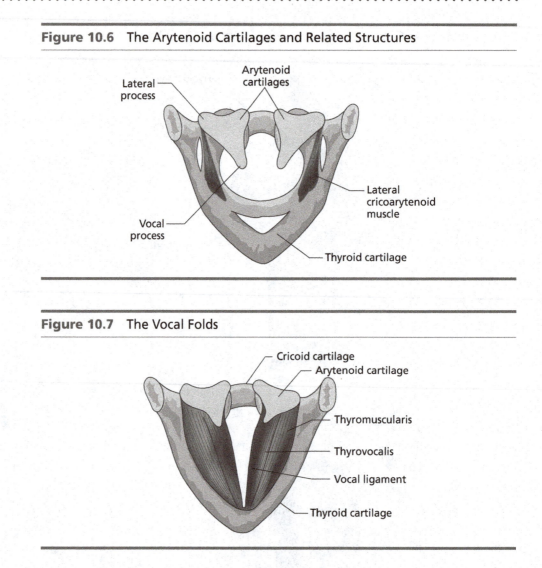

Figure 10.7   The Vocal Folds

at the angle of the thyroid, extend posteriorly along the inner sides of the thyroid, and attach to the vocal processes of the arytenoids. As indicated in Figure 10.7, each vocal fold extends into the opening of the larynx like a shelf. The space between the folds is called the *glottis*. The glottis varies in width, depending on which laryngeal muscles contract and how much they contract. During normal breathing, the glottis is relatively wide open. When a speaker whispers, the front part of the glottis closes but the posterior portion remains open. During full voice, the folds are closed along their entire length, and the glottis disappears.

Making the Voice Generator *Work*

Muscles in the larynx allow the speaker to open and close the vocal folds, and the muscles making up the vocal folds allow the speaker to make the folds tense or relax. These adjustments are basic to producing the voice. Muscles that have both of their attachments within the larynx itself are *intrinsic muscles* of the larynx. These are the muscles primarily responsible for the adjustments necessary for voice production. The extrinsic muscles, with one attachment in the larynx and the other attachment outside the larynx, move the entire structure up and down, but these adjustments have little to do with generating voice. This section, therefore, focuses on those intrinsic muscles most directly involved in opening and closing the vocal folds.

The muscles whose primary responsibility is to open the vocal folds are called *abductors*. To *abduct* means to move or pull away from the middle. In the case of laryngeal function, the abductors pull the vocal folds away from each other, opening the glottis between them. Those muscles primarily responsible for closing the vocal folds are called *adductors*, which means that they move the vocal folds toward the middle, effectively closing the glottis.

The muscles of abduction are the *posterior cricoarytenoid* muscles (Figure 10.8). As is true of most muscles of the body, the name itself identifies the points of attachment. These muscles originate on both sides of the posterior plate of the cricoid cartilage and attach to the lateral or muscular processes of the arytenoid cartilages. When these muscles contract, they pull the arytenoids in a manner that causes them to rotate, opening the folds attached to their vocal processes.

Adduction of the vocal folds is accomplished by contraction of the paired *lateral cricoarytenoid* muscles and the *interarytenoid* muscles (Figure 10.9).

Figure 10.8 The Action of the Posterior Cricoarytenoid Muscles: Abduction

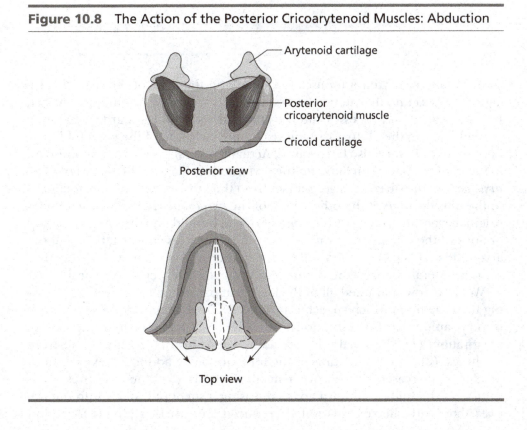

Arytenoid cartilage

Posterior cricoarytenoid muscle

Cricoid cartilage

Posterior view

Top view

Figure 10.9   The Interarytenoid Muscles: Transverse and Oblique (Rear View)

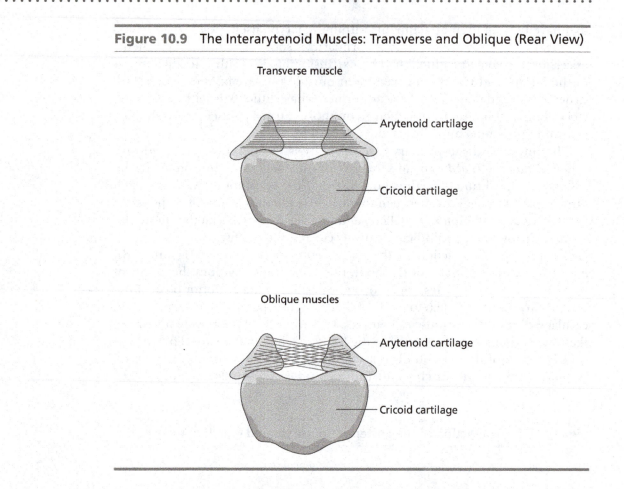

The lateral cricoarytenoid muscles originate on the sides of the cricoid carti-lage and insert into the lateral processes of the arytenoids. When they contract, they pull the vocal processes and the attached vocal folds toward the middle, partially closing the glottis. To achieve complete closure of the vocal folds, the interarytenoids must also be involved. Actually, several interarytenoid muscles, as the name implies, run between the arytenoid cartilages. The *transverse inter-arytenoid*, an unpaired muscle, courses from the outside edge of one arytenoid to the outside edge of the other. Each of the two *oblique interarytenoid* muscles originates on the lower outside edge of one arytenoid and attaches to the top or apex of the other. When the interarytenoid muscles contract, they pull the arytenoid cartilages and the vocal folds together, and when they work together with the lateral cricoarytenoid muscles, they completely close the vocal folds.

We have now examined all of the laryngeal parts that are active in generat-ing the tone upon which speech is produced. The laryngeal tone is the result of very rapid vocal fold vibrations. Consider what happens in a single cycle of vibration: (1) The vocal folds are adducted to restrict the flow of air from the lungs; (2) At the same time as the folds are being adducted, exhalation is producing increased air pressure beneath the folds; (3) When this pressure is sufficient, the folds are blown apart, releasing a small puff of air into the tra-chea above; (4) This release results in reduced pressure beneath the folds; and

(5) The reduction of air pressure combined with the elasticity of the folds forces the folds to snap back together, ready to be blown apart again when the pressure builds up. This five-step sequence is repeated 120 to 145 times per second in adult males, and 200 to 260 times per second in adult females (Zemlin, 1990).

Pitch changes are accomplished by varying the length and mass of the folds. In general, pitch rises when there is an increase in length and a decrease in mass, adjustments that result in more rapid vocal fold vibrations. The tone produced by the larynx is most often called the *glottal* or *laryngeal tone*. It sounds like the combination of a hum and a buzz until it is shaped by the resonating cavities of the neck and head and eventually broken up by the articulators into the speech sounds we combine into words and sentences.

Resonation

The next speech process is resonation. Have you ever blown over the top of a partially filled bottle of pop? The sound you hear results from the size and shape of the resonating cavity, in this case the space in the bottle above the pop. If you drink more of the pop and blow over the top again, the tone will change. The change is the result of a larger and, depending on bottle shape and the amount of pop remaining, differently shaped resonating cavity. In other words, if the tone fed into the bottle remains constant but the size and shape of the resonating cavity within the bottle change, the resulting tones will change. In general, the larger the resonating cavity, the lower the perceived pitch of the tone, because the larger cavity will reinforce the lower frequencies in the original tone. Resonance in speech, therefore, is the process whereby certain frequencies in the laryngeal tone are reinforced or emphasized, depending on the size and shape of the speech resonators, including the pharynx, mouth, and nasal cavities (Figure 10.10). Although a bottle's resonating cavity has a

Figure 10.10   The Resonating Cavities

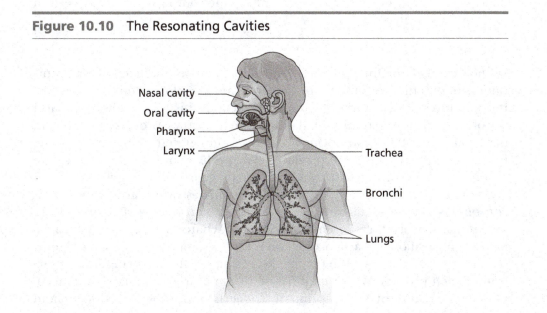

fairly limited range of adjustments, the resonating cavities for speech are capable of seemingly limitless adjustments.

Although resonation is important for shaping all speech sounds, it is particularly important for vowels. The primary characteristic differentiating vowels from consonants is that they are open sounds, produced with a relatively free flow of air. There is very little constriction anywhere in the vocal tract when a vowel is produced. Say the following sounds aloud: /p/, /t/, /k/. Notice that the airflow is actually stopped and released on these sounds. Now say /s/, /f/, and /u/. Notice that the flow of air continues, but it is constricted. Now produce a few vowels aloud such as /e/, /o/, and /i/. There is little restriction of airflow in the mouth. Now try producing a constant laryngeal tone and simply change the size and shape of your mouth by opening it wide and narrowing the opening, by lifting the tongue and lowering it without touching anything, and by moving the tongue forward and pulling it back. These are the kinds of adjustments we make to produce different vowels. When we produce a vowel like the /i/ in *feet*, we create a narrow, high, front-of-the-mouth resonating cavity. When we produce a vowel like the /a/ in *father*, we shape a wide, low, back-of-the-mouth cavity. Notice that the /i/ sounds higher in pitch than the /a/, even though the laryngeal tone remains the same. Keep in mind that we have considered changes only in the mouth. The pharynx, which connects the trachea and the mouth, is a muscular structure capable of many adjustments, and it is constantly changing its shape during speech, adding subtle resonated qualities to the laryngeal tone.

It is generally understood that the nasal cavities are opened for resonation only for the production of the consonants *m*, *n*, and *ng*. We actually experience some nasal resonation on vowels in words containing these consonants because we cannot close off the nasal cavities quickly enough to eliminate the nasal quality. You may also have noticed that there is a nasal quality in some dialects of American English, particularly in the southern and southwestern parts of the country.

Articulation

We now come to the final process of speech, articulation, which is most simply understood as the breaking up of the airstream into the sounds of speech by the structures of the mouth. It should be clear at this point, however, that it is not possible to separate articulation from the other processes of speech, particularly resonation, with which it is closely integrated. Although it is true, for example, that vowels are primarily the products of resonation, they are also the products of articulatory adjustments, especially varying jaw openings and tongue manipulations. We most commonly associate articulation with consonants, but as has already been noted, the consonants *m*, *n*, and *ng* are very much the products of nasal resonance. Whatever separation we make between resonation and articulation, therefore, is somewhat arbitrary and must be understood as an effort to emphasize and clarify the most important function of each process. With that purpose in mind, it is reasonable and accurate to note that resonation is primarily concerned with vowel production and articulation is primarily concerned with consonant production, although each process is involved in the production of all speech sounds.

The articulators include the teeth, tongue, lips, alveolar ridge, hard palate, soft palate (velum), and jaw (Figure 10.11). Notice that some of these structures can move and others are fixed. The tongue, lips, soft palate, and jaw can move, but not at the same speeds. The tongue is capable of relatively rapid movements, but the soft palate moves very slowly. The soft palate is the muscular tissue at the posterior end of the roof of the mouth. For all of the sounds of speech except /m/, /n/, and /y/, it lifts up and back to close off the opening between the mouth and the nasal cavities. The alveolar ridge is the bony shelf in which the upper teeth are set. The hard palate is the bony portion of the roof of the mouth. These structures and the teeth do not move. Another way to understand articulation, therefore, is that the mobile articulators move toward and away from, and sometimes make contact with, the fixed articulators. These adjustments account for how most, but not all, speech sounds are articulated, because the sounds /k/, /g/, and /ŋ/ involve contacts between the back of the tongue and the soft palate, two mobile articulators.

The Four Processes in *Review*

Now that we have examined each process as a separate part of the anatomy and physiology of speech, we will consider how they work together in the simple production of the word *be*.

A speaker inhales by contracting the diaphragm and the muscles of the thorax, which has the effect of increasing the volume of the thorax in the vertical, side-to-side, and front-to-back dimensions. This increase in volume creates reduced pressure in the lungs, which expand along with the expanding thorax. Air comes into the lungs until the pressure in the lungs equals the pressure

Figure 10.11 The Articulators

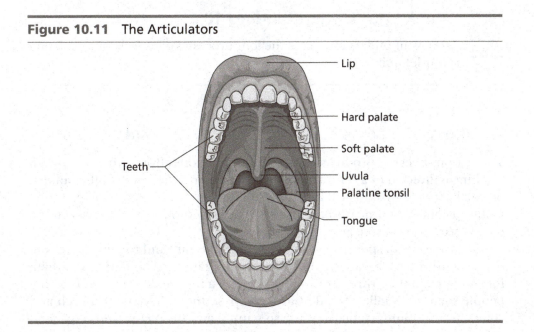

outside the body. The speaker then exhales by relaxing most of the muscles of inhalation and contracting the muscles of exhalation in a prolonged and controlled manner. These actions push a column of air out of the lungs, through the trachea, and into the larynx.

Because both sounds in the word *be* require vocal fold vibration, the speaker contracts the adductor muscles to bring the vocal folds together. As the column of air is pushed through the folds by the forces of exhalation, the folds vibrate, creating a disturbance in the particles of air that we refer to as the *glottal* or *laryngeal tone*. The now-vibrating column of air passes out of the larynx into the pharynx.

The speaker adjusts the *resonators*, including the pharynx, mouth, and nasal cavities, to shape the laryngeal tone according to the characteristics of the sounds being produced. In producing *be*, for example, the speaker will lift the soft palate to close off the nasal cavities because the sounds in the word do not receive nasal resonance. The speaker closes the lips to stop the flow of air and then quickly releases this closure to *articulate* the /b/ sound and, at the same time, raises the tongue toward the front part of the hard palate to create the high, narrow resonating chamber for the /i/. The vocal folds vibrate throughout the entire production.

You should once again be impressed with the complexity of these adjustments and the speed at which they occur. The human anatomy has been ideally developed for the production of speech, and the physiology involved occurs so naturally and effortlessly that we make these rapid, intricate adjustments thousands upon thousands of times every day without giving them a conscious thought.

Check Your Understanding 10.1

Assess your understanding of the four processes of speech by completing this brief quiz.

The Brain: The Computer Center for Speech and Language

The reason speech is produced with so little conscious effort is that the speech machine is directed by a central nervous system unmatched in any other animal on earth. Some physiological functions in humans and in all animals are automatic, of course. Our hearts beat and we breathe without any conscious efforts on our part, whether we are awake or asleep.

The behaviors of speech and language are voluntary and require more conscious control than breathing, but they require far less direct attention than, for example, putting thread through the eye of a needle. Remember, too, that people sometimes talk while they are asleep, so the behaviors of speech and language are voluntary, but they are so natural and instinctive and require so little effort that we can sometimes talk in our sleep. This would not be possible without the complex and highly reliable nervous system that serves as a kind of computer center for speech and language.

A detailed description of neuroanatomy and neurophysiology is beyond the scope of this book, but for our purposes, we will focus on the major features of the human nervous system, and especially on those parts that are most directly related to speech, language, and hearing.

The nervous system can be arbitrarily divided into two major divisions: (1) central nervous system; and (2) peripheral nervous system. The *central nervous system* (Figure 10.12) includes the brain and the spinal cord. The brain is divided into halves called the right and left *cerebral hemispheres*, the *brain stem*, and the *cerebellum*. The brain is encased in the skull, and the spinal cord is surrounded by the bony *vertebral column*, sometimes called the *spinal column*.

The *peripheral nervous system* consists of all the cranial and spinal nerves that carry information to the brain in the form of sensations such as hearing, pain, or temperature, and information from the brain in the form of motor commands to the muscles of the body.

The most basic anatomical unit of the nervous system is the *neuron*. There are millions of neurons in the body, which are organized into complex networks or circuits. Any message carried anywhere in the nervous system is carried by the tiny neuron.

Figure 10.12   The Central Nervous System

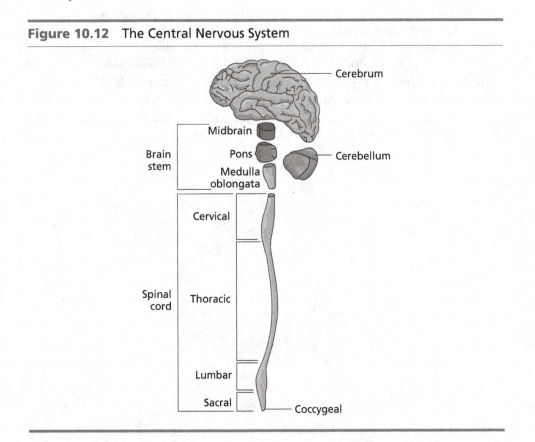

Speech and Language Functions of the Brain

Even though the speech and language functions of the brain are not fully understood, we have been able to identify certain areas of the cerebral hemispheres that have primary responsibilities for this uniquely human range of behaviors. What follows is a brief overview of the information researchers have gathered over the years about those structures they believe are most closely associated with speech and language functions. Be forewarned: because this is only an overview and intentionally introductory in nature, we will focus only on the most obvious relevant structures.

The Cerebrum: Left and Right Cerebral Hemispheres

The *cerebrum*, the largest portion of the brain, is incompletely divided into two hemispheres. The two halves of the cerebrum are connected by a large band of neural fibers known as the *corpus callosum*, a structure that serves as a major communication pathway between the two hemispheres. Although we cannot generalize left and right hemispheric functions for all people, it is appropriate to indicate that in most people the left hemisphere has greater responsibilities for speech and language activities than the right. Three areas of the left hemisphere and a bundle of neural fibers (Figure 10.13) are of particular interest: *Wernicke's area*, *Broca's area*, the *motor cortex*, and the *arcuate fasciculus*. Wernicke's area is primarily concerned with the comprehension and formulation of language. Language information is transmitted to Broca's area from Wernicke's area via a bundle of neural fibers called the *arcuate fasciculus*. The term *fasciculus* refers to a bundle of nerve fibers that share a common origin, termination, and function. In Broca's area, language information is organized into the appropriate articulatory motor sequences for speech. These motor commands are then transmitted to the motor cortex. The neural messages

---

Figure 10.13 Left Cerebral Hemisphere

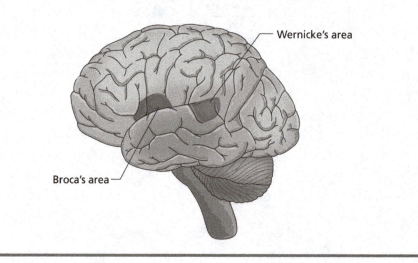

Wernicke's area

Broca's area

carrying speech and language information are eventually sent to the speech musculature along special pathways that will be described in the next section.

The right hemisphere is less involved with speech and language than the left, but it does contribute to the processing of emotional content that often underlies speech and language. There is also evidence that the melodic patterns we superimpose on speech when we sing are associated with right hemispheric functions (Blumstein & Cooper, 1974; Knox & Kimura, 1970).

The suggestion here is that functions of the hemispheres are highly specialized, and although areas in each hemisphere do seem to have specific functions, it is important to understand that there is significant integration of the functions of the cerebrum. For example, we have noted that emotional processing is associated with the right hemisphere, and language and speech functions are associated with the left hemisphere. It should be immediately clear, however, that we can communicate emotional messages through speech and language only if the two hemispheres interact with each other in a manner that allows us to integrate emotional messages into language form, which are then expressed in meaningful speech.

Motor Speech Control

How do we get our speech and language messages from the cerebrum to the muscles of speech? Once thoughts are formulated and put into language form, the cerebrum sends the motor messages of speech along a complex neural network of special pathways within the central nervous system. The information contained in these pathways ultimately reaches the various motor portions of the cranial and spinal nerves that constitute the peripheral nervous system. The peripheral nerves are connected to the muscles of the body and are the final pathways over which the messages will be delivered.

It may help to think of this process of getting motor commands from the cerebrum to the structures of speech as being analogous to a relay race. The "runners" that will be the initial carriers of information in this complicated delivery system are the many neurons that make up specialized pathways in the central nervous system. Positioned at strategic locations within the nervous system are the other runners or neurons that make up the cranial and spinal nerves of the peripheral nervous system. Once the communication plan is developed, the runners of the central nervous system are given complex messages, which they carry to the runners of the peripheral nervous system by way of the special pathways. Upon reaching the stations where the peripheral nervous system runners are waiting, the messages are passed on and carried by those runners to the muscles of the body that must be activated to produce the message in its final form—speech.

Central Nervous System Pathways: The Beginning of the Relay Race

One of the special pathways of the central nervous system is called *pyramidal* because the tiny neurons that give rise to this system have cell bodies shaped like pyramids. This part of the system has direct input into the motor cranial and spinal nerves that represent the second leg in the relay race to the structures of speech. The pyramidal pathway controls refined, intricate movements in structures such as the lips and tongue. This kind of control is crucial to an activity like speech, which is the product of complex, precise, and delicately integrated motor adjustments.

The *extrapyramidal* system has a more *indirect* connection to the motor cranial and spinal nerves than the pyramidal system, and it is responsible for providing commands for more gross and unskilled motor activities such as those involved in postural adjustment. The act of writing provides a simple example of the difference between pyramidal and extrapyramidal responsibilities. When you write, the extrapyramidal tract gets your hand to the paper, and the pyramidal tract controls the fine motor skills necessary for you to write on that paper. In the context of our relay race analogy, the runners in the extrapyramidal system stop at a number of locations within the central nervous system to gather additional information in order to make the necessary adjustments to provide a background against which the pyramidal system makes its more precise, finely tuned movements.

The cerebellum coordinates the activities controlled by the pyramidal and extrapyramidal systems. It is constantly receiving sensory information about the status of the muscles and limbs of the body and monitors the motor commands being sent along the pyramidal and extrapyramidal pathways. Using this steady flow of information to and from the central nervous system, the cerebellum makes crucial adjustments in commands to ensure that the final motor products are performed s accurately as possible.

Peripheral Nervous System Pathways: The Relay Race Continues

The commands that have been formulated in the cerebral hemispheres, carried through the central nervous system along the pyramidal and extrapyramidal pathways, and fine-tuned by the cerebellum are now passed to the message carrier that will run along the pathways of the cranial and spinal nerves that comprise the peripheral nervous system.

There are 12 pairs of *cranial nerves*. Some of these nerves carry only sensory information, some carry only motor information, and others are mixed and carry both sensory and motor information. Only six of the cranial nerves are concerned with motor speech (Figure 10.14).

There are 31 pairs of *spinal nerves*, and they are all mixed; that is, they carry both sensory and motor information. More than half of these nerves control the muscles of respiration. Because, as we observed earlier in this chapter, controlled and prolonged exhalation is crucial to speech production, these nerves make important contributions to the speech machine.

The Relay Race in Review: Instant Replay

There is much that is not understood about the nervous system in general and much that is not known about the functions related to speech and language. We do know, however, that the nervous system is organized in a hierarchical manner. That is, at some levels in the system, information is developed, refined, and integrated as it works its way to the speech musculature.

Figure 10.14 Pyramidal Fibers Serving Motor Cranial Nerves of Speech

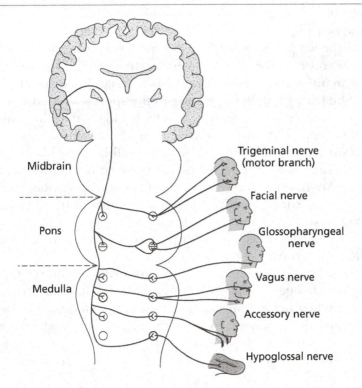

Using the relay race analogy, we can now summarize the process. At the highest level in the system, the cerebrum, thoughts are developed and language to express those thoughts is formulated. The message is carried by runners along the pyramidal and extrapyramidal pathways of the central nervous system. These runners carry the message through the cerebellum, which fine-tunes the motor commands, before they hand off the message to other runners that carry the message along the pathways of the cranial and spinal nerves involved in speech. The race ends when the commands reach the muscles of the speech structures, which contract in patterns producing strings of sounds that are a direct translation of the original thought.

In continuous speech, of course, the relay race is infinitely more complicated than this summary indicates because new thoughts, new language forms, and new motor messages are being sent, monitored, and fine-tuned constantly. The nervous system carries so much information so quickly with such tremendous efficiency that it makes the Internet look like a slow-moving freeway during rush hour.

Check Your Understanding 10.2

Assess your understanding of the brain as the center of speech and language by completing this brief quiz.

The Ear: An Energy Transformer

It is impossible to understand speech as a physiological process without considering the hearing mechanism that allows us to receive speech and monitor our own speech productions. You will quickly appreciate the importance of hearing if you consider how a child learns to talk. She does not buy a *How to Talk* manual, nor does she enroll in Human Speech 101 at the local university. She learns to talk by *listening* to the speech around her. If a child has any significant deficit in hearing, it is highly likely that the acquisition of speech will be impaired. At the other end of the age spectrum, a normally speaking adult who loses hearing later in life will not lose language but may experience some deterioration in speech because he cannot hear his own productions. Articulation may not be as precise as it once was, for example, and there may be some nasality on speech sounds that are not supposed to have nasal resonance. The point is simple but important. Hearing is as crucial to normal speech as any other part of the complete anatomical and physiological speech package.

The human hearing mechanism is an extraordinary energy transformer, and tracing the changes in energy forms is one of the best ways to understand the parts of the hearing system and how they are related to one another. For the sake of convenience, we will consider the three traditional anatomical divisions of the ear—*outer, middle,* and *inner*—but it is important to note that the outer and middle ears function together to transform acoustic energy into mechanical energy.

The Outer Ear

Sound travels to the outer ear (see Figure 10.15) in the form of sound waves that, as we noted in Chapter 1, are disturbances of air particles characterized by compressions and rarefactions. These waves are caught by the *pinna*, the visible fleshy part of the ear attached to the side of the head. The pinna contributes minimally to our ability to hear, but it does serve to direct sound waves into the *external auditory meatus* or ear canal. This canal is slightly curved, about an inch long and a quarter of an inch across, dimensions that make it a resonator specifically tuned to the frequencies of speech sounds. At the end of the canal is the *tympanic membrane* or eardrum, which serves as the boundary between the outer and middle ears.

The Middle Ear

In the middle ear (see Figure 10.16), the tympanic membrane is semitransparent and is usually pearl gray when it is healthy. The center of the membrane is pulled in because it is attached to one of the tiny bones in the middle ear. The tympanic membrane absorbs the acoustic energy of sound waves and transforms it into mechanical energy, which is the vibration of a solid material.

The tiny bones in the middle ear, called the *ossicles*, are the *malleus* (hammer), *incus* (anvil), and *stapes* (stirrup). The malleus is the largest ossicle, and its "handle" is attached to the center of the tympanic membrane. The middle

Figure 10.15   The Outer Ear

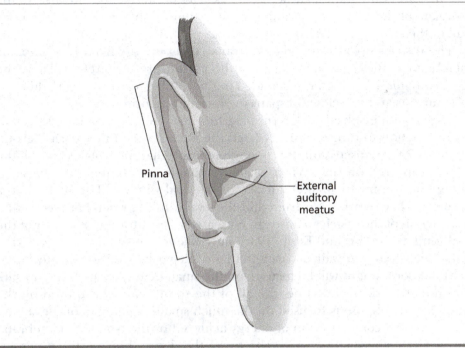

Figure 10.16   The Middle Ear

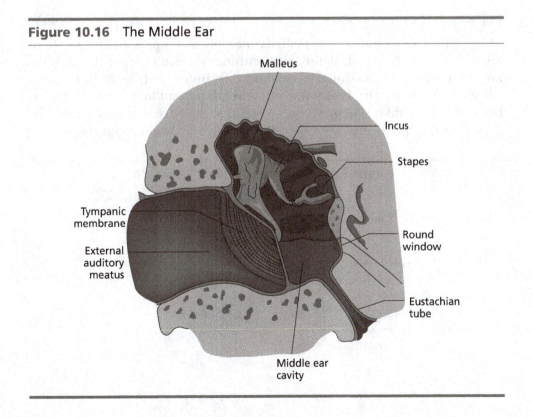

ossicle is the incus, which is attached to the innermost ossicle, the stapes. The bottom part of the stapes, known as the *footplate* because of its similarity to the footplate of the stirrup of a saddle, fits into an oval-shaped hole in the bony wall of the inner ear called the *oval window*.

The ossicles operate together in transferring energy from the tympanic membrane to the oval window and, for this reason, are often referred to as the *ossicular chain*. This chain is suspended in the air-filled cavity of the middle ear by ligaments and muscles and spans the cavity like a bridge.

The physics involved in determining how the ossicular chain and the eardrum function to transfer energy from the outer to the inner ear is beyond the scope of this discussion. It is enough to know that the ossicles take all the energy captured on the surface of the tympanic membrane and focus this energy on the much smaller surface of the oval window. The surface area difference between the eardrum and the oval window, when coupled with a lever action of the ossicles, causes an increased concentration of energy at the oval window. Perkins and Kent (1986) have likened this to a woman wearing spike heels trying to walk across a wet lawn. Regardless of how petite she is, her total body weight will be focused on the small heels, causing them to sink into the ground. In the same way, all of the sound energy captured on the tympanic membrane is focused on the much smaller footplate of the stapes. The increased concentration of energy achieved by the tympanic membrane and the ossicular chain is necessary to set the dense fluids of the inner ear into motion.

The Inner Ear

Although the inner ear is very small, its anatomy is complex and its functions are not fully understood. Before we continue to trace hearing through the inner ear, we need to examine its anatomy. The inner ear (Figure 10.17) actually serves two functions. It contains structures important to hearing, of course, but it also contains a system we use to maintain balance or equilibrium. The structures of equilibrium are called the *semicircular canals*. Even though the

Figure 10.17   The Inner Ear in Relation to Middle Ear Structures

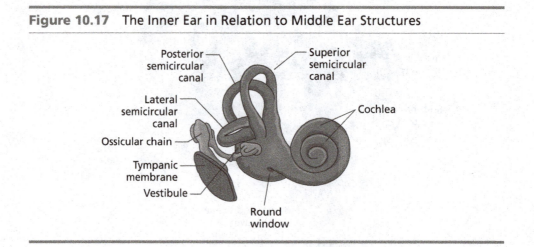

Posterior semicircular canal

Superior semicircular canal

Lateral semicircular canal

Cochlea

Ossicular chain

Tympanic membrane

Vestibule

Round window

inner ear has two functions, the divisions are connected and share the same fluid system.

The inner ear is encased in the temporal bone of the skull. The division containing the organs of hearing is called the *cochlea*, a structure that coils about two and a half times around a cone-shaped bone called the *modiolus*. The nerve pathways from the cochlea feed into the modiolus where they merge into the *auditory nerve*, which carries hearing messages to the brain.

Figure 10.18 shows a cross section of the cochlea. Imagine that we have uncoiled the cochlea, laid it lengthwise, and cut it. This figure shows what you would see if you looked through the cochlea as you might look through a pipe. Remember that everything you see here continues along the length of the structure. The cochlea is actually a bony tube containing two membranes that divide the tube into three sections: the *scala vestibule, scala media*, and *scala tympani*. The scala vestibule and scala media are separated by *Reissner's membrane*, and the scala media and scala tympani are separated by the *basilar membrane*. All three of these divisions are filled with fluid. The scala vestibule and scala tympani, which are connected at the top of the cochlea through a small opening called the *helicotrema*, are filled with fluid called *perilymph*. The fluid in the scala media is called *endolymph*.

The *organ of Corti*, sometimes called the *essential* or *end organ* of hearing, is situated along the length of basilar membrane. It consists of thousands of tiny auditory nerve receptors with *hair cells* that are the delicate final endings of the auditory nerve. These receptors and their hair cells are arranged into one inner row and three outer rows along the basilar membrane. A jellylike structure called the *tectorial membrane* hangs suspended over the tops of these highly sensitive hair cells. The tectorial membrane is a relatively free-floating membrane that responds to movements in the fluid of the scala media.

Figure 10.18   Cross Section of the Cochlea

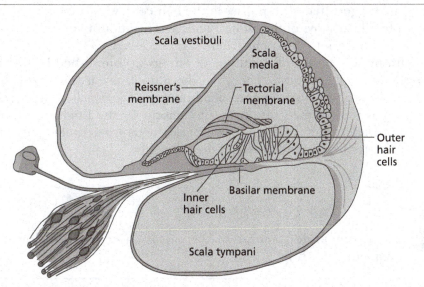

The oval window, which is occupied by the footplate of the stapes, serves as the communicating link between the middle ear and the scala vestibuli of the inner ear. The *round window* is located below the oval window and is adjacent to the scala tympani section of the inner ear. Sound vibrations enter the cochlea through the oval window. When the stapes pushes into the oval window, the mechanical energy of the ossicles is transformed into hydraulic energy in the form of fluid motion. The pressure of this motion is relieved by the round window, which moves toward the middle ear as the footplate of the stapes moves inward toward the inner ear.

There is some uncertainty about what happens next. We do know that motion of the fluids in the inner ear causes the tectorial membrane to move in a manner that somehow excites the hair cells, triggering neural impulses. The net result is that the hydraulic energy of the fluids is transformed into neural energy, which is carried by the peripheral pathways of the auditory nerve to the brain.

Tracing the Pathway of Hearing: A Brief Summary

To summarize the hearing mechanism, we will follow a sound wave through the system and note the major structures of hearing along the way.

The sound wave is captured by the pinna, directed into the external auditory meatus, and strikes the surface of the tympanic membrane, setting it into vibration. This vibration is carried by the ossicles across the middle ear cavity and is focused on the footplate of the stapes in the oval window. The inward movement of the stapes sets the perilymph of the scala vestibuli into motion, which causes Reissner's membrane to move, which then causes motion in the endolymph of the scala media. The motion of the endolymph causes movement of the tectorial membrane and movement along the basilar membrane. The motion finally makes its way along the scala tympani to the round window, which bulges slightly into the middle ear cavity. The motion of the tectorial membrane triggers neural responses in the hair cells, which are connected to the peripheral pathways of the auditory nerve. The auditory nerve carries the hearing information to the brain, where it is processed.

Finally, notice the transformations of energy accomplished by the hearing mechanism. The acoustic energy of the sound wave is transformed into mechanical energy by the tympanic membrane and the ossicles. This mechanical energy is transformed into hydraulic energy by the fluids of the inner ear. The hydraulic energy is eventually transformed into neural energy by the action of the tectorial membrane and the hair cells.

Check Your Understanding 10.3

Assess your understanding of the ear as an energy transformer by completing this brief quiz.

SUMMARY

We have now examined the anatomy and physiology, albeit briefly and superficially, of the structures that make up the speech machine. It is a complex system of systems, each part precisely and efficiently integrated with every other part and directed by a reliable and constantly adapting central nervous system. Humans are born with all this equipment, and we quickly and easily adapt it for expressing language through speech.

▥ Surfing the Web

If you are interested in exploring topics discussed in this appendix in more detail, process one or more of the following relevant terms into a search engine.

anatomy of human respiration for speech production

physiology of human respiration for speech production

anatomy of human phonation for speech production

physiology of human phonation for speech production

anatomy of human vocal resonance

physiology of human vocal resonance

anatomy of human articulation of speech sounds

physiology of human articulation of speech sounds

central nervous system and speech production

left cerebral hemisphere and speech production

right cerebral hemisphere and speech production

motor control during speech

anatomy of the human ear

hearing pathways from ear to brain

▥ Chapter Review 10.1

1. Identify and define the four processes of speech production.
2. Discuss the integration of respiration, phonation, resonation, and articulation in the production of speech.
3. Explain the main structures and their functions for respiration: the power source for speech.
4. Describe the role of the vocal folds in phonation: using the larynx to generate voice.
5. Report on the process of resonation: shaping the cavities of the speech mechanism to modify the tones of speech.
6. Identify and describe the structures and process of articulation: using the structures of the mouth to produce the sounds of speech.
7. Trace the human nervous system: linking the brain to the muscles of speech.
8. Describe the ear: moving sound waves from the pinna to the brain.

Glossary

Accent   Variations in pronunciation of sounds, modulation of pitch or tone, and prominence of syllables or words during speech.

Accommodation   Cognitive process whereby new schemes are created for information that does not fit existing schemes.

Account   Spontaneous description of an event or experience without prompting from an adult.

Adaptations   Changes children make to their schemes in order to fit into and function within their environment when experiencing cognitive conflict, achieved through *assimilation* or *accommodation*.

Additive approach   Strategy whereby teachers add to an existing curriculum to take cultures other than the dominant culture into account by expanding content and introducing culturally related concepts, themes, and perspectives without altering the basic structure of the curriculum.

Additive bilingual environment   Environment in which children are encouraged to retain their first language and to embrace their native culture while learning the majority language and also embracing a second culture.

Additive conjunctive relation   Connects two or more sentences, clauses, or parts of clauses by adding more information to what is already there (*and, in addition, also,*); the first conjunctive relation developed by children.

Adjectival   Word or phrase that modifies a noun and can be an adjective (*pretty, tall*), an ordinal (*second, last*), or a quantifier (*one, couple, few*).

Adverbial   Word that describes or changes the meaning of a verb or verb phrase, but it also qualifies adjectives, other adverbs, and clauses. Adverbs often end in *-ly* and answer *wh-* questions, such as *how, when, where,* and *why.*

Adverbial conjuncts   Adverb that connects two clauses and demonstrates addition (*furthermore, equally important*), a time sequence (*simultaneously, after a while*), contrast (*in spite of, regardless*), comparison (*likewise, also*), or other relationships.

Adverbial disjuncts   Clause that expresses information about the speaker's attitude towards the content of the sentence, possibly intended to focus attention on the speaker's purpose, apart from or in addition to the communication ("*To be quite honest with you,* you're making a mistake").

Adversative conjunctive relation   Coordinating conjunctions used to express comparisons or contrasts with regard to the main clause of the sentence (e.g., *but, yet, still, however, although*).

Age of acquisition effect   As new learning occurs, this phenomenon allows the neural network to retain its plasticity and its stability in word representations so that word learning increases efficiently across time. This effect is associated with the tendency for words that are learned earlier to show faster retrieval during naming and reading tasks than words learned later.

Agent   Words that refer to things that cause action.

Agentive   Grammatical form that denotes the doer of a given action, often (but not always) accomplished by adding an *-er* to a verb in order to change it into a noun (e.g., a person who teaches is a teach*er*).

Allophone   One speech sound among a set of sounds used to pronounce a single *phoneme.*

Alveolar ridge   Thickened bone protuberance on the roof of the mouth just behind the upper teeth.

Anaphoric reference   Type of reference in which a pronoun is used to refer to something in a preceding utterance.

Analytic level   Reading level that activates a reader's deep processing of the information.

Anticipatory coarticulation   Feature or characteristic of a speech sound is anticipated during the production of a preceding speech sound.

Arbitrariness   Idea that there is nothing inherent in a spoken word to account for its meaning, no limitation to what language can describe, and no explicit or necessary connection between sounds used and the message being sent; Charles Hockett's eighth "design feature" of language.

Arcuate fasciculus   Bundle of nerve fibers that serves as the neural pathway to connect the expressive (i.e., Broca's area) and receptive (i.e., Wernicke's area) language areas to each other.

Articulation disorder A disorder in the use of the speech mechanism to form the necessary place, manner, and voicing of sounds.

Aspiration Release of air on the production of phonemes during speech.

Assimilation Cognitive process whereby a new stimulus is fitted into an existing schema.

Assimilation processes Form of simplification during speech in which one sound takes on the identity (or some of the characteristics) of another sound.

Attrition Process by which a dominant first language fades, and a second language becomes dominant.

Autism spectrum disorder Group of developmental disabilities, with an onset before 36 months of age, that can cause significant social, communication, and behavioral challenges.

Auxiliary verb "Helping" verb, such as *be, do,* or *have,* that accompanies a main verb and expresses tense, aspect, modality, voice, or emphasis.

Aversive stimulus Warning that there will be an unpleasant consequence for a particular behavior.

Babbling Combinations of vowel- and consonant-like sounds produced without meaning.

Bilingual first language acquisition Process of acquiring two languages from birth and becoming competent in both languages at a relatively equal rate.

Bilingual second language acquisition Process of acquiring one language before exposure to a second language.

Book-sharing activities Reading activity in which caregivers engage in interactive reading with a child.

Bound morpheme Morphemes that are attached to words and cannot stand alone (e.g., possessive form of -*s*).

Broadcast transmission Idea that the sound of speech is heard in all directions but listeners interpret it as coming from one specific direction; Charles Hockett's second "design feature" of language.

Broca's area Region in the frontal lobe of the left hemisphere of the brain associated with language production (expressive language), specifically the role of assigning and organizing the motor sequences for the sounds of speech.

Case grammar Semantic theory developed by Charles Fillmore to explain the importance of semantics and its influence on the form of language; a form of generative grammar that describes the deep structure of sentences in terms of the relation of a verb to a set of semantic cases.

Causal conjunctive relation One clause expresses an action or state of being, and the other clause provides a reason or describes the effect.

Causality Understanding that people, objects, or events can have an effect on other people, objects, or events.

Centering Organizational narrative structure that involves building a story around a central theme with each item or action in the narrative being connected to the central theme by an attribute that is related to the theme.

Cerebrovascular accident Stroke; damage to the brain due to a lack of blood flow and oxygen.

Chaining Instructional procedure that involves reinforcing individual responses occurring in a sequence to form a complex behavior; organizational narrative structure that involves ordering events so that one event logically follows the preceding event.

Chunking Process of placing words into categories based on their semantic relationships.

Classical conditioning Variation of conditioned learning in which an originally neutral stimulus is repeatedly paired with an unconditioned stimulus that elicits a desired response.

Cluttering A disorder that involves both speech and language errors including sound omissions and distortions, irregular rate and lack of pausing, poor awareness and self-monitoring, incomplete phases, and disorganization in the construction and execution of verbal information.

Coarticulation During rapid speech, a speech sound is influenced by, and becomes more like, a preceding or following speech sound.

Code mixing Combinations of words or phrases from more than one language.

Communication Sending and receiving information, ideas, feelings, or messages.

Communicative context Situation in which a communicative event takes place.

Comparative adjective Adjective used to compare one noun to another noun; occurs through the addition of the suffix -*er.*

Comparative level Reading level that requires a reader to use all the other reading levels to reflect on information from multiple sources in order to compare meanings.

Conductive hearing loss Hearing loss that occurs due to poor transmission of information from the outer or middle ear to the inner ear, with the most common causes being fluid in the middle ear, malformations of the outer ear, impacted cerumen, perforation or inflammation of the tympanic membrane, or poor functioning of the tiny bones of the middle ear (malleus, incus, and stapes).

Conjoining Process of combining and joining language constructions.

Consolidation phase Second phase of writing development in which a child writes strings of words using the same vocabulary and rules of grammar used in his own speech.

Consonant clusters Group of two or more consonant sounds that come before, after, or between vowels.

Contingent responding Parent's prompt response to a child's behavior or verbalization.

Contracted verb Reduction or shortening of a pronoun and verb phrase (e.g., *he's* running).

Contributions approach Strategy whereby teachers include information on selected heroes and holidays from a range of cultures, and they focus on a few specific characteristics of these cultures while maintaining the existing curriculum.

Controlled attention Capacity to maintain and hold relevant information, especially when there are internal or external distractions or interferences in the environment.

Conversational repair Revision, clarification, or repetition of a message to increase the chances of successful communication.

Conversations Forms of interactive communication between two or more people.

Cooing Production of vowel-like sounds and brief consonant-like sound during the first few months.

Copula verb Word used to link the subject and predicate of a sentence; main verb.

Creole Language that develops as a result of contact between two groups that do not know each other's language.

Creolist theory Hypothesis which suggests that African American Vernacular English is a complicated hybrid derived from several African languages and Portuguese, Dutch, French, and English as a result of the early contact between Africans and Europeans.

Cross-linguistic studies Research about language or language development that looks for universal patterns among various languages.

Cultural curriculum Knowledge students must learn regarding the world that is shared at particular grade levels, regardless of cultural backgrounds of individual students.

Cultural hearths Five places along the eastern and southern coasts of the United States from which most regional dialects have evolved: Boston, Philadelphia, tidewater Virginia, Charleston, and New Orleans.

Customary production Average age of a group of children at which a particular phoneme is produced with more than 50% accuracy in at least two word positions.

Decontextualized Devoid of situation or context.

Decreolization Process by which a creole language becomes increasingly similar to the language of the dominant culture.

Deep structure In Chomsky's transformational grammar, the underlying syntactic structure of a sentence generated by *phrase-structure rules.*

Deictic gestures Use of pointing, showing, or reaching for something to call attention to or indicate an object or event.

Deictic word pairs Words bound to either a linguistic or an extralinguistic context for their interpretation that specify identity, spatial, or temporal location from the perspective of a speaker or listener in the context in which the message occurs (*here/there, this/that,* and *I/you*).

Deixis Phenomenon in which understanding the meaning of certain words and phrases in an utterance requires contextual information; message interpretation depends on extralinguistic contexts, such as who is speaking, time, place, location, and gestures of the speaker.

Delayed imitation More complex form of *imitation* whereby an action or behavior is repeated some time after the model.

Delta stimulus Signal indicating that reinforcement will not follow a particular response.

Derivational morpheme Morphemes added to the beginning (e.g., *re-, un-*) and end (e.g., *-ly, -un*) of words; prefixes and suffixes.

Determiner First unit in a noun phrase that is an article (*a, the*), a possessive pronoun (*my, his, her*), a demonstrative pronoun (*this, that, these, those*), or a qualifier (*some, most, any*).

Developing readers Individuals who are not yet reading independently, but read for meaning using the text, illustrations, letter/sound associations, and their own knowledge of print conventions to sample, predict, and confirm printed words.

Developmental disability   Broad term used when a disability occurs prior to the age of 22 and is associated with mental or physical impairments.

Dialect   Any given variety of a language shared by a group of speakers.

Differentiation phase   Third stage of writing development in which students' writing becomes differentiated from the way they talk through the use of more sophisticated grammar; this stage continues for many people throughout their lives.

Directional reception   Listener can compare the loudness and timing of sound reaching each ear and can determine the direction from where the sound is coming; Charles Hockett's second "design feature" of language.

Disappearance   When an object has been present, but then disappears; words used to express this relationship may be *bye-bye.*

Discreteness   Idea that each language is limited to a finite or discrete number of sounds. Furthermore, each sound used in one or more human languages has very specific characteristics and can be placed in distinct categories that differentiate them from one another; Charles Hockett's ninth "design feature" of language.

Discriminative stimulus   Stimulus, such as a cue, that provides information about what to do.

Displacement   Human ability to refer to things in space and time and communicate about things that are not currently present; Charles Hockett's 10th "design feature" of language.

Distancing   Ability to use an abstract symbol or word to represent the real object. Language is the way humans represent people, places, and things in thought and interactions.

Distinctive feature approach   View that speech sounds comprise characteristics of place of articulation, manner of articulation, and voicing.

Dual language system hypothesis   Concept that a child who is exposed to two languages from birth uses two separate language systems from the very beginning and does not go through stages in which a conjoined language system is gradually differentiated into two language systems.

Duality of patterning   The restricted number of sounds in a given language can be combined in an infinite number of ways to produce an infinite variety of words, which in turn are combined again

to make meaningful sentences; Charles Hockett's 12th "design feature" of language.

Early phonemic stage   Second stage of spelling development in which a child often only attends to the first letter of a word, uses consonants but excludes vowels, and thinks that other letters typically have no correspondence to the remaining segments of the target word.

Echolalia   Imitation or repetition of words, phrases, or whole sentences spoken by another person.

Embedding   Placing new strings of words within already existing constructions.

Emergent readers   Individuals who are not yet reading, but are just beginning to grasp the basic concepts of books and print and developing alphabetical knowledge and phonological awareness skills.

Equilibrium   Cognitive process to maintain a balance between existing schemata (*assimilation*) and the creation of new schemata (*accommodation*).

Event sequence   Order or sequence of events taking place in a story.

Existence   When an object is present in a child's immediate environment and the child is attending to it; words used to express this relationship may be *this, that,* and *there.*

Expansion   An adult's repetition of what a child has said, adding additional words and/or structure to the utterance.

Expressive elaboration   Use of components including introductory information, background information, and evaluations (emphasis and meaning) to generate more creative and meaningful narratives.

Expressive language   Producing and conveying communicative messages through speaking, writing, signing, or gestures.

Extension   When an adult repeats a child's utterance adding additional words, structure, and new information to the utterance.

Fast mapping   Act of learning a new concept after limited exposure, commonly used by young children when acquiring language.

Figurative language   Non-literal form of language used to describe something by comparing it with something else (e.g., idioms, similes, metaphors, and irony).

Financial/material capital   Objects that have value, but do not do anything alone (e.g., money); wealth of the individual within a society.

First words A child's initial words that convey meaning in a purposeful, consistent, and specific way.

Focused chain A form of narrative where the same character remains the focus; there is an emergence of cause/effect, temporal relationships, weak plot, and character motivation; and the ending may not be logical.

Functional disorder Disorder in which there is a failure to identify a pathology of an organ system after using the best diagnostic procedures and technologies available.

Functional core hypothesis Idea that children do not categorize things according to perceptual attributes (e.g., shapes and size), but rather develop meanings of early words based on their actions if they are animate objects, or on the objects performed on them if they are inanimate objects; children form concepts by viewing objects in terms of the whole, not a sum of parts or features.

Fully resonant nuclei Vowel and consonant sounds with a full range of frequencies and resonant characteristics.

Gerund Verbal or non-finite verb form (based on a verb and expresses action or a state of being) that ends in *ing* and functions as a noun.

Glossing Repeating what a child says during collection of a language sample to capture the precise utterance for transcription accuracy.

Grammatical ellipsis When speakers delete or withhold information that they assume listeners already possess.

Graphophonemic awareness Ability to match letters to individual sounds.

Heaps Unrelated statements connected by a common originating stimulus where information is simply chained together in an additive fashion without a meaningful sequence.

Hidden curriculum Expectations teachers have for student behavior.

Horizontal expansion Adding semantic features to one's definitions of a word to create a greater understanding and use of a word in common situations with greater differentiation of it from other words.

Human capital Collective skills, knowledge, or other intangible assets of individuals that can be used to create economic value. These skills are influenced by culture and are affected by parent and societal beliefs about age, gender, and birth order.

Idioms Commonly used combination of words that has a figurative meaning, which is separate from the literal meaning or definition of the actual words in the phrase (e.g., "The cat's out of the bag").

Illocutionary act Purpose or motive underlying an utterance.

Illocutionary stage Time between 8 and about 12 months of age when infants begin to use gestures and combine these with vocalizations to express a range of specific and recognizable communicative functions.

Imitation Duplication of models one hears and sees.

Incidence Number of new cases of a disorder.

Independent readers Readers who confidently and competently read on their own and when they are alone, pay little conscious attention to the details of printed words but rather focus on constructing and maintaining meaning.

Indexicality Pragmatic feature of language referring to the circumstances or context in which a communicative message takes place; situational context is important in establishing meaning in our communicative attempts.

Indirect request Expression of desire or inclination requiring the receiver of a request to use an inference (*I am very thirsty*).

Inflection Change in a word created by adding a grammatical morpheme.

Inflectional morpheme Suffixes that change the meaning of words by marking grammatical adjustments for things such as plurality, possession, and verb tense.

Information processing theory Theory that examines the sequence and execution of cognitive events, focusing on how individuals attend, encode, relate, store, and retrieve information, particularly for language acquisition purposes.

Informative Providing information.

Initiator Word or phrase that precedes a *determiner* and places a limit on the noun (*only, all, both, just*).

Inspectual level Reading level at which a reader quickly scans reading materials to determine the main ideas.

Instructional conversation Teaching format that involves engaging, informal discussion about a designated topic between students and teacher in which ideas are explored.

Integration phase Fourth and final stage of writing development in which writers develop a *style* that reflects their own personality, makes them unique, and allows them to express varying moods and attitudes in their writing; not all individuals will reach this stage.

Intellectual disability Significant limitations in intelligence as determined by an IQ test score below 70, and limitations in adaptive behavior.

Intelligibility Degree to which speech can be understood.

Interchangeability Anything that people are able to hear, they are also able to reproduce through spoken language; Charles Hockett's fourth "design feature" of language.

Interlanguage Type of language hybrid that combines rules from a dominant language, rules from a second language, and rules a child invents to bridge any gaps between the two.

Intersubjectivity Term to conceptualize the psychological relationship between individuals.

Invented spellings Stage of spelling development in which young children use their best judgments about spelling words using visual memory and sounding-out strategies.

IRE model The initiate-response-evaluate (IRE) model of questioning; a traditional teacher-directed question-and-answer session to check for factual knowledge or fast recall whereby the teacher *initiates* a question, the student *responds*, and the teacher then *evaluates* the answer.

Ironic compliment Negative statement intended to mean something positive.

Ironic criticism Positive statement with the intent to mean something negative.

Irony Use of words to express something other than or opposite to the literal meaning.

Irregular verb Verb form that indicates an action took place in the past, but does not follow conventional past tense (*-ed*) morphology rules (e.g., *ran, sat*).

Jargon babbling Final stage of babbling, also known as conversational babbling, in which productions are distinguished by melodic patterns and have many of the characteristics of real speech such as rhythm, stress, rate variations, and intonational contours.

Joint attention Shared focus of two individuals (e.g., caregiver and child) on each other or on an object or event; joint reference.

Joint reference Shared focus on the same object or event at the same time.

Language System of arbitrary, established symbols and rule-governed structures used for communication that change over time; conventionalized sounds, signs, gestures, or symbols that have shared and understood meanings.

Language acquisition device (LAD) Concept of the nativist theory of language that humans are born with the innate "device" for acquiring language.

Language acquisition support structure (LASS) Concept of the interactionist view that language acquisition is a product of children's early social interactions with the important people in their life.

Language of academic subjects or curriculum Specific vocabulary and manners of discourse associated with education and academics.

Language of behavior management Traditional type of language used by teachers to establish who is allowed to talk, what one is allowed to say, and how one is allowed to say it in a classroom environment.

Language of personal identity Language that is necessary for people to express themselves to others and develop a sense of self.

Learnability Idea that learning occurs when people's innate capacity for learning, a learning environment, and some stimulus for learning that comes from learners themselves are combined, suggesting that cognitive structures interact with experience to produce learning.

Learning disability Broad term used to designate difficulties in acquiring spoken language, written language, and mathematical skills; disorder is presumed to be due to neurological causes and not due to other causes, such as sensory loss, motor conditions, environment, and cultural differences.

Legally blind Visual acuity that is 20/200 or less in the better eye, or having a 20-degree visual field.

Letter–name stage Third stage of spelling development in which a child represents vowels as well as consonants with letters whose names sound like the speech sounds they are assumed to represent.

Limited capacity hypothesis Theory that children have the innate ability to acquire one language completely, but do not have the ability to acquire two or more languages simultaneously without suffering some reduction in competence in one or both languages.

Literal level Level of reading at which a student focuses on word meanings and the relationships between ideas conveyed in the paragraph.

Locutionary act Producing an utterance using words via speaking, signing, or using assistive technology.

Locutionary stage Time around 12 months and older when a child begins using words to communicate.

Logical sequences Organization of narrative information or components into a temporal order of related ideas.

Low vision Some functional use of eyesight ranging from a moderate to severe impairment.

Manner of articulation Description of how a consonant sound is produced, such as a *stop, fricative,* or *nasal.*

Marginal babbling Early form of babbling in which an infant strings together single consonants and vowels that are made in a row, such as "a, a, a," and "da, da, da."

Marked sounds Sounds that occur less frequently in languages of the world and develop later because they are more difficult to produce.

Mastered sounds Sounds that a child can consistently produce accurately.

Mathetic Relating to science or learning.

Mean length of utterance Calculation of the average number of morphemes a child produces in a representative sample of utterances.

Means/ends Conceptual extension of causality; the understanding that there are ways (means) to attain a goal (end).

Metalinguistics Ability to think about the language and manipulate the components of language, such as counting syllables and sounds in words.

Mirror neurons Specialized neurons whose activity has been found to represent actions that can be used not only for imitating actions but also to recognize and determine differences in the actions of others; neurons that "mirror" the behavior of others, as though the observer itself were acting. It has been proposed that problems with the mirror neural system may underlie cognitive disorders, particularly in children with autism.

Mixed hearing loss Combination of conductive and sensorineural hearing loss.

Modal Type of auxiliary verb used to indicate the attitude or mood of the verb that it precedes (e.g., *must, will, should*).

Modality Characteristics of sentences such as verb tense or the expression of negation or interrogation.

Modulations of meaning Children learn to expand on noun and verb phrases in order to create distinct meanings with words in sentences.

Morpheme Smallest grammatical unit in a language that conveys meaning.

Morphophonemic alteration Speech sound change that occurs when the shape of the base morpheme is changed (e.g., the final sound in the word *public* is the *k* sound, but when *public* becomes *publicity*, that *k* becomes an *s* sound).

Motherese Also known as parentese, it is a general style used by adults when talking to young children, often characterized by higher pitch, a "cooing" intonation, and simplified or shortened words.

Motor cortex Region of the cerebral cortex involved in the planning, control, and execution of voluntary movements which sends the neural messages to carry speech and language information to the muscles involved in producing speech.

Multicultural education Idea that all students regardless of gender, race, culture, social class, religion, or exceptionality should experience educational equality in the school.

Muscle tension dysphonia Voice disorder in which the larynx in strained due to inappropriate or excessive use of the muscles above and around the vocal folds.

Naming deficit Brief period during which a child (typically 18-20 months) experiences short-term difficulty with word recall. Thought to occur due to the densely packed representations stored in memory during rapid vocabulary growth which produce competition in word selection, or because the child's words are undergoing reorganization, causing confusion about words that have strong semantic relationships.

Narrative A story; an account of events or experiences.

Narrative discourse Type of written or verbal communication that involves telling a story, typically involving a sequential order of events.

Natural sounds Sounds common to all languages and that emerge first in developing children.

Neurogenic voice disorders Variety of conditions related to muscle control and innervations of the muscles involved in respiration, phonation, resonation, and articulation.

Nonexistence An object is expected to be present or occur, but is not, or an action is expected to occur, but does not; words used to express this relationship may be *all gone* or *no*.

Noun phrase Group of words containing a noun and words that describe or modify the noun.

Object Words that refer to things receiving action.

Object permanence Knowledge that objects exist in time and space even if you can't see or act on them.

Object specification Semantic relation of using *and* to connect a clause that describes or elaborates on the subject of the preceding clause; linking subjects and objects appropriately in a listing sense.

Objective pronoun Personal pronoun that acts as the object of a sentence and receives the action of the verb (e.g., *me, her, him, them*).

Open words Words that can be used alone and in combination with other open words, in combination with *pivot words*, and in either the first or second position of two-word utterances.

Operant Any behavior whereby frequency can be affected by the responses following it.

Order of mention When a child learning language interprets a sentence according to the order of the phrases, rather than the meaning of the phrases; concept that in the normal thought process, a cause is identified before its effect is considered.

Organic disorder Disorder caused by a demonstrable pathology of an organ system.

Organization Natural tendency of the mind to organize information into related, interconnected structures, with a scheme being the most basic structure.

Overextension When a child uses a word or concept too broadly, (e.g., calling all four-legged animals "doggie").

Parentese Also known as motherese, it is a general style used by adults when talking to young children, often characterized by higher pitch, a "cooing" intonation, and simplified or shortened words.

Passive transformation Changing the surface structure of a sentence so that the grammatical subject receives the verb's action; example: "The ball was hit by the boy."

Perception Processes by which an individual selects, organizes, integrates, and interprets sensory stimuli.

Perlocutionary act Effect a locutionary act might have on a listener, which may or may not be consistent with the speaker's communicative intention.

Perlocutionary stage Time between birth and about eight months of age during which infants respond in a reflexive manner to their environment and are not signaling any communication intent other than crying and nonspecific use of face and body.

Phoneme Speech sound; the smallest contrastive unit in the sound system of a particular language.

Phonics Relationship between the speech sound, syllable, or word to its orthographic letters.

Phonological awareness Ability to focus on and understand the sound structure of language.

Phonological disorder Underlying disorder in establishing and using the appropriate rules for sounds and their combinations, characterized by difficulty mastering where to use speech sounds in order to make words sound different from each other.

Phonological encoding Human ability to process rapidly paced speech and impose a phonemic (sound) identity to incoming speech sounds which are then analyzed; the structure of words is then determined, and the code for each word is stored, along with its meaning, in long-term, semantic memory.

Phonology Study of speech sounds and the rules that determine how sounds can be sequenced into syllables and words in a language.

Phonotactics Rules that govern the permissible arrangements of sounds in a given language.

Phrase Combination of words that are related to one another; serves a grammatical purpose, but does not contain both a subject and a predicate.

Phrase structure rules Universal rules for all languages, associated with Chomsky's transformational grammar, that describe the underlying relationships of words and phrases.

Pidgin Language that usually develops for the purpose of allowing groups with different languages to trade or communicate, and includes a combination of both languages, beginning as an informal language consisting mostly of nouns and many gestures and eventually becoming more formal.

Pivot-open grammar Proposed primitive form of grammar which suggests that children have two classes of words: *open* and *pivot*; concept used to explain the structure behind two-word phrases often used by children.

Pivot words Words that cannot be used alone or combined with other pivot words but can be used in conjunction with almost any other word a child has learned, and are used in either the first or second position of two-word utterances.

Place of articulation Point of contact where an obstruction occurs in the vocal tract when producing a consonant, helping to give a consonant its distinctive sound.

Plasticity Dynamic flexibility and adaptability of the human brain to change—physically, functionally, and chemically—throughout life, and as individuals constantly learn.

Play Child-directed activities that provide children with opportunities for learning.

Plural Noun form used to denote that there are two or more of something.

Possessive Noun form used to denote ownership, marked by adding an *'s* to the end of a noun, or an apostrophe after plural nouns.

Postmodifier Adjective phrase that comes after a noun ("The man *who called last night* is my uncle").

Poverty threshold Minimum level of income based on the size of the family unit and updated each year by the U.S. Census Bureau to use for statistical estimates of the number of Americans living in poverty.

Pragmatics Component of language regarding the ability to functionally use language in social contexts; the rules for social language needed to establish and maintain relationships with others.

Preparation phase First stage of writing development in which a child is learning to form letters.

Prephonemic stage First stage of spelling development in which children scribble, inconsistently form letters, and string letters together with little awareness that letters represent phonemes or speech sounds.

Present progressive Verb form that indicates an action is taking place right now.

Presupposition Assumption that speakers make concerning what their listener knows about the subject of their conversation.

Prevalence Total number of cases of a disorder/disease in a population at a particular time.

Prevarication Ability of humans to intentionally deceive others in their communications.

Primary auxiliary verb Verb that usually accompanies or helps the main verb by expressing or making distinctions in mood, voice, aspect, and tense.

Primary motor strip Area in the frontal lobe of the brain, also known as the precentral gyrus or primary motor cortex, involved in the planning and execution of motor movements, including swallowing and speech.

Primitive narrative Story-telling during a child's third and fourth years that includes a central character, topic, or setting. Children may discuss characters' facial expressions or body postures.

Primitive speech act Child's use of a word, a change in prosodic pattern, or a gesture to communicate.

Principle of minimal distance Concept that the preceding noun closest to the verb is treated as the subject of the sentence.

Print-concept knowledge Knowledge of the rule-governed organizational properties of print, including being able to show the front of the book, the title, the difference between pictures and print, left-to-right and top-to-bottom directionality for reading, and the concepts of letter and first letter in a word.

Print interest A child's realization that oral language can be represented by print, or written language.

Print referencing During reading, when a caregiver highlights and points out basic elements of print to direct a child's attention to the forms, features, and functions of written language.

Private speech A child speaks to himself to help him think through a problem and guide him through actions first aloud, and then with development, silently.

Productivity Human ability to create an infinite variety of novel and unique messages from a previously existing finite collection of sounds; Charles Hockett's 11th "design feature" of language.

Pronoun Word that takes the place of a noun or noun phrase.

Proposition Characteristics of a sentence such as the relationship between nouns and verbs; the content of a meaningful, declarative sentence.

Protodeclarative Primitive speech act used to establish social interaction and direct a caregiver's attention; use of a gesture (sometimes paired with a vocalization) to gain attention to an object or event.

Protoimperative Primitive speech act used as a request for objects or actions as well as to control and manipulate the behaviors of others.

Protonarratives Young children's early recounts or storytelling in temporal-causal sequences.

Prototype hypothesis Idea that children rely on both perceptual features and functions of words to develop early meanings; children build mental models of a conceptual category—an ideal or representative example (prototype) that other members of this group must resemble.

Proverb Popular, wise saying or a precise statement of truth.

Psychogenic stuttering Onset of stuttering associated with a specific, identifiable psychological trauma.

Psychogenic voice disorders Hoarseness or complete loss of the voice without physical cause, but rather due to severe emotional trauma or conflict.

Punishment Consequence used to cause a behavior to occur with less frequency.

Quasi-resonant nuclei Sounds that have a low pitch and a muffled resonance quality (e.g., grunting, crying, reflexive fussing, and vegetative sounds).

Rapid fading Speech signals are transitory and a listener can only receive specific auditory information at the time it is spoken; Charles Hockett's third "design feature" of language.

Reading fluency Ability to decode printed words in texts with accuracy and speed appropriate to age, grade, and exposure to reading instruction.

Receptive language Listening to and understanding what is communicated; the ability to comprehend a message.

Recounts The narration or telling of past events or experiences.

Recurrence When an object reappears or an event happens again; words used to express this relationship may be *more* or *another*.

Recursion Human ability to use acquired knowledge to create language, imagine what others may be thinking, engage in mental time travel to the past and the future, think about and gain understanding of *self*, and relate to a divine being in the development and demonstration of spirituality.

Reduplicated babbling More specific term for *babbling* involving repeated consonant/vowel (CV) syllables (e.g., "mamama")

Reflexiveness Human ability to use language to think and talk about language; also referred to as *metalinguistic ability*.

Regional dialect A variety of language used by people living in a restricted geographic area and distinguished by features of vocabulary, grammar, and pronunciation from other regional variations.

Regular verb Verb form that indicates an action took place in the past (e.g., *danced, looked*).

Reinforcement Consequence used to cause a behavior to occur with greater frequency.

Relational words Words that identify relationships among people, objects, and events; these words reflect a child's understanding of space, time, amount, dimensions, and kinship.

Relevance Pertinence, timeliness, or usefulness of a conversational topic.

Reliability Degree of confidence that a language sample represents a child's typical language production.

Representation Ability to think about things or use words without having to act on them directly.

Representational gestures Signify some features of an object or its function; have meaning independent of the objects (e.g., holding a fist to the ear to mean "telephone").

Retentive coarticulation When a preceding sound affects a sound that follows.

Revoicing Student-led format in which a teacher facilitates learning by promoting student discussion, acknowledging responses, and posing questions to prompt further thought; repeating part or all of a student's utterance or response and asking the student to verify whether the interpretation is correct.

Rich interpretation Using context to help determine the meanings of a child's utterances.

Saliency Perceptual relevance; a pronounced feature.

Scaffolding Support given during the learning process that is tailored to the needs of the individual and gradually removed to promote independent learning.

Schema Cognitive structure that helps children process, identify, organize, and store information.

School or classroom curriculum Conceptualized rules about who talks to whom and when these interactions should occur in a classroom environment, as well as the attitudes and values of teachers regarding the expectations of how to use language in the classroom.

Self-organizing neural network Interconnected neural system, in which learning in one language domain, such as the sound system, cannot help but affect other language domains, such as grammar;

network involved in the learning, storing, organizing, and retrieving of information.

Self-regulated writing Proactive and self-directed process of writing in which a writer takes into account aspects such as the audience and the literary style most appropriate to convey the message.

Semantic feature hypothesis Idea that the order of appearance of words in the course of a child's language acquisition is governed by the type and complexity of the semantic features they contain.

Semanticity Ability to use human speech to convey particular messages, and the idea that speech is needed in most cases to ensure the specificity of messages; Charles Hockett's seventh "design feature" of language.

Semantics Component of language regarding the meaning and interpretation of language; the use of vocabulary to construct ideas through relationships between words.

Semantic-syntactic rules Underlying rules for combining words and grammar to produce meaningful utterances; concept that emphasizes that meaning precedes and influences form.

Sensorineural hearing loss Hearing loss caused by damage to the auditory nervous system, due to heredity, infection, trauma, exposure to toxins, or repeated exposure to loud noise. The damage may be located in the cochlea of the inner ear, in the auditory nerve, at various points along the auditory pathway, or in the primary auditory cortex in the temporal lobe of the brain.

Sentence Grammatical unit consisting of one or more words meaningfully grouped to express a statement, question, exclamation, request, command, or suggestion; a grammatical unit consisting of a noun and verb phrase.

Shading Changing the topic of conversation by deriving a new topic from the immediately previous topic so that some continuity in the conversational flow is maintained.

Shape bias Tendency of young children learning common nouns to generalize on the basis of shape, rather than material, color, or texture.

Shaping Developing a behavior through small steps that gradually approximate the target behavior.

Signature tunes Rhythmic characteristic of *motherese*, which is more regular than adult speech, resulting in what some researchers describe as a *singsong cadence*.

Simultaneous acquisition Process by which a child learns two languages at once during early childhood.

Slow mapping Gradual process over time of expanding, reorganizing, and fine-tuning word meanings as words are acquired and the relationship between words develops along with cognition and linguistic attainments.

Social action approach Educational strategy that leads students, through their increased understanding of cultural diversity, to make decisions about how best to address social issues affected by cultural differences and encouraging students to actually take action to solve problems that are created by cultural differences.

Social-cultural capital Resources available to individuals based on group membership, relationships inside and outside of the group, and networks of influence and support in combination with access to forms of knowledge, skills, education, advantages, and attitudes necessary to gain social and economic mobility.

Social interactionism Explanation of language acquisition in which both environmental and biological factors are important in the process; however, the role of social interaction between the developing child and the linguistically knowledgeable adults is emphasized.

Social-material capital Nonfinancial social assets that promote social mobility beyond economic means (e.g., education, intellect, dress).

Social-political capital Expected combined or economic benefits taken from the preferential treatment and cooperation between individuals and groups.

Socioeconomic status (SES) Position of an individual on a hierarchical social-economic scale that measures factors such as education, income, type of occupation, and place of residence.

Sound waves Fluctuation of pressure passed through some medium (e.g., air or water), composed of frequencies within the range of hearing.

Specialization Idea that speech is a specialized human function (made apparent by the anatomy of human speech organs and the human ability to exhibit some control over these organs), is specifically designed for communication, and serves no other purpose; Charles Hockett's sixth "design feature" of language.

Specific language impairment Term used to categorize a childhood language disorder that is *not* accompanied by deficits in hearing, intelligence, neurological functions, or motor function.

Speech Oral expression of language.

Standard dialect Variety of a language spoken by people of relatively high status who have economic, political, social, and educational power.

Story grammar Knowledge about general structure of stories and how to ask oneself important questions while reading stories to facilitate comprehension.

Stuttering Speech disorder characterized by disruptions in the flow of speech by involuntary repetitions and prolongations of sounds, syllables, words, or phrases as well as involuntary silent pauses or blocks in which sound is unable to be produced.

Subjective pronoun Personal pronoun (e.g., *I, he, she, they*) that acts as the subject of the sentence and performs the action of the verb.

Substantive words Words that refer to objects or events that have perceptual or functional features in common (e.g., *doggie, horsie, truck*).

Substitution processes Form of language simplification in which children use phonemes within their developmental level as substitutes for sounds they are not able to use consistently.

Subtractive bilingual environment Environment in which children who speak a minority language gives up their minority language when acquiring the majority language, and in this process, give up their culture.

Successive bilingualism (or acquisition) The consecutive development of two (or more) languages.

Superlative adjective Adjective used to compare three or more nouns; occurs through the addition of the suffix *-est.*

Suprasegmental Features of speech, such as stress, pitch, and duration, that accompany individual speech sounds, words, and sentences.

Surface structure In Chomsky's transformational grammar, the outward form of a sentence, which is derived from *deep structures* by a series of *transformations.*

Syllable structure Arrangement of vowels and consonants that make up a single syllable.

Symbolic play A play activity in which objects or actions are used to represent other objects and actions.

Syntagmatic-paradigmatic shift Change in a child's processing and organization of words to reflect more adult-like patterns of organizing words into classes, rather than by syntactic relationships (e.g., syntagmatic relationship: "cat-meows"; paradigmatic relationship: "cat-animal").

Syntax Rules that govern the ways in which words combine to form phrases, clauses, and sentences; sentence structure.

Telegraphic speech Simplified manner of speech during the early years of language acquisition using the most important content words for expressing ideas lacking appropriate grammar and inflection.

Temporal conjunctive relation Expresses aspects and relations of time to discuss one event that follows another in time.

Text comprehension Goal of reading instruction that focuses on deriving meaning from texts through employment of cognitive and dialogic strategies.

Theory of mind Cognitive ability to designate mental states—beliefs, intents, desires, knowledge, and so on—to oneself and others, and to understand that others have different mental states than oneself.

Topic-associating narrative Story that connects two or more different events that share a common theme, in which each episode in the narrative might have different characters, and the stories might occur in different places and times.

Topic-based narrative Story centered on single characters or on single events having clearly defined chronologies.

Topic collaborating Strategy whereby one conversational partner matches the topic of the other conversational partner.

Total feedback Speakers have the ability to hear themselves speak, and through this, receive feedback allowing them to make constant adjustments so that output is as finely tuned as possible for conveying accurate thoughts. This feedback also provides control for the mechanics of speech so that speech errors are caught and corrected or even anticipated and avoided; Charles Hockett's fifth "design feature" of language.

Traditional transmission Idea that speech is instinctive in humans and the capacity for language acquisition is genetic; however, the details of a language, including vocabulary and structural rules, are learned; Charles Hockett's 13th and last "design feature" of language.

Transformation approach Education strategy that fundamentally changes an existing curriculum by redesigning it to allow students to understand, appreciate, and value concepts, issues, events, and themes from the perspectives of a representative range of ethnic and cultural groups.

Transformational generative grammar Linguistic theory, developed by Noam Chomsky, that attempts to account for the infinite number of grammatical sentences possible in a language. This theory suggests that language is processed at two levels, *deep* and *surface.*

Transformations Nonuniversal rules or conventions that describe a language's deep structure and surface structure.

Transitional stage Fourth and last stage of spelling development in which children may try a number of spelling strategies, including using a particular spelling they saw in print, applying rules for spelling they observed, and continuing to rely on letter–name spellings and sounding-out strategies to spell words.

Traumatic brain injury Sudden trauma to the brain that causes injury.

True narrative Story that focuses on a true plot, character development, a sequence of events, and a definite resolution of the central conflict or problem.

Underextension When a child uses a word too narrowly (e.g., only calling golden retrievers "doggie"); not applying a new word to things that are included in the meaning of that word.

Underground curriculum Styles of language used during the school day appropriate for interactions with peers.

Unitary language system hypothesis Concept that children who are exposed to two languages from birth in the first stage of language development actually function with a single language that is a hybrid of two distinctly different languages, a hybrid that includes vocabulary and grammatical rules from both languages.

Valid The degree to which a language sample measures what it is suppose to measure: the child's expressive language.

Variegated babbling More complex form of *babbling* involving more complex combinations of consonant and vowel syllables (e.g., "madagaba")

Verb phrase Group of words that contains a verb and possibly other supporting or qualifying words.

Vernacular dialect Native, nonstandard variety of language from a specific population.

Vertical expansion Developing an understanding of the deeper meanings of words by taking a known word and breaking it down into categories.

Vocables Consistent patterns of sounds, unique to individual children, used in reference to particular things or situations; also referred to as *phonetically consistent forms, performatives,* or *protowords.*

Vocabulary instruction One reading comprehension strategy shown to improve reading achievement.

Vocal-auditory channel Idea that standard human language occurs as a vocal type of communication in which air is forced through the vocal folds of the larynx, breaking the vibrating air stream into sounds of speech, which are organized into words and sentences and perceived through a listener's ears; Charles Hockett's first "design feature" of language.

Vocal play Process by which infants "play" and experiment with their voices by changing the loudness, pitch, rate, and quality (e.g., squeals, grunts, raspberries).

Voicing Use of vocal fold vibration to produce all vowel sounds and certain consonant sounds.

Vowel processes Simplification of vowel sounds due to a child's tendency to produce vowels in the center of the oral cavity, making it neither high/low nor front/back, which results in vowels that are either too high or low or made too far in front or back of the intended target; a process more common for children with hearing loss.

Wernicke's area Region in the temporal lobe of the left hemisphere of the brain associated with language comprehension (receptive language).

Whole-word templates Idea that the organizing principle in early phonological development is whole words, not features or segments.

Word retrieval Ability to recall stored information, or known words, from long-term memory.

Word storage Process of creating a permanent record of encoded information of a specific word in memory.

Working memory System that actively holds and allows for the voluntary, focused, and exclusive processing and maintenance of task-relevant information.

Zone of proximal development Range of abilities a child can perform with assistance, but cannot yet perform independently.

References and Suggested Readings

Abbs, J., Gracco, V., & Cole, K. (1984). Control of multimovement coordination: Sensorimotor mechanisms in speech motor programming. *Journal of Motor Behaviors, 16,* 195.

Abercrombie, D. (1967). *Elements of general phonetics.* Edinburgh: University Press.

Abrahamsen, E., & Rigrodsky, S. (1984). Comprehension of complex sentences in children at three levels of cognitive development. *Journal of Psycholinguistic Research, 13,* 333–350.

Ackerman, B. P. (1983). Form and function in children's understanding of ironic utterances. *Journal of Experimental Child Psychology, 35,* 487–508.

Acredolo, L., & Goodwyn, S. (1998). *Baby signs.* Chicago: Contemporary Books.

Ad Hoc Committee on Service Delivery in the Schools, American Speech–Language–Hearing Association. (1993). Definitions of communication disorders and variations. *American Speech-Language-Hearing Association, 35*(3) (Suppl. 10), 40–41.

Adams, M. J. (1990). *Beginning to read: Thinking and learning about print—A summary.* Austin, TX: Center for the Study of Reading.

Ahktar, N. (2002). Relevance and early word learning. *Journal of Child Language, 29,* 677–686.

Ahktar, N., Dunham, F., & Dunham, P. (1991). Directive interactions and early vocabulary development: The role of joint attentional focus. *Journal of Child Language, 18,* 41–49.

Ainsworth, S., & Fraser, J. (Eds.). (1988). *If your child stutters: A guide for parents* (3rd ed.). Memphis, TN: Speech Foundation of America.

Akmajian, A., Demers, R., & Harnish, R. (1984). *Linguistics: An introduction to language and communication.*, London: MIT Press.

Alamargot, D., & Chanquoy, L. (2001). *Through the models of writing.* Dordrecht, the Netherlands: Kluwer.

Albright, K., & O'Neal, J. (1998). The newborn with hearing loss: Detection in the nursery. *Pediatrics, 102,* 142–146.

Al-Issa, I. (1969). The development of word definition in children. *Journal of Genetic Psychology, 114,* 25–28.

Allen, H., & Linn, M. (Eds.). (1986). *Dialect and language variation.* Orlando, FL: Academic Press.

Alterac, M., & Saroha, E. (2007). Lifetime prevalence of learning disability among U.S. children. *Pediatrics, 119,* (Suppl. 1), S77–S83.

Altwerger, B., Diehl-Faxon, J., & Dockstader-Anderson, K. (1985). Read-aloud events as meaning construction. *Language Arts, 62,*(5), 476–484.

Ambrose, S. E., VanDam, M., & Moeller, M. P. (2012). *Relationships between linguistic input, television exposure, and the language development of toddlers with hearing loss.* Presentation at the Symposium on Research in Child Language Disorders, University of Wisconsin-Madison. Retrieved from http://www.lenafoundation.org/pdf/Ambrose-SRCLD.PDF

American Academy of Pediatrics. Committee on Public Education, American Academy of Pediatrics: children, adolescents, and television. *Pediatrics, 107*(2), 423-426.

American Association on Intellectual and Developmental Disabilities. (2013). FAQ on intellectual disabilities. Retrieved from www.aaidd.org/content_104.cfm

American Foundation for the Blind. (2013). *Glossary of Eye Conditions.* Retrieved from www.afb.org/section.aspx?FolderID=2&SectionID=93

American Speech–Language–Hearing Association (ASHA). (2008a). Communication facts: Special populations: Autism—2008 edition. Retrieved from http://asha.org/Research/reports/autism

American Speech–Language–Hearing Association. (ASHA). (2008b). *Incidence and prevalence of communication disorders in hearing loss in children*—2008 edition. Retrieved from http://www.nsslha.org/research/reports/children.htm

American Speech–Language–Hearing Association (ASHA). (2010). *Communication facts: Special populations: Traumatic Brain Injury—2010 Edition.* Retrieved from http://www.asha.org/Researh/reports/tbi

Ames, L. (1966). Children's stories. *Genetic Psychological Monographs, 73,* 307–311.

Anderson, S. R. (2010). How many languages are there in the world? Linguistic Society of America

Brochure Series: Frequently Asked Questions. Linguistic Society of America. www.linguisticsociety. org/sites/default/files/how-many-languages.pdf

Anderson, S. R. (2004). *Doctor Doolittle's delusion: Animals and the uniqueness of human language.* New Haven, CT: Yale University Press.

Andrews, G. (1984). The epidemiology of stuttering. In R. F. Curlee & W. H. Perkins (Eds.), *Nature and treatment of stuttering: New directions.* San Diego, CA: College Hill Press.

Anglin, J. (1985). The child's expressible knowledge of word concepts: What preschoolers can say about the meanings of some nouns and verbs. In K. E. Nelson (Ed.), *Children's language* (Vol. 5, pp. 77–127). Hillsdale, NJ: Erlbaum.

Anglin, J. (1993). Vocabulary development: A morphological analysis. *Monographs of the Society for Research in Child Development, 58*(10), Serial No. 238.

Anglin, J. (1995, April). *Word knowledge and the growth of potentially knowable vocabulary.* Paper presented at the biennial meeting of the Society for Research in Child Development, Indianapolis, IN.

Applebee, A. (1978). *The child's concept of story.* Chicago: University of Chicago Press.

Applebee, A., Langer, J., & Mullis, I. (1988). *Who reads best? Factors related to reading achievement in grades 3, 7, and 11.* Princeton, NJ: National Assessment of Educational Progress, Educational Testing Service.

Aram, D. (1991). Comments on specific language impairment as a clinical category. *Language, Speech, and Hearing Services in Schools, 22,* 84–87.

Archibald, L. M. D., & Gathercole, S. E. (2006). Short-term and working memory in specific language impairment. *International Journal of Language and Communication Disorders, 41*(6), 675–693.

Aronson, A. (1985). *Clinical voice disorders* (2nd ed.). New York: Thieme-Stratton.

Aslin, R., Pisoni, D., & Jusczyk, P. (1983). Auditory development and speech perception in infancy. In M. Haith & J. Campos (Eds.), *Handbook of child psychology: Vol. 2. Infancy and developmental psychobiology.* New York: Wiley.

Attanasio, J. (1987). A case of late-onset or acquired stuttering in adult life. *Journal of Fluency Disorders, 12,* 287–290.

Aukett, R., Ritchie, J., & Mill, K. (1988). Gender differences in friendship patterns. *Sex Roles, 19,* 57–66.

Austin, J. (1962). *How to do things with words.* London: Oxford University Press.

Autism Science Foundation. (2013).

Baddeley, A. (1986). *Working memory.* New York: Oxford University Press.

Baddeley, A. D. (1996). Exploring the central executive. *Quarterly Journal of Experimental Psychology: Human Experimental Psychology, 49*(1), 5–28.

Baddeley, A. D., & Logie, R. H. (1999). Working memory: The multiple component model. In A. Miyake & P. Shah (Eds.), *Models of working memory: Mechanisms of active maintenance and executive control* (pp. 28–61). New York: Cambridge University Press.

Bailey, G., & Maynor, N. (1989). The divergence controversy. *American Speech, 64,* 12–13.

Baillargeon, R. (1987). Object permanence in three-and-a-half and four-and-a-half-month-old infants. *Developmental Psychology, 23,* 655–664.

Baillargeon, R., & DeVos, J. (1991). Object permanence in young infants: Further evidence. *Child Development, 62,* 1227–1246.

Baillargeon, R., DeVos, J., & Graber, M. (1989). Location memory in eight-month-old infants in a non-search AB task: Further evidence. *Cognitive Development, 4,* 345–367.

Baillargeon, R., Graber, M., DeVos, J., & Black, J. (1990). Why do young infants fail to search for hidden objects? *Cognition, 36,* 255–284.

Bakeman, R., Adamson, L., Konner, M., & Barr, R. (1990). !Kung infancy: The social context of object exploration. *Child Development, 61,* 794–809.

Baker, L., Mackler, K., Sonnenschein, S., & Serpell, R. (2001). Parents' interactions with their first-grade children during story-book reading and elations with subsequent home reading activity and reading achievement. *Journal of School Psychology, 39,* 415–438.

Baker, L., Scher, D., & Mackler, K. (1997). Home and family influences on motivations for reading. *Educational Psychologist, 32,* 69–82.

Baldie, B. (1976). The acquisition of the passive voice. *Journal of Child Language, 3,* 331–348.

Banks, J. (1999). Multicultural education in the new century. *School Administrator, 56,* 4–7.

Banks, J., & Banks, C. (1997). *Multicultural education: Issues and perspectives* (3rd ed.). Boston: Allyn & Bacon.

Barlow, S., & Abbs, J. (1978, November). *Some evidence of auditory feedback contributing to the ongoing control of speech production.* Paper presented at the American Speech and Hearing Association Convention, San Francisco.

Barnes, S., Gutfreund, M., Satterly, D., & Wells, G. (1983). Characteristics of adult speech which predict children's language development. *Journal of Child Language, 10,* 65–84.

Barrago, N. (1983). *Visual handicaps & learning.* Austin, Texas: Exceptional Resources.

Barrett, M., Harris, M., & Chasin, J. (1991). Early lexical development and maternal speech: A comparison of children's initial and subsequent uses of words. *Journal of Child Language, 18,* 21–40.

Barsky-Firsker, L., & Sun, S. (1998). Universal newborn hearing screenings: A three-year experience. *Pediatrics, 99*(6): 2, 3.

Barth, R., & Kinder, B. (1988). A theoretical analysis of sex differences in same-sex friendship. *Sex Roles, 19,* 349–363.

Bartlett, C. (1982). Learning to write: Some cognitive and linguistic components. In R. Shuy (Ed.), *Linguistics and literacy series* (No. 2). Washington, DC: Center of Applied Linguistics.

Bartolucci, G., Pierce, S., Streiner, D., & Eppel, P. (1976). Phonological investigation of verbal autistic and intellectual disability subjects. *Journal of Autism and Childhood Schizophrenia, 6,* 303–316.

Bartoshuk, A. (1964). Human neonatal cardiac responses to sound: A power function. *Psychodynamic Science, 1,* 151–152.

Bashir, A., & Scavuzzo, A. (1992). Children with language disorders: Natural history and academic success. *Journal of Learning Disabilities, 25*(1), 53–65.

Bashir, A., & Singer, B. D. (2006). Assisting students in becoming self-regulated writers. In Ukrainetz, T. (Ed.), *Contextualized language intervention: Scaffolding prek-12 literacy achievement* (pp. 565–598). Eau Claire, WI: Thinking Publications.

Bateman, H., & Mason, R. (1984). *Applied anatomy and physiology of the speech and hearing mechanism.* Springfield, IL: Charles C. Thomas.

Bates, E. (1979). *The emergence of symbols: Cognition and communication in infancy.* New York: Academic Press.

Bates, E., & MacWhinney, B. (1982). Functionalist approaches to grammar. In E. Wanner & L. Gleitman (Eds.), *Language acquisition: The state of the art* (pp. 173–218). Cambridge, MA: Harvard University Press.

Bates, E., & MacWhinney, B. (1987). Competition, variation, and language learning. In B. MacWhinney (Ed.), *Mechanisms of language acquisition.* Hillsdale, NJ: Erlbaum.

Bates, E. & Marchman, V. A. (1988). What is and is not universal in language acquisition. In F. Plum (Ed.), *Language, communication, and the brain* (pp. 19–38). New York: Raven Press.

Bates, E., & Snyder, L. (1987). The cognitive hypothesis in language development. In I. Uzgiris & J. Hunt (Eds.), *Infant performance and experience: New findings with the ordinal scale.* Urbana: University of Illinois Press.

Bates, E., Benigni, L., Bretherton, I., Camaioni, L., & Volterra, V. (1977). From gesture to the first word: On cognitive and social prerequisites. In M. Lewis & L. Rosenblum (Eds.), *Interaction, conversation, and the development of language.* New York: Wiley.

Bates, E., Benigni, L., Bretherton, I., Camaioni, L., & Volterra, V. (1979). *The emergence of symbols: Cognition and communication in infancy.* New York: Academic Press.

Bates, E., Bretherton, I., & Snyder, L. (1988). *From first words to grammar: Individual differences and dissociable mechanisms.* New York: Cambridge University Press.

Bates, E., Bretherton, I., Beeghly-Smith, M., & McNew, S. (1983). Social basis of language development: A reassessment. In H. Reese & L. Lipsitt (Eds.), *Advances in child development and behavior* (Vol. 16, pp. 8–75). New York: Academic Press.

Bates, E., Bretherton, I., Snyder, L., Shore, C., & Volterra, V. (1980). Vocal and gestural symbols at 13 months. *Merrill-Palmer Quarterly, 26,* 407–423.

Bates, E., Bretherton, L., Shore, C., & McNew, S. (1983). Names, gestures and objects: The role of context in the emergence of symbols. In K. Nelson (Ed.), *Children's language* (Vol. 4). Hillsdale, NJ: Erlbaum.

Bates, E., Camaioni, L., & Volterra, V. (1975). The acquisition of performatives prior to speech. *Merrill-Palmer Quarterly, 21,* 205–224.

Bates, E., Camaioni, L., & Volterra, V. (1975). The acquisition of performatives prior to speech. *Merrill-Palmer Quarterly, 21,* 205–216.

Bates, E., Marchman, V., Thal, D., Fenson, L., Dale, P., Reznick, J., Reilly, J., & Hartung, J. (1994). Developmental and stylistic variation in the composition of early vocabulary. *Journal of Child Language, 21,* 85–123.

Bates, E., Reilly, J., Wulfeck, B., Dronkers, N., Opie, M., Fension, J., Kriz, S., Jeffries, R., Miller, L., & Herbst, K. (2001). Differential effects of unilateral lesions on language production in children and adults. *Brain and Language, 79*(2), 223–265. Retrieved from http://dxdoi.org/10.1006/brin .2001.2482.

Battles, D. (1983). Social dialects. *American Speech–Language–Hearing Association, 25,* 23–24.

Bauer, D., Goldfield, R., & Reznick, J. (2002). Alternative approaches to analyzing individual difference in the rates of early vocabulary development. *Applied Psycholinguistics, 22,* 313–335.

Baumgartner, J., & Duffy, J.R. (1997). Psychogenic stuttering in adults with and without neurologic disease. *Journal of Medical Speech-Language Pathology, 5*(2), pp. 75-96.

Baumwell, L., Tamis-LeMonda, C., & Bornstein, M. (1997). Maternal verbal sensitivity and child language comprehension. *Infant Behavior and Development, 20,* 247–258.

Beals, D. E., & Snow, C. E. (1994). "Thunder is when the angels are upstairs bowling": Narratives and explanations at the dinner table. *Journal of Narrative and Life History, 4,* 331–352.

Beauchamp, G.K., & Mennella, J.A. (2009). Early flavor learning and its impact on later feeding behavior, *Journal of Pediatric Gastroenterology & Nutrition, 48(p),* S25-30. DOI: 10.1097/MPG.0b013e31819774a5

Beaumont, S. (1995). Adolescent girls' conversations with mothers and friends: A matter of style. *Discourse Processes, 20,* 109–132.

Bebout, L., & Arthur, B. (1992). Cross-cultural attitudes toward speech disorders. *Journal of Speech and Hearing Research, 35,* 45–52.

Bedore, L. (1999). The acquisition of Spanish. In O. Taylor & L. Leonard (Eds.), *Language acquisition across North America: Cross-cultural and cross-linguistic perspectives* (pp. 157–208). San Diego, CA: Singular.

Bedore, L. (2004). Morphosyntactic development. In B. Goldstein (Ed.), *Bilingual language development and disorders in Spanish-English speakers.* Baltimore: Brookes.

Behrend, D., Rosengren, K., & Perlmutter, M. (1992). The relation between private speech and parental interactive style. In R. Diaz & L. Berk (Eds.), *Private speech: From social interaction to self-regulation.* Hillsdale, NJ: Erlbaum.

Bell-Berti, F. (1975). Control of pharyngeal cavity size for English voiced and voiceless stops. *Journal of the Acoustical Society of America, 57,* 456–461.

Bench, J. (1969). Audio-frequency and audio-intensity discrimination in the human neonate. *International Audiology, 8,* 615–625.

Benedict, H. (1979). Early lexical development: Comprehension and production. *Journal of Child Language, 6,* 183–200.

Benelli, B., Arcuri, L., & Marchesini, G. (1988). Cognitive and linguistic factors in the development of word definitions. *Journal of Child Language, 15,* 619–635.

Benelli, B., Belacchi, C., Gini, G., & Lucangeli, D. (2006). "To define means to say what you know about things": The development of definitional skills as metalinguistic acquisition. *Journal of Child Language, 33,* 71–97.

Bennett, R. (1981). *Types of literature.* Lexington, MA: Ginn.

Bennett-Kaster, T. (1986). Cohesion and predication in child narrative. *Journal of Child Language, 13,* 353–370.

Bergeson, T., & Trehub, S. E. (2007). Signature tunes in mother's speech to infants. *Infant Behavior & Development, 30,* 648–654.

Berk, L. (1992). Children's private speech: An overview of theory and the status of research. In R. Diaz & L. Berk (Eds.), *Private speech: From social interaction to self-regulation.* Hillsdale, NJ: Erlbaum.

Berk, L., & Landau, S. (1993). Private speech of learning disabled and normally achieving children in classroom academic and laboratory contexts. *Child Development, 64,* 556–571.

Berk, L., & Spuhl, S. (1995). Maternal interaction, private speech, and task performance in preschool children. *Early Childhood Research Quarterly, 10,* 145–169.

Berko-Gleason, J., & Greif, E. (1983). Men's speech to young children. In B. Thorne, C. Kramerae, & N. Henley (Eds.), *Language, gender, and society.* Rowley, MA: Newbury House.

Berko-Gleason, J., Hay, D., & Cain, L. (1988). Social and affective determinants of language acquisition. In M. L. Rice & R. L. Schiefelbusch (Eds.), *The teachability of language* (pp. 171–186). Baltimore: Brookes.

Bernhardt, B., & Stemberger, J. P. (1998). *Handbook of phonological development from the perspective of constraint-based nonlinear phonology.* San Diego, CA: Academic Press.

Bernstein, D. (1989). Language development: The preschool years. In D. Bernstein & E. Tiegerman (Eds.), *Language and communication disorders in children* (2nd ed.). Upper Saddle River, NJ: Merrill/Prentice Hall.

Bernthal, J., & Bankson, N. (1993). *Articulation and phonological disorders.* Upper Saddle River, NJ: Prentice Hall.

Bernthal, J., & Bankson, N. (2004). *Articulation and phonological disorders* (5th ed.). Boston: Allyn & Bacon.

Berti, F., & Hirose, H. (1975). Palatal activity in voicing distinctions: A simultaneous fiberoptic and electromyographic study. *Journal of Phonetics, 3,* 69–74.

Bhatia, T., & Ritchie, W. (1999). The bilingual child: Some issues and perspectives. In W. C. Ritchie & T. Bhatia (Eds.), *Handbook of child language acquisition* (pp. 569–646). San Diego, CA: Academic Press.

Bialystok, E. (1986). Factors in the growth of linguistic awareness. *Child Development, 57,* 498–510.

Bialystok, E. (1988). Levels of bilingualism and levels of linguistic awareness. *Developmental Psychology, 24,* 560–567.

Bialystok, E. (1997). Effects of bilingualism and biliteracy on children's emerging concepts of print. *Developmental Psychology, 33,* 429–440.

Bialystok, E. (1999). Cognitive complexity and attentional control in the bilingual mind. *Child Development, 70,* 636–644.

Bialystok, E. (2001). *Bilingualism in development: Language, literacy, and cognition.* New York: Cambridge University Press.

Bialystok, E. (2001). *Bilingualism in development: Language, literacy, and cognition.* Cambridge, England: Cambridge University Press.

Bialystok, E. (2007). Acquisition of literacy in bilingual children: A framework for research. *Language Learning, 57*(Suppl. 1), 45–77.

Bialystok, E., Luk, G., & Kwan, E. (2005). Bilingualism, biliteracy, and learning to read: Interactions among languages and writing systems. *Scientific Studies of Reading, 9,* 43–61.

Bialystok, T. (1992). Attentional control in children's metalinguistic performance and measures of field independence. *Developmental Psychology, 28,* 654–664.

Biemiller, A. (1970). The development of the use of graphic and contextual information as children learn to read. *Reading Research Quarterly, 6,* 75–96.

Billow, R. (1975). A cognitive developmental study of metaphor comprehension. *Developmental Psychology, 11,* 415–423.

Bishop, D., & Adams, C. (1992). Comprehension problems in children with specific language impairment: Literal and inferential meaning. *Journal of Speech and Hearing Research, 35,* 119–129.

Bishop, D. V. M., North, T., & Donlan, C. (1995). Genetic basis of specific language impairment: Evidence from a twin study. *Developmental Medicine and Child Neurology, 37,* 56–71.

Bivens, J., & Berk, L. (1990). A longitudinal study of the development of elementary school children's private speech. *Merrill-Palmer Quarterly, 36,* 443–463.

Bjorkqvist, K., Lagerspetz, K., & Kaukiainen, A. (1992). Do girls manipulate and boys fight? Developmental trends in regard to direct and indirect aggression. *Aggressive Behavior, 18,* 117–127.

Blache, S. (1978). *The acquisition of distinctive features.* Baltimore: University Park Press.

Blake, J., & deBoysson-Bardies, B. (1992). Patterns of babbling: A cross-linguistic study. *Journal of Child Language, 19,* 51–74.

Bless, D., & Miller, J. (1972, November). *Influence of mechanical and linguistic factors on lung volume events during speech.* Paper presented at the American Speech and Hearing Association Convention, San Francisco.

Bloodstein, O. (1979). *Speech pathology, an introduction.* Boston: Houghton Mifflin.

Bloodstein, O. (1990). On pluttering, skivering, and floggering: A commentary. *Journal of Speech and Hearing Disorders, 55,* 392–393.

Bloodstein, O. (1993). *Stuttering: The search for a cause and cure.* Boston: Allyn & Bacon.

Bloodstein O. (1995). *A handbook on stuttering* (5th ed.). San Diego, CA: Singular.

Bloom, K., Borod, J., Obler, L., & Gerstman, L. (1992). Impact of emotional content on discourse production in patients with unilateral brain damage. *Brain and Language, 42,* 153–164.

Bloom, L. (1970). *Language development: Form and function of emerging grammars.* Cambridge, MA: MIT Press.

Bloom, L. (1973). *One word at a time: The use of single-word utterances before syntax.* The Hague: Mouton.

Bloom, L. (1974). Talking, understanding, and thinking. In R. Schiefelbusch & L. Lloyd (Eds.), *Language perspectives: Acquisition, retardation and intervention.* Baltimore: University Park Press.

Bloom, L., & Lahey, M. (1978). *Language development and language disorders.* New York: Wiley.

Bloom, L., Lahey, P., Hood, L., Lifter, K., & Fiess, K. (1980). Complex sentences: Acquisition of syntactic connectors and the semantic relations they encode. *Journal of Child Language, 7,* 235–262.

Bloom, L., Miller, P., & Hood, L. (1975). Variation and reduction as aspects of competence in language development. In A. Pick (Ed.), *Minnesota Symposia* on Child Psychology (Vol. 9, pp. 3–55). Minneapolis: University of Minnesota Press.

Bloom, L., Rocissano, L., & Hood, L. (1976). Adult–child discourse: Developmental interaction between information processing and linguistic interaction. *Cognitive Psychology, 8,* 521–552.

Bloom, L., Tackeff, J., & Lahey, M. (1984). Learning "to" in complement constructions. *Journal of Child Language, 11,* 391–406.

Blumenfeld, H., & Eisenfeld, L. (2006). Does a mother singing to her premature baby affect feeding in the neonatal intensive care unit? *Clinical Pediatrics, 45,* 65–70.

Blumstein, S., & Cooper, W. (1974). Hemispheric processing of intonational contours. *Cortex, 10,* 146–158.

Bohannon, J. (1982). Close encounters of the primate kind. *American Journal of Primatology, 3,* 353–358.

Bohannon, J., & Hirsch-Pasek, K. (1984). Do children say as they're told? A new perspective on motherese. In L. Feagans, C. Garvey, & R. Golinkoff (Eds.), *The origins and growth of communication* (pp. 176–195). Norwood, NJ: Ablex.

Bohannon, J., & Warren-Leubecker, A. (1988). Recent developments in child-directed speech: You've come a long way, baby-talk. *Language Science, 10,* 89–110.

Bohannon, J., & Warren-Leubecker, A. (1989). Theoretical approaches to language acquisition. In J. Berko-Gleason (Ed.), *The development of language* (pp. 167–213). Columbus, OH: Merrill/Prentice Hall.

Boone, D. R., McFarlane, S. C., Von Berg, S. L., & Zraick, R. I. (2010). *The voice and voice therapy* (8th ed.). New York: Allyn & Bacon.

Booth, A. E., Waxman, S. R., & Huang, Y. T. (2005). Conceptual information permeates word learning in infancy. *Developmental Psychology, 41,* 491–505.

Borden, G. (1980). Use of feedback in established and developing speech. In N. Lass (Ed.), *Speech and language advances in basic research and practice* (Vol. 3). New York: Academic Press.

Borden, G., & Harris, K. (1984). *Speech science primer* (2nd ed.). Baltimore: Williams & Wilkins.

Bornstein, M. H., Hahn, C. S., & Haynes, O. M. (2004). Specific and general language performance across early childhood: Stability and gender considerations. *First Language, 24,* 267–304.

Bosch, L., & Sebastian-Galles, N. (2001). Early language differentiation in bilingual infants. In J. Cenoz & F. Genesee (Eds.), *Trends in bilingual acquisition* (pp. 71–94). Amsterdam: John Benjamins.

Boudreau, D. (2008). Narrative abilities: Advances in research and implications for clinical practice. *Topics in Language Disorders, 28*(2), 99–114.

Bower, T. (1977). *The perceptual world of the child.* Cambridge, MA: Harvard University Press.

Bowerman, M. (1978). Systematizing semantic knowledge: Changes over time in the child's organization of word meaning. *Child Development, 49,* 977–987.

Bowerman, M. (1978). The acquisition of word meaning: An investigation into some current conflicts. In N. Waterson & C. Snow (Eds.), *The development of communication.* New York: Wiley.

Bowerman, M. (1982). Reorganizational processes in lexical and syntactic development. In E. Wanner & L. Gleitman (Eds.), *Language acquisition: The state of the art* (pp. 319–346). Cambridge: Cambridge University Press.

Bowman, B. (1989). Educating language-minority children: Challenges and opportunities. *Phi Delta Kappan, 71,* 118–120.

Boyd, F. B., & Brock. C. H. (Eds.). (2004). *Multicultural and multilingual literacy and language: Contexts and practices.* New York: Guilford Press.

Bradley, R. H., & Corwyn, R. F. (2002). Socioeconomic status and child development, *Annual Review of Psychology, 53,* 371–399.

Braine, M. (1963). The ontogeny of English phrase structure: The first phrase. *Language, 39,* 1–13.

Branigan, G. (1979). Some reasons why successive single word utterances are not. *Journal of Child Language, 6,* 411–421.

Brazelton, T., & Cramer, B. (1990). *The earliest relationship: Parents, infants, and the drama of early attachment.* Reading, MA: Addison-Wesley.

Bredin-Oja, S.L. & Fey, M. (2014). Children's responses to telegraphic and grammatically complete prompts to imitate. *American Journal of Speech-Language Pathology, 23,* 15-26. Doi10.1044/1058-0360(2013/12-0155)

Brent, M., & Siskin, J. (2001). The role of exposure to isolated words in early vocabulary development. *Cognition, 81,* B33–B44.

Bretherton, I. (1988). How to do things with one word: The ontogenesis of intentional message-making in infancy. In M. Smith & J. Locke (Eds.), *The emergent lexicon: The child's development of a linguistic vocabulary.* San Diego, CA: Academic Press.

Bretherton, I., Fritz, J., Zahn-Waxler, C., & Ridgeway, D. (1986). Learning to talk about emotions: A functionalist perspective. *Child Development, 57,* 529–548.

Brewer, W., & Stone, J. (1975). Acquisition of spatial antonym pairs. *Journal of Experimental Child Psychology, 19,* 299–307.

Bridger, W. (1961). Sensory habituation and discrimination in the human neonate. *American Journal of Psychiatry, 117,* 991–996.

Brinton, B., & Fujiki, M. (1984). Development of topic manipulation skills in discourse. *Journal of Speech and Hearing Research, 27,* 350–358.

Brinton, B., & Fujiki, M. (1989). *Conversational management with language-impaired children: Pragmatic assessment and intervention.* Rockville, MD: Aspen.

Brinton, B., Fujiki, M., Loeb, D., & Winkler, E. (1986). Development of conversational repair strategies in response to requests for clarification. *Journal of Speech and Hearing Research, 29,* 75–81.

Broderick, J. (1975). *Modern English linguistics.* New York: Crowell.

Brown, J. (1975). On the neural organization of language: Thalamic and cortical relationships. *Brain and Language, 2,* 18–30.

Brown, R. (1973). *A first language: The early stages.* Cambridge, MA: Harvard University Press.

Brown, R., & Bellugi, U. (1964). Three processes in the child's acquisition of syntax. *Harvard Educational Review, 34,* 133–151.

Brown, R., Cazden, C., & Bellugi, U. (1969). The child's grammar from I to III. In J. Hill (Ed.), *Minnesota symposia on child psychology* (Vol. 2). Minneapolis: University of Minnesota Press.

Brownell, H., Gardner, H., Prather, P., & Marino, G. (1995). Language, communication, and the right hemisphere. In H. Kirshner (Ed.), *Handbook of neurological speech and language disorders* (pp. 325–349), New York: Marcel Dekker.

Bruner, J. (1975). The ontogenesis of speech acts. *Journal of Child Language, 2,* 1–19.

Bruner, J. (1978). Learning the mother tongue. *Human Nature, 1,* 42–49.

Bruner, J. (1981). The social context of language acquisition. *Language and Communication, 1,* 155–178.

Bruner, J. (1983). *Child's talk: Learning to use language.* New York: Norton.

Bruner, J. (1983). *Child's talk: Learning to use language.* Oxford, Eng.: Oxford University Press.

Brutten, G., & Shoemaker, D. (1967). *The modification of stuttering.* Upper Saddle River, NJ: Prentice Hall.

Bryant, R. E., MacLean, M., Bradley, L. L., & Crossland, J. (1990). Rhyme and alliteration, phoneme detection, and learning to read. *Developmental Psychology, 26,* 429–438.

Bryen, D. (1978). *Variant English: An introduction to language variation.* Upper Saddle River, NJ: Merrill/Prentice Hall.

Bryen, D. (1982). *Inquiries into child language.* Boston: Allyn & Bacon.

Bryne, R. W., & Whiten, A. (1990). Tactical deception in primates: The 1990 database. *Primate Report, 27,* 10.

Bushnell, I., Sai, F., & Mullin, J. (1989). Neonatal recognition of the mother's face. *British Journal of Developmental Psychology, 7,* 3–15.

Butler, A., & Turbill, J. (1987). *Towards a reading—writing classroom.* Portsmouth, NH: Heinemann.

Butterfield, E. C., Hacker, D. J., & Albertson, L. R. (1996). Environmental, cognitive and metacognitive influences on text revision. *Educational Psychology Review, 8*(3), 239–297.

Butterworth, G., & Morissette, P. (1996). Onset of pointing and the acquisition of language in infancy. *Journal of Reproductive and Infant Psychology, 14,* 219–231.

Byrne, B., & Fielding-Barnsley, R. (1998). Phonemic awareness and letter knowledge in the child's acquisition of the alphabetic principle. *Journal of Educational Psychology, 81,* 313–321.

Calvin, W., & Ojemann, G. (1980). *Inside the brain.* New York: New American Library.

Camera, L. (2015) Wanted: Bilingual Teachers. *Education Reporter, October.* Retrieved at http://www.usnews.com/news/articles/2015/10/16/us-faces-shortage-of-bilingual-teachers. February 5, 2017.

Cameron-Faulkner, T., Leiven, L., & Tomasello, M. (2003). A construction based analysis of child-directed speech. *Cognitive Science, 27,* 843–873.

Campbell, A., & Namy, L. (2003). The role of social referential context and verbal and nonverbal symbol learning. *Child Development, 74,* 549–563.

Campbell, L. (1993). Maintaining the integrity of home linguistic varieties: Black English vernacular. *American Journal of Speech–Language Pathology, 2,* 11–12.

Campbell, L. (1994). Discourse diversity and Black English vernacular. In D. Ripich & N. Creaghead (Eds.), *School discourse problems* (2nd ed.). San Diego, CA: Singular.

Canter, G. (1971). Observations on neurogenic stuttering: A contribution to differential diagnosis. *British Journal of Disorders of Communication, 6*, 139–143.

Canterbury, D. R., Dixon, C. L., & Gish, K. D. (1981). Hearing loss in Alaska. *Journal of the American Audiology Society, 17*, 18–24.

Carey, S. (1978). The child as word learner. In M. Halle, J. Bresnan, & G. Miller (Eds.), *Linguistic theory and psychological reality*. Cambridge, MA: MIT Press.

Carey, S., & Bartlett, E. (1978). Acquiring a single new word. *Papers and Reports on Child Language Development, 15*, 17–29.

Carger, C. (1997). Attending to new voices. *Educational Leadership, 54*, 39–43.

Carlson, S. M., & Meltzoff, A. N. (2008). Bilingual experience and executive functioning in young children. *Developmental Science, 11*(2), 282–298.

Carpenter, K. (1991). Later rather than sooner: Extralinguistic categories in the acquisition of Thai classifiers. *Journal of Child Language, 18*, 93–113.

Carrell, P. (1981). Children's understanding of indirect requests: Comparing child and adult comprehension. *Journal of Child Language, 8*, 329–345.

Carroll, J. (1981). Twenty-five years of research on foreign language aptitude. In K. C. Diller (Ed.), *Individual differences and universals in language learning aptitude*. Rowley, MA: Newbury House.

Carroll, S. (1999). Putting "input" in its proper place. *Second Language Research, 15*, 337–388.

Carroll, S. (2001). *Input and evidence*. Amsterdam: John Benjamins.

Carrow, E. (1973). *Test of auditory comprehension of language*. Austin, TX: Urban Research Group.

Carter, A. (1975). The transformation of sensorimotor morphemes into words: A case study of the development of "more" and "mine." *Journal of Child Language, 2*, 233–250.

Carver, C. (1987). *American regional dialects: A word geography*. Ann Arbor: University of Michigan Press.

Caselli, M. (1990). Communicative gestures and first words. In V. Bolterra & C. Erting (Eds.), *From gesture to sign in hearing and deaf children* (pp. 56–67). New York: Springer.

Caskey, M., Stephens, B., Tucker, R., & Vohr, B. (2011). Importance of parent talk on the development of preterm infant vocalizations. *Pediatrics, 128*(5). Retrieved from pediatrics.aappublications.org/content/128/5/910.full

Catts, H.W., & Kamhi, A.G. (Eds.) (2005). *The connections between language and reading disabilities*. New Jersey: Lawrence Erlbaum Associates, Inc.

Catts, H.W., Kamhi, A.G., & Adolf, S.M. (2012). Causes of reading disability. In A.G., Kamhi, & H.W. Catts (Eds.), *Language and reading disabilities* (pp. 77–111). Boston: Pearson.

Cazden, C. (1968). The acquisition of noun and verb inflection. *Child Development, 39*, 433–438.

Cazden, C. (1988). *Classroom discourse: The language of teaching and learning*. Portsmouth, NH: Heinemann.

Center on Addiction and Substance Abuse (2005). *Substance abuse and the American woman*. New York: Columbia University Press.

Chafe, W. (1970). *Meaning and the structure of language*. Chicago: University of Chicago Press.

Chall, J. S. (1983). *Learning to read: The great debate*. New York: Wiley.

Chall, J. S. (1996). *Stages of reading development* (2nd ed.). New York: McGraw-Hill.

Champion, T., & Mainess, K. (2003). Typical and disordered narration in African American children. In A. McCabe & L. S. Bliss (Eds.), *Patterns in narrative discourse: A multicultural lifespan approach* (pp. 55–70). Boston: Allyn & Bacon.

Chan, Y. L., & Marinellie, S. A. (2008). Definitions of idioms in preadolescents, adolescents, and adults. *Journal of Psycholinguistic Research, 37*, 1–20.

Chang-Rodriguez, E. (1991). *Latin America, her civilization and culture*. New York: HarperCollins.

Chapman, R. (1978). Comprehension strategies in children. In J. Kavanaugh & W. Strange (Eds.), *Speech and language in the laboratory, school, and clinic*. Cambridge, MA: MIT Press.

Chapman, R., & Miller, J. (1975). Word order in early two- and three-word utterances: Does production precede comprehension? *Journal of Speech and Hearing Research, 18*, 355–371.

Chapman, R., Paul, R., & Wanska, S. (1981). Syntactic structures in simple sentences. In J. Miller (Ed.), *Assessing language production in children: Experimental procedures*. Baltimore: University Park Press.

Chapman, R., Streim, N., Crais, E., Salmon, D., Strand, E., & Negri, N. (1992). Child talk: Assumptions of a developmental process model for early language learning. In R. Chapman (Ed.), *Processes in language acquisition and disorders*. St. Louis, MO: Mosby-Year Book.

Cheng, L. (1987, June). Cross-cultural and linguistic considerations in working with Asian populations. *American Speech–Language–Hearing Association, 29*(6), 33–38.

Cherry, L., & Lewis, M. (1976). Mothers and two-year-olds: A study of sex-differentiated aspects of verbal interaction. *Developmental Psychology, 12,* 278–282.

Chiat, S. (1986). Personal pronouns. In P. Fletcher & M. Garman (Eds.), *Language acquisition* (2nd ed.). New York: Cambridge University Press.

Childers, J., & Tomasello, M. (2002). Two-year-olds learn novel nouns, verbs, and conventional actions from massed or distributed exposures. *Developmental Psychology, 38,* 967–978.

Childs, C., & Greenfield, P. M. (1982). Informal modes of learning and teaching: The case of Zinacanteco weaving. In N. Warren (Ed.), *Advances in cross-cultural psychology* (Vol. 2). London: Academic Press.

Choi, S. (1988). The semantic development of negation: A cross-linguistic longitudinal study. *Journal of Child Language, 15,* 517–531.

Chomsky, C. (1969). *The acquisition of syntax in children from 5 to 10.* Cambridge, MA: MIT Press.

Chomsky, N. (1957). *Syntactic structures.* The Hague: Mouton.

Chomsky, N. (1965). *Aspects of a theory of syntax.* Cambridge, MA: MIT Press.

Chomsky, N. (1968). *Language and mind.* New York: Harcourt, Brace & World.

Chomsky, N., & Halle, M. (1968). *The sound patterns of English.* New York: Harper & Row.

Christakis, D. A., Gilkerson, J., Richards, J. A., Zimmerman, F. J., Garrison, M. M., Xu, D., Gray, S., & Yapanel, U. (2009). Audible television and decreased adult words, infant vocalization, and conversational turns. *Archives and Pedriatrics & Adolescent Medicine, 163*(6), 554–558.

Ciscero, C. A., & Royer, J. M. (1995). The development and cross-language transfer of phonological awareness. *Contemporary Educational Psychology, 20,* 275–303.

Clark, E. (1973). What's in a word? On the child's acquisition of semantics in his first language. In T. Moore (Ed.), *Cognitive development and the acquisition of language.* New York: Academic Press.

Clark, E. (1975). Knowledge, context, and strategy in the acquisition of meaning. In D. Dato (Ed.), *Developmental psycholinguistics: Theory and application.* Washington, DC: Georgetown University Press.

Clark, E., & Sengul, C. (1978). Strategies in the acquisition of deixis. *Journal of Child Language, 5,* 457–475.

Clark, H., & Chase, W. (1972). On the process of comparing sentences against pictures. *Cognitive Psychology, 3,* 472–517.

Clayton, N. S., Bussey, T. J., & Dickinson, A. (2003). Can animals recall the past and plan for the future? *Nature Reviews Neuroscience, 4,* 685–691.

Clements, G. (1985). The geometry of phonological features. *Phonology Yearbook, 2,* 225–252.

Clements, G. N., & Keyser, S. J. (1983). *CV phonology.* Cambridge, MA: MIT Press.

Cleveland, A., & Striano, T. (2007). The effects of joint attention on object processing in four- and nine-month-old infants. *Infant Behavior & Development, 30,* 499–504.

Clifton, R., Graham, R., & Hatton, H. (1968). Newborn heart-rate response and response habituation as a function of stimulus duration. *Journal of Experimental Child Psychology, 6,* 265–278.

Coballes-Vega, C. (1992). Considerations in teaching culturally diverse children. Retrieved from ERIC Digest (ED 341648).

Coggins, T. (1979). Relational meaning encoded in two-word utterances of Stage I Down's syndrome children. *Journal of Speech and Hearing Research, 22,* 166–178.

Cole, P., & Taylor, O. (1990). Performance of working class African-American children on three tests of articulation. *Language, Speech, Hearing Services in Schools, 21,* 171–176.

Collier, V. (1987). Age and rate of acquisition of second language for academic purposes. *TESOL Quarterly, 21,* 617–641.

Collier, V. (1987/1988). The effect of age on acquisition of a second language for school. *Forum, 2,* Winter.

Conture, E. (1990). *Stuttering* (2nd ed.). Upper Saddle River, NJ: Prentice Hall.

Conture, E. (2001). *Stuttering, its nature, diagnosis, and treatment.* Boston: Allyn & Bacon.

Conture, E., & Kelly, E. (1991). Young stutterers' nonspeech behaviors during stuttering. *Journal of Speech and Hearing Research, 34,* 1041–1056.

Corballis, M. C. (2007). The uniqueness of human recursive thinking: The ability to think about thinking may be the critical attribute that distinguishes us from all other species. *American Scientist, 95*(3), 240–249.

Coriat, I. (1933). Psychoanalytic concept of stammering. *Nervous Child, 2*, 167–171.

Corrigan, R. (1975). A scalogram analysis of the development of the use and comprehension of "because" in children. *Child Development, 46*, 195–201.

Corsaro, W. (1979). Young children's conception of status and role. *Sociology of Education, 52*, 46–50.

Crago, M., Eriks-Brophy, A., Pesco, D., & McAlpine, L. (1997). Culturally based miscommunication in classroom interaction. *Language, Speech, and Hearing Services in Schools, 28*, 245–254.

Craig, H. (1993). Social skills of children with specific language impairment: Peer relationships. *Language, Speech, and Hearing Services in Schools, 24*, 206–215.

Craig, H., & Evans, J. (1991). Turn exchange behaviors of children with normally developing language: The influence of gender. *Journal of Speech and Hearing Research, 34*, 866–878.

Craig, H., & Gallagher, T. (1983). Adult–child discourse: The conversational relevance of pauses. *Journal of Pragmatics, 7*, 347–360.

Craig, H., & Washington, J. (2002). Oral language expectations for African American preschoolers and kindergartners. *American Journal of Speech–Language Pathology, 11*, 59–70.

Craig, H., Connor, C., & Washington, J. (2003). Early positive predictors of later reading comprehension for African American students: A preliminary investigation. *Language, Speech, and Hearing Services in Schools, 34*, 31–43.

Craig, H., Washington, J., & Thompson-Porter, C. (1998). Average c-unit lengths in the discourse of African American children from low-income, urban homes. *Journal of Speech, Language, and Hearing Research, 41*, 433–444.

Craik, F., & Lockhart, R. (1972). CHARM is not enough: Comments on Eich's model of cued recall. *Psychological Review, 93*, 360–364.

Crais, E. (1990). World knowledge to word knowledge. *Topics in Language Disorders, 10*, 45–62.

Crais, E. (1992). Fast mapping: A new look at word learning. In R. Chapman (Ed.), *Processes in language acquisition and disorders.* St. Louis: Mosby–Year Book.

Crais, E., Douglas, D. D., & Campbell, C. C. (2004). The intersection of the development of gestures and intentionality. *Journal of Speech, Language, and Hearing Research, 47*, 678–694.

Creaghead, N., Newman, P., & Secord, W. (Eds.). (1989). *Assessment and remediation of articulatory and phonological disorders* (2nd ed.). Upper Saddle River, NJ: Merrill/Prentice Hall.

Cross, T. (1978). Mother's speech and its association with rate of linguistic development in young children. In N. Waterson & C. Snow (Eds.), *The development of communication.* New York: Wiley.

Crowe Hall, B. (1991). Attitudes of fourth and sixth graders toward peers with mild articulation disorders. *Language, Speech, Hearing Services in Schools, 22*, 334–340.

Crystal, D. (1986). Prosodic development. In P. J. Fletcher & M. Garman (Eds.), *Studies in first language development* (pp. 174–197). New York: Cambridge University Press.

Crystal, D., Fletcher, P., & Garman, M. (1976). *The grammatical analysis of language disability: A procedure for assessment and remediation.* London: Arnold.

Cummins, J. (1989). A theoretical framework for bilingual special education. *Exceptional Children, 56*, 111–119.

Cummins, J. (1989). *Empowering minority students.* Sacramento: California Association for Bilingual Education.

Cummins, J. (1999). BICS and CALP: Clarifying the distinction. U.S. Department of Education, Retrieved from www.eric.ed.gov/ERICWebPortal/search/ED438551

Cummins, J. (2000). *Language, power and pedagogy: Bilingual children in the crossfire.* Clevedon, England: Multilingual Matters.

Curlee, R., & Perkins, W. (Eds.). (1984). *Nature and treatment of stuttering: New directions.* San Diego, CA: College-Hill.

Curlee, R., & Siegel, G. (Eds.). (1997). *Nature and treatment of stuttering: New directions.* Boston: Allyn & Bacon.

Current Population Reports. (1990). *1990 census of population and housing.* Washington, DC: U.S. Census Bureau. Retrieved from http://www.census.gov/cdrom/lookup

Current Population Survey (1994, March). *Hispanic origin.* Washington, DC: U.S. Census Bureau. Retrieved from http://www.census.gov/population

Curtis, S., Katz, W., & Tallal, P. (1992). Delay versus deviance in the language acquisition of language-impaired children. *Journal of Speech and Hearing Research, 35*, 373–383.

Cutting, L. E., & Denckla, M. B. (2003). Attention: Relationship between attention-deficit hyperactivity disorder and learning disabilities. In H. L. Swanson, K. R. Harris, & S. Graham (Eds.), *Handbook of Learning Disabilities* (pp. 125–139). New York: Guilford Press.

D'Odorico, L. (1984). Nonsegmental features in prelinguistic communications: An analysis of some types of infant cry and noncry vocalizations. *Journal of Child Language, 11,* 17–27.

D'Odorico, L., Cassibba, R., & Salerni, N. (1997). Temporal relationships between gaze and vocal behavior in prelinguistic and linguistic communication. *Journal of Psycholinguistic Research, 26,* 539–556.

Dale, P., & Crain-Thoreson, C. (1993). Pronoun reversals: Who, when, and why? *Journal of Child Language, 20,* 573–589.

Dale, P. S., Price, T. S., Bishop, D. V. M., & Plomin, P. (2003). Outcomes of early language delay: I. Predicting persistent and transient language difficulties at 3 and 4 years. *Journal of Speech, Language, and Hearing Research, 46,* 544–560.

Daly, D. (1993). Cluttering: The orphan of speech-language pathology. *ASHA, 2,* 6–8.

Daly, D. A., & Cantrelle, R. P. (2006). *Cluttering: Characteristics identified as diagnostically significant by 60 fluency experts.* Paper presented at the Fifth International Fluency Association World Congress on Disorders of Fluency, Dublin, Ireland.

Dapretto, M., Davies, M. S., Pfeifer, J. H., Scott, A. A., Sigman, M., Bookheimer, S. Y., & Iacoboni, M. (2005). Understanding emotions in others: mirror neuron dysfunction in children with autism spectrum disorders. Retrieved from http://www.nature.com/natureneuroscience/reprintsandpermissions/; doi:10.1038/nn1611

Darley, F., Aronson, A., & Brown, J. (1975). *Motor speech disorders.* Philadelphia: Saunders.

Davis, B., & MacNeilage, P. (1990). Acquisition of correct vowel production: A quantitative case study. *Journal of Speech and Hearing Research, 33,* 16–27.

Davis, G. (1993). *A survey of adult aphasia* (2nd ed.). Upper Saddle River, NJ: Prentice Hall.

DeCasper, A. J., Lecanuet, J. P., Busnel, M. C., Granier-Deferre, C., & Maugeais, R. (1994). Fetal reactions to recurrent maternal speech. *Infant Behavior and Development, 17*(2), 159–164.

de Houwer, A. (1990). *The acquisition of two languages from birth: A case study.* Cambridge, MA: Harvard University Press.

de Houwer, A. (1995). Bilingual language acquisition. In P. Fletcher & B. MacWhinney (Eds.), *Handbook of child language* (pp. 219–250). Oxford, England: Basil Blackwell.

de Houwer, A. (1998). Environmental factors in early bilingual development: The role of parental beliefs and attitudes. In G. Extra & L. Verhoeven (Eds.), *Bilingualism and migration* (pp. 75–95). Berlin: Mouton de Gruyter.

de l'Etoile, S. K. (2006). Infant behavioral responses to infant-directed singing and other material interactions. *Infant Behavior & Development, 29,* 456–470.

de Villiers, J., & de Villiers, P. (1973). A cross-sectional study of the acquisition of grammatical morphemes in child speech. *Journal of Psycholinguistic Research, 2,* 267–278.

Deák, G. O., Walden, T. A., Kaiser, M. Y., & Lewis, A. (2008). Driven from distraction: How infants respond to parents' attempts to elicit and re-direct their attention. *Infant Behavior & Development, 31,* 34–50.

DeCasper, A., & Fifer, W. (1980). Of human bonding: Newborns prefer their mothers' voices. *Science, 208,* 1174–1176.

DeCasper, A., & Spence, M. (1986). Prenatal maternal speech influences newborns' perception of speech sounds. *Infant Behavior and Development, 9,* 133–150.

Delgado-Gaitan, C. (2001). *The power of community: Mobilizing for family and schooling.* Lanham, MD: Rowman & Littlefield.

Dell, G. S. (1990). Effects of frequency and vocabulary type on phonological speech errors. *Language and Cognitive Processes, 5,* 313–349.

Demers, R. A. (1988). *Linguistics and animal communication.* New York: Cambridge University Press.

Denes, P., & Pinson, E. (1993). *The speech chain* (2nd ed.). New York: Freeman.

DePaulo, B., & Bonvillian, J. (1978). The effect on language development of the special characteristics of speech addressed to children. *Journal of Psycholinguistic Research, 7,* 189–211.

Devescovi, A., Caselli, M. C., Marchione, D., Pasqualetti, P., Reilly, J., & Bates, E. (2005). A cross-linguistic study of the relationship between grammar and lexical development. *Journal of Child Language, 32,* 759–786.

deVilliers, J., & deVilliers, P. (1978). *Language acquisition*. Cambridge, MA: Harvard University Press.

Diebold, A. (1968). The consequences of early bilingualism in cognitive and personality formation. In E. Norbeck, D. Price-Williams, & W. M. McCord (Eds.), *The study of personality: An interdisciplinary appraisal* (pp. 218–245). New York: Holt, Rinehart & Winston.

Diesendruck, G., & Bloom, P. (2003). How specific is the shape bias? *Child Development, 74,* 168–178.

Dillard, J. (1973). *Black English: Its history and usage in the United States.* New York: Vintage.

Dimond, S., & Beaumont, J. (1974). Experimental studies of hemispheric function in the human brain. In S. Dimond & J. Beaumont (Eds.), *Hemispheric function in the human brain.* New York: Wiley.

Dixon, J. A., & Foster, D. H. (1997). Gender and hedging: From sex differences to situated practice. *Journal of Psycholinguistic Research, 26,* 89–107.

Doake, D. (1995). *Literacy learning: A revolution in progress.* Bothell, WA: Wright Group.

Dodd, B., & Carr, A. (2003). Young children's letter-sound knowledge. *Language, Speech, and Hearing Services in Schools, 34,* 128–137.

Dodd, B., Holm, A., Hua, Z., & Crosbie, S. (2003). Phonological development: A normative study of British-speaking children. *Clinical Linguistics and Phonetics, 17*(8), 617–643.

Donnellan, A., & Kilman, B. (1986). Behavioral approaches to social skill development in autism. In E. Schopler & G. Mesibov (Eds.), *Social behavior in autism.* New York: Plenum.

Dopke, S. (1992). *One parent one language: An interactional approach.* Amsterdam: John Benjamins.

Dopke, S. (2000). The interplay between language-specific development and cross-linguistic influence. In S. Dopke (Ed.), *Cross-linguistic structures in simultaneous bilingualism* (pp. 79–103). Amsterdam: John Benjamins.

Dore, J. (1974). A pragmatic description of early language development. *Journal of Psycholinguistic Research, 3,* 343–350.

Dore, J. (1975). Holophrases, speech acts, and language universals. *Journal of Child Language, 2,* 21–40.

Draper, P., & Cashdan, E. (1988). Technological change and child behavior among the !Kung. *Ethnology, 27,* 339–365.

Duffy, G., & Roehler, L. (1981). *Building reading skills: Level 4.* Evanston, IL: McDougal, Little.

Dunst, C. (1980). *Clinical and educational manual for use with the Uzgiris and Hunt scales of infant psychological development.* Baltimore: University Park Press.

Durgunoğlu, A. Y. (1998). Acquiring literacy in English and Spanish in the United States. In A. Y. Durgunoğlu & L. Verhoeven (Eds.), *Literacy development in a multilingual context: Cross-cultural perspectives* (pp. 135–145). Mahwah, NJ: Erlbaum.

Durgunoğlu, A. Y., Nagy, W. E., & Hancin-Bhatt, B. J. (1993). Cross-language transfer of phonological awareness. *Journal of Educational Psychology, 85,* 453–465.

Durkin, D. (1980). *Teaching young children to read.* Boston: Allyn & Bacon.

Dykstra, J., Babatos-DeVito, M. G., Irvin, D. W., Boyd, B. A., Hume, K. A., & Odem, S. L. (2012). Using the Language Environment Analysis (DENA) system in preschool classrooms with children with autism spectrum disorders. Retrieved from http://www.lenafoundation.org/pdf/Dykstra

Dyson, A. (1983, April). *Early writing as drawing: The developmental gap between speaking and writing.* Paper presented at the American Educational Research Association Convention, Montreal, Canada.

Dyson, A. T. (1988). Phonetic inventories of two- and three-year-old children. *Journal of Speech and Hearing Disorders, 53,* 89–93.

Ebeling, K., & Gelman, S. (1994). Children's use of context in interpreting "big" and "little." *Child Development, 65,* 1178–1192.

Edelsky, C. (1977). Acquisition of an aspect of communicative competence: Learning what it means to talk like a baby. In S. Ervin & C. Mitchell-Kernan (Eds.), *Child discourse.* New York: Academic Press.

Edmonsten, N., & Thane, N. (1992). Children's use of comprehension strategies in response to relational words: Implications for assessment. *American Journal of Speech-Language Pathology, 1,* 30–35.

Edwards, W., and Winford, D. (1991). *Verb phrase patterns in Black English and Creole.* Detroit, MI: Wayne State University Press.

Egland, G. (1970). *Speech and language problems: A guide for the classroom teacher.* Upper Saddle River, NJ: Prentice Hall.

Ehrenreich, B. (1981). The politics of talking in couples. *Ms, 5,* 43–45, 86–89.

Eimas, P., Siqueland, E., Jusczyk, P., & Vigorito, J. (1971). Speech perception in infants. *Science, 171,* 303–306.

Eisenberg, A. R. (1985). Learning to describe past experiences in conversation. *Discourse Rocesses , 8,* 177–204.

Eisenberg, R. (1976). *Auditory competence in early life: The roots of communicative-behavior.* Baltimore: University Park Press.

Elias, C., & Berk, L. (2002). Self-regulation in young children: Is there a role for sociodramatic play? *Early Childhood Research Quarterly, 17,* 1–17.

Elkins, J. (2007, September–October). Learning disabilities: Bringing fields and nations together. *Journal of Learning Disabilities, 40*(5), 392–399.

Ellis, A. W., & Morrison, C. M. (1998). Real age-of-acquisition effects in lexical retrieval. *Journal of Experimental Psychology: Learning, Memory, and Cognition, 24,* 515–523.

Ely, R. (2005). Language and literacy in the school years. In J. Berko-Gleason (Ed.), *The development of language* (6th ed., pp. 396–429). Boston: Allyn & Bacon.

Ely, R., & Berko-Gleason, J. (1995). Socialization across contexts. In P. Fletcher & B. MacWhinney (Eds.), *Handbook of child language* (pp. 251–270). Oxford: Blackwell.

Ely, R., Berko-Gleason, J., & McCabe, A. (1996). "Why didn't you talk to your Mommy, honey?" Gender differences in talk about past talk. *Research on Language and Social Interaction, 29,* 7–25.

Emerson, H. (1979). Children's comprehension of "because" in reversible and nonreversible sentences. *Journal of Child Language, 6,* 279–300.

Emerson, H., & Gekoski, W. (1976). Interactive and categorical grouping strategies and the syntagmaticparadigmatic shift. *Child Development, 47,* 1116–1125.

Engle, P. L., Castle, S., & Menon, P. (1996). Child development: vulnerability and resilience. *Social Science and Medicine, 43*(5), 621–635.

Ervin, S. (1961). Changes with age in the verbal determinants of word-association. *American Journal of Psychology, 74,* 361–372.

Ervin-Tripp, S. (1977). From conversation to syntax. *Papers and Reports in Child Language Development, 13,* 11–21.

Ervin-Tripp, S. (1977). Wait for me roller-skate. In S. Ervin-Tripp & C. Mitchell-Kernan (Eds.), *Child discourse.* New York: Academic Press.

Ervin-Tripp, S. (1979). Children's verbal turn-taking. In E. Ochs & B. Schieffelin (Eds.), *Developmental pragmatics.* New York: Academic Press.

Ervin-Tripp, S., & Gordon, D. (1986). The development of requests. In R. Schiefelbusch (Ed.), *Language competence: Assessment and intervention.* San Diego, CA: College-Hill.

Ervin-Tripp, S., O'Connor, M., & Rosenberg, J. (1987). Language and power in the family. In C. Kramerae & M. Schulz (Eds.), *Language and power.* Urbana: University of Illinois Press.

Escamilla, K. (1993). Integrating Mexican-American history and culture into the social studies classroom. In L. Gronlund (Ed.), *Striving for excellence: The national education goals* (Vol. 2, pp. 53–54). Washington, DC: Educational Resources Information Center.

Everett, D. (2005). Cultural constraints on grammar and cognition in Pirahã: Another look at the design features of human language. *Current Anthropology, 46*(4), 621–646.

Ewing-Cobbs, L., Fletcher, J., & Leven, H. (1985). In M. Ylvisaker (Ed.), *Head injury rehabilitation: Children and adolescents.* Austin, TX: PRO-ED.

Ezell, H. K., Justice, L. M., & Parsons, D. (2000). Enhancing the emergent literacy skills of preschoolers with communication disorders: A pilot investigation. *Child Language Teaching and Therapy, 16,* 121–140.

Fadiga, L., & Craighero, L. (2006). Hand actions and speech representation in Broca's area. *Cortex, 42*(4), 486–490.

Fantz, R. (1964). Visual experience in infants: Decreased attention to familiar patterns relative to novel ones. *Science, 146,* 668–670.

Farrar, M. (1990). Discourse and the acquisition of grammatical morphemes. *Journal of Child Language, 17,* 607–624.

Farrar, M. J., Ashwell, S., & Maag, L. (2005). The emergence of phonological awareness: Connections to language and theory of mind development. *First Language, 25*(2), 157–172.

Fasold, R. (1984). *The sociolinguistics of society.* London: Basil Blackwell.

Fawcett, A., & Nicolson, R. (1995). Persistence of phonological awareness deficits in older children with dyslexia. *Reading and Writing: An Interdisciplinary Journal, 7,* 361–376.

Fay, W., & Schuler, A. (1980). *Emerging language in autistic children.* Baltimore: University Park Press.

Fazio, B. B., Naremore, R. C., & Connell, P. (1996). Tracking children from poverty at risk for specific language impairment: A 3-year longitudinal study. *Journal of Speech and Hearing Research, 39*, 611–624.

Fein, D. (1983). The prevalence of speech and language impairments. *American Speech–Language–Hearing Association, 25*, 37.

Fenson, L., Bates, E., Dale, P., Goodman, J., Reznick, J. S., & Thal, D. (2000). Measuring variability in early child language: Don't shoot the messenger. *Child Development, 71*, 323–328.

Fenson, L., Dale, P. S., Esznick, J. S., Bates, E., Thal, D. J., & Pethick, S. J. (1994). Variability in early communicative development. *Monographs of the Society for Research in Child Development, 59* (Serial No. 242).

Ferguson, C. (1978). Learning to pronounce: The earliest stages of phonological development in the child. In F. Minifie & L. Lloyd (Eds.), *Communicative and cognitive abilities—Early behavioral assessment.* Baltimore: University Park Press.

Fernald, A. (1985). Four-month-old infants prefer to listen to motherese. *Infant Behavior and Development, 8*, 181–195.

Fernald, A. (1994). Human maternal vocalizations to infants as biologically relevant signals: An evolutionary perspective. In P. Bloom (Ed.), *Language acquisition: Core readings.* Cambridge, MA: MIT Press.

Fernald, A., & Morikawa, H. (1993). Common themes and cultural differences in Japanese and American mothers' speech to infants. *Child Development, 64*, 637–656.

Fey, M. (1986). *Language intervention with young children.* San Diego, CA: College-Hill.

Fey, M. (1992). Articulation and phonology: Inextricable constructs in speech pathology. *Language, Speech, and Hearing Services in Schools, 23*, 225–232.

Fields, M., & Spangler, K. (1995). *Let's begin reading right: Developmentally appropriate beginning literacy* (3rd ed.). Upper Saddle River, NJ: Prentice Hall.

Fifer, W.P. (1994). The role of mother's voice in the organization of brain function in the newborn. *Acta Paediatrica, 83*(s397), 86–93.

Figueroa, R. (1989). Psychological testing of linguistic-minority students: Knowledge gaps and regulations. *Exceptional Children, 56*, 145–152.

Fillmore, C. (1968). The case for case. In E. Bach & R. Harmas (Eds.), *Universals in linguistic theory.* New York: Holt, Rinehart & Winston.

Fisher, S. E., Vargha-Khadem, F., Watkins, K. E., Monaco, A. P., & Pembray, M. E. (1998). Localisation of a gene implicated in a severe speech and language disorder. *Nature Genetics, 18*, 168–170.

Flavell, J. H. (1977). *Concept development.* Upper Saddle River, NJ: Prentice Hall.

Flavell, J. H. (1985). *Cognitive development* (2nd ed.). Upper Saddle River, NJ: Prentice Hall.

Flavell, J. H., (2004). Theory-of-mind development: Retrospect and prospect. *Merrill-Palmer Quarterly, 50*(3) 274–290.

Fogel, P. T. (2008). *Foundations of communication sciences and disorders.* Clifton Park, NY: Cengage Learning.

Folger, J., & Chapman, R. (1978). A pragmatic analysis of spontaneous imitations. *Journal of Child Language, 5*, 25–38.

Fontanella de Weinberg, M. (1992). *Spanish in America.* Madrid: Mapfre.

Forbes, J., & Poulin-DuBois, D. (1997). Representational change in young children's understanding of familiar verb meaning. *Journal of Child Language, 24*, 389–406.

Foster, S. (1986). Learning topic management in the preschool years. *Journal of Child Language, 13*, 231–250.

Foy, J., & Mann, V. (2003). Home literacy environment and phonological awareness in preschool children: Differential effects for rhyme and phoneme awareness. *Applied Psycholinguistics, 24*, 59–88.

Francis, W. (1987). *Dialectology: An introduction.* New York: Longman.

Frauenglass, M., & Diaz, R. (1985). Self-regulatory functions of children's private speech: A critical analysis of recent challenges to Vygotsky's theory. *Developmental Psychology, 21*, 357–364.

Freedman, D. (1964). Smiling in blind infants and the issue of innate vs. acquired. *Journal of Child Psychology and Psychiatry, 5*, 171–184.

Freeley, A. (1993). *Argumentation and debate: Critical thinking for reasoned decision making.* Belmont, CA: Wadsworth.

Freund, H. (1966). *Psychopathology and the problems of stuttering.* Springfield, IL: Charles C. Thomas.

Friedlander, D., & Martinson, K. (1996). Effects of mandatory basic education for adult AFDC recipients. *Educational Evaluation and Policy Analysis, 13*, 327–337.

Fritzel, B. (1969). The velopharyngeal muscles in speech: An electromyographic and cinefluorographic study. *Acta Otolaryngology* (Stockholm), Suppl. 250.

Galaburda, A., & Sanides, F. (1980). Cytoarchitectonic organization of the human auditory cortex. *Journal of Comparative Neurology, 190,* 597–610.

Gallagher, T. (1977). Revision behaviors in the speech of normal children developing language. *Journal of Speech and Hearing Research, 20,* 303–318.

Gallagher, T. (1981). Contingent query sequences within adult–child discourse. *Journal of Child Language, 8,* 51–62.

Gallup, G. G., Jr. (1982). Self-awareness and the emergence of mind in primates. *American Journal of Primatology, 2*(3), 237–248.

Gardner, H. (1983). *Frames of mind: The theory of multiple intelligences.* New York: Basic Books.

Gardner, R., & Gardner, B. (1969). Teaching sign language to a chimpanzee. *Science, 165,* 664–672.

Gardner, R., & Gardner, B. (1971). Two-way communication with a chimpanzee. In A. Schrier & F. Stollnitz (Eds.), *Behavior of nonhuman primates* (Vol. 4, pp. 117–184). New York: Academic Press.

Gardner, R., & Gardner, B. (1975). Early signs of language in child and chimpanzee. *Science, 187,* 752–753.

Garvey, C., & Berninger, G. (1981). Timing and turn taking in children's conversations. *Discourse Processes, 4,* 27–57.

Gathercole, V. (1985). "Me has too much hard questions": The acquisition of the linguistic mass-count distinction in "much" and "many." *Journal of Child Language, 12,* 395–415.

Gelman, S., Coley, J., Rosengran, K., Hartman, E., & Pappas, A. (1998). Beyond labeling: The role of maternal input in the acquisition of richly structured categories. *Monographs of the Society for Research in Child Development, 63*(253).

Gelman, S., Croft, W., Fu, P., Clausner, T., & Gottfried, G. (1998). Why is a pomegranate an *apple*? The role of shape, taxonomic relatedness, and prior lexical knowledge in children's overextensions of *apple* and *dog. Journal of Child Language, 25,* 267–291.

Genesee, F. (1976). The role of intelligence in second language learning. *Language Learning, 26,* 267–280.

Genesee, F. (1989). Early bilingual development: One language or two? *Journal of Child Language, 16,* 161–179.

Genesee, F. (2003). Rethinking bilingual acquisition. In J. M. de Waele (Ed.), *Bilingualism: Challenges and directions for future research* (pp. 158–182). Clevedon, England: Multilingual Matters.

Genesee, F., Nicoladis, E., & Paradis, J. (1995). Language differentiation in early bilingual development. *Journal of Child Language, 22,* 611–631.

Genesee, F., Paradis, J., & Crago, M. (2004). *Dual language development and disorders: A handbook on bilingualism and second language learning.* Baltimore: Brookes.

Gentner, D. (1982). Why nouns are learned before verbs: Linguistic relativity versus natural partitioning. In S. Kuczaj (Ed.), *Language development: Vol. 2. Language, thought, and culture.* Hillsdale, NJ: Erlbaum.

Gentner, T. Q., Fenn, K. M., Margoliash, D., & Nusbaum, H. C. (2006). Recursive syntactic pattern learning by songbirds. *Nature, 440,* 1204–1207.

Gershkoff-Stowe, L., & Hahn, E. R. (2007). Fast mapping skills in the developing lexicon. *Journal of Speech, Language, and Hearing Research, 50,* 682–697.

Gershkoff-Stowe, L., & Smith, L. B. (1997). A curvilinear trend in naming errors as a function of early vocabulary growth. *Cognitive Psychology, 34*(1), 37–71.

Gertner, B., Rice, M. L., & Hadley, P. A. (1994). Influence of communicative competence on peer preferences in a preschool classroom. *Journal of Speech and Hearing Research, 37,* 913–923.

Geschwind, N. (1982). Specializations of the brain. In W. Wang (Ed.), *Human communication: Language and its psycho-biological bases* (pp. 110–119). San Francisco: Freeman.

Gibbs, R. W., Jr. (2000). Irony in talk among friends. *Metaphor and Symbol, 15,* 5–27.

Gibson, E., & Levin, H. (1975). *The psychology of reading.* Cambridge, MA: MIT Press.

Gilbertson, M., & Bramlett, R. (1998). Phonological awareness screening to identify at-risk readers: Implications for practitioners. *Language, Speech and Services in Schools, 2,* 109–116.

Gilkerson, J., & Richards, J. A. (2008). *The power of talk* (2nd ed.). Infoture Technical Report ITR-01–2. Boulder, CO: LENA Foundation.

Gilligan, C. (1982). *In a different voice: Psychological theory and women's development.* Cambridge, MA: Harvard University Press.

Ginsberg, G., & Kilbourne, B. (1988). Emergence of vocal alternation in mother/infant interchanges. *Journal of Child Language, 15,* 221–235.

Girolametto, L., Weitzman, E. & Greenberg, J. (2003). Training day care staff to facilitate children's language, *American Journal of Speech-Language Pathology, 12,* 299–311. Doe:10.1044/1058-0360(2003/076)

Gleitman, L., & Wanner, E. (1982). Language acquisition: The state of the state of the art. In E. Wanner & L. Gleitman (Eds.), *Language acquisition: The state of the art.* Cambridge, MA: Harvard University Press.

Gleitman, L., Newport, E., & Gleitman, H. (1984). The current status of the motherese hypothesis. *Journal of Child Language, 11,* 43–79.

Goehl, H., & Kaufman, P. (1984). Do the effects of adventitious deafness include disordered speech? *Journal of Speech and Hearing Disorders, 49,* 58–64.

Goetz, P. J. (2003). The effects of bilingualism on theory of mind development. *Bilingualism: Language and Cognition, 6,* 1–15.

Goldfield, B. (2000). Nouns before verbs in comprehension vs. production: The view from pragmatics. *Journal of Child Language, 27,* 501–520.

Goldfield, B., & Reznick, J. (1990). Early lexical acquisitions: Rate, content, and the vocabulary spurt. *Journal of Child Language, 17,* 171–183.

Goldsmith, J. A. (1990). *Autosegmental and metrical phonology.* Oxford, England: Blackwell.

Goldstein, B. A. (Ed.). (2004). *Bilingual development and disorders in Spanish-English speakers.* Baltimore: Brookes.

Goldstein, M. H., & Schwade, J. A. (2008). Social feedback to infants' babbling facilitates rapid phonological learning. *Psychological Science, 19*(5), 515–523.

Goldstein, M., King, A., & West, M. (2003). Social interaction shapes babbling: Testing parallels between birdsong and speech. *Proceedings of the National Academy of Sciences, 100,* 8030–8035.

Golinkoff, R., Hirsh-Pasek, K., Cauley, K., & Gordon, L. (1987). The eyes have it: Lexical and syntactic comprehension in a new paradigm. *Journal of Child Language, 14,* 23–45.

Gollnick, D., & Chin, P. (1991). Multicultural education for exceptional children. Retrieved from ERIC Digest (ED 333620).

Goodman, K. (1976). Behind the eye: What happens in reading. In H. Singer & R. Ruddell (Eds.), *Theoretical models and processes of reading* (2nd ed.). Newark, DE: International Reading Association.

Goodman, K. (1986). *What's whole in whole language?* Richmond Hill, Canada: Scholastic-TAB Publications.

Goodsitt, J., Morse, P., VerHoeve, J., & Cowan, N. (1984). Infant speech recognition in multisyllabic contexts. *Child Development, 55,* 903–910.

Gopnik, A., & Choi, S. (1990). Language and cognition. *First Language, 10,* 199–216.

Gopnik, A., & Meltzoff, A. (1984). Semantic and cognitive development in 15- to 21-month-old children. *Journal of Child Development, 11,* 495–513.

Gopnik, A., & Meltzoff, A. (1986). Relations between semantic and cognitive development in the one-word stage: The specificity hypothesis. *Child Development, 57,* 1040–1053.

Gopnik, A., & Meltzoff, A. (1987). The development of categorization in the second year and its relation to other cognitive and linguistic developments. *Child Development, 58,* 1523–1531.

Gordon, D., & Ervin-Tripp, S. (1984). The structure of children's requests. In R. Schiefelbusch & J. Pickar (Eds.), *The acquisition of communicative competence.* Baltimore: University Park Press.

Gorlin, R. J., Toriello, H. V., & Cohen, M. M. (1995). *Hereditary hearing loss and its syndromes.* New York: Oxford University Press.

Gorski, P.C. (2015). Multicultural curriculum reform: Stages of Multicultural Curriculum transformation. EdChange.org.Retrievedfrom www.edchange.org/multicultural/curriculum/steps.

Graves, D. (1979). What children show us about revision. *Journal of Language Arts, 56,* 312–319.

Graves, D. (1983). *Writing: Teachers and children at work.* Portsmouth, NH: Heinemann.

Greenfield, P. (1978). Informativeness, presupposition, and semantic choice in single-word utterances. In N. Waterson & C. Snow (Eds.), *The development of communication.* New York: Wiley.

Greenfield, P., & Savage-Rumbaugh, S. (1984). Perceived variability and symbol use: A common language-cognition interface in children and chimpanzees (*Pan troglodytes*). *Journal of Comparative Psychology, 2,* 201–218.

Greenfield, P., & Smith, J. (1976). *The structure of communication in early language development.* New York: Academic Press.

Greenman, G. (1963). Visual behavior of newborn infants. In A. Solnit & S. Provence (Eds.), *Modern perspectives in child development.* New York: Hallmark.

Greenwald, C., & Leonard, L. (1979). Communicative and sensorimotor development in Down's syndrome children. *American Journal of Mental Deficiency, 84,* 296–303.

Greif, E., & Berko-Gleason, J. (1980). Hi, thanks, and goodbye: More routine information. *Language in Society, 9,* 159–166.

Greif, E., & Berko-Gleason, J. (1980). Hi, thanks, and goodbye: Some more routine information. *Language and Society, 9,* 159–166.

Grieser, D. L., & Kuhl, P. (1988). Maternal speech to infants in a tonal language: Support for universal prosodic features in motherese. *Developmental Psychology, 24,* 14–20.

Grimes, B. (Ed.). (1996). *Ethnologue: Languages of the world* (13th ed.). Dallas, TX: Summer Institute of Linguistics.

Grimm, H. (1975, September). *Analysis of short-term dialogues in 5–7- year-olds: Encoding of intentions and modifications of speech acts as a function of negative feedback loops.* Paper presented at the Third International Child Language Symposium, London.

Gropen, J., Pinker, S., Hollander, M., & Goldberg, R. (1991). Syntax and semantics in the acquisition of locative verbs. *Journal of Child Language, 19,* 115–151.

Grosjean, F. (1998). Studying bilinguals: Methodological and conceptual issues. *Language and Cognition, 1,* 131–149.

Grossman, I. (1983). *Classification in intellectual disability.* Washington, DC: American Association on Mental Deficiency.

Grunwell, P. (1981). The development of phonology: A descriptive profile. *First Language, 3,* 161–191.

Guitar, B. (1998). *Stuttering: An integrated approach to its nature and treatment* (2nd ed.). Baltimore: Williams & Wilkins.

Gulati, S., & Kalra, V. (2003). Stroke in children. *Indian Journal of Pediatrics, 70*(8), 639–648.

Gundloch, R. (1981). On the nature and development of children's writing. In C. Frederiksen & J. Dominic (Eds.), *Writing: The nature, development, and teaching of written communication* (Vol. 2). Hillsdale, NJ: Erlbaum.

Gutierrez, V. (2004). Narrative development and disorders in bilingual children. In B. Goldstein (Ed.), *Bilingual language development and disorders in Spanish-English speakers.* Baltimore: Brookes.

Gutierrez-Clellen, V., & Dreiter, J. (2003). Understanding child bilingual acquisition using parent and teacher reports. *Applied Psycholinguistics, 24,* 267–288.

Guttentag, R. E., Haith, M. M., Goodman, G. S., & Hauch, J. (1984). Semantic processing of unattended words in bilinguals: A test of the input switch mechanism. *Journal of Verbal Learning and Verbal Behavior, 23,* 178–188.

Haaf, R., & Bell, R. (1967). A facial dimension in visual discrimination by human infants. *Child Development, 38,* 893–899.

Haas, A. (1979). The acquisition of genderlect. *Annals of the New York Academy of Sciences, 327,* 101–113.

Haas, A., & Owens, R. (1985). *Preschoolers' pronoun strategies: You and me make us.* Paper presented at the annual convention of the American Speech-Language-Hearing Association.

Haight, W., & Miller, P. (1993). *Pretending at home: Early development in a sociocultural context.* Albany: SUNY Press.

Hailman, J. S., & Ficken, M. S. (1986). Combinatorial animal communication with computable syntax: Chick-a-dee calling qualifies as "language" by structural linguistics. *Animal Behavior, 34,* 1899–1901.

Haith, M. (1976, July). *Organization of visual behavior at birth.* Paper presented at the 21st International Congress of Psychology, Paris, France.

Hakes, D. (1980). *The development of metalinguistic abilities in children.* Berlin: Springer.

Hakes, D. (1982). The development of metalinguistic abilities: What develops? In S. Kuczaj (Ed.), *Language development: Vol. 2. Language, thought and culture.* Hillsdale, NJ: Erlbaum.

Hakuta, K. (1986). *Mirror of language: The debate on bilingualism.* New York: Basic Books.

Hakuta, K. (1990). *Bilingualism and bilingual education: Research perspective.* Washington, DC: National Clearinghouse on Bilingual Education.

Hakuta, K. (1994). Distinguishing among proficiency, choice, and attitudes in questions about language for bilinguals. In G. Lamberty & C. Garcia Coll (Eds.), *Puerto Rican women and children: Issues in health, growth and development* (pp. 191–209). New York: Plenum Press.

Hakuta, K., & D'Andrea, D. (1992). Some properties of bilingual maintenance and loss in Mexican background high-school students. *Applied Linguistics, 13*(1), 72–99.

Hakuta, K., & Diaz, R. (1985). The relationship between degree of bilingualism and cognitive ability. In K. Nelson (Ed.), *Children's language* (Vol. 5, pp. 319–344). Mahwah, NJ: Erlbaum.

Hakuta, K., & Garcia, E. (1989). Bilingualism and education. *American Psychologist, 44,* 374–379.

Hakuta, K., & McLaughlin, B. (1996). Bilingualism and second language learning: Seven tensions that define the research. In D. Berliner & R. Calfee (Eds.), *Handbook of educational psychology* (pp. 603–621). New York: Macmillan.

Hakuta, K., Ferdman, B., & Diaz, R, (1989). *Bilingualism and cognitive development: Three perspectives and methodological implications.* Los Angeles: University of California.

Hakuta, K., Goto Butler, Y., & Witt, D. (2000). *How long does it take English, learners to attain proficiency?* Policy Report 2000–1. Davis: University of California Linguistic Minority Research Institute. Retrieved from http://www.stanford.edu/hakuta/Docs/HowLong.pdf

Halliday, M. (1975). *Learning how to mean: Explorations in the development of language.* New York: Arnold.

Halperin, M. (1974). Developmental changes in the recall and recognition of categorized word lists. *Child Development, 45,* 144–151.

Ham, R. (1990). *Therapy of stuttering, preschool through adolescence.* Upper Saddle River, NJ: Prentice Hall.

Hammer, C., & Weiss, A. (1999). Guiding language development: How African American mothers and their infants structure play interactions. *Journal of Speech, Language, and Hearing Research, 42,* 1219–1233.

Hammer, C., & Weiss, A. (2000). African American mothers' views on their infants' language-development and language-learning environment. *American Journal of Speech-Language Pathology, 9,* 1226–140.

Hammer, C., Miccio, A., & Rodriquez, B. (2004). Bilingual language acquisition and the child socialization process. In B. Goldstein (Ed.), *Bilingual language development and disorders in Spanish-English speakers.* Baltimore: Brookes.

Hammer, C., Miccio, A., & Wagstaff, D. (2003). Home literacy experiences and their relationship to bilingual preschoolers' developing English literacy abilities: An initial investigation. *Language, Speech, and Hearing Services in Schools, 34,* 20–30.

Hannah, A., & Murachver, T. (1999). Gender and conversational style as predictors of conversational behavior. *Journal of Language and Social Psychology, 18,* 153–174.

Harbaugh, M. (1990). Celebrating diversity. *Instructor, 100,* 45–48.

Harding, C. (1983a). Acting with intention: A framework for examining the development of intention. In L. Feagans, C. Garvey, & R. Golinkoff (Eds.), *The origins and growth of communication.* Norwood, NJ: Ablex.

Harding, C. (1983b). Setting the stage for language acquisition: Communication development in the first year. In R. Golinkoff (Ed.), *The transition from prelinguistic to linguistic communication.* Hillsdale, NJ: Erlbaum.

Harris, G. (1992). American Indian cultures: A lesson in diversity. In D. E. Battle, (Ed.), *Communication disorders in multicultural populations* (pp. 78–107). Boston: Andover Medical.

Harris, M., Yeeles, C., Chasin, J., & Oakley, Y. (1995). Symmetries and asymmetries in early lexical comprehension and production. *Journal of Child Language, 22,* 1–18.

Harste, J., Woodward, V., & Burke, C. (1984). *Language stories and literacy lessons.* Portsmouth, NH: Heinemann.

Hart, B., & Risley, T. R. (1995). *Meaningful differences in the everyday experiences of young American children.* Baltimore: Brookes.

Haskill, A. M., & Tyler, A. A. (2007). A comparison of linguistic profiles in subgroups of children with specific language impairment. *American Journal of Speech-Language Pathology, 16,* 209–221.

Haskins, J., & Butts, H. (1973). *The psychology of black language.* New York: Harper & Row.

Hauser, M. D. (2007). When males call, females listen: Sex differences in responsiveness to rhesus monkey, *Macaca mulatta,* copulation calls. *Animal Behavior, 73*(6), 1059–1065.

Hauser, M. D., Chomsky, N., & Fitch, W. T. (2002). The faculty of language: What is it, who has it, and how did it evolve? *Science, 298,* 1569–1579.

Hayes, B. (1988). Metrics and phonological theory. In R. Newmeyer (Ed.), *Linguistics: The Cambridge Survey. II. Linguistic Theory: Extensions and implications* (pp. 220–249). Cambridge, England: Cambridge University Press.

Hayes, R. A., & Slater, A. (2008). Three-month-old's detection of alliteration in syllables. *Infant Behavior & Development, 31,* 153–156.

Hayne, H., Boniface, J., & Barr, R. (2000). The development of declarative memory in human infants: Age-related changes in deferred imitation. *Behavioral Neuroscience, 114,* 77–83.

Hayne, H., Rovee-Collier, C., & Perris, E. (1987). Categorization and memory retrieval by three-month-olds. *Child Development, 58,* 750–767.

Heath, S. (1982a). Toward an ethnohistory of writing in American education. In M. Whiteman (Ed.), *Writing: The nature, development and teaching of written composition* (Vol. 1). Hillsdale, NJ: Erlbaum.

Heath, S. (1982b). Questioning at home and at school: A comparative study. In G. D. Spindler (Ed.), *Doing the ethnography of schooling.* New York: Holt, Rinehart & Winston.

Heath, S. (1983). *Ways with words: Language, life, and work in communities and classrooms.* Cambridge: Cambridge University Press.

Heath, S. (1986a). Separating "things of the imagination" from life: Learning to read and write. In W. Teale & E. Sulzby (Eds.), *Emergent literacy.* Norwood, NJ: Ablex.

Heath, S. (1986b). Taking a cross-cultural look at narratives. *Topics in Language Disorders, 7*(1), 84–94.

Hegde, M. (2004). *Introduction to communicative disorders* (3rd ed.). Austin, TX: PRO-ED.

Hedge, M., & Maul, C. A. (2006). *Language disorders in children: An evidence-based approach to assessment and treatment.* Boston: Pearson Allyn & Bacon.

Heilmann, J., Miller, J.F., Nockerts, A., & Dunaway, C. (2010). Properties of the narrative scoring scheme using narrative retells in your school-age children. *American Journal of Speech Language Pathology, 19,* 154–166.

Herbert, J., Gross, J., & Hayne, H. (2006). Age-related changes in deferred imitation between 6 and 9 months of age. *Infant Behavior & Development, 29,* 136–139.

Herdina, P., & Jessner, U. (2002). *A dynamic model of multilingualism: Changing the psycholinguistic perspective.* Clevedon, England: Multilingual Matters.

Herman, J. (1996). *"Grenouille, where are you?" Cross-linguistic transfer in bilingual kindergarteners learning to read.* Unpublished doctoral dissertation, Harvard University, Cambridge, MA.

Herman, L. (1981). Cognitive characteristics of dolphins. In L. Herman (Ed.), *Cetacean behavior* (pp. 363–429). New York: Wiley.

Herman, L., & Forestell, P. (1985). Reporting presence or absence of named objects by a language-trained dolphin. *Neuroscience and Biobehavioral Reviews, 9,* 667–681.

Herman, L., Hovancik, J., Gory, J., & Bradshaw, G. (1989). Generalization of visual matching by a bottle-nosed dolphin (*Tursiops truncates*): Evidence for invariance of cognitive performance with visual and auditory materials. *Journal of Experimental Psychology Animal Behavior Processes, 15,* 124–136.

Hertrich, I., & Ackermann, H. (1994). Acquired stuttering in Parkinson syndrome. *Journal of Fluency Disorders, 19,* 179.

Hickey, T. (1993). Identifying formulas in first language acquisition. *Journal of Child Language, 20,* 27–41.

Hilke, D. (1988). Infant vocalizations and changes in experience. *Journal of Child Language, 15,* 1–15.

Hirsh-Pasek, K., Treiman, R., & Schneiderman, M. (1984). Brown and Hanlon revisited: Mother's sensitivity to ungrammatical forms. *Journal of Child Language, 11,* 81–88.

Hixon, T. (1987). Respiratory function in speech. In T. Hixon (Ed.), *Respiratory function in speech and song.* Boston: College-Hill.

Hobbs, J. (Ed.) (1987a). *Cleft lip and cleft palate from birth to three years.* Pittsburgh, PA: American Cleft Palate Educational Foundation.

Hobbs, J. (Ed.) (1987b). *Cleft lip and cleft palate: The child from three to twelve years.* Pittsburgh, PA: American Cleft Palate Educational Foundation.

Hockett, C. (1960). The origin of speech. *Scientific American, 203,* 89–97.

Hodgkinson, H. (1998). Demographics of diversity for the 21st century. *Education Digest, 64,* 4–7.

Hodson, B., & Paden, E. (1991). *Targeting intelligible speech* (2nd ed.). Austin, TX: PRO-ED.

Hoff, E., & Naigles, L. (2002). How children use input to acquire a lexicon. *Child Development, 73,* 418–433.

Hoff-Ginsberg, E. (1986). Function and structure in maternal speech: Their relation to the child's development of syntax. *Developmental Psychology, 22,* 155–163.

Hoff-Ginsberg, E. (1990). Maternal speech and the child's development of syntax: A further look. *Journal of Child Language, 17,* 85–89.

Hoff-Ginsberg, E., & Shatz, M. (1982). Linguistic input and the child's acquisition of language. *Psychological Bulletin, 92,* 3–26.

Hoffman, K. A. (1982). *Speech sound acquisition and natural process occurrence in the continuous speech of three-to-six-year-old children.* Unpublished master's thesis. University of Wisconsin–Madison.

Hoffman, P. (1990). Spelling, phonology, and the speech-language pathologist: A whole language perspective. *Language, Speech, Hearing Services in Schools, 21,* 238–243.

Hoffner, C., Cantor, J., & Badzinski, D. (1990). Children's understanding of adverbs denoting degree of likelihood. *Journal of Child Language, 17,* 217–231.

Hohensee, J., & Derman-Sparks, L. (1992). Implementing anti-bias curriculum in early childhood programs. Retrieved from ERIC Digest (ED 35114692).

Hoit, J., Hixon, T., Watson, P., & Morgan, W. (1990). Speech breathing in children and adolescents. *Journal of Speech and Hearing Research, 33,* 51–69.

Hollien, H. (1960a). Some laryngeal correlates of vocal pitch. *Journal of Speech and Hearing Research, 3,* 52–58.

Hollien, H. (1960b). Vocal pitch variations related to changes in vocal fold length. *Journal of Speech and Hearing Research, 3,* 150–156.

Hood, L., & Bloom, L. (1979). What, when, and how about why: A longitudinal study of early expressions of causality. *Monographs of the Society for Research in Child Development, 44.*

Horgan, D. (1978). The development of the full passive. *Journal of Child Language, 5,* 65–80.

Horgan, D. (1981). Rate of language acquisition and noun emphasis. *Journal of Psycholinguistic Research, 10,* 629–640.

Horst, J. S., & Samuelson, L. K. (2008). Fast mapping but poor retention by 24-month-old infants. *Infancy, 13*(2), 128–157.

Houston, P. (1999). The accelerating change of American diversity. *School Administrator, 56,* 6–7.

Hsu, H., & Jeng, S. (2007). Two-month-olds' attention and affective response to maternal still face: A comparison between term and preterm infants in Taiwan. *Infant Behavior & Development, 31,* 194–206.

Hudson, J. A. (1990). The emergence of autobiographic memory in mother/child conversation. In R. Fivush & J. A. Hudson (Eds.), *Knowing and remembering in young children* (pp. 166–196). Cambridge, Eng.: Cambridge University Press.

Hudson, J. A., & Shapiro, L. R. (1991). From knowing to telling: The development of scripts, stories, and personal narratives. In A. McCabe & C. Peterson (Eds.), *Developing narrative structure* (pp. 89–136). Hillsdale, NJ: Erlbaum.

Hughes, D., McGillivray, L., & Schmidek, M. (1997). *Guide to narrative language: Procedures for assessment.* Eau Claire, WI: Thinking Publications.

Hughes, M., & Grieve, R. (1980). On asking children bizarre questions. *First Language, 1,* 149–160.

Hulit, L. (1989). A stutterer like me. *Journal of Fluency Disorders, 14,* 209–214.

Hulit, L. (2004). *Straight talk on stuttering* (2nd ed.). Springfield, IL: Charles C. Thomas.

Hulit, L., & Wirtz, L. (1994). The association of attitudes toward stuttering with selected variables. *Journal of Fluency Disorders, 19,* 247–267.

Hummer, P., Wimmer, H., & Antes, G. (1993). On the origins of denial. *Journal of Child Language, 20,* 607–618.

Hutchinson, J., & Putnam, A. (1974). Aerodynamic aspects of sensory deprived speech. *Journal of the Acoustical Society of America, 56,* 1612–1617.

Huttenlocher, J. (1974). The origins of language comprehension. In R. Soslo (Ed.), *Theories in cognitive psychology: The Loyola symposium.* New York: Wiley.

Huttenlocher, J., Haight, W., Bryk, A., Seltzer, M., & Lyons, T. (1991). Early vocabulary growth: Relation to language input and gender. *Developmental Psychology, 27,* 236–248.

Huxley, R. (1970). The development of the correct use of subject personal pronouns in two children. In G. Flores d'Arcais & W. Levelt (Eds.), *Advances in psycholinguistics.* Amsterdam: North-Holland.

Ingram, D. (1971). Transitivity in child language. *Language, 47,* 888–910.

Ingram, D. (1974a). Phonological rules in young children. *Journal of Child Language, 1,* 49–64.

Ingram, D. (1974b). The relationship between comprehension and production. In R. Schiefelbusch & L. Lloyd (Eds.), *Language perspectives—Acquisition, retardation, and intervention.* Baltimore: University Park Press.

Ingram, D. (1976). *Phonological disability in children.* London: Arnold.

Ingram, D. (1989). *First language acquisition: Method, description and explanation.* Cambridge: Cambridge University Press.

Ingram, D. (1991). *Phonological disability in children* (2nd ed.). San Diego, CA: Singular.

Ingram, D., Christensen, D., Veach, S., & Webster, B. (1980). The acquisition of word-initial fricatives and affricates in English by children between 2 and 6 years. In G. Yeni-Komshian, J. Kavanaugh, & C. Ferguson (Eds.), *Child phonology: Vol. 2. Production.* New York: Academic Press.

Institute of Education Sciences, National Center for Education Statistics. Table 204.30: Children 3 to 21 years old served under Individuals with Disabilities Education Act (IDEA), Part B, by type of disability: Selected years, 1976–77 through 2011–12. Retrieved from https://nces.ed.gov/programs/digest/d13/tables/dt13_204.30.asp March 18, 2017.

International Reading Association, Division of Research and Policy. (2002). Summary of the (U.S.) National Reading Panel Report, *Teaching children to read* (pp. 1–19). Retrieved from http://www.reading.org/general/CurrentResearch/Reports/NationalReadingPanelReport.aspx

Isshiki, N. (1959). Regulatory mechanism of the pitch and volume of voice. *Otorhinolaryngology Clinic* (Kyoto), *52*, 1065.

Isshiki, N. (1964). Regulatory mechanisms of voice intensity variation. *Journal of Speech and Hearing Research, 7,* 17–29.

Isshiki, N., & Ringel, R. (1964). Air flow during the production of selected consonants. *Journal of Speech and Hearing Research, 7,* 233–244.

Jackendoff, R., & Pinker, S. (2005). The nature of language faculty and its implications for evolution of language (reply to Fitch, Hauser, and Chomsky). *Cognition, 97*(2), 211–225.

Jackson-Maldonado, D. (2004). Verbal morphology and vocabulary in monolinguals and emergent bilinguals. In B. Goldstein (Ed.), *Bilingual language development and disorders in Spanish-English speakers,* Baltimore: Brookes.

Jackson-Maldonado, D., Thal, D., Marchman, V., Bates, E., & Gutierrez-Clellen, V. (1993). Early lexical development in Spanish-speaking infants and toddlers. *Journal of Child Language, 20,* 523–549.

Jaffe, J., Stern, D., & Perry, C. (1973). "Conversational" coupling of gaze behavior in prelinguistic human development. *Journal of Psycholinguistic Research, 2,* 321–330.

Jakobson, R. (1949). On the identification of phonemic entities. *Travaux du Cercle Linguistique de Prague, 5,* 205–213.

Jakobson, R. (1968). *Child language, aphasia, and phonological universals* (A. R. Keiler, Trans.). The Hague: Mouton.

Jakobson, R., Fant, G., & Halle, M. (1952). *Preliminaries to speech analysis: The distinctive features and their correlates.* Cambridge, MA: MIT Press.

James, C. (1996). A cross-linguistic approach to language awareness. *Language Awareness, 3 & 4,* 201–209.

James, S. (1980). *Language and sensorimotor cognitive development in the young child.* Paper presented at the annual convention of the New York Speech–Language–Hearing Association, New York City.

James, S. (1990). *Normal language acquisition.* Austin, TX: PRO-ED.

James, S., & Kahn, L. (1982). Grammatical morpheme acquisition: An approximately invariant order? *Journal of Psycholinguistic Research, 11,* 381–388.

James, S., & Seebach, M. (1982). The pragmatic function of children's questions. *Journal of Speech and Hearing Research, 25,* 2–11.

Janik, V. (2000). Whistle matching in bottlenose dolphins. *Science, 289,* 1355–1357.

Jay, T. (1992). *Cursing in America.* Philadelphia: Benjamins.

Jensen, P., Williams, W., & Bzoch, K. (1975, November). *Preference of young infants for speech vs. nonspeech stimuli.* Paper presented at the annual American Speech and Hearing Association convention, Washington, DC.

Jessner, U. (2006). *Linguistic awareness in multilinguals: English as a third language.* Edinburgh: Edinburgh University Press.

Jessner, U. (2008). A DST model of multilingualism and the role of metalinguistic awareness. *The Modern Language Journal, 92,* 270–283.

Jia, G., & Aaronson, D. (2003). A longitudinal study of Chinese children and adolescents learning English in the United States. *Applied Psycholinguistics, 24,* 131–161.

Jia, G., Aaronson, D., & Wu, Y. (2002). Long-term language attainment of bilingual immigrants: Predictive variables and language group differences. *Applied Psycholinguistics, 23,* 599–621.

Johnson, B. (1996). *Language disorders in children: An introductory clinical perspective.* Clifton Park, NY: Cengage Learning.

Johnson, C., & Anglin, J. (1995). Qualitative developments in the content and form of children's definitions. *Journal of Speech and Hearing Research, 38,* 612–629.

Johnson, N. S., & Mandler, J. M. (1980). A tale of two structures: Underlying and surface forms in stories. *Poetics, 9,* 51–66.

Johnson, W. (1946). *People in quandaries*. New York: Harper.

Johnson, W., & Moeller, D. (1967). *Speech-handicapped school children* (3rd ed.). New York: Harper & Row.

Johnston, J. (1982). Narratives: A new look at communication problems in older language disordered children. *Language, Speech and Hearing Services in Schools, 13*, 144–155.

Johnston, J. (1984). Acquisition of locative meanings: "Behind" and "in front of." *Journal of Child Language, 11*, 407–422.

Jusczyk, P. W. (1997). *The discovery of spoken language*. Cambridge, MA: MIT Press.

Justice, L. M., & Ezell, H. K. (2000). Enhancing children's print and word awareness through home-based intervention. *American Journal of Speech-Language Pathology, 9*, 257–269.

Justice, L. M., & Ezell, H. K. (2001). Written language awareness in preschool children from low-income households: A descriptive analysis. *Communication Disorders Quarterly, 22*, 123–134.

Justice, L. M., & Ezell, H. K. (2002). Use of storybook reading to increase print awareness in at-risk children. *American Journal of Speech-Language Pathology, 11*, 17–29.

Justice, L. M., & Ezell, H. K. (2004). Print referencing: An emergent literacy enhancement strategy and its clinical applications. *Language, Speech, and Hearing Services in Schools, 35*, 185–193.

Justice, L. M., Bowles, R. P., & Skibbe, L. E. (2006). Measuring preschool attainment of print-concept knowledge: A study of typical and at-risk three- to five-year-old children using item response theory. *Language, Speech, and Hearing Services in Schools, 37*, 224–235.

Kaderavek, J., & Sulzby, E. (2000). Narrative production by children with and without specific language impairment: Oral narratives and emergent readings. *Journal of Speech, Language, and Hearing Research, 43*, 34–49.

Kahane, J., & Folkins, J. (1984). *Atlas of speech and hearing anatomy*. Upper Saddle River, NJ: Prentice Hall.

Kail, R. (1984). *The development of memory in children* (2nd ed.). New York: Freeman.

Kamhi, A. (1981). Developmental vs. difference theories of intellectual disability: A new look. *American Journal of Mental Deficiency, 86*, 1–7.

Kamhi, A. G. (1997). Three perspectives on comprehension: Implications for assessing and treating comprehension problems. *Topics in Language Disorders, 17*(3), 62–74.

Kamhi, A. G., & Catts, H. (1986). Toward an understanding of developmental language and reading disorders. *Journal of Speech and Hearing Disorders, 51*, 337–347.

Kane, M. J., & Engle, R. W. (2002). The role of prefrontal cortex in working-memory capacity, executive attention, and general fluid intelligence: An individual-differences perspective. *Psychonomic Bulletin and Review, 9*, 637–671.

Kaplan, P., Bachorowski, J., Smoski, M., & Hudenko, W. (2002). Infants of depressed mothers, although competent learners, fail to learn in response to their own mothers' infant-directed speech. *Psychological Science, 13*, 268–271.

Karrass, J., Braungart-Rieker, J., Mullins, J., & Lefever, J. (2002). Processes in language acquisition: The roles of gender, attention, and maternal encouragement of attention over time. *Journal of Child Language, 29*, 519–543.

Kay Raining-Bird, E., & Chapman, R.S. (1998). Partial representations and phonological selectivity in the comprehension of 13- to 16-month-olds. *First Language, 18*, 105-127.

Kaye, K. (1977). Towards the origin of dialogue. In H. Schaffer (Ed.), *Studies in mother–child interaction*. London: Academic Press.

Kaye, K. (1979). Thickening thin data: The maternal role in developing communication and language. In M. Bullowa (Ed.), *Before speech*. New York: Cambridge University Press.

Kaye, K. (1980). Why we don't talk "baby talk" to babies. *Journal of Child Language, 7*, 489–507.

Kay-Raining Bird, E., & Chapman, R. S. (1998). Partial representation and phonological selectivity in the comprehension of 13- to 16-month-olds. *First Language, 18*, 105–127.

Keenan, E., & Schieffelin, B. (1976). Topic as a discourse notion: A study of topic in the conversation of children and adults. In C. Li (Ed.), *Subject and topic: A new typology of language*. New York: Academic Press.

Keil, F. C. (2008). The shape of things to come: The future of the shape bias controversy. *Developmental Science, 11*(2), 216–222.

Keller, H., Otto, H., Lamm, B., Yovsi, R. D., & Kärtner, J. (2007). The timing of verbal/vocal communications between mothers and their infants: A longitudinal cross-cultural comparison. *Infant Behavior & Development, 31*, 217–226.

Kellogg, R. (1994). *The psychology of writing*. New York: Oxford University Press.

Kelly, C., & Dale, P. (1989). Cognitive skills associated with the onset of multiword utterances. *Journal of Speech and Hearing Research, 32,* 645–656.

Kelly, S. (2001). Broadening the units of analysis in communication: Speech and nonverbal behaviors in pragmatic comprehension. *Journal of Child Language, 28,* 325–349.

Kelso, J., Tuller, B., & Harris, K. (1983). A dynamic pattern perspective on the control and coordination of movement. In P. MacNeilage (Ed.), *The production of speech.* New York: Springer.

Kemp, C. (2001). *Metalinguistic awareness in multilinguals: Implicit and explicit grammatical awareness and its relationship with language experience and language attainment.* Unpublished doctoral thesis, University of Edinburgh, Scotland.

Kemper, S. (1984). The development of narrative skills: Explanations and entertainments. In S. Kuczaj (Ed.), *Discourse development: Progress in cognitive development research.* New York: Springer.

Kemper, S., & Edwards, L. (1986). Children's expression of causality and their construction of narratives. *Topics in Language Disorders, 7,* 11–20.

Kent, R. (1984). Brain mechanisms of speech and language with special reference to emotional interactions. In R. Naremore (Ed.), *Language science: Recent advances.* San Diego, CA: College-Hill.

Kerbel, D., & Grunwell, R. (1997). Idioms in the classroom: An investigation of language unit and mainstream teachers' use of idioms. *Child Language Teaching and Therapy, 13*(2), 113–123.

Kessen, W., Levine, J., & Wendrich, K. (1979). The imitation of pitch in infants. *Infant Behavior and Development, 2,* 93–100.

Klatsky, R., Clark, E., & Macken, M. (1973). Asymmetries in the acquisition of polar adjectives: Linguistic conceptual? *Journal of Experimental Child Psychology, 16,* 32–46.

Klecan-Acker, J., & Kelty, K. (1990). An investigation of the oral narratives of normal and language-learning disabled children. *Journal of Childhood Communication Disorders, 13,* 207–216.

Klee, T. (1985). Role of inversion in children's question development. *Journal of Speech and Hearing Research, 28,* 225–232.

Klein, P., & Meltzoff, A. (1999). Long-term memory, forgetting, and deferred imitation in 12-month-old infants. *Developmental Science, 2,* 102–113.

Klima E., & Bellugi-Klima, U. (1971). Syntactic regularities in the speech of children. In A. Bar-Adon & W. Leopold (Eds.), *Child language: A book of readings.* Upper Saddle River, NJ: Prentice Hall.

Klima, E., & Bellugi, U. (1966). Syntactic regularities in the speech of children. In J. Lyons & R. Wales (Eds.), *Psycholinguistic papers.* Edinburgh, Scotland: Edinburgh University Press.

Knox, C., & Kimura, D. (1970). Cerebral processing of nonverbal sounds in boys and girls. *Neuropsychologia, 8,* 227–237.

Kobasigawa, A. (1974). Utilization of retrieval cues by children in recall. *Child Development, 45,* 127–134.

Kobasigawa, A. (1997). Retrieval strategies in the development of memory. In R. Kail & J. W. Hagen (Eds.), *Perspectives in the development of memory and cognition* (pp. 177–201). Hillsdale, NJ: Erlbaum.

Kobasigawa, A., & Mason, P. L. (1982). Use of multiple cues by children in memory retrieval situations. *Journal of General Psychology, 107,* 195–201.

Koelsch, S., & Siebel, W. A. (2005). Towards a neural basis of music perception. *Trends in Cognitive Science, 9,* 578–584.

Kohnert, K (2004). Processing skills in early sequential bilinguals. In B. Goldstein (Ed.), *Bilingual language development and disorders in Spanish-English speakers.* Baltimore: Brookes.

Kohnert, K., & Bates, E. (2002). Balancing bilinguals, II: Lexical comprehension and cognitive processing in children learning Spanish and English. *Journal of Speech, Language, and Hearing Research, 45,* 347–359.

Kohnert, K., Bates, E., & Hernandez, A. (1999). Balancing bilinguals: Lexical-semantic production and cognitive processing in children learning Spanish and English. *Journal of Speech, Language, and Hearing Research, 42,* 1400–1413.

Krafft, K., & Berk, L. (1998). Private speech in two preschools: Significance of open-ended activities and make-believe play for verbal self-regulation. *Early Childhood Research Quarterly, 13,* 637–658.

Krauss, R., & Glucksberg, S. (1977). Social and nonsocial speech. *Scientific American, 236,* 100–105.

Krcmar, M., Grela, B., & Lin, K. (2007). Can toddlers learn vocabulary from television? An experimental approach. *Media Psychology, 10,* 41–63.

Kroll, B. (1981). Developmental relationships between speaking and writing. In B. Kroll & R. Vann (Eds.), *Exploring speaking–writing relationships: Connections and contrasts.* Urbana, IL: National Council of Teachers of English.

Kuczaj, S. A., & Kirkpatrick, V. M. (1993). Similarities and differences in human and animal language research: Toward a comparative psychology of language. In H. Roitblat, L. Herman, & P. Nachtigall (Eds.), *Language and communication: Comparative perspectives* (pp. 45–63). Hillsdale, NJ: Erlbaum.

Kuehn, D., Lemme, M., & Baumgartner, J. (Eds.). (1989). *Neural bases of speech, hearing, and language.* Boston: College-Hill.

Kuhl, P.K. (2000). A new view of language acquisition. *Proceedings of the National Academy of Sciences, 97*(22) 11850-11857.

Kurland, B., & Snow, C. (1997). Longitudinal measurement of growth in definitional skill. *Journal of Child Language, 24,* 603–625.

Kuykendall, M., & Fahey, K. R. (2000). The development of written language. In K. R. Fahey & D. K. Reid (Eds.), *Language development, differences, and disorders* (pp. 135–173). Austin, TX: PRO-ED.

Labov, W. (1966). *The social stratification of English in New York City.* Washington, DC: Center for Applied Linguistics.

Labov, W. (1972). *Language in the inner city: Studies in the Black English vernacular.* Philadelphia: University of Pennsylvania Press.

Ladefoged, P. (1971). *Preliminaries to linguistic phonetics.* Chicago: University of Chicago Press.

Landau, B., & Gleitman, L. (1985). *Language and experience: Evidence from the blind child.* Cambridge, MA: Harvard University Press.

Lane, V., & Molyneaux, D. (1992). *The dynamics of communicative development.* Upper Saddle River, NJ: Prentice Hall.

Langdon, H. W., & Cheng, L. L. (1992). *Hispanic children and adults with communication disorders.* Gaithersburg, MD: Maryland: Aspen.

Langdon, H. W., & Merino, B. J. (1992). Acquisition and developmental of a second language in the Spanish speaker. In H. W. Langdon & L. L. Cheng (Eds.), *Hispanic children and adults with communication disorders* (pp. 132–159). Baltimore: Aspen.

Larkins, P. (1985). *Speech-language pathology update.* Rockville, MD: American Speech–Language–Hearing Association.

Lass, N., Ruscello, D., Schmitt, J., Pannbacker, M., Orlando, M., Dean, K., Ruziska, J., & Bradshaw, K. (1992). Teachers' perceptions of stutterers. *Language, Speech, Hearing Services in Schools, 23,* 78–81.

Lazar, R. T., Warr-Leeper, G. A., Nicholson, C. B., & Johnson, S. (1989). Elementary school teachers' use of multiple meaning expressions. *Language, Speech, and Hearing Services in Schools, 20,* 420–430.

Leaper, C. (1991). Influence and involvement in children's discourse: Age, gender, and partner effects. *Child Development, 62,* 797-811.

Lebrun, Y., Leleux, C., Rousseau, J., & Devreux, F. (1983). Acquired stuttering. *Journal of Fluency Disorders, 8,* 323–330.

Legerstee, M., & Barillas, Y. (2003). Sharing attention and pointing to objects at 12 months: Is the intentional stance implied? *Cognitive Development, 18,* 91–110.

Legerstee, M., & Markova, G. (2008). Variations in 10-month-old infant imitation of people and things. *Infant Behavior & Development, 31,* 81–91.

Lemish, D., & Rice, M. (1986). Television as a talking picture book: A prop for language acquisition. *Journal of Child Language, 13,* 251–274.

Lempert, H. (1990). Acquisition of passives: The role of patient animacy, salience, and lexical accessibility. *Journal of Child Language, 17,* 677–696.

Lenneberg, E. (1964). A biological perspective of language. In E. Lenneberg (Ed.), *New directions in the study of language.* Cambridge, MA: MIT Press.

Lenneberg, E. (1967). *Biological foundations of language.* New York: Wiley.

Leonard, L. (1987). Is specific language impairment a useful construct? In S. Rosenberg (Ed.), *Advances in applied psycholinguistics* (Vol. 1). Cambridge, England: Cambridge University Press.

Leonard, L. B. (1998). *Children with specific language impairment.* Cambridge, MA: MIT Press.

Leonard, L., & Loeb, D. (1988). Government-binding theory and some of its implications: A tutorial. *Journal of Speech and Hearing Research, 31,* 515–524.

Leonard, L., Wilcox, J., Fulmer, K., & Davis, A. (1978). Understanding indirect requests: An investigation of children's comprehension of pragmatic meanings. *Journal of Speech and Hearing Research, 21,* 528–537.

Leske, M. (1981a). Prevalence estimates of communicative disorders in the U.S.: Speech disorders. *American Speech–Language–Hearing Association, 23,* 217–225.

Leske, M. (1981b). Prevalence estimates of communicative disorders in the U.S.: Language, hearing and vestibular disorders. *American Speech–Language–Hearing Association, 23,* 229–237.

Levelt, W. J. M. (1989). *Speaking: From intention to articulation.* Cambridge, MA: MIT Press.

Lewis, B. A., & Thompson, L. A. (1992). A study of developmental speech and language disorders in twins. *Journal of Speech and Hearing Research, 35,* 1086–1094.

Lewis, M. (1951). *Infant speech: A study of the beginnings of language.* New York: Humanities Press.

Lewis, R. (1996). Interference in short-term memory: The magical number two (or three) in sentence processing. *Journal of Psycholinguistic Research, 25,* 93–121.

Li, P. (2003). Language acquisition in a self-organizing neural network model. In P. Quinlan (Ed.), *Connectionist models of development: Developmental processes in real and artificial neural networks* (pp. 115–149). New York: Psychology Press.

Li, P. (2004). Early lexical development in a self-organizing neural network, *Neural Networks, 17,* 1345–1362.

Liberman, M. (1975). *The intonational system of English.* Unpublished doctoral dissertation, Massachusetts Institute of Technology, Cambridge.

Liberman, M., & Prince, A. (1977). On stress and linguistic rhythm. *Linguistic Inquiry, 8,* 249–336.

Lieberman, P. (1975). *On the origins of language: An introduction to the evolution of human speech.* Series in Physical Anthropology. New York: Macmillan.

Liebman, M. (1991). *Neuroanatomy made easy and understandable* (4th ed.). Rockville, MD: Aspen.

Lillard, A. (2001). Pretending, understanding pretense, and understanding minds. In. S. Reifel (Ed.), *Theory in context and out: Play and culture studies* (Vol. 3, pp. 233–254). Westport, CT: Ablex.

Ling, D. (1972). Acoustic stimulus duration in relation to behavioral responses of newborn infants. *Journal of Speech and Hearing Research, 15,* 567–571.

Liszkowski, U., Albrecht, K., Carpenter, M., & Tomasello, M. (2008). Infants' visual and auditory communication when a partner is or is not visually attending. *Infant Behavior & Development, 31,* 157–167.

Liszkowski, U., Carpenter, M., & Tomasello, M. (2007). Reference and attitude in infant pointing. *Journal of Child Language, 34,* 1–20.

Liszkowski, U., Carpenter, M., Henning, A., Striano, J., & Tomasello, M. (2004). Twelve-month-olds point to share attention and interest. *Developmental Science, 7*(3), 297–307.

Litowitz, B. (1977). Learning to make definitions. *Journal of Child Language, 4,* 289–304.

Lochman, J. E., & Szczepanski, R. G. (1999). Externalizing conditions. In V. L. Schwean & D. H. Saklofske (Eds.), *Handbook of psychosocial characteristics of exceptional children* (pp. 219–246). New York: Kluwer Academic/Plenum.

Lonigan, C. J. (2004, October). *Development and promotion of emergent literacy: An evidence-based perspective.* Paper presented at the Early Literacy Development Conference, Niagara Falls, Canada.

Lowe, R. J. (1994). *Phonology: Assessment and intervention applications in speech pathology.* Baltimore: Williams & Wilkins.

Lubker, J. (1968). An electromyographic-cinefluorographic investigation of velar function during normal speech production. *Cleft Palate Journal, 5,* 1–18.

Lund, N., & Duchan, J. (1988). *Assessing children's language in naturalistic contexts.* Upper Saddle River, NJ: Prentice Hall.

Lundgren, K., Helm-Estabrooks, N., & Klein, R. (2010). Stuttering following acquired brain damage: A review of the literature. *Journal of Neurolinguistics, 23*(5), pp. 447–454.

Lynch, M., Oller, K., & Steffens, M. (1989). Development of speech-like vocalizations in a child with congenital absence of cochleas: The case of total deafness. *Applied Psycholinguistics, 10,* 315–333.

Macartney, S. (2011). *Child Poverty in the United States 2009 and 2010: Selected Race Groups and Hispanic Origin.* American Community Survey Briefs, November, 2011) Retrieved from www.census.gov/prod/2011pubs/acsbr10-05.pdf

Mackay, M.T., & Gordon, A. (2007). Stroke in children. *Australian Family Physician, 36*(11), 896–902.

MacNeilage, P. (1970). Motor control of serial ordering of speech. *Psychological Review, 77,* 182–196.

MacWhinney, B. (1987). *Mechanisms of language acquisition.* Hillsdale, NJ: Erlbaum.

MacWhinney, B. (2001). Lexicalist connectionism. In P. Broeder & J. M. Murre (Eds.), *Models of language acquisition: Inductive or deductive approaches* (pp. 9–32). Oxford: Oxford University Press.

MacWhinney, B., & Bates, E. (1978). Sentential devices for conveying givenness and newness: A cross-cultural developmental study. *Journal of Verbal Learning and Verbal Behavior, 17,* 539–558.

Maess, B., Koelsch, S., Gunter, T. C., & Friederici, A. D. (2001). Musical syntax is processed in Boca's area: An MEG study. *Nature Neuroscience, 4,* 540–545.

Mahecha, N. (2003). Typical and disordered child narration in Spanish-speaking children. In A. McCabe & L. S. Bliss (Eds.), *Patterns of narrative discourse: A multicultural lifespan approach* (pp. 73–90). Boston: Allyn & Bacon.

Mahoor, M.H., Mattson, W.I., Anderson, D.R., & Messinger, D.S. (2011). Analysis of eye gaze pattern of infants at risk of autism spectrum disorder using Markov models. Applications of Computer Vision (WACV) IEEE Workshop. DOI: 10.1109/WACV.2011.571151

Mahr, G., & Leith, W. (1992). Psychogenic stuttering of adult onset. *Journal of Speech and Hearing Research, 35,* 283–286.

Makau, J. (1990). *Reasoning and communication: Thinking critically about arguments.* Belmont, CA: Wadsworth.

Maltz, D., & Borker, R. (1982). A cultural approach to male–female miscommunication. In J. J. Gumperz (Ed.), *Language and social identity.* Cambridge: Cambridge University Press.

Mandler, J. (1992a). The foundations of conceptual thought in infancy. *Cognitive Development, 7,* 273–285.

Mandler, J. (1992b). How to build a baby: II. Conceptual primitives. *Psychological Review, 99,* 587–604.

Maneva, B., & Genesee, F. (2002). Bilingual babbling: Evidence for language differentiation in dual language acquisition. In B. Skarabela, S. Fish, & A.-H. Do (Eds.), *Proceedings of the 26th Boston University Conference on Language Development* (pp. 383–392). Somerville, MA: Cascadilla Press.

Manning, M., & Baruth, L. (1996). *Multicultural education of children and adolescents* (2nd ed.). Boston: Allyn & Bacon.

Maratsos, M. (1974). When is a high thing the big one? *Developmental Psychology, 10,* 367–375.

Marchman, V., & Bates, E. (1991). *Vocabulary size and composition as predictors of morphological development* (Technical Report No. 9103). University of California, San Diego: Center for Research in Language.

Marchman, V., & Bates, E. (1994). Continuity in lexical and morphological development: A test of the critical mass hypothesis. *Journal of Child Language, 21,* 339–366.

Marcos, H. (1987). Communicative function of pitch range and pitch direction in infants. *Journal of Child Language, 14,* 255–268.

Marin, O., Schwartz, M., & Saffran, E. (1979). Origins and distribution of language. In M. Gazzaniga (Ed.), *Handbook of behavioral neurobiology.* New York: Plenum.

Marinellie, S. A., & Chan, Y. (2006). The effect of word frequency on noun and verb definitions: A developmental study. *Journal of Speech, Language, and Hearing Research, 49,* 1001–1021.

Marsh, G., Friedman, M., Welch, V., & Desberg, P. (1981). A cognitive-developmental theory of reading acquisition. In G. McKinnon & T. Weller (Eds.), *Reading research: Advances in theory and practice.* New York: Academic Press.

Martin, H., McConkey, R., & Martin, S. (1984). From acquisition theories to intervention strategies: An experiment with mentally handicapped children. *British Journal of Disorders of Communication, 19,* 3–14.

Martin, R. (1997). "Girls don't talk about garages!": Perceptions of conversations in same- and cross-sex friendships. *Personal Relationships, 4,* 115–130.

Masataka, N. (1992). Pitch characteristics of Japanese maternal speech to infants. *Journal of Child Language, 19,* 213–223.

Masataka, N. (1993). Effects of contingent and noncontingent maternal stimulation on the vocal behavior of three- to four-month-old Japanese infants. *Journal of Child Language, 20,* 303–312.

Mason, J. (1989). *Reading and writing connections.* Boston: Allyn & Bacon.

Mason, J. A., & Herrmann, K. R. (1998). Universal infant hearing screening by automated auditory brainstem response measurement. *Pediatrics, 101,* 221–228.

Massey, A. (1996). Cultural influences on language assessment and intervention. In A. Kamhi, K. Pollock, & J. Harris (Eds.), *Communication development and disorders in African American children: Research, assessment, and intervention.* Baltimore: Brookes.

Mattingly, J. (1972). Reading the linguistic process and linguistic awareness. In J. Kavanagh & J. Mattingly (Eds.), *Language by ear and by eye.* Cambridge, MA: MIT Press.

Mavlov, L. (1994). Mechanisms of fluency disorders in neocerebellar dysarthria and premotor articulatory apraxia. *Journal of Fluency Disorders, 19,* 192–193.

Maxwell, M., & Meisser, M. J. (1997). *Teaching English in middle and secondary schools.* Englewood Cliff, NJ: Prentice Hall.

May, P. A., Hymbaugh, K. J., Aase, J. M., & Samet, J. M. (1984). Epidemiology of fetal alcohol syndrome among American Indians of the southwest. *Social Biology, 30*(4), 374–387.

McCabe, A. (1996). *Chameleon readers: Teaching children to appreciate all kinds of good stories.* New York: McGraw-Hill.

McCabe, A. (1997). Developmental and cross-cultural aspects of children's narration. In M. Bamberg (Ed.), *Narrative development: Six approaches* (pp. 137–174). Mahwah, NJ: Erlbaum.

McCabe, A., & Peterson, C. (1985). A naturalistic study of the production of causal connectives by children. *Journal of Child Language, 12,* 145–159.

McCabe A., & Peterson, C. (1991). Getting the story: A longitudinal study of parental styles in eliciting narratives and developing narrative skill. In A. McCabe & C. Peterson (Eds.), *Developing narrative structure* (pp. 217–253). Hillsdale, NJ: Erlbaum.

McCarthy, L. (1988). Feature geometry and dependency: A review. *Journal of Phonetics, 43,* 84–108.

McCathren, R., Warren, S., & Yoder, P. (1996). Prelinguistic predictors of later language development. In K. Cole, P. Dale, & D. Thal (Eds.), *Assessment of communication and language.* Baltimore: Brookes.

McCormick, L. (1990). Bases for language and communication development. In L. McCormick & R. Schiefelbusch (Eds.), *Early language intervention: An introduction* (2nd ed.). Upper Saddle River, NJ: Prentice Hall.

McCormick, L. (1990). Sequences of language and communication development. In L. McCormick & R. Schiefelbusch (Eds.), *Early language intervention: An introduction* (2nd ed.). Upper Saddle River, NJ: Merrill/Prentice Hall.

McCune, L. (1993). The development of play as the development of consciousness. In M. H. Bornstein & A. O'Reilly (Eds.), *New directions for child development* (No. 59, pp. 67–79). San Francisco: Jossey-Bass.

McDonough, L. (2002). Basic-level nouns: First learned but misunderstood. *Journal of Child Language, 29,* 357–377.

McGregor, K., Friedman, R., Reilly, R., & Newman, R. (2002). Semantic representation and naming in young children. *Journal of Speech, Language, and Hearing Research, 45,* 332–346.

McGurk, H., & McDonald, J. (1976). Hearing lips and seeing voices. *Nature, 264,* 746–748.

McKeough, D. (1982). *The coloring review of neuroscience.* Boston: Little, Brown.

McLaughlin, B. (1978). *Second-language acquisition in childhood.* Mahwah, NJ: Erlbaum.

McLeod, S. (2007). *The international guide to speech acquisition.* Clifton Park, NY: Cengage Learning.

McLeod, S., van Doorn, J., & Reed, V. A. (2001). Normal acquisition of consonant clusters. *American Journal of Speech–Language Pathology, 10,* 99–110.

McNeil, D. (1970). *The acquisition of language: The study of developmental psycholinguistics.* New York: Harper & Row.

McTear, M. (1985). *Children's conversation.* Oxford: Blackwell.

McTear, M., & Conti-Ramsden, G. (1991). *Pragmatic disability in children.* San Diego, CA: Singular.

Meadows, D., Elias, G., & Bain, J. (2000). Mother's ability to identify infants' communicative acts. *Journal of Child Language, 27,* 393–406.

Mehan, H. (1979). *Learning lessons.* Cambridge, MA: Harvard University Press.

Mehan, H. (1984). Language and schooling. *Sociology of Education, 57,* 174–183.

Meltzoff, A. (1988a). Imitation of televised models by infants. *Child Development, 59,* 1221–1229.

Meltzoff, A. (1988b). Infant imitation after a 1-week delay: Long-term memory for novel acts and multiple stimuli. *Developmental Psychology, 24,* 470–476.

Meltzoff, A., & Moore, M. (1999). Persons and representations: Why infant imitation is important for theories of human development. In J. Nadel & G. Butterworth (Eds.), *Imitation in infancy* (pp. 9–35). Cambridge: Cambridge University Press.

Meltzoff, A. N. (1995). Understanding the intentions of others: Re-enactment of intended actions by 18-month-old children. *Development Psychology, 31,* 838–850.

Menyuk, P. (1968). The role of distinctive features in children's acquisition of phonology. *Journal of Speech and Hearing Research, 11,* 138–146.

Menyuk, P. (1969). *Sentences children use.* Cambridge, MA: MIT Press.

Menyuk, P. (1971). *The acquisition and development of language.* Upper Saddle River, NJ: Prentice Hall.

Menyuk, P. (1977). *Language and maturation.* Cambridge, MA: MIT Press.

Merchant, K., "How Men And Women Differ: Gender Differences in Communication Styles, Influence Tactics, and LeadershipStyles" (2012).CMC Senior Theses.Paper 513. http://scholarship.claremont.edu/cmc_theses/513.

Merino, B. J. (1992). Acquisition of syntactic and phonological features in Spanish. In H. W. Langdon & L. L. Cheng (Eds.), *Hispanic children and adults with communication disorders* (pp. 57–91). Baltimore: Aspen.

Mervis, C., & Mervis, C. (1988). Role of adult input in young children's category evolution: An observational study. *Journal of Child Language, 15*, 257–272.

Messinger, D., & Fogel, A. (1998). Give and take: The development of conventional infant gestures. *Merrill-Palmer Quarterly, 44*, 566–590.

Miccio, A., Hammer, C., & Toribio, A. (2002). Linguistics and speech-language pathology: Combining research efforts toward improved interventions for bilingual children. In J. Alatis, H. Hamilton, & A.-H. Tan (Eds.), *Georgetown University Round Table on Languages and Linguistics 2000: Linguistics, language and the profession* (pp. 234–250). Washington, DC: Georgetown University Press.

Michaels, S. (1981). "Sharing time": Children's narrative styles and differential access to literacy. *Language and Society, 10*, 423–442.

Michaels, S. (1990). Person hood and personal identify. *Journal of Philosophy, 87*, 71–92.

Michaels, S. (1991). The dismantling of narrative. In A. McCabe & C. Peterson (Eds.), *Developing narrative structure* (pp. 303–352) Norwood, NJ: Ablex.

Miikkulainen, R. (1993). *Subsymbolic natural language processing: An integrated model of scripts, lexicon, and memory.* Cambridge, MA: MIT Press.

Miikkulainen, R. (1997). Dyslexic and category-specific aphasic impairments in a self-organizing feature map model of the lexicon. *Brain and Language, 59*, 334–366.

Miller, C. (2006). Developmental relationships between language and theory of mind. *American Journal of Speech-Language Pathology, 15*, 142–154.

Miller, G., & Gildea, P. (1987). How children learn words. *Scientific American, 257*, 94–99.

Miller, J. (1981). *Assessing language production in children: Experimental procedures.* Baltimore: University Park Press.

Miller, J., & Chapman, R. (1981). The relation between age and mean length of utterance in morphemes. *Journal of Speech and Hearing Research, 24*, 154–161.

Miller, J., Chapman, R., Branston, M., & Reichle, J. (1980). Language comprehension in sensorimotor stages 5 and 6. *Journal of Speech and Hearing Research, 4*, 1–12.

Miller, J., Chapman, R., Branston, M., & Reichle, J. (1980). Language comprehension in sensorimotor stages V and VI. *Journal of Speech and Hearing Research, 23*, 284–311.

Miller, L. (1990). The roles of language and learning in the development of literacy. *Topics in Language Disorders, 10*, 1–23.

Miller, P., & Sperry, L. (1988). Early talk about the past: The origins of conversational stories of personal experience. *Journal of Child Language, 15*, 293–315.

Miller, S., & Madison, C. (1984). Public school voice clinics. I: A working model. *Language, Speech and Hearing Services in Schools, 15*, 51–57.

Milligan, K., Atkinson, L., Trehub, S. E., Benoit, D., & Poulton, L. (2003). Maternal attachment and the communication of emotion through song. *Infant Behavior & Development, 26*, 1–13.

Millikan, C., & Darley, F. (1967). *Brain mechanisms underlying speech and language.* New York: Grune & Stratton.

Minami, M., & McCabe, A. (1991). Haiku as a discourse regulation device: A stanza analysis of Japanese children's personal narratives. *Language and Society, 20*, 577–599.

Minami, M., & McCabe, A. (1995). Rice balls and bear hunts: Japanese and North American family narrative patterns. *Journal of Child Language, 22*, 423–445.

Mirenda, P., & Donnellan, A. (1986). Effects of adult interaction style on conversational behavior in students with severe communication problems. *Language, Speech, and Hearing Services in Schools, 17*, 126–141.

Mirmiran, M., Maas, Y.G.H., & Ariagno, R. L. (2003). Development of fetal and neonatal sleep and circadian rhythms. *Sleep Medicine Reviews, 7*(4), 321-334.

Missall, K. N., Carta, J. J., McConnell, S. R., Walker, D., & Greenwood, C. (2008). Using individual growth and developmental indicators to measure early language and literacy. *Infants & Young Children, 21*(3), 241–253.

Mitchell, P., & Kent, R. (1990). Phonetic variation in multisyllabic babbling. *Journal of Child Language, 17*, 247–265.

Mitchell-Kernan, C., & Kernan, K. (1977). Pragmatics of directive choice among children. In

C. Mitchell-Kernan & S. Ervin-Tripp (Eds.), *Child discourse*. New York: Academic Press.

Mithum, M. (1989). The acquisition of polysynthesis. *Journal of Child Language, 16*, 285–312.

Moerk, E. (1975). Verbal interactions between children and their mothers during the preschool years. *Developmental Psychology, 11*, 788–794.

Moerk, E. (1977). *Pragmatic and semantic aspects of early language development*. Baltimore: University Park Press.

Moerk, E. (1983). *The mother of Eve—As a first language teacher*. Norwood, NJ: Ablex.

Moerk, E. (1989). The LAD was a lady and the tasks were ill-defined. *Developmental Review, 9*, 21–57.

Moll, K., & Daniloff, R. (1971). Investigation of the timing of velar movements during speech. *Journal of the Acoustical Society of America, 50*, 678–684.

Moon, C., Bever, T., & Fifer, W. (1992). Canonical and non-canonical syllable discrimination by two-day-old infants. *Journal of Child Language, 19*, 1–17.

Moon, C., Lagercrantz, H., Kuhl, P.K. (2013). Language experienced in utero affects vowel perception after birth: a two-country study. *Acta Pediatrica, 102*(2) 156–160. DOI: 10.1111/apa.12098

Moore, K. (2001). Framework for understanding the intergenerational transmission of poverty and well-being in developing countries. Chronic Poverty Research Center, International Development Department, The University of Birmingham. Retrieved from www.chronicpoverty.org/uploads/publication_files/WP08_Moore.pdf

Moore, K., & Meltzoff, A. (1978). Object permanence, imitation, and language development in infancy: Toward a neo-Piagetian perspective on communicative development. In F. Minifie & L. Lloyd (Eds.), *Communicative and cognitive abilities—Early behavioral assessment*. Baltimore: University Park Press.

Morgan, J., & Travis, L. (1989). Limits on negative information in language input. *Journal of Child Language, 16*, 531–552.

Morton, N. E. (1991). Genetic epidemiology of hearing impairment. *Annals of the New York Academy of Science, 630*, 16–31.

Mowrer, D. (1990). *Methods of modifying speech behaviors* (2nd ed.). Prospect Heights, IL: Waveland.

Mowrer, O. (1952). Speech development in the young child: The autism theory of speech development and some clinical applications. *Journal of Speech and Hearing Disorders, 17*, 263–268.

Mueller, E. (1972). The maintenance of verbal exchanges between young children. *Child Development, 43*, 930–938.

Mueller, E., Bleier, M., Krakow, J., Hegedus, K., & Cournoyer, P. (1977). The development of peer verbal interaction among two-year-old boys. *Child Development, 48*, 284–287.

Muir, D., & Field, J. (1979). Newborn infants orient to sounds. *Child Development, 50*, 431–436.

Mulac, A., Bradac, J.J. & Gibbons, P. (2001). Empirical support for the gender-as-culture hypothesis: An intercultural analysis of male/female language differences. *Human Communication Research, 27*, 121-152.

Muma, J., & Zwycewicz-Emory, C. (1979). Contextual priority: Verbal shift at seven? *Journal of Child Language, 6*, 301–311.

Murray, A., Johnson, J., & Peters, J. (1990). Fine tuning of utterance length to preverbal infants: Effects on later language development. *Journal of Child Language, 17*, 511–525.

Myhill, D., & Jones, S. (2007). More than just error correction: Students' perspectives on their revision processes during writing. *Written Communication, 24*(4), 323–343.

Nagafuchi, M. (1994). Acquired stuttering due to damage to the left premotor area. *Journal of Fluency Disorders, 19*, 195.

Nagy, W., Diakidoy, I., & Anderson, R. (1991). *The development of knowledge of derivational suffixes*. Technical Report N. 536, Center for the Study of Reading. Champaign: University of Illinois at Urbana-Champaign.

Nagy, W., Diakidoy, I., & Anderson, R. (1993). The acquisition of morphology: Learning the contribution of suffixes to the meanings of derivatives. *Journal of Reading Behavior, 25*, 155–170.

Nagy, W., Herman, P., & Anderson, R. (1985). Learning words from context. *Reading Research Quarterly, 22*, 233–253.

Naigles, L. (1990). Children use syntax to learn verb meanings. *Journal of Child Language, 17*, 357–374.

Nakata, T., & Trehub, S. E. (2004). Infants' responsiveness to maternal speech and singing. *Infant Behavior & Development, 27*, 455–464.

Nakazima, S. (1975). Phonemicization and symbolization in language development. In E. Lenneberg & E. Lenneberg (Eds.), *Foundations of language: Vol. 1. A multidisciplinary approach*. New York: Academic Press.

Naremore, R. (1980). Language variation in a multicultural society. In T. Hixon, L. Shriberg, & J. Saxman (Eds.), *Introduction to communication disorders.* Upper Saddle River, NJ: Prentice Hall.

Naremore, R., & Hopper, R. (1990). *Children learning language* (3rd ed.). New York: Harper & Row.

Nathani, S., Ertmer, J., & Stark, R. E. (2006). Assessing vocal development in infants and toddlers. *Clinical Linguistics and Phonetics, 20*(5), 351–369.

National Committee on Learning Disabilities. (1991). Learning disabilities: Issues on definition. *American Speech–Language–Hearing Association, 33*(Suppl. 5), 18–20.

National Institute for Literacy. (n.d.). *Frequently asked questions.* Retrieved from http://www.nifl.gov/nifl/faqs.html

National Institute of Child Health and Human Development (NICHD). (2000). *Teaching children to read: An evidence-based assessment of the scientific research literature on reading and its implications for reading instruction* (NIH Publication No. 00–4769). Report of the National Reading Panel. Washington, DC: U.S. Government Printing Office.

National KIDS COUNT (2015). Children in Poverty By Race and Ethnicity. Retrieved from http://datacenter.kidscount.org/data/tables/44-children-in-poverty-by-race-and-ethnicity#detailed/1/any/false/573,869,36,868,867/10,11,9,12,1,185,13/324,323

National KIDS COUNT Children in Single-Parent Families by Race retrieved from http://datacenter.kidscount.org/data/tables/107-children-in-single-parent-families-by#detailed/1/any/false/573,869,36,868,867/10,11,9,12,1,185,13/432,431

National Reading Association Division of Research and Policy. (2002). Summary of the (U.S.) National Reading Panel Report, *Teaching Children to Read.* Retrieved from http://www.reading.org/Libraries/Reports_and_Standards/nrp_summary.sflb.ashx

Nazzi, T., Bertoncini, J., & Mehler, J. (1998). Language discrimination by newborns: Toward an understanding of the role of rhythm. *Journal of Experimental Psychology: Human Perception and Performance, 24,* 756–766.

Negus, V. (1962). *The comparative anatomy and physiology of the larynx.* New York: Hafner.

Nelson, K. (1973). Structure and strategy in learning to talk. *Monographs of the Society for Research in Child Development, 38*(Serial No. 149).

Nelson, K. (1974). Concept, word and sentence: Interrelations in acquisition and development. *Psychological Review, 31,* 267–285.

Nelson, K. (1986). *Event knowledge.* New York: Academic Press.

Nelson, N. (1985). Teacher talk and children listening—Fostering a better match. In C. Simon (Ed.), *Communication skills and classroom success: Assessment of language-learning disabled children.* San Diego, CA: College-Hill.

Nelson, N. (1986). Individual processing in classroom settings. *Topics in Language Disorders, 6,* 13–27.

Nelson, N. (1989). Curriculum-based language assessment and intervention. *Language, Speech, and Hearing Services in Schools, 20,* 170–184.

Nelson, N. (1993). *Childhood language disorders in context: Infancy through adolescence.* New York: Macmillan.

Nelson, N. W. (2010). *Language and literacy disorders: Infancy through adolescence.* Boston: Allyn & Bacon.

Nelson, N. W., & Friedman, K. K. (1988). *Development of the concept of story in narratives written by older children.* Unpublished paper. Kalamazoo: Western Michigan University.

Netsell, R., Kent, R., & Abbs, J. (1980). The organization and reorganization of speech movement. *Society of Neuroscience Abstracts, 6,* 462.

Newcombe, N., & Zaslow, M. (1981). Do I1-year-olds hint? A study of directive forms in the speech of I2-year-old children to adults. *Discourse Processes, 4,* 239–252.

Newport, E. (1976). Motherese: The speech of mothers to young children. In N. Castellan, D. Pisoni, & G. Potts (Eds.), *Cognitive theory* (Vol. 2). Hillsdale, NJ: Erlbaum.

Newschaffer, C. J., Falb, M. D., & Gurney, J. G. (2005). National autism prevalence trends from United States special education data. *Pediatrics, 115*(3), e277–e282.

Nicoladis, E., & Genesee, F. (1996a). A longitudinal study of pragmatic differentiation in young bilingual children. *Language Learning, 46*(3), 439–464.

Nicoladis, E., & Genesee, F. (1996b). Word awareness in second language learners and bilingual children. *Language Awareness, 5*(2), 80–89.

Nicoladis, E., & Secco, G. (2000). Productive vocabulary and language choice. *First Language, 20*(58), 3–28.

Nicolaides, P., & Appleton, R. E. (1996). Stroke in children. *Developmental Medicine & Child Neurology,*

38(2), 172–180.

Nilsen, A. (1977). Sexism in children's books and elementary teaching materials. In A. Nilsen, H. Bosmajian, H. L. Gershuny, & J. P. Stanley (Eds.), *Sexism and language.* Urbana, IL: National Council of Teachers of English.

Nippold, M. (1990). Concomitant speech and language disorders in stuttering children: A critique of the literature. *Journal of Speech and Hearing Disorders, 55,* 51–60.

Nippold, M. A. (1998). *Later language development: The school-age and adolescent years.* Austin, TX: PRO-ED.

Nippold, M. A., Moran, C., & Schwarz, I. E. (2001). Idiom understanding in preadolescents: Synergy in action. *American Journal of Speech-Language Pathology, 10,* 169–179.

Nippold, M., & Duthie, J. (2003). Mental imagery and idiom comprehension: A comparison of school-age children and adults. *Journal of Speech, Language, and Hearing Research, 46,* 788–799.

Nippold, M., & Haq, F. (1996). Proverb comprehension in youth: The role of concreteness and familiarity. *Journal of Speech and Hearing Research, 39*(1), 166–176.

Nippold, M., & Martin, S. (1989). Idiom interpretation in isolation versus context: A developmental study with adolescents. *Journal of Speech and Hearing Research, 32,* 59–66.

Nippold, M., & Sullivan, M. (1987). Verbal and perceptual analogical reasoning and proportional metaphor comprehension in young children. *Journal of Speech and Hearing Research, 30,* 367–376.

Nippold, M., Allen, M., & Kirsch, D. (2001). Proverb comprehension as a function of reading proficiency in preadolescents. *Language, Speech, and Hearing Services in Schools, 32,* 90–100.

Nippold, M., Hegel, S., Sohlberg, M., & Schwarz, I. (1999). Defining abstract entities: Development in pre-adolescents, adolescents, and young adults. *Journal of Speech, Language, and Hearing Research, 42,* 473–481.

Nippold, M., Martin, S., & Erskine, B. (1988). Proverb comprehension in context: A developmental study with children and adolescents. *Journal of Speech and Hearing Research, 31,* 19–28.

Nippold, M., Schwarz, I., & Undlin, R. (1992). Use and understanding of adverbial conjuncts. *Journal of Speech and Hearing Research, 35,* 108–118.

Nippold, M., Taylor, C., & Baker, J. (1995). Idiom understanding in Australian youth: A cross-cultural comparison. *Journal of Speech, Language, and Hearing Research, 39,* 442–447.

Nippold, M., Uhden, L., & Schwarz, I. (1997). Proverb explanation through the lifespan: A developmental study of adolescents and adults. *Journal of Speech, Language, and Hearing Research, 40,* 245–253.

Nippold, M., Ward-Lonergan, J. M., & Fanning, J. L. (2005). Persuasive writing in children, adolescents, and adults: A study of syntactic, semantic, and pragmatic development. *Language, Speech, and Hearing Services in Schools, 36,* 125–138.

No Child Left Behind Act (NCLB), P. L. 107-110, 115 Stat. 1425, 20 U.S.C, 6301 *et seq.* (2001).

Nold, E. (1981). Revising. In C. Frederiksen & J. Dominic (Eds.), *Writing: The nature, development, and teaching of written communication* (Vol. 2). Hillsdale, NJ: Erlbaum.

Numes, T., Bryant, P., & Bindman, M. (2006). The effects of learning to spell on children's awareness of morphology. *Reading and Writing, 19,* 767–787.

O'Hanlon, L., & Roseberry-McKibbin, C. (2004). Strategies for working with children from low-income backgrounds. *ADVANCE for Speech-Language Pathologists and Audiologists. 14*(6), 12–20.

O'Reilly, A. (1995). Using representations: Comprehension and production of actions with imagined objects. *Child Development, 66,* 999–1010.

Oakes, L., Madole, K., & Cohen, L. (1991). Infants' object examining: Habituation and categorization. *Cognitive Development, 6,* 377–392.

Oller, D. (1980). The emergence of the sounds of speech in infancy. In G. Yeni-Komshian, J. Kavanagh, & C. Ferguson (Eds.), *Child phonology: Vol. 1. Production.* New York: Academic Press.

Oller, D. K. (2000). *The emergence of speech capacity.* Hillsdale, NJ: Erlbaum.

Oller, D., & Eilers, R. (1988). The role of audition in infant babbling. *Child Development, 59*(2), 441–449.

Oller, D., Eilers, R., Bull, D., & Carney, A. (1985). Prespeech vocalizations of a deaf infant: A comparison with normal metaphonological development. *Journal of Speech and Hearing Research, 28,* 47–62.

Ornstein, R., & Thompson, R. (1984). *The amazing brain.* Boston: Houghton Mifflin.

Owens, R. (1990). Development of communication, language, and speech. In G. Shames & E. Wiig (Eds.), *Human communication disorders: An introduction* (3rd ed.). Upper Saddle River, NJ: Prentice Hall.

Owens, R. (1991). *Language disorders: A functional approach to assessment and intervention.* Upper Saddle River, NJ: Merrill/Prentice Hall.

Owens, R. (1995). *Language disorders: A functional approach to assessment and intervention* (2nd ed.). Boston: Allyn & Bacon.

Owens, R. (2004). *Language disorders: A functional approach to assessment and intervention* (4th ed.). Boston: Allyn & Bacon.

Owens, R. (2016). *Language development: An introduction* (9th ed.). Boston: Pearson.

Padilla, A., & Liebman, E. (1975). Language acquisition in the bilingual child. *Bilingual Review, 2*(1, 2), 34–55.

Padilla, A., & Lindholm, K. (1984). Child bilingualism: The same old issues revisited. In J. Martinez & R. Mendoza (Eds.), *Chicano psychology* (pp. 369–408). Orlando, FL: Academic Press.

Pannbacker, M. (1992). Some common myths about voice therapy. *Language, Speech, Hearing Services in Schools, 23*, 12–19.

Papousek, M. (2007). Communication in early infancy: An area of intersubjective learning. *Infant Behavior & Development, 30*, 258–266.

Paradis, J., Nicoladis, E., & Genesee, F. (2000). Early emergence of structural constraints on code-mixing: Evidence from French-English bilingual children. In F. Genesee (Ed.), *Bilingualism: Language and cognition* (pp. 245–261). Cambridge, MA: Harvard University Press.

Park, J., Turnbull, A. P., & Turnbull, H. R. III. (2002). Impacts of poverty on quality of life in families with disabilities. *Exceptional Children, 68*, 151–170.

Parlee, M. (1979). Conversational politics. *Psychology Today, 5*, 48–56.

Parsons, C. (1980). *The effect of speaker age and listener compliance and noncompliance on the politeness of children's request directives.* Unpublished doctoral dissertation, Southern Illinois University, Carbondale.

Pass, S. (2007). When constructivists Jean Piaget and Lev Vygotsky were pedagogical collaborators: A viewpoint from a study of their communications. *Journal of Constructivist Psychology, 20*, 277–282.

Paul, R. (1981). Analyzing complex sentence development. In J. Miller (Ed.), *Assessing language production in children: Experimental procedures.* Baltimore: University Park Press.

Paul, R. (1987). Communication in autism. In D. J. Cohen & A. M. Donnellan (Eds.), *Handbook of autism and pervasive developmental disorders.* New York: Wiley.

Paul, R. (1990). Comprehension strategies: Interactions between world knowledge and the development of sentence comprehension. *Topics in Language Disorders, 10*(3), 63–75.

Paul, R. (2007). *Language disorders from infancy through adolescence: Listening, Speaking, reading, writing, and communicating* (3rd ed.). St. Louis, MO: Elsevier Mosby.

Paul, R., & Jennings, P. (1992). Phonological behavior in toddlers with slow expressive language development. *Journal of Speech and Hearing Research, 35*, 99–107.

Paul, R. & Norbury, C.F. (2012). *Language disorders from infancy through adolescence.* 4th ed. St. Louis, Missouri: Elsevier.

Payne, A. C., Whitehurst, G. J., & Angell, A. L. (1994). The role of home literacy environment in the development of language ability in preschool children from low-income families. *Early Childhood Research Quarterly, 9*, 427–440.

Payne, R. K. (2003). *A framework for understanding poverty* (4th ed.). Highlands, TX: Aha! Process.

Pea, R., & Kurland, D. (1987). Cognitive technologies for writing. *Review of Research in Education, 14*, 277–326.

Pearson, B. (1998). Assessing lexical development in bilingual babies and toddlers. *International Journal of Bilingualism, 29*3). Lexical development in bilingual infants and toddlers: Comparison to monolingual norms. *Language Learning, 43*, 93–120.

Pearson B., Fernandez, S., & Oller, D. (1995). Cross-language synonyms in the lexicons of bilingual infants: One language or two? *Journal of Child Language, 22*, 345–368.

Pearson, B., Fernandez, S., Lewedag, V., & Oller, D. (1997). Input factors in lexical learning of bilingual infants (ages 10 to 30 months). *Applied Psycholinguistics, 18*, 41–58.

Pence Turnbull, K.L. & Justice, L.M. (2008). *Language development from theory to practice* (2nd ed). Boston, MA: Pearson.

Pence, K. L., & Justice, L. M. (2008). *Language development from theory to practice.* Upper Saddle River, NJ: Pearson.

Penman, R., Cross, T., Milgrom-Friedman, J., & Meares, R. (1983). Mothers' speech to prelingual infants: A pragmatic analysis. *Journal of Child Language, 10*, 17–34.

Pepper, J., & Weitzman, E. (2004). *It takes two to talk: A practical guide for parents of children with language delays.* (4th ed.) The Hanen Program ®, A Hanen Centre Publication.

Perconti, P. (2002). Context-dependence in human and animal communication. *Foundations of Science, 7*(3), 341–362.

Perera, K. (1986). Language acquisition and writing. In P. Fletcher & M. Garman (Eds.), *Language acquisition* (2nd ed.). New York: Cambridge University Press.

Perfetti, C., & Goodman, D. (1970). Semantic constraint on the decoding of ambiguous words. *Journal of Experimental Psychology, 86,* 420–427.

Perkins, W. (1978). *Human perspectives in speech and language disorders.* St. Louis, MO: Mosby.

Perkins, W. (1990). What is stuttering? *Journal of Speech and Hearing Disorders, 55,* 370–382.

Perkins, W., & Kent, R. (1986). *Functional anatomy of speech, language, and hearing: A primer.* Boston: College-Hill.

Perlmann, R., & Berko-Gleason, J. (1994). The neglected role of fathers in children's communicative development. *Seminars in Speech and Language, 14,* 314–324.

Peterson, C. (1990). The who, when and where of early narratives. *Journal of Child Language, 17,* 433–455.

Peterson, C., & McCabe, A. (1983). *Developmental psycholinguistics: Three ways of looking at a child's narrative.* New York: Plenum.

Peterson, C., & McCabe, A. (1990). Linking children's connective use and narrative microstructure. In A. McCabe & C. Peterson (Eds.), *Developing narrative structure.* Hillsdale, NJ: Erlbaum.

Petitto, L. (1984). *From gesture to symbol: The relationship between form and the meaning in the acquisition of personal pronouns in American Sign Language.* Unpublished doctoral dissertation, Harvard University, Cambridge, MA.

Petitto, L. (1985a). *"Language" in the prelinguistic child* (Technical Report No. 4). Montreal: McGill University, Department of Psychology.

Petitto, L. (1985b, October). *On the use of prelinguistic gestures in hearing and deaf children.* Paper presented at the 10th Annual Boston University Conference on Language Development, Boston.

Petitto, L. (1986). *From gesture to symbol: The relationship between form and the meaning in the acquisition of personal pronouns in American Sign Language.* Bloomington: Indiana University Linguistics Club Press.

Petitto, L. (1987). On the autonomy of language and gesture: Evidence from the acquisition of personal pronouns in American Sign Language. *Cognition, 27*(1), 1–52.

Petitto, L. (1988). "Language" in the prelinguistic child. In F. Kessel (Ed.), *Development of language and language researchers: Essays in honor of Roger Brown* (pp. 187–221). Hillsdale, NJ: Erlbaum.

Petitto, L. A., Holowka, S., Sergio, L. E., & Ostry, D. (2001). Language rhythms in baby hand movements. *Nature, 413,* 35–36. doi: 10.1038/35092613

Petitto, L., & Marentette, P. (1990, October). *The timing of linguistic milestones in sign language acquisition: Are first signs acquired earlier than first words?* Paper presented at the 15th Annual Boston University Conference on Language Development, Boston.

Petitto, L., & Marentette, P. (1991, April). The timing of linguistic milestones in sign and spoken language acquisition. In L. Petitto (Chair), *Are the linguistic milestones in signed and spoken language acquisition similar or different?* Symposium conducted at the Biennial Meeting of the Society for Research in Child Development, Seattle.

Petitto, L., Katerelos, M., Levy, B., Gauna, K., Tetreault, K., & Ferraro, V. (2001). Bilingual signed and spoken language acquisition from birth: Implications for the mechanism underlying early bilingual language acquisition. *Journal of Child Language, 28,* 453–496.

Petrovich-Bartell, N., Cowan, N., & Morse, P. (1982). Mothers' perceptions of infant distress vocalizations. *Journal of Speech and Hearing Research, 25,* 371–376.

Pew Hispanic Center/Kaiser Family Foundation (2002). *2002 national survey of Latinos: Summary of findings.* Update: March 2004. Washington, DC. Retrieved from http://www.kff.org or www.pewhispanic.org

Pexman, P. M., & Glenwright, M. (2007). How do typically developing children grasp the meaning of verbal irony? *Journal of Neurolinguistics, 20,* 178–196.

Phillips, J. (1973). Syntax and vocabulary of mothers' speech to young children: Age and sex comparisons. *Child Development, 44,* 182–185.

Piaget, J. (1926). *Language and thought of the child.* London: Routledge & Kegan Paul.

Piaget, J. (1952). *Origins of intelligence in children.* New York: International Universities Press.

Piaget, J. (1954). *The construction of reality in the child.* New York: Basic Books.

Piaget, J. (1963). *The origins of intelligence in children.* New York: Norton.

Piaget, J. (1966). Time perception in children. In J. Frazer (Ed.), *The voices of time.* New York: Braziller.

Pinker, S. (1979). Formal models of language learning. *Cognition, 7,* 217–283.

Pinker, S. (1984). *Language, learnability and language development.* Cambridge, MA: Harvard University Press.

Pinker, S. (1987). The bootstrapping problem in language acquisition. In B. MacWhinney (Ed.), *Mechanisms of language acquisition* (pp. 399–439). Hillsdale, NJ: Erlbaum.

Pinker, S., & Prince, A. (1988). On language and connectionism: Analysis of a parallel distributed processing model of language acquisition. *Cognition, 28,* 73–193.

Polka, L., & Sundara, M. (2003). Word segmentation in monolingual and bilingual infant learners of English and French. In M. J. Sole, D. Recasens, & J. Romero (Eds.), *Proceedings of the International Congress of Phonetic Sciences, 15,* 1021–1024.

Pollio, M. R., & Pollio, H. R. (1974). The development of figurative language in school children. *Journal of Psycholinguistic Research, 3,* 185–201.

Poole, I. (1934). Genetic development of articulation of consonant sounds in English. *Elementary English Review, 11,* 159–161.

Portes, A., & Rumbaut, R (2001). *Legacies: The story of the immigrant second generation.* Berkeley and Los Angeles: University of California Press.

Prather, E., Hedrick, D., & Kern, C. (1975). Articulation development in children aged two to four years. *Journal of Speech and Hearing Disorders, 40,* 179–191.

Preece, A. (1987). The range of narrative forms conversationally produced by young children. *Journal of Child Language, 14,* 353–373.

Preisser, D. A., Hodson, B. W., & Paden, E. P. (1988). Developmental phonology: 18–29 months. *Journal of Speech and Hearing Disorders, 53,* 125–130.

Premack, D. (2007). Human and animal cognition: Continuity and discontinuity. *PNAS, 104*(35) 13861-13867. Available at www.pnas.org/cgi/doi/10.1073/pnas.0706147104

Prutting, C. (1979). Process: The action of moving forward progressively from one point to another on the way to completion. *Journal of Speech and Hearing Disorders, 44,* 3–30.

Putnam, A., & Ringel, R. (1979). Oral sensation and perception. In W. Williams & D. Goulding (Eds.), *Articulation and learning.* Springfield, IL: Charles C. Thomas.

Qi, C. H., & Kaiser, A. P. (2004). Problem behaviors of low-income children with language delays: An observation study. *Journal of Speech, Language, and Hearing Research, 47,* 595–609.

Qualls, C. (1998). *Figurative language comprehension in younger and older African Americans.* Unpublished doctoral dissertation, City University of New York.

Qualls, C., & Harris, J. (1999). Effects of familiarity on idiom comprehension in African American and European American fifth graders. *Language, Speech, and Hearing Services in Schools, 30,* 141–151.

Quay, S. (2008). Dinner conversations with a trilingual two-year old: Language socialization in a multilingual context. *First Language, 28*(1), 5–33.

Quigley, S., & King, C. (1982). The language of deaf children and youth. In S. Rosenberg (Ed.), *Handbook of applied psycholinguistics: Major thrusts of research and theory* (pp. 429–475). Hillsdale, NJ: Erlbaum.

Ramirez, A. (1992). *The Spanish of the United States: The language of the Hispanics.* Madrid: Mapfre.

Rathmann, C., Mann, W., & Morgan, G. (2007). Narrative structure and narrative development in deaf children. *Deafness Education International, 9*(4), 187–196.

Ratner, N. (1988). Patterns of parental vocabulary selection in speech to very young children. *Journal of Child Language, 15,* 481–492.

Read, C. (1981). Writing is not the inverse of reading for young children. In C. Frederiksen & J. Dominic (Eds.), *Writing: The nature, development, and teaching of written communication.* Hillsdale, NJ: Erlbaum.

Redclay, E., Haist, F., & Courchesne, E. (2008). Functional neuroimaging of speech perception during a pivotal period in language acquisition. *Developmental Sciences, 11*(2), 237–252.

Reddy, V., Chisholm, V., Forrester, D., Conforti, M., & Maniatopoulou, D. (2007). Facing the perfect contingency: Interactions with the self at 2 and 3 months. *Infant Behavior & Development, 30,* 195–212.

Reed, V. (Ed.). (1986). *An introduction to children with language disorders.* New York: Macmillan.

Rees, N. (1972). The role of babbling in the child's acquisition of language. *British Journal of Disorders in Communication, 4,* 17–23.

Rees, N. (1975). Imitation and language development: Issues and clinical implications. *Journal of Speech and Hearing Disorders, 40*, 339–350.

Reich, P. (1986). *Language development.* Upper Saddle River, NJ: Prentice Hall.

Reid, D. (1998). Scaffolding: A broader view. *Journal of Learning Disabilities, 31*, 386–396.

Reid, D. (2000). Discourse in classrooms. In K. R. Fahey & D. K. Reid (Eds.), *Language development, differences, and disorders.* Austin, TX: PRO-ED.

Reid, D. K. (2000). The development of discourse: Conversations, stories, and explanations. In K. R. Fahey & D. K. Reid (Eds.), *Language development, differences, and disorders* (pp. 39–77). Austin, TX: PRO-ED.

Reid, V. M., Striano, T., Kaufman, J., & Johnson, M. H. (2004). Eye gaze cueing facilitates neural processing of objects in 4-month-old infants. *NeuroReport, 15*, 2553–2555.

Ricciardelli, L. (1992). Bilingualism and cognitive development in relation to threshold theory. *Journal of Psycholinguistic Research, 21*, 301–316.

Ricciardelli, L. (1993). Two components of metalinguistic awareness: Control of linguistic processing and analysis of linguistic knowledge. *Applied Psycholinguistics, 14*, 349–367.

Rice, M. (1983). Contemporary accounts of the cognitive/language relationship: Implications for speech-language clinicians. *Journal of Speech and Hearing Disorders, 48*, 347–359.

Rice, M., Buhr, J., & Nemeth, C. (1990). Fast mapping word-learning abilities of language-delayed preschoolers. *Journal of Speech and Hearing Disorders, 55*, 33–42.

Richards, M. (1980). Adjective ordering in the language of young children: An experimental investigation. *Journal of Child Language, 6*, 253–277.

Richey, K. D. (2008). The building blocks of writing: Learning to write letters and spell words. *Reading and Writing, 21*, 27–47.

Richmond, V., & Gorham, J. (1988). Language patterns and gender role orientation among students in grades 3–12. *Communication Education, 37*, 142–149.

Rickard Liow, S. J., & Poon, K. K. L. (1998). Phonological awareness in multilingual Chinese children. *Applied Psycholinguistics, 19*, 339–362.

Rideout, V., & Hamel, E. (2006, May). *The media family: Electronic media in the lives of infants, toddlers, preschoolers and their parents.* Retrieved June 25, 2006, from http://www.kff.org/entmedia/upload/7500/pdf.

Ripich, D., & Creaghead, N. (Eds.). (1994). *School discourse problems* (2nd ed.). San Diego, CA: Singular.

Rispoli, M. (2003). Changes in the nature of sentence production during the period of grammatical development. *Journal of Speech, Language, and Hearing Research, 46*, 818–830.

Ritter, H., & Kohonen, T. (1989). Self-organizing semantic maps. *Biological Cybernetics, 61*, 241–254.

Ritvo, E., & Freeman, B. (1978). National Society for Autistic Children definition of the syndrome of autism. *Journal of Autism and Childhood Schizophrenia, 8*, 162–167.

Rizzolatti, G. & Arbib, M. (1998a). From grasping to speech: Imitation might provide a missing link. *Trends in Neurosciences, 22*(4), 151–152.

Rizzolatti, G., & Arbib, M. A. (1998b). Language within our grasp. *Trends in Neuroscience, 21*(5), 188–194.

Rizzolatti, G., Fadiga, L., Gallese, V., & Fogassi, L. (1996). Premotor cortex and the recognition of motor actions. *Cognitive Brain Research, 3*(2), 131–141.

Roach, E. S. (2000). Stroke in children. *Current Treatment Options in Neurology, 2*, 295–303.

Robb, M. P., & Bleile, K. M. (1994). Consonant inventories of young children from 8 to 25 months. *Clinical Linguistics and Phonetics, 8*, 295–320.

Robb, M., & Saxman, J. (1990). Syllable durations of preword and early word vocalizations. *Journal of Speech and Hearing Research, 33*, 585–593.

Robbins, J. (1988). Employers' language expectations and nonstandard dialect speakers. *English Journal, 77*, 22–24.

Roberts, K. (1988). Retrieval of a basic-level category in prelinguistic infants. *Developmental Psychology, 24*, 21–27.

Robertson, K., & Murachver, T. (2003). Children's speech accommodation to gendered language styles. *Journal of Language and Social Psychology, 22*, 321–333.

Robinson, E. (1981). The child's understanding of inadequate messages and communication failures: A problem of ignorance or egocentrism? In W. P. Dickson (Ed.), *Children's oral communication skills.* New York: Academic Press.

Robinson, E. J., Haigh, S. N., & Pendle, J. E. C. (2008). Children's working understanding of the knowledge gained from seeing and feeling. *Developmental Science, 11*(2), 299–305.

Robinson, G. L., & Acevedo, M. C. (2001). Infant reactivity and reliance on mother during emotion challenges: Prediction of cognition and language skills in a low-income sample. *Child Development, 72,* 402–415.

Rodino, A., Gimbert, C., Perez, C., & McCabe, A. (1991). *Getting your point across: Contrastive sequencing in low-income African-American and Latino children's personal narratives.* Paper presented at the Sixteenth Annual Boston University Conference on Language Development, Boston.

Rogoff, B. (1990). *Apprenticeship in thinking.* New York: Oxford University Press.

Rogow, S. M. (1982). Rhythms and rhymes: Developing communication in very young blind and multihandicapped children. *Child: Care, Health, and Development, 8,* 249–260.

Rollins, P. (2003). Caregivers' contingent comments to 9-month-old infants: Relationship with later language. *Applied Psycholinguistics, 24,* 221–234.

Romaine, S. (1995). *Bilingualism* (2nd ed.). Oxford: Blackwell.

Rondal, J., & Cession, A. (1990). Input evidence regarding the semantic bootstrapping hypothesis. *Journal of Child Language, 17,* 711–717.

Roodenburg, P.J., Wladimiroff, J.W., van Es, A., & Prechti, H.F.R. (1991). Classification and quantificative aspects of fetal movements during the second half of normal pregnancy. *Early Human Development, 25*(1), 19–35. Doi: 10.1016/0378-3782(91)90203-F

Roseberry-McKibben, C. (2007). The impact of environmental factors on language development. In C. Roseberry-McKibben, *Language disorders in children: A multicultural and case perspective* (pp. 347–394). Boston, MA: Pearson.

Roseberry-McKibben, C., Brice, A., & O'Hanlon, L. (2005). Serving English language learners in public school settings: A national survey. *Language, Speech, and Hearing Services in Schools, 36,* 48–61.

Rosetti, L. (2001). *Communication intervention: Birth to three.* Clifton Park, NY: Cengage Learning.

Roth, C., Aronson, A., & Davis, L. (1989). Clinical studies in psychogenic stuttering of adult onset. *Journal of Speech and Hearing Disorders, 54,* 634–646.

Ruben, R.J. (2009). Redefining the survival of the fittest: Communication disorders in the 21st Century. The Laryngoscope, 110:241. Doi: 10.1097/00005537-200002010-00010

Rumbaugh, D., & Beran, M. (2003). Language acquisition by animals. In L. Nadel (Ed.), *Encyclopedia of cognitive science.* London: Macmillan.

Rumelhart, D. (1977). Toward an interactive model of reading. In S. Dornic (Ed.), *Attention and performance* (Vol. 1). Hillsdale, NJ: Erlbaum.

Ruscello, D., St. Louis, K., & Mason, N. (1991). School-aged children with phonologic disorders: Coexistence with other speech/ language disorders. *Journal of Speech and Hearing Research, 34,* 236–242.

Rvachew, S. (2006). Longitudinal predictors of implicit phonological awareness skills. *American Journal of Speech-Language Pathology, 15,* 165–178.

Ryan, J. (1974). Early language development: Towards a communicational analysis. In P. Richards (Ed.), *The integration of a child into a social world.* London: Cambridge University Press.

Ryder, N., & Leinonen, E. (2003). Use of context in question answering by three-, four-, and five-year-old children. *Journal of Psycholinguistic Research, 32,* 397–416.

Sachs, J. (1982). "Don't interrupt!": Preschoolers' entry into ongoing conversations. In C. Johnson & C. Thew (Eds.), *Proceedings of the Second International Congress for the Study of Child Language* (Vol. 1, pp. 344–356). Washington, DC: University Press of America.

Sachs, J. (1989). Communication development in infancy. In J. Berko-Gleason (Ed.), *The development of language.* Upper Saddle River, NJ: Merrill/ Prentice Hall.

Sachs, J., Lieberman, P., & Erickson, D. (1973). Anatomical and cultural determinants of male and female speech. In R. Schuy & R. Fasold (Eds.), *Language attitudes: Current trends and prospects.* Washington, DC: Georgetown University Press.

Samuelson, L. K., & Bloom, P. (2008). The shape of controversy: What counts as an explanation of development: Introduction to the special section. *Developmental Science, 11*(2), 183–184.

Samuelson, L. K., & Horst, J. S. (2008). Confronting complexity: Insights from the details of behavior over multiple timescales. *Developmental Science, 11*(2), 209–215.

Samuelson, L., & Smith, L. (1998). Memory and attention make smart word learning: An alternative account of Akhtar, Carpenter, and Tomasello. *Child Development, 69,* 94–104.

Sander, E. (1972). When are speech sounds learned? *Journal of Speech and Hearing Disorders, 37,* 55–63.

Sanders, L., Neville, H., & Woldorff, M. (2002). Speech segmentation by native and nonnative speakers: The use of lexical, syntactic, and stress-pattern cues. *Journal of Speech, Language, and Hearing Research, 45*, 519–530.

Sause, E. (1976). Computer content analysis of sex differences in the language of children. *Journal of Psycholinguistic Research, 5*, 311–324.

Savage-Rumbaugh, E. (1987). A new look at ape language: Comprehension of vocal speech and syntax. In D. Leger (Ed.), *The Nebraska symposium on motivation.* Lincoln: University of Nebraska Press.

Savage-Rumbaugh, E. (1990). Verbal communication in the chimpanzee. In N. Krasnegor, D. Rumbaugh, R. Schiefelbusch, & M. Studdert-Kennedy (Eds.), *Biobehavioral foundations of language development.* Hillsdale, NJ: Erlbaum.

Savage-Rumbaugh, E., MacDonald, K., Sevcik, R., Hopkins, W., & Rubert, E. (1986). Spontaneous symbol acquisition and communicative use by pygmy chimpanzees (*Pan paniscus*). *Journal of Experimental Psychology, General, 115*, 211–235.

Savage-Rumbaugh, E., Sevcik, R., Brakke, K., & Rumbaugh, D. (1990). Symbols: Their communicative use, combination, and comprehension by bonobos (*Pan paniscus*). In L. Lipsitt & C. Rovee-Collier (Eds.), *Advances in infancy research.* Norwood, NJ: Ablex.

Savage-Rumbaugh, S., Shanker, S., & Taylor, T. (1998). *Ape language and the human mind.* New York: Oxford University Press.

Saxe, G. G. (1988). Candy selling and math learning. *Educational Researcher, 17*, 14–21.

Saywitz, K., & Cherry-Wilkinson, L. (1982). Age-related differences in metalinguistic awareness. In S. Kuczaj (Ed.), *Language development: Vol. 2. Language, thought and culture.* Hillsdale, NJ: Erlbaum.

Schafer, G., & Plunkett, J. (1998). Rapid word learning by 15-month-olds under tightly controlled conditions. *Child Development, 69*, 309–320.

Schappert, S. M. (1992). Office visits for otitis media: United States, 1975–90. *Advance Data 13*(137), 17.

Scheerenberger, R. (1987). *A history of mental retardation.* Baltimore: Brookes.

Scherer, N., & Olswang, L. (1984). Role of mothers' expansions in stimulating children's language production. *Journal of Speech and Hearing Research, 27*, 387–396.

Schiff-Myers, N. (1992). Considering arrested language development and language loss in the assessment of second language learners. *Language, Speech, and Hearing Services in Schools, 23*, 28–33.

Schlesinger, I. (1971). Production of utterances and language acquisition. In D. Slobin (Ed.), *The ontogenesis of grammar.* New York: Academic Press.

Schlesinger, I. (1977). The role of cognitive development and linguistic input in language acquisition. *Journal of Child Language, 4*, 153–169.

Schneider, E. (1989). *American earlier Black English.* Tuscaloosa: University of Alabama Press.

Schober-Peterson, D., & Johnson, C. (1989). Conversational topics of four-year-olds. *Journal of Speech and Hearing Research, 32*, 857–870.

Schober-Peterson, D., & Johnson, C. (1991). Nondialogue speech during preschool interactions. *Journal of Child Language, 18*, 153–170.

Schoenbrodt, L., Kumin, L., & Sloan, J. M. (1997). Learning disabilities existing concomitantly with communication disorders. *Journal of Learning Disability, 30*(3), 264–281.

Schön, D., Boyer, M., Moreno, S., Besson, M., Peretz, I., & Kilinsky, R. (2008). Songs as an aid for language acquisition. *Cognition, 106*, 975–983.

Schultz, T., & Horibe, F. (1974). The development of the appreciation of verbal jokes. *Developmental Psychology, 10*, 13–20.

Schusterman, R. (1986). Cognition and intelligence of dolphins. In R. Schusterman, J. Thomas, & F. Wood (Eds.), *Dolphin cognition and behavior: A comparative approach* (pp. 137–139). Hillsdale, NJ: Erlbaum.

Schwartz, R., & Leonard, L. (1984). Words, objects, and actions in early lexical acquisition. *Journal of Speech and Hearing Research, 27*, 119–127.

Scollon, R., & Scollon, S. (1981). *Narrative, literacy and face in interethnic communication.* Norwood, NJ: Ablex.

Scott, C. (1984). Adverbial connectivity in conversations of children 6 to 12. *Journal of Child Language, 11*, 423–452.

Scott, C. (1987). *Summarizing text: Context effects in language disordered children.* Paper presented at the First International Symposium on Specific Language Disorders in Children, University of Reading, England.

Scott, C. (1988a). Producing complex sentences. *Topics in Language Disorders, 8*(2), 44–62.

Scott, C. (1988b). Spoken and written syntax. In M. A. Nippold (Ed.), *Later language development: Ages nine through nineteen* (pp. 49–95). Austin, TX: PRO-ED.

Scott, C., & Ringel, R. L. (1971). Articulation without oral sensory control. *Journal of Speech and Hearing Research, 14*, 804–818.

Searle, J. (1965). What is a speech act? In M. Black (Ed.), *Philosophy in America*. New York: Allen & Unwin, Cornell University Press.

Searle, J. (1969). *Speech acts*. Cambridge, England: Cambridge University Press.

Searle, J. (1975). *Indirect speech acts*. In P. Cole & J. L. Morgan (Eds.), *Syntax and semantics 3: Speech acts*. New York: Academic Press.

Searle, J. (1976). The classification of illocutionary acts. *Language in Society, 5*, 1–24.

Sekiyama, K., & Burnham, D. (2008). Impact on language and development of auditory-visual speech perception. *Developmental Science, 11*(2), 306–320.

Senecal, M. (1997). The differential effect of storybook reading on preschooler's acquisition of expressive and receptive vocabulary. *Journal of Child Language, 24*, 123–128.

Shames, G. H., Wiig, E. H., & Secord, W. A. (1998). *Human communication disorders: An introduction* (5th ed.). Boston: Allyn & Bacon.

Shames, G., & Rubin, H. (Eds.). (1986). *Stuttering: Then and now*. Upper Saddle River, NJ: Merrill/Prentice Hall.

Shatz, M., & O'Reilly, A. (1990). Conversational or communicative skill? A reassessment of two-year-olds' behavior in miscommunication episodes. *Journal of Child Language, 17*, 131–146.

Shatz, M., Wellman, H., & Silber, F. (1983). The acquisition of mental verbs: A systematic investigation of the first reference to mental state. *Cognition, 14*, 301–321.

Sherman, T. (1985). Categorization skills in infants. *Child Development, 56*, 1561–1573.

Shewan, C. (1988). *ASHA work force study: Final report*. Rockville, MD: American Speech–Language–Hearing Association.

Shewan, C., & Malm, K. (1990). The prevalence of speech and language impairments. *American Speech–Language–Hearing Association, 32*, 108.

Shipley, K., Maddox, M., & Driver, J. (1991). Children's development of irregular past tense verb forms. *Language, Speech, and Hearing Services in Schools, 22*, 115–122.

Shipley, K. G., & McAfee, J. G. (2009). *Assessment in speech-language pathology: A resource manual* (4ᵗʰ ed). Delmar, Cengage Learning, Clifton Park, New Jersey.

Short, D. J., & Fitzsimmons, S. (2006). Double the work: Challenges and solutions to acquiring language and academic literacy for adolescent English language learners. Alliance for Excellent Education. Retrieved from www.all4ed.org/files/DoubleWork.pdf

Siegel, G., Cooper, M., Morgan, J., & Renneise-Sarshad, R. (1990). Imitation of intonation by infants. *Journal of Speech and Hearing Research, 33*, 9–15.

Silverman, E., & Zimmer, C. (1975). Incidence of chronic hoarseness among school-age children. *Journal of Speech and Hearing Disorders, 40*, 211–215.

Silverman, F. (1996). *Stuttering and other fluency disorders* (2nd ed.). Boston: Allyn & Bacon.

Sinclair, A. (1986). Metalinguistic knowledge and language development. In I. Kurkz, G. W. Shugar, & J. H. Danks (Eds.), *Knowledge and language*. Amsterdam: North-Holland.

Singh, L., Morgan, J., & Best, C. (2002). Infants' listening preferences: Baby talk or happy talk? *Infancy, 3*, 365–394.

Singh, S. (1976). *Perceptual correlates of distinctive feature systems*. Washington, DC: Howard University Press.

Singh, S., & Polen, S. (1972). Use of distinctive feature model in speech pathology. *Acta Symbolica, 3*, 17–25.

Skinner, B. F. (1957). *Verbal behavior*. Upper Saddle River, NJ: Prentice Hall.

Skinner, P., & Shelton, R. (Eds.). (1985). *Speech, language and hearing*. New York: Wiley.

Sloat, C., Taylor, S. H., & Hoard, J. E. (1978). *Introduction to phonology*. Englewood Cliffs, NJ: Prentice Hall.

Slobin, D. (1978). Cognitive prerequisites for the development of grammar. In L. Bloom & M. Lahey (Eds.), *Readings in language development*. New York: Wiley.

Slobin, D. (1986). Cross-linguistic evidence for the language-making capacity. In D. Slobin (Ed.), *The cross-linguistic study of language acquisition: Theoretical issues*. Hillsdale, NJ: Erlbaum.

Smith, B., Brown-Sweeney, S., & Stoel-Gammon, C. (1989). A quantitative analysis of reduplicated and variegated babbling. *First Language, 9*, 175–189.

Smith, K. E., Landry, S. H., & Swank, P. R. (2000). Does the content of mothers' verbal stimulation explain differences in children's development of verbal and nonverbal cognitive skills: *Journal of School Psychology, 38*, 27–49.

Smith, L. B., Jones, S. S., Landau, B., Gershkoff-Stowe, L., & Samuelson, L. K. (2002). Object name learning provides on-the-job training for attention. *Psychological Science, 13*, 13–19.

Smitherman, G. (1994). *Black talk, words and phrases from the hood to the amen corner.* New York: Houghton Mifflin.

Snow, C. (1977). The development of conversation between mothers and babies. *Journal of Child Language, 4*, 1–22.

Snow, C. (1990). The development of definitional skill. *Journal of Child Language, 17*, 697–710.

Snow, C. (1991). The theoretical basis for relationships between language and literacy development. *Journal of Research in Childhood Education, 6*, 5–10.

Snow, C. (1999). Social perspectives on the emergence of language. In B. MacWhinney (Ed.), *The emergence of language* (pp. 257–276). Mahwah, NJ: Erlbaum.

Snow, C., & Dickinson, D. (1991). Skills that aren't basic in a new conception of literacy. In A. Purves & E. Jennings (Eds.), *Literate systems and individual lives. Perspectives on literacy and schooling.* Albany: SUNY Press.

Snow, C., Burns, M., & Griffin, P. (Eds.). (1998). *Preventing reading difficulties in young children.* Washington, DC: National Academy Press.

Snow, C. E., Tabors, P. O., & Dickinson, K. K. (2001). Language development in the preschool years. In D. K. Dickinson & P. O. Tabors (Eds.), *Beginning literacy with language: Young children learning at home and school* (pp. 1–25). Baltimore: Brookes.

Snow, C., Perlmann, R., Berko-Gleason, J., & Hooshyar, N. (1990). Developmental perspectives on politeness: Sources of children's knowledge. *Journal of Pragmatics, 14*, 289–305.

Snowling, M.J. (2000). *Dyslexia* (2nd ed.). Malden: Blackwell Publishing.

Snyder, L. (1978). Communicative and cognitive abilities and disabilities in the sensorimotor period. *Merrill-Palmer Quarterly, 24*, 161–180.

Sosa, A.V. (2016). Association of the type of toy used during play with the quantity and quality of parent-child communication. *JAMA Pediatrics, 170*(2), 132-137. Doe:101001/jamapediatrics.2015.3753.

Spector, C. (1990). Linguistic humor comprehension of normal and language-impaired adolescents. *Journal of Speech and Hearing Disorders, 55*, 533–541.

St. Louis, K., & Rustin, L. (1992). Professional awareness of cluttering. In F. Myers & K. St. Louis (Eds.), *Cluttering: A clinical perspective,* (pp. 23–35). Leicester, England: Far Communications.

Staats, A. (1971). Linguistic-mentalistic theory versus an explanatory S-R learning theory of language development. In D. Slobin (Ed.), *The ontogenesis of grammar.* New York: Academic Press.

Staats, C., & Staats, A. (1957). Meaning established by classical conditioning. *Journal of Experimental Psychology, 54*, 74–80.

Stampe, D. (1969). The acquisition of phonetic representation. In *Papers from the fifth regional meeting of the Chicago Linguistic Society* (pp. 433–444). Chicago: Chicago Linguistic Society.

Stampe, D. (1973). *A dissertation on natural phonology.* Unpublished doctoral dissertation, University of Chicago.

Stampe, D. (1979). *A dissertation on natural phonology.* New York: Garland.

Stanovich, K. (1980). Toward an interactive-compensatory model of individual differences in the development of reading fluency. *Reading Research Quarterly, 16*, 32–71.

Stanovich, K. (2000). *Progress in understanding reading: Scientific foundations and new frontiers.* New York: Guilford Press.

Stark, R. (1978). Features of infant sounds: The emergence of cooing. *Journal of Child Language, 5*, 1–12.

Stark, R. (1979). Prespeech segmental feature development. In P. Fletcher & M. Garman (Eds.), *Language acquisition.* New York: Cambridge University Press.

Stark, R. (1980). Stages of speech development in the first year of life. In G. Yeni-Komshian, J. Kavanagh, & C. Ferguson (Eds.), *Child phonology: Vol. 1. Production.* New York: Academic Press.

Stark, R. (1981). Infant vocalizations: A comprehensive view. *Infant Mental Health Journal, 2*, 118–128.

Stark, R. (1986). Prespeech segmental feature development. In P. Fletcher & M. Garman (Eds.), *Language acquisition: Studies in first language acquisition.* New York: Cambridge University Press.

Stark, R. (1989). Temporal patterning of cry and non-cry sounds in the first eight months of life. *First Language, 9*, 107–136.

Stark, R., & Tallal, P. (1988). *Language, speech, and reading disorders in children: Neuropsychological studies.* San Diego, CA: College-Hill.

Stark, R., Bernstein, L., & Demorest, M. (1993). Vocal communication in the first 18 months of life. *Journal of Speech and Hearing Research, 36*(3), 548–558.

Stark, R. E., Bernstein, L. E., & Demorest, M. E. (1983). Vocal communication in the first 18 months of life. *Journal of Speech and Hearing Research, 36*, 548–558.

Starkweather, C. (1987). *Fluency and stuttering*. Upper Saddle River, NJ: Prentice Hall.

Starkweather, C., & Givens-Ackerman, J. (1997). *Stuttering*. Austin, TX: PRO-ED.

Stein, N. (1979). How children understand stories. In L. Katz (Ed.), *Current topics in early childhood education* (Vol. 2). Norwood, NJ: Ablex.

Stein, N. (1982). What's in a story: Interpreting the interpretations of story grammars. *Discourse Processes 5*, 319–335.

Stein, N., & Albro, E. (1997). Building complexity and coherence: Children's use of goal-structured knowledge in telling stories. In M. Banberg (Ed.), *Narrative development: Six approaches* (pp. 5–44). Mahwah, NJ: Erlbaum.

Stein, N., & Glenn, C. (1979). An analysis of story comprehension in elementary school children. In R. Freedle (Ed.), *New directions in discourse processing*. Norwood, NJ: Ablex.

Stein, N., & Policastro, M. (1984). The concept of story: A comparison between children's and teachers' viewpoints. In H. Mandl, N. Stein, & T. Trabasso (Eds.), *Learning and comprehension of text*. Hillsdale, NJ: Erlbaum.

Stemberger, J. (1993). Vowel dominance in overregularizations. *Journal of Child Language, 20*, 503–521.

Stemberger, J. P. (1989). Speech errors in early child language production. *Journal of Memory and Language, 28*, 164–188.

Stemberger, J. P., & MacWhinney, B. (1986). Frequency and the lexical storage of regularly inflected forms. *Memory and Cognition, 14*, 17–26.

Stern, D. (1977). *The first relationship*. Cambridge, MA: Harvard University Press.

Sternberg, R. (1979). Developmental patterns in the encoding and combination of logical connectives. *Journal of Experimental Child Psychology, 28*, 469–468.

Sternberg, R. (1987). Most vocabulary is learned from context. In M. G. McKeown & M. E. Curtis (Eds.), *The nature of vocabulary acquisition* (pp. 89–105). Hillsdale, NJ: Erlbaum.

Stine, E., & Bohannon, J. (1983). Imitation, interactions and acquisition. *Journal of Child Language, 10*, 589–604.

Stockman, I. J. (1999). Semantic development of African American children. In O. L. Taylor & L. B. Leonard (Eds.), *Language acquisition across North America* (pp. 61–108). San Diego, CA: Singular.

Stoel-Gammon, C. (1985). Phonetic inventories, 15–24 months: A longitudinal study. *Journal of Speech and Hearing Research, 28*, 505–512.

Stoel-Gammon, C. (1987). Phonological skills of 2-year-olds. *Language, Speech, and Hearing Services in Schools, 18*, 323–329.

Stoel-Gammon, C. (1988). Prelinguistic vocalizations of hearing-impaired and normally hearing subjects: A comparison of consonantal inventories. *Journal of Speech and Hearing Disorders, 53*, 302–315.

Stoel-Gammon, C. (1990). Down syndrome: Effects on language development. *American Speech–Language–Hearing Association, 32*, 42–44.

Stoel-Gammon, C., & Cooper, J. A. (1984). Patterns of early lexical and phonological development. *Journal of Child Language, 11*, 247–271.

Stoel-Gammon, C., & Dunn, C. (1985). *Normal and disordered phonology in children*. Baltimore: University Park Press.

Stoel-Gammon, C., & Otomo, K. (1986). Babbling development of hearing-impaired and normally hearing subjects. *Journal of Speech and Hearing Disorders, 51*, 33–41.

Storkel, H. L., & Morrisette, M. L. (2002). The lexicon and phonology: Interactions in language acquisition. *Language, Speech & Hearing Services in Schools, 33*(1), 24–37.

Striano, T., & Bertin, E. (2005). Relation among joint attention skills in 5- to 10-month-old infants. *British Journal of Developmental Psychology, 23*, 1–11.

Stromswold, K. (1998). Genetics of spoken language disorders. *Human Biology, 70*, 297–324.

Strong, C. & Shaver, J. (1991). Stability and cohesion in the speech narratives of language-impaired and normally developing children. *Journal of Speech and Hearing Research, 34*, 95–111.

Subtelny, J., Oya, N., & Subtelny, J. (1972). Cineradiographic study of sibilants. *Folia Phoniatrics* (Basel, Switzerland), *24*, 30–50.

Sue, D., Arredona, P., & McDavis, R. (1992). Multicultural counseling competencies and standards: A call to the profession. *Journal of Counseling and Development, 70*, 477–486.

Sugarman, S. (1978). A description of communicative development in the prelanguage child. In I. Markova (Ed.), *The social context of language*. New York: Wiley.

Suhor, C. (1988). "English only" movement emerging as a major controversy. *Educational Leadership, 46*, 80–81.

Sullivan, J., & Horowitz, F. (1983). The effects of intonation on infant attention: The role of the rising intonation contour. *Journal of Child Language, 10*, 521–534.

Sulzby, E. (1981). *Kindergartners begin to read their own compositions*. Final report to the Research Foundation of the National Council of Teachers of English. Urbana, IL: Research Foundation of the National Council of Teachers of English.

Suskind, D., Leffel, K., Hernandez, M., Sapolich, S., Suskind, E., Kirkham, E., & Meehan, P. (2013, February). An exploratory study of "qualitative linguistic feedback": Effect of LENA feedback on adult language production. *Communication Disorders Quarterly.* doi:10.1177/1525740112473146

Sussman, F. (1999). *More than words: A guide to helping parents promote communication and social skills in children with autism spectrum disorder.* (3ʳᵈ ed.) Hanen Centre®

Sussman, H. (1979). Evidence for left hemisphere superiority in processing movement-related tonal signals. *Journal of Speech and Hearing Research, 22,* 224–235.

Sutter, J., & Johnson, C. (1990). School-age children's metalinguistic awareness of grammaticality in verb form. *Journal of Speech and Hearing Disorders, 33,* 84–95.

Sutton-Smith, B. (1986). The development of fictional narrative performances. *Topics in Language Disorders, 7*(1), 1–10.

Swacher, M. (1975). The sex of the speaker as a sociolinguistic variable. In B. Thorne & N. Henley (Eds.), *Language and sex: Difference and dominance.* Rowley, MA: Newbury House.

Swank, L. K. (1994). Phonological coding abilities: Identification of impairments related to phonologically based reading problems. *Topics in Language Disorders, 14*(2), 56–71.

Swanson, H. L, & Saez, L. (2003). Memory difficulties in children and adults with learning disabilities. In H. L. Swanson, K. R. Harris, & S. Graham (Eds.), *Handbook of learning disabilities* (pp. 182–212). New York: Guilford Press.

Swartz, K., & Hall, A. (1972). Development of relational concepts and word definition in children five through eleven. *Child Development, 43,* 239–244.

Swettenham, J., Baron-Cohen, S., Charman, T., Cox, A., Baird, G., Drew, A., Ress, L., & Wheelwright, S. (1998). The frequency and distribution of spontaneous shifts between social and non-social stimuli in autistic, typically developing, and nonautistic developmentally delayed infants. *Journal of Child Psychology and Psychiatry, 39*(5), 747–753.

Swingley, D. (2010). Fast-mapping and slow-mapping in children's word learning. *Language Learning and Development, 6,* 179–183.

Swinney, D. A., & Cutler, A. (1979). The access and processing of idiomatic expressions. *Journal of Verbal Learning and Verbal Behavior, 18,* 523–534.

Swisher, L., & Demetras, M. (1985). The expressive language characteristics of autistic children compared with intellectual disability or specific language-impaired children. In E. Schopler & G. B. Mesibov (Eds.), *Communication problems in autism.* New York: Plenum.

Tabors, P. (1997). *One child, two languages: A guide for preschool educators of children learning English as a second language.* Baltimore: Brookes.

Tadic, V., Pring, L., & Dale, N. (2010). Are language and social communication intact in children with congenital visual impairment at school age? *Journal of Child Psychology & Psychiatry, 51*(6), 696–705.

Tager-Flusberg, H. (1985). The conceptual basis for referential word meaning in children with autism. *Child Development, 56,* 1167–1178.

Tager-Flusberg, H., & Calkins, S. (1990). Does imitation facilitate the acquisition of grammar? Evidence from a study of autistic, Down syndrome, and normal children. *Journal of Child Language, 17,* 591–606.

Tallal, P., Stark, R., & Mellits, D. (1985). Identification of language-impaired children on the basis of rapid perception and production skills. *Brain and Language, 25,* 314–322.

Tannen, D. (1990). *You just don't understand: Women and men in conversation.* New York: Morrow.

Tannen, D. (1994). *Talking from 9 to 5—Women and men in the workplace: Language, sex, and power.* New York: Avon.

Tannen, D. (1994a). *Gender and discourse.* New York: Oxford University Press.

Tannen, D. (1994b). *Talking from 9 to 5: How women's and men's conversational styles affect who gets heard, who gets credit, and what gets done at work.* London: Virago.

Task Force on Newborn and Infant Hearing. (1999). Newborn and infant hearing loss: Detection and intervention. *Pediatrics, 103*(2), 527–530.

Taylor, O. (1972). An introduction to the historical development of Black English: Some implications for American education. *Language, Speech, and Hearing Services in the Schools, 3,* 5–15.

Taylor, O. (1990). Language and language differences. In G. Shames & E. Wiig (Eds.), *Human communication disorders* (3rd ed.). Upper Saddle River, NJ: Merrill/Prentice Hall.

Taylor, O. (Ed.). (1986). *Nature of communication disorders in culturally and linguistically diverse populations.* San Diego, CA: College-Hill.

Taylor, O., & Clarke, M. (1994). Communication disorders and cultural diversity: A theoretical framework. *Seminars in Speech and Language, 15,* 103–113.

Taylor, O. L., & Leonard, L. B. (1999). *Language acquisition across America.* San Diego, CA: Singular.

Teale, W. (1988). Developmentally appropriate assessment of reading and writing in the early childhood classroom. *Elementary School Journal, 89*(2), 173–183.

Templin, M. (1957). Certain language skills in children: Their development and interrelationships. *Institute of Child Welfare Monographs* (Vol. 26). Minneapolis: University of Minnesota Press.

Terrace, H. (1980). *Nim: A chimpanzee who learned sign language.* New York: Knopf.

Terrace, H., Pettito, L., Saunder, R., & Bever, J. (1979). Can an ape create a sentence? *Science, 206,* 891–902.

Terrell, S. (1983). Effects of speaking Black English upon employment opportunities. *ASHA, 25,* 27–29.

Terrell, S., & Terrell, F. (1993). African-American cultures. In D. E. Battles (Ed.), *Communication disorders in multicultural populations.* Stoneham, MA: Butterworth-Heinemann.

Thelen, E., & Smith, L. B. (1994). *A dynamic systems approach to the development of cognition and action.* Cambridge, MA: MIT Press.

Thorne, B., Kramerae, C., & Henley, N. (Eds.). (1983). *Language, gender, and society.* Rowley, MA: Newbury House.

Tiegerman, E. (1989). The cognitive bases in language development. In D. Berstein & E. Tiegerman (Eds.), *Language and communication disorders in children* (2nd ed.). Upper Saddle River, NJ: Merrill/Prentice Hall.

Tomasello, M. (1999). Social cognition before the revolution. In P. Rochat (Ed.), *Early social cognition: Understanding others in the first months of life* (pp. 301–314). Mahwah, NJ: Erlbaum.

Tomasello, T. (2003). *Constructing a Language: A Usage-Based Theory of Language Acquisition.* Cambridge, MA: Harvard University Press.

Tomasello, M., Conti-Ramsden, G., & Ewert, B. (1990). Young children's conversations with their mothers and fathers: Differences in breakdown and repair. *Journal of Child Language, 17,* 115–130.

Tomasello, M., Striano, T., & Rochat, P. (1999). Do young children use objects as symbols? *British Journal of Developmental Psychology, 17,* 563–584.

Tomblin, J. B., & Buckwalter, P. R. (1998). Heritability of poor language achievement among twins. *Journal of Speech, Language, and Hearing Research, 41,* 188–199.

Torrey, J. (1979). Reading that comes naturally: The early reader. In T. Waller & G. MacKinnon (Eds.), *Reading research: Advances in theory and practice.* New York: Academic Press.

Toubbeh, J. (1985). Handicapping and disabling conditions in native American populations. *American Rehabilitation, 11*(1), 3–9.

Trainor, L. J., & Desjardins, R. N. (2002). Pitch characteristics of infant-directed speech affect infants' ability to discriminate vowels. *Psychological Bulletin and Review, 9,* 335–340.

Trainor, L. J., Austin, C. M., & Desjardins, R. N. (2000). Is infant-directed speech prosody a result of the vocal expression of emotion? *Psychological Science, 11,* 188–195.

Trehub, S. (1976). The discrimination of foreign speech contrasts by infants and children. *Child Development, 47,* 466–472.

Trehub, S. E. (2001). Musical predispositions in infancy. In R. J. Zatorre & I. Peretz (Eds.), *The biological foundations of music. Annals of the New York Academy of Sciences* (Vol. 930, pp. 1–16). New York: New York Academy of Sciences.

Trehub, S. E., Hill, D. S., & Kamenetsky, S. B. (1997). Parents sung performances for infants. *Canadian Journal of Experimental Psychology, 51,* 385–396.

Trehub, S. E., Trainor, L. J., & Unyk, A. M. (1993). Maternal singing in cross-cultural perspective. *Infant Behavior & Development, 16,* 285–295.

Trehub, S., Schellenberg, G., & Hill, D. (1997). The origins of music perception and cognition: A developmental perspective. In I. Deliege & J. Sloboda (Eds.), *Perception and cognition of music* (pp. 103–128). Hove, Eng.: Psychology Press.

Trevarthen, C. (1979). Communication and cooperation in early infancy: A description of primary intersubjectivity. In M. Bullowa (Ed.), *Before speech.* New York: Cambridge University Press.

Trotter, R. (1983, August). Baby face. *Psychology Today, 17*(8), 14–20.

Tucker, D. (1981). Lateral brain function, emotion and conceptualization. *Psychological Review, 89,* 19–46.

Tunmer, W. E., & Cole, P. G. (1991). Learning to read: A metalinguistic act. In C. S. Simon (Ed.), *Communication skills and classroom success* (pp. 386–402). Eau Claire, WI: Thinking Publications.

Tyack, D., & Ingram, D. (1977). Children's production and comprehension of questions. *Journal of Child Language, 4*, 211–224.

Tyack, P. (2000). Dolphins whistle a signature tune. *Science, 289*, 1310–1311.

Tye-Murray, N. (2004). *Foundations of aural rehabilitation: Children, adults, and their family members* (2nd ed.). Clifton Park, NJ: Thomson Delmar Learning.

U.S. Bureau of the Census. (1990). Populations and housing unit counts for identified American Indian areas and Alaska native villages. *1990 census population general population characteristics.* Washington, DC: U.S. Department of Commerce Series PC 90–1B.

U.S. Bureau of the Census. (1995). *Statistical Brief, Housing of American Indians on reservations.* Retrieved from http://www.census.gov/apsd/www/statbrief/sb95_9.pdf

U.S. Bureau of the Census (2000). Update April, 2001. *Languages spoken at home.* Retrieved October 25, 2004 from http://www.census.gov

U.S. Bureau of the Census. (2007). *American community survey reports 2004. The American community—Hispanics.* Retrieved from http://www.census.gov/prod/2007pubs/acs-03.pdf

U.S. Bureau of the Census. (2009). *America's Families and Living Arrangements: 2007.* Retrieved from www.census.gov/population/www/socdemo/hh-fam/p20-561.pdf

U.S. Bureau of the Census. (2012a). *USA Statistics in Brief—Race and Hispanic Origin.* Retrieved from http:www.census.gov/compendia/statab/2012/files/racehisp.html

U.S. Bureau of the Census. (2012b). *Facts for Features: Hispanic Heritage Month 2012.* Retrieved from http://www.census.gov/newsroom/releases/archives/facts_for_featurees_specialeditions/cb12-ff19.html

U.S. Bureau of the Census. (2015). Figure 6. Poverty Rates by Age and Sex: 2015. Retrieved from https://www2.census.gov/programs-surveys/demo/visualizations/p60/256/figure6.pdf

U.S. Bureau of the Census. (2017). *Poverty Thresholds.* Retrieved March 3, 2017 from https://www.census.gov/data/tables/time-series/demo/income-poverty/historical-poverty-thresholds.html

U.S. Department of Education. (2005). *To ensure the free appropriate public education of all Americans: Twenty-seventh annual report to Congress on the implementation of the Individuals with Disabilities Education Act.* Retrieved from http://www.ed.gov/about/reports/annaul/osep/2005/partb-c/index.html

U.S. Department of Health and Human Services. (2012). *2012 HHS Poverty Guidelines.* Retrieved from aspe.hhs.gov/poverty/12poverty.shtml

U.S. Department of Labor, Bureau of Labor Statistics (2010). Data retrieval: Labor Force Statistics (CPS). Accessed on May 29, 2013 from http://www.bls.gov/webapps/legacy/cpsatab6.htm

Ukrainetz, T., Justice, L., Kaderavek, J., Eisenberg, S., Gillam, R., & Harm, H. (2005). The development of expressive elaboration in fictional narratives. *Journal of Speech, Language, and Hearing Research, 48*(6), 1363–1377.

Vaidyanathan, R. (1988). Development of forms and functions of interrogatives in children: A language study of Tamil. *Journal of Child Language, 15*, 533–549.

Vaidyanathan, R. (1991). Development of forms and functions of negation in the early stages of language acquisition: A study of Tamil. *Journal of Child Language, 18*, 51–60.

Van Camp, G., & Smith, R.J.H. (1991). Hereditary hearing loss homepage. Retrieved from http://hereditaryhearingloss.org

van der Lely, H. K. J., & Stollwerck, L. (1996). A grammatical specific language impairment in children: An autosomal dominant inheritance? *Brain and Language, 52*(3), 484–504.

Van Keulen, J., Weddington, G., & DeBose, C., (1998). *Speech, language, learning, and the African American child.* Boston: Allyn & Bacon.

van Kleeck, A. (1990). Emergent literacy: Learning about print before learning to read. *Topics in Language Disorders, 10*, 25–45.

van Kleeck, A., & Scheule, C. (1987). Precursors to literacy: Normal development. *Topics in Language Disorders, 7*, 13–31.

van Kleeck, A., Gillam, R. B., Hamilton, L., & McGrath, C. (1997). The relationship between middle-class parents' book-sharing discussions and their preschoolers' abstract language development. *Journal of Speech, Language, and Hearing Research, 40*, 1261–1271.

Van Kleeck, A., Schwarz, A.L., Fey, M., Kaiser, A., Miller, J., & Weitzman, E. (2010). Should we use telegraphic or grammatical input in the early stages of language development with children who have language impairments? A meta-analysis of the research and expert opinion. *American Journal of Speech-Language Pathology, 19,* 3-21. Doi:10.1044/1058-0360(2009/08-0075

Van Riper, C. (1964). *Speech correction, principles and methods* (4th ed.). Upper Saddle River, NJ: Prentice Hall.

Van Riper, C. (1973). *The treatment of stuttering.* Upper Saddle River, NJ: Prentice Hall.

Van Riper, C. (1992). *The nature of stuttering* (2nd ed.). Prospect Heights, IL: Waveland.

Van Riper, C., & Erickson, R. (1996). *Speech correction: An introduction to speech pathology and audiology* (9th ed.). Boston: Allyn & Bacon.

Vance, M., Stackhouse, J., & Wells, B. (2005). Speech production skills in children aged 3-7 years. *International Journal of Language and Communication Skills, 40*(1), 29-48.

Vanevery, H., & Rosenberg, S. (1970). Semantics, phrase structure and age as variables in sentence recall. *Child Development, 41,* 853–859.

Vellutino, F. (1974). *Dyslexia: Theory and research.* Cambridge, MA: MIT Press.

Vellutino, F. (1979) Alternative conceptualization of dyslexia: Evidence in support of a verbal-deficit hypothesis. *Harvard Educational Review, 47,* 334–354.

Vihman, M. (1996). *Phonological development: The origins of language in the child.* Cambridge, MA: Blackwell.

Vihman, M. M., & Croft, W. (2007). Phonological development: Toward a "radical" templatic phonology. *Linguistics, 45,* 683–725.

Vihman, M. M., Ferguson, C. A., & Elbert, M. (1986). Phonological development from babbling to speech: Common tendencies and individual differences. *Applied Psycholinguistics, 7,* 3–40.

Vihman, M. M, & Greenlee, M. (1987). Individual differences in phonological development: Ages one and three years. *Journal of Speech and Hearing Research, 30,* 503–521.

Volterra, V., & Taeschner, T. (1978). The acquisition and development of language by bilingual children. *Journal of Child Language, 5,* 311–326.

Von Frisch, K. (1967). *The dance language and orientation of bees* (L. E. Chadwick, Trans.). Cambridge, MA: Belknap.

von Raffler-Engle, W. (1973). The development from sound to phoneme in child language. In C. Ferguson & D. Slobin (Eds.), *Studies of child language development.* New York: Holt, Rinehart & Winston.

Vygotsky, L. (1986). *Thought and language* (A. Kozuhn, Trans.). Cambridge, MA: MIT Press. (Original work published 1934.)

Vygotsky, L. S. (1962). *Language and thought.* Cambridge, MA: Harvard University Press.

Wadsworth, B. (1971). *Piaget's theory of cognitive development.* New York: McKay.

Wagner, R. K., Torgeson, J. K., Rashotte, C., Hecht, S., Barker, T., Burgess, S., Donohue, J., & Garon, T. (1997). Changing relations between phonological processing abilities and word-level reading as children develop from beginning to skilled readers: A 5-year longitudinal study. *Developmental Psychology, 33,* 468–479.

Walker, M. (1999). The acquisition of African American English: Social-cognitive and cultural factors. In O. Taylor & L. Leonard (Eds.), *Language acquisition across North America: Cross-cultural and cross-linguistic perspectives.* San Diego, CA: Singular.

Walker, S. (2001). Cognitive, linguistic, and social aspects of adults' noun definitions. *Journal of Psycholinguistic Research, 30,* 147–161.

Wall, M., & Meyers, F. (1984). *Clinical management of childhood stuttering.* Baltimore: University Park Press.

Wallach, G. P., & Miller, L. (1988). *Language intervention and academic success.* Boston: College Hill/Little, Brown.

Warren, S.F. (2015). Right from birth: Eliminating the talk gap in young children. LENA Research Foundattion website. https:www.LENA.org/research/, Accessed January 1, 2017.

Warren, S.F., Gilkerson, J., Richards, J.A., Oller, D.K., Xu, D., Yapanel, U., Gray, S. (2010). What Automated vocal analysis reveals about the vocal production and language learning environment of young children with autism. *J Autism Dev Disord* DOI 10.1007/s10803-009-0902-5.

Warren-Leubecker, A. (1982). *Sex differences in speech to children.* Unpublished master's thesis, Georgia Institute of Technology, Atlanta.

Warren-Leubecker, A., & Bohannon, J. (1984). Intonation patterns in child-directed speech: Mother–father differences. *Child Development, 55,* 1379–1385.

Warren-Leubecker, A., & Bohannon, J. (1989). Pragmatics: Language in social contexts. In

J. Berko-Gleason (Ed.), *The development of language* (2nd ed.). Upper Saddle River, NJ: Merrill/Prentice Hall.

Washington, J., & Craig, H. (1994). Dialectal forms during discourse of poor, urban, African American preschoolers. *Journal of Speech, Language, and Hearing Research, 41,* 618–626.

Washington, J., & Craig, H. (2002). Morphosyntactic forms of African American English used by young children and their caregivers. *Applied Psycholinguistics, 23,* 209–231.

Waterman, P., & Schatz, M. (1982). The acquisition of personal pronouns and proper names by an identical twin pair. *Journal of Speech and Hearing Research, 25,* 149–154.

Waterson, N. (1971). Child phonology: A prosodic view. *Journal of Linguistics, 7,* 179–211.

Waterson, N. (1981). A tentative developmental model of phonological representation. In T. Myers, J. Laver, & J. Anderson (Eds.), *The cognitive representation of speech.* Amsterdam: North-Holland.

Watson, J. (1924). *Behaviorism.* Chicago: University of Chicago Press.

Watson, M. M., & Scukancec, G. P. (1997). Phonological changes in the speech of two-year-olds: A longitudinal investigation. *Infant-Toddler Intervention, 7,* 67–77.

Weaver, C. (1994). *Reading process and practice: From sociopsycholinguistics to whole language.* Portsmouth, NH: Heinemann.

Wehren, A., DeLisi, R., & Arnold, M. (1981). The development of noun definition. *Journal of Child Language, 8,* 165–175.

Weiss, C., Gordon, M., & Lillywhite, H. (1987). *Clinical management of articulatory and phonologic disorders* (2nd ed.). Baltimore: Williams & Wilkins.

Weiss, D. (1964). *Cluttering.* Upper Saddle River, NJ: Prentice Hall.

Weiss, D. (1967). Similarities and differences between cluttering and stuttering. *Folia Phoniatrica, 19,* 98–104.

Wellman, B., Case, I., Mengert, E., & Bradbury, D. (1931). *Speech sounds of young children.* University of Iowa Studies in Child Welfare. Iowa City: University of Iowa Press.

Wellman, H., & Estes, D. (1987). Children's early use of mental verbs and what they mean. *Discourse Processes, 16,* 141–156.

Wellman, H., & Lempers, J. (1977). The naturalistic communicative abilities of two-year-olds. *Child Development, 48,* 1052–1057.

Wells, G. (1979). Learning and using the auxiliary verb in English. In V. Lee (Ed.), *Language development.* New York: Wiley.

Wells, G. (1985). *Language development in the preschool years.* New York: Cambridge University Press.

Wells, G. (1986). *The meaning makers: Children learning language and using language to learn.* Portsmouth, NH: Heinemann.

Werker, J., & Tees, R. (1984). Cross-language speech perception: Evidence for perceptual reorganization during the first year of life. *Infant Behavior and Development, 7,* 49–64.

Wertsch, J. (1991). *Voices of the mind: A sociocultural approach to mediated action.* Cambridge, MA: Harvard University Press.

Wertsch, J., & Tulviste, P. (1992). L. S. Vygotsky and contemporary developmental psychology. *Developmental Psychology, 28,* 548–557.

West, C., & Garcia, A. (1988). Conversational shift work: A study of topical transitions between women and men. *Social Problems, 35,* 551–571.

Westby, C. (1980). Assessment of cognitive and language abilities through play. *Language, Speech, and Hearing Services in Schools, 11,* 154–168.

Westby, C. (1994). The effects of culture on genre, structure and style of oral and written texts. In G. P. Wallach & K. G. Butler (Eds.), *Language learning disabilities in school-age children and adolescents* (pp. 180–213). Boston: Allyn & Bacon.

Westby, C. (2006). There's more to passing than knowing the answers: Learning to do school. In T. A. Ukrainetz (Ed.), *Contextualizing language intervention: Scaffolding PreK–12 literacy achievement* (pp. 319–388). Eau Claire, WI: Thinking Publications.

Wetherby, A. (1986). Ontogeny of communicative functions in autism. *Journal of Autism and Developmental Disorders, 16,* 295–316.

Wexler, K., & Culicover, P. (1980). *Formal principles of language acquisition.* Cambridge, MA: MIT Press.

White, T., Power, M., & White, S. (1989). Morphological analysis: Implications for teaching and understanding vocabulary growth. *Reading Research Quarterly, 24,* 283–304.

Whitehurst, G., & Lonigan, C. (2001). Emergent literacy: Development from prereaders to readers. In S. B. Neuman & D. K. Dickinson (Eds.), *Handbook of early literacy research* (Vol. 1, pp. 11–29). New York: Guilford Press.

Whitehurst, G., & Vasta, R. (1975). Is language acquired through imitation? *Journal of Psycholinguistic Research, 4*, 37–59.

Whorf, B. (1956). *Language, thought, and reality.* New York: Wiley.

Wiener, F., Lewnau, L., & Erway, E. (1983). Measuring language competency in speakers of Black American English. *Journal of Speech and Hearing Disorders, 48*, 76–84.

Wiggins, M., Gabbard, S., Thompson, N., Goberis, D., & Yoshinaga-Itano, C. (2012). The school to home link: Summer preschool and parents. Seminars in Speech and Language, *33*(04), 290-296. DOE: 10.1055/s-0032-1326919

Wilbur, R. (2003). What studies of sign language tell us about language. In M. Marschark & P. Spencer (Eds.), *The handbook of deaf studies, language, and education* (pp. 332–346). Oxford, Eng.: Oxford University Press.

Wilde, S. (1992). *You kan red this! Spelling and punctuation for whole language classrooms, K–6.* Portsmouth, NH: Heinemann.

Wilhelm, R. (1994). Exploring the practice–rhetoric gap: Current curriculum for African-American history month in some Texas elementary schools. *Journal of Curriculum and Supervision, 9*, 217–233.

Wilkinson, L., Calculator, S., & Dollaghan, C. (1982). Ya wanna trade—just for awhile: Children's requests and responses to peers. *Discourse Processes, 5*, 161–176.

Williams, R., & Wolfram, W. (1977). *Social dialects: Difference versus disorder.* Rockville, MD: American Speech–Language–Hearing Association.

Willis, F., & Williams, S. (1976). Simultaneous talking in conversation and the sex of speakers. *Perceptual and Motor Skills, 43*, 1067–1070.

Wilson, D. (1979). *Voice problems in children* (2nd ed.). Baltimore: Williams & Wilkins.

Wilton, A. P. (2011). Implications of parent-child interactions for early language development of young children with visual impairments. *Insight: Research & Practice in Visual Impairment & Blindness, 4*(3), 139–147.

Wing, C., & Scholnick, E. (1981). Children's comprehension of pragmatic concepts expressed in "because," "although," "if" and "unless." *Journal of Child Language, 8*, 347–365.

Wingate, M. (1997). *Stuttering: A short history of a curious disorder.* Westport, CT: Bergin & Garvey.

Winitz, H. (1988). *Human communication and its disorders: A review.* Norwood, NJ: Ablex.

Winsboro, B., & Solomon, I. (1990). Standard English vs. the American dream. *Educational Digest, 56*, 51–52.

Wolf, C. D., & Bell, M. A. (2007). Sources of variability in working memory in early childhood: A consideration of age, temperament, language, and brain electrical activity. *Cognitive Development, 22*, 431–455.

Wolf, M., & Dickenson, D. (1989). From oral to written language: Transitions in the school years. In J. Berko-Gleason (Ed.), *The development of language* (2nd ed.). Upper Saddle River, NJ: Merrill/Prentice Hall.

Wolff, P. (1969). The natural history of crying and other vocalizations in early infancy. In B. Foss (Ed.), *Determinants of infant behavior IV.* London: Methuen.

Wolfram, W., & Christian, D. (1989). *Dialects and education: Issues and answers.* Upper Saddle River, NJ: Prentice Hall.

Wong Fillmore, L. (1979). Individual differences in second language acquisition. In C. Fillmore, D. Kempler, & W. S.-Y. Wang (Eds.), *Individual differences in language ability and language behavior* (pp. 203–227). San Diego, CA: Academic Press.

Wong Fillmore, L. (1983). The language learner as an individual: Implications of research on individual differences for the ESL teacher. In M. Clarke & J. Handscombe (Eds.), *On TESOL "82: Pacific perspectives on language learning and teaching* (pp. 157–173). Washington, DC: Teachers of English to Speakers of Other Languages.

Wood, D. (1989). Social interaction as tutoring. In M. Bornstein & J. Bruner (Eds.), *Interaction in human development.* Hillsdale, NJ: Erlbaum.

Woodward, A. L., Markham, E. M., & Fitzsimmons, C. M. (1994). Rapid word learning in 13- and 18-month-olds. *Developmental Psychology, 30*, 553–566.

Wootten, J., Merkin, S., Hood, L., & Bloom, L. (1979, March). *Wh-questions: Linguistic evidence to explain the sequence of acquisition.* Paper presented at the biennial meeting of the Society for Research in Child Development, San Francisco.

World Health Organization (WHO). (2001). *International Classification of Functioning, Disability and Health* (WHO/ICF). Geneva, Switzerland. Retrieved from www.who.int/classification/icf

Xu, D., Richards, J. A., Gilkerson, J., Warren, S. F., & Oller, D. K. (2010). *Automatic identification of children at risk for autism spectrum disorder using audio recordings.* [Poster]. Retrieved from http://www.lenafoundation.org/pdf/IMFAR-2010-PosterAutism-Screen.pdf

Xu, F., & Pinker, S. (1995). Weird past tense forms. *Journal of Child Language, 22,* 531–556.

Yairi, E., & Grinager A. N. (2004). *Early childhood stuttering.* Austin, TX: Pro-Ed.

Yopp, H. K. (1992). Developing phonemic awareness in young children. *The Reading Teacher, 45,* 696–703.

Yopp, H. K., & Yopp, R. H. (2000). Supporting phonemic awareness development in the classroom. *The Reading Teacher, 54,* 130–143.

Zachary, W. (1978). Ordinality and interdependence of representation and language development in infants. *Child Development, 49,* 681–687.

Zebrowski, P. M. (2003, July). Developmental stuttering. *Pediatric Annals, 32*(7), 453–458.

Zemlin, W. (1988). *Speech and hearing science, anatomy and physiology* (3rd ed.). Upper Saddle River, NJ: Prentice Hall.

Zemlin, W. (1990). Anatomy and physiology of speech. In G. Shames & E. Wiig (Eds.), *Human communication disorders* (3rd ed.). Upper Saddle River, NJ: Merrill/Prentice Hall.

Zentella, A. (2002). Latina languages and identities. In M. Suarez-Orozco & M. A. Paez (Eds.), *Latinos: Remaking America* (pp. 321–338). Berkeley: University of California Press.

Zera, D. A., & Lucian, D. G. (2001). Self-organization and learning disabilities: A theoretical perspective for the interpretation and understanding of dysfunction. *Learning Disabilities Quarterly, 24*(2), 107–118.

Zipke, M. (2007). The role of metalinguistic awareness in the reading comprehension of sixth and seventh graders. *Reading Psychology, 28,* 375–396.

ZUKOW-GOLDRING, P. (2001). Perceiving referring actions: Latino and Euro-American infants and caregivers comprehending speech. In K. Nelson, A. Aksu-Koc, & C. Johnson (Eds.), *Children's Language* (Vol. 11, pp. 140–163). Mahwah, NJ: Erlbaum.

Zuniga, M. (2004). Families with Latino roots. In E. Lynch & M. Hanson (Eds.), *Developing cross-cultural competence* (3rd ed., pp. 179–198). Baltimore: Brookes.

Name Index

Subject Index

A

accents, 260, 322, 344–45, 361–62

accommodation, 65–66, 157

accuracy, 18, 31, 79, 143, 185, 308, 321, 337, 342

acoustics characteristics, 6, 23, 100, 102

acquisition, 27–33, 35–41, 43–61, 66–68, 83–84, 110–11, 113–15, 129–30, 211, 249–50, 252–53, 258–63, 274–77, 335–37, 382–85

  effect, 31

  formula, 40

  process, 25, 28, 48, 52, 56, 129, 307

acts

  illocutionary, 56–57

  locutionary, 56–57

  perlocutionary, 56–57

action words, 163, 165, 192

activation, 31, 72, 147–48

activities, 39–40, 69, 71, 73–74, 76–78, 87, 90, 92, 121, 183, 227, 229, 242–44, 307, 412

adaptations, 34, 64–65, 124, 286, 360

adjectivals, 215–16, 227

adjectives, 157, 188, 214, 216, 230–32, 234, 245, 290–93, 366, 371, 387

adolescence, 39, 66, 88, 221, 262, 276, 278, 284, 291, 296, 306, 321, 381

adult speakers, 15, 224, 238, 241, 294

adult word count (AWC), 135–136, 138, 140, 143, 145

adult words, 137, 141, 178, 332

adverbs, 39, 170, 188, 217, 233–34, 276, 290, 292–94, 296–97

adverbial conjuncts, 39, 170, 217, 233, 293–94, 296–97

adverbs, 188, 234, 276, 290, 292–94

affricates, 327, 329, 334–35, 342, 366

African American English (AAE), 345–50, 353, 356

African Americans, 116, 133, 270, 302, 345, 347, 349

agents, 73, 78, 107, 162, 170, 172–73, 178, 190, 192, 250, 276, 286

aggression, 12, 298

air, 7, 10, 23–24, 88, 284, 304, 327–29, 393–94, 396–400, 404, 406–8

air particles, 24–25, 408, 414

alliteration, 123, 178, 304, 307

alveolar ridge, 7, 14, 325, 327, 341, 395, 407

ambiguities, 277, 290, 305

American Academy of Pediatrics, 142

American Association on Intellectual and Developmental Disabilities (AAIDD), 377

American English, 15, 282, 325, 345, 347, 349, 406

American Speech-Language-Hearing Association, 364

anaphoric references, 213, 239

anatomy, 282, 394, 407, 416

animals, 8–22, 28, 30, 34, 39–40, 55, 84, 90, 193, 198–99, 201–2, 204–5, 277, 279–80, 408

approximations, 40, 42, 74, 310, 314

arbitrariness, 11, 14–15, 108

arcuate fasciculus, 29, 410

arms, 24, 70, 221

arrangements, 5, 11, 63, 157, 189, 338

art, 7–8, 20, 27, 237, 290, 294–95, 327, 341–42, 347–48, 353, 370–71, 382, 385–86, 393–95, 405–8

arytenoid cartilage, 402–4

Asian English (AE), 345, 353–56

ASL (American Sign Language), 33, 375

assimilation, 65–66, 157, 338–39

associations, 103–4, 226

attention

  joint, 98, 108, 125–26, 129, 133, 142, 155–56, 376

  selective, 108, 110

attitudes, 117, 216, 265, 272, 294, 296, 320, 344

attributes, 93, 120, 172, 192, 226, 291, 329

auditory cues, 147, 278

auditory nerve, 375, 417–18

auditory nervous system, 375

auditory processing, 103

auditory stimulation, 97

autism spectrum disorder (ASD), 30–31, 143, 379–80, 391

autoclitics, 43–44

autosegmental theory, 342

auxiliary

  contractible, 187–88, 204–5, 210–12, 214–20, 227–29, 231, 245–48, 348, 353, 355

  uncontractible, 187, 211, 245

auxiliary verbs, 210, 214–17, 219–20, 227–29, 231, 246–48, 353

  secondary, 215

awareness, 72, 111, 123, 155, 237–38, 244, 267–68, 303–5, 307, 324, 342, 369, 387

  graphophonemic, 316–17

  metalinguistic, 111, 259, 303, 305–6

B

babbling, 56, 76, 78, 128, 150–53, 158–59, 168, 234, 314, 331–33, 335

  reduplicated, 150–52

balance, 65–66, 399, 416

behaviorists, 28, 40, 45, 50, 58, 61

behavior management, 42, 271, 273

behaviors

  coded, 28

  cognitive, 51

  goal-oriented, 73, 75

  human, 40, 222, 278, 373

  learned, 41, 61, 129

  means/ends, 74

  non-linguistic, 176

  nonverbal, 4, 156

  pretending, 82

  sensorimotor, 74

  sensory, 74